MIGRAINE

MIGRAINE

Third Edition

David W. Dodick, MD, FRCP
Mayo Clinic College of Medicine
Scottsdale, AZ

Stephen D. Silberstein, MD, FRCP
Thomas Jefferson University
Philadelphia, PA

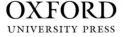

OXFORD
UNIVERSITY PRESS

OXFORD
UNIVERSITY PRESS

Oxford University Press is a department of the University of Oxford. It furthers
the University's objective of excellence in research, scholarship, and education
by publishing worldwide. Oxford is a registered trade mark of Oxford University
Press in the UK and certain other countries.

Published in the United States of America by Oxford University Press
198 Madison Avenue, New York, NY 10016, United States of America.

© Oxford University Press 2016

First Edition published in 1994
Second Edition published in 2002

Library of Congress Cataloging-in-Publication Data
Dodick, David, author.
Migraine / David W. Dodick, Stephen D. Silberstein.—3rd edition.
p. ; cm.—(Contemporary neurology series ; 91)
Preceded by: Migraine : manifestations, pathogenesis, and management / Robert A. Davidoff. 2nd ed. 2002.
Includes bibliographical references and index.
ISBN 978–0–19–979361–7 (alk. paper)
I. Silberstein, Stephen D., author.   II. Davidoff, Robert A., 1934—. Migraine. Preceded by (work):   III. Title.
IV. Series: Contemporary neurology series ; 91. 0069-9446
[DNLM: 1. Migraine Disorders. W1 CO769N v.91 2015 / WL 344]
RC392
616.8'4912—dc23
2014050057

9 8 7 6 5 4 3 2 1
Printed by Walsworth, USA

Contents

Chapter 1

Migraine Symptoms and Diagnosis

INTRODUCTION

Migraine is a disabling neurologic disorder characterized by recurrent attacks of premonitory symptoms, headache, gastrointestinal and neurologic symptoms, and in some patients, aura.[1–6] The term "migraine" is derived from the Greek word *hemicrania*, introduced by Galen in approximately 200 A.D.[7] The physical examination, neurologic examination, and laboratory studies are usually normal and serve to exclude other, more ominous causes of headache. The diagnosis of migraine has been facilitated by the development and publication of the International Classification of Headache Disorders (ICHD-1, ICHD-2, and ICHD-3 β),[8] which provide criteria for a total of six subtypes of migraine (see Table 1.1).[6] In this chapter, we review the clinical features of migraine and then discuss classification and diagnosis.

PHASES AND CLINICAL FEATURES OF MIGRAINE

The migraine attack can be divided into four phases: the premonitory phase or prodrome, which occurs hours or days before the headache; the aura, which consists of neurologic symptoms that immediately precede or accompany the headache; the headache phase,

1

Table 1.1 **ICHD-3 β Migraine Classification**

1. **Migraine**
 1.1 Migraine without aura
 1.2 Migraine with aura
  1.2.1 Migraine with typical aura
   1.2.1.1 Typical aura with headache
   1.2.1.2 Typical aura without headache
  1.2.2 Migraine with brainstem aura
  1.2.3 Hemiplegic migraine
   1.2.3.1 Familial hemiplegic migraine
    1.2.3.1.1 FHM 1
    1.2.3.1.2 FHM 2
    1.2.3.1.3 FHM 3
    1.2.3.1.4 FHM other loci
   1.2.3.2 Sporadic hemiplegic migraine
  1.2.4 Retinal migraine
 1.3 Chronic migraine
 1.4 Complications to migraine
  1.4.1 Status migrainosus
  1.4.2 Persistent aura without infarction
  1.4.3 Migrainous infarction
  1.4.4 Migraine triggered seizures
 1.5 Probable migraine
  1.5.1 Probable migraine without aura
  1.5.2 Probable migraine with aura
 1.6 Episodic syndromes that may be associated with migraine
  1.6.1 Recurrent gastrointestinal disturbance
1.6.1.1 Cyclical vomiting syndrome
1.6.1.2 Abdominal migraine
  1.6.2 Benign paroxysmal vertigo
  1.6.3 Benign paroxysmal torticollis

comprising headache and associated symptoms; and the postdrome (Table 1.2). Migraine without aura consists of at least the headache phase, and in most patients, the premonitory phase, the postdrome, or both. The relationship between the aura and the headache phase may vary between patients and even within the same patient (Figure 1.1). Migraine with aura consists of at least the aura and the headache and may also include the premonitory and postdromal phases. If aura occurs in the absence of headache, the disorder is termed "migraine aura without headache."

Table 1.2 **Phases of the Migraine Attack**

 I. Premonitory phase
 II. Aura
 III. Headache
 IV. Postdrome

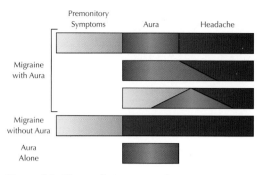

Figure 1.1. Phases of migraine attack.

Premonitory Phase (Prodrome)

The prodrome consists of psychological, neurologic, or general (constitutional, autonomic) symptoms in various combinations (see Table 1.3).[9–11] More than 70% of migraineurs experience premonitory phenomena hours to days before headache onset. Psychological symptoms include anxiety, depression, euphoria, irritability, restlessness, mental slowness, hyperactivity, fatigue, and drowsiness. Neurologic phenomena include photophobia, phonophobia, difficulty concentrating, and hyperosmia. General symptoms include a stiff neck, a cold feeling, yawning, sluggishness, increased thirst, increased urination, nausea, anorexia, diarrhea, constipation, fluid retention, and food cravings. [11,12] Evolutive and non-evolutive premonitory features are sometimes distinguished. The evolutive features start approximately 6 hours before the attack, gradually increase in intensity, and often culminate in the attack; a dopaminergic mechanism has been suggested.[13,14] Non-evolutive features precede the attack by up to 48 hours. Premonitory symptoms are common; Blau[9] found them in 28/50 migraineurs, while Isler[10] found them in 65/100 migraineurs, with equal frequency in migraine with or without aura.

Quintela et al. studied migraine premonitory symptoms using a questionnaire that was given to 100 migraineurs by their general physician. Premonitory symptoms were those experienced the day before the headache started, only if the symptoms were not present during a pain-free period. Premonitory symptoms were experienced by 84% of subjects

Table 1.3 **Premonitory Features of Migraine (Prodrome)**

Psychological	Neurological	General
Depression	Difficulty concentrating	Anorexia
Drowsiness	Dysphasia	Cold feeling
Euphoria	Hyperosmia	Diarrhea or constipation
Hyperactivity	Phonophobia	Fluid retention
Irritability	Photophobia	Food cravings
Restlessness	Yawning	Sluggishness
Talkativeness		Stiff neck
		Thirst
		Urination

during the first attack. Anxiety (46%), phonophobia (44%), irritability (42%), unhappiness and yawning (40%), and asthenia (38%) were the commonest symptoms; they were more frequent in subjects who had migraine with aura. Patients on preventive medications showed a decreased frequency of premonitory symptoms. Headache severity was associated with the presence of premonitory symptoms. Premonitory symptoms were quite consistent after three attacks. Almost two-thirds of the symptoms were noticed in at least two of three attacks; more than half were repeated in three of three attacks.[15]

Griffin et al.[11] used electronic diaries in a 3-month multicenter study to record non-headache symptoms before, during, and after a migraine attack. They recruited subjects who reported non-headache symptoms that they believed predicted headache in at least two of three attacks. Symptoms were entered in the diaries by patient initiation and through prompted entries at random times during the day. Data recorded included non-headache symptoms occurring during all three phases of the migraine, prediction of the attack from premonitory symptoms, general state of health, and action taken to prevent the headache. Of the 120 patients who were recruited, 97 provided usable data. Patients correctly predicted migraine headaches from 72% of diary entries with premonitory symptoms. The commonest premonitory symptoms were feeling tired and weary (72% of attacks with warning features), having difficulty concentrating (51%), and a stiff neck (50%). Premonitory nausea (24%), photophobia (49%), and phonophobia (38%) continued into the headache and postdrome phases. Subjects who functioned poorly in the premonitory phase were the most likely

to correctly predict their headaches. When premonitory symptoms were present, 72% of patients experienced a migraine headache within 72 hours. The majority of symptoms occurred throughout all three phases. Except for yawning, hunger or food cravings, and increased energy, the majority of premonitory symptoms became commoner in the headache phase. Griffin et al. did not ascertain the background prevalence of these symptoms interictally, but interictal tiredness was 22% in Quintela's study.

Aura

The migraine aura comprises focal neurologic phenomena that precede or accompany an attack. Most aura symptoms develop over 5–20 minutes and usually last less than 60 minutes. [5] The aura can be characterized by visual, sensory, or motor phenomena, and may also involve language or brainstem disturbances (Table 1.4). If it occurs, the headache usually begins within 60 minutes of the end of the aura. In one prospective study, the headache followed the aura only 80% of the time. [16] If the headache is delayed, most patients do not return to a normal sense between the end of the aura and the onset of the headache. Patients may experience symptoms, including anxiety or fears, other alterations in mood, disturbances of speech or thought, or detachment from the environment or from other people. The headache may begin before or simultaneously with the aura, the aura may occur in isolation, or, rarely, auras occur repeatedly. This may occur many times an hour for as long as several months. It has been termed "migraine aura status," but other organic causes must be

Table 1.4 **Aura**

Visual: scotomata; photopsia or phosphenes; geometric forms; fortification spectra; objects may rotate, oscillate, or shimmer; brightness appears often very bright

Visual hallucinations or distortions: metamorphopsia; macropsia; zoom or mosaic vision

Sensory: paresthesias, often migrating, often lasting for minutes (cheiro-oral), can become bilateral

Olfactory hallucinations

Motor: weakness or ataxia

Language: dysarthria or aphasia

Delusions and disturbed consciousness: déjà vu, multiple conscious trance-like states

considered.[17] Sacks described two variants of aura status: one characterized by recurring visual scotomata and the other characterized by repetitive sensory auras.[18] Patients may experience more than one type of aura, with a progression from one symptom to another. Most patients with a sensory aura also have a visual aura (see Figure 1.1).[19]

Visual aura is the commonest of the neurologic events; it occurs in 99% of patients who have an aura, and it often has a hemianopic distribution. The aura may consist of photopsia (the sensation of unformed flashes of light before the eyes), or scotoma (partial loss of sight) [20–23], or the almost diagnostic aura of migraine, the fortification spectrum. [21,23]

Auras vary in their complexity. Elementary visual disturbances include scotomata, simple flashes (phosphenes), specks, or geometric forms. They may move across the visual field and sometimes cross the midline. Shimmering or undulations in the visual field may also occur and may be described by patients as "heat waves." These "minor visual disorders" are more likely to occur during than before the headache.[24] Because they are bilateral they are believed to arise from the occipital cortex. More complicated auras include teichopsia (Greek: town wall and vision) or the fortification spectrum, the most characteristic visual aura of migraine. The fortification spectrum consists of an arc of scintillating lights, usually but not always beginning near the point of fixation, forming into a herringbone-like pattern that expands to encompass an increasing portion of a visual hemifield. It migrates across the visual field with a scintillating edge

of often zigzag, flashing, or occasionally colored phenomena. The visions of Hildegard of Bingen, an eleventh-century abbess have been attributed in part to her migrainous auras. Characteristic of the visions that she and other visionary prophets, including Ezekiel (Ezekiel 1:1–28) experienced, were working, boiling, or fermenting lights.

Visual distortions and hallucinations, speculated to represent Lewis Carroll's descriptions in Alice in Wonderland, can occur. These phenomena are commoner in children, are usually followed by a headache, and are characterized by a complex disorder of visual perception that may include metamorphopsia, micropsia, macropsia, and zoom or mosaic vision [18,25]. Nonvisual symptoms can occur; these include complex difficulties in the perception and use of the body (apraxia and agnosia), speech and language disturbances, states of double or multiple consciousness associated with *déjà vu* or *jamais vu*, and elaborate dreamy, nightmarish, trance-like, or delirious states. Olfactory hallucinations may also occur.[26]

Paresthesias characterize the second commonest aura and occur in about one-third of migraines with aura. They are typically cheirooral, with numbness starting in the hand, migrating up the arm, and then jumping to involve the face, lips, and tongue.[27] The leg is occasionally involved.[28] As with visual auras (with positive, followed by negative, symptoms), paresthesias may be followed by numbness and, in a few cases, loss of position sense. Paresthesias begin bilaterally or become bilateral in half of patients. Sensory auras rarely occur in isolation and usually follow a visual aura. Patients may experience more than one type of aura, with a progression from one symptom to another. Most patients with a sensory aura also have a visual aura.[19]

Motor symptoms occur in as many as 18% of patients, often in association with sensory symptoms;[16] however, true weakness is rare and is always unilateral.[28] Sensory ataxia is often reported as weakness;[28] hyperkinetic movement disorders, including chorea, have been reported. Aphasic auras have been reported in 17%–20% of patients.[16,28] However, since patients are rarely examined during an aura, many of the reported cases may be dysarthria and not aphasia.[28] Young et al. characterized the clinical features of 24 patients with non-familial migraine with unilateral motor symptoms (MUMS) and compared these features with those of migraine without weakness (48 matched controls). The symptoms of MUMS were fairly characteristic. Motor symptoms begin with the onset of pain or worsen as the pain intensifies. Motor symptoms are usually accompanied by sensory symptoms. Ninety-two percent of patients had a march of motor and sensory symptoms. Patients with MUMS always had weakness involving the arm subjectively, and both arm and leg objectively. A give-way character was always present. Only 17% of patients with MUMS reported facial weakness; 58% reported persistent interictal weakness. A rostrocaudal march of motor and sensory symptoms was common. Visual symptoms can be positive or negative. Other common neurologic symptoms include non-specific language disturbances and dizziness. Weakness was ipsilateral to unilateral headache in two-thirds of the patients. Compared with controls, patients with MUMS had similar pain intensities, but were more likely to report other migrainous symptoms, including allodynia. Thirty-eight percent of patients with MUMS were told they had had a stroke, and 17% believed they had had a stroke despite normal brain imaging. Patients with MUMS reported fewer affective disorders and more adjustment disorders than controls, and had similar Beck Depression Inventory (BDI) scores. Except for the distinction between true and give-way weakness, many patients with MUMS fulfill the ICHD-2 criteria for hemiplegic migraine. As patients will not report the difference between true weakness and give-way weakness, and as distinguishing give-way and true weakness on examination may be difficult,[29,30] some reports of sporadic hemiplegic migraine likely include patients with MUMS.[31]

Headache

A migraine headache is typically unilateral, throbbing, moderate to marked in severity, and aggravated by routine physical activity. Not all of these features are required by the ICHD: pain may be bilateral and throbbing or unilateral and non-throbbing. The headache of migraine can occur at any time of the day or night, but occurs most frequently on arising in the morning.[24] The onset is usually gradual; the pain peaks and then subsides, and usually

lasts less than 24 hours, with a range of 4–72 hours in adults and 2–48 hours in children.[5] The headache is bilateral in 40% and unilateral in 60% of cases; it consistently occurs on the same side in 20% of patients.[24] Migraineurs whose headaches alternate sides do not develop more consistently lateralized headaches with the passage of time (see Figure 1.2).

The pain varies greatly in intensity, ranging from annoying to incapacitating, although most migraineurs report at least moderate pain.[32] The pain has a throbbing quality, particularly when severe, but can be tight or bandlike.[24] During an attack, pain may move from one part of the head to another and may radiate down the neck into the shoulder. The pain is commonly aggravated by physical activity or simple head movement. Patients prefer to lie down in a dark, quiet room. Many patients have scalp tenderness during or after the headache. This tenderness may involve the head and neck and may prevent the patient from lying on the affected side.[33]

Olesen looked at the clinical features of 750 patients seen with an acute migraine attack at the Copenhagen Acute Headache Clinic. Forty-seven percent of patients had pulsating pain; 42% had pressing pain; and 11% had other types of pain quality. Unilateral pain was seen in 56% of patients and bilateral pain in 44%. Half the patients had interictal headaches. In

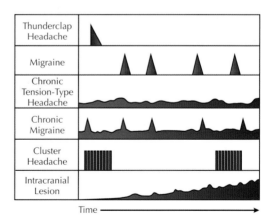

Figure 1.2. Time course of different headache types. Thunderclap headache is of sudden onset. Migraine is of more gradual onset and occurs less than 15 days/month. CTTH is low grade and near daily. Transformed (chronic) migraine is migraine that occurs more than 15 days/month. Cluster headache consists of attacks of high-frequency short-duration attacks. Intracranial lesions tend to gradually worsen.

patients with severe pain, the quality was significantly more often pulsating. Patients with bioccipital headache had significantly fewer visual disturbances than did patients whose pain was in other locations (see Figure 1.3).[34]

Many migraineurs have headache profiles that do not meet the IHS criteria for migraine. [34] Some are ICHD 1.6 probable migraine, missing one criterion; others are shorter and less severe and often meet the IHS criteria for episodic tension-type headache (TTH). Some patients note that their headache begins as a TTH and builds into a "migraine."[34,35] We believe these phenomenologic TTHs are all migrainous in nature, have more migraine features than TTH features, and, unlike typical TTH occurring in non-migraineurs, respond to specific migraine drugs.[36–38]

Kelman described the pain characteristics of the acute migraine attack in 1283 migraine patients. Headache character (throbbing, aching, pressure, stabbing scaled grade 0 to 3 [0 = none; 1 = mild; 2 = moderate; 3 = severe]); intensity (for average, minimum, and maximum intensity headaches, scaled 0 to 10); lifetime duration; frequency per month; duration in minutes (for average, minimum, maximum duration headaches); time of onset of headache (morning, afternoon, evening, night, anytime); aggravation of headache with activity (scaled 0 to 3); percentage recurrence; and time to recurrence were recorded.

Of the 1283 patients, 874 were classified as ICHD migraine, 524 as episodic, 350 as chronic, and 409 as probable migraine. The time of headache onset was morning in 18.7% of patients, afternoon in 13.5%, evening in 4.0%, during the night in 9.4%, and "anytime" in 54.3%. The median time to peak headache was greater in migraine than probable migraine (90 minutes vs. 60 minutes; $p < .01$). The average headache duration was 29.2 hours (mean) and 24.0 hours (median). Headache character (greater than grade 1) was throbbing (73.5%), aching (73.8%), pressure (75.4%), and stabbing (42.6%), with significantly more throbbing in migraine than in probable migraine (73.5% vs. 63.2%; $p < .01$) and more aching in chronic than in episodic migraine (65.4% vs. 63.1%; $p < .05$). Headache was increased by activity in 90.2% of patients, grade 1 in 13.8%, grade 2 in 30.8%, and grade 3 in 45.5%.[39]

Migraineurs may also experience short-lived jabs of pain, lasting for seconds, occurring between more characteristic migraine attacks (so-called idiopathic stabbing headache). The pain is described as an "ice pick," "needle," "nail," "jabs and jolts," or "pinprick" headache, and occurs in about 40% of migraineurs.

Rarely, head pain in migraine extends to involve the maxillary or mandibular region of the face; sometimes isolated facial pain is the only and atypical presentation of migraine. The prevalence of these fairly unusual symptoms is widely unknown. Yoon et al. estimated the prevalence of facial pain in migraine in a population-based sample of 517 migraine patients in Germany. In 46 cases (8.9%), migraine pain involved the head and the lower half of the face. Patients with facial pain suffer more trigemino-autonomic symptoms than migraine patients (47.8% vs. 7.9%; $p < 0.001$). In one case, isolated facial pain without headache was the leading symptom of migraine. These results demonstrate that facial pain is not unusual in migraine, while isolated facial migraine is extremely rare.[40]

Associated Phenomena

Migraine attacks are characteristically accompanied by associated symptoms that often contribute to migraine-related disability. Their type and prevalence are detailed in Table 1.5. Gastrointestinal disturbances are often the most distressing symptoms. Anorexia is common, but food cravings can occur; nausea occurs in 90% of patients and vomiting in about one-third.[24,34,41] Gastroparesis contributes to gastrointestinal distress and poor absorption of oral medication.[42–44] Diarrhea occurs in about 16% of patients.[24,34,45–47] Many migraineurs have enhanced sensory perception or sensitivity manifested by photophobia, phonophobia, and osmophobia, and seek a dark, quiet room.[24,48] Others will have lightheadedness and vertigo.[49] Premonitory symptoms, such as exhilaration, agitation, fatigue, lethargy, disorientation, hypomania, anger, rage, or depression, can continue into the headache. Constitutional, mood, and mental changes are almost universal. Blurry vision, nasal stuffiness, pallor or redness, and sensations of heat, cold, or sweating may occur. Fluid retention can develop hours to days before the headache. Frank edema may precede, accompany, or follow the headache, with resolution of

Table 1.5 **Prevalence of Associated Symptoms in the Migraine Attack**

Reference	Study Type	No. of Patients	Nausea	Vomiting	Photophobia	Phonophobia	Visual Disturbances	Dizziness
Selby & Lance, 1960	C	500	87	55	82	NR	41	72
Lance & Anthony, 1966	C	500	93	55	49	NR	33	NR
Olesen, 1978	C	750	86	47	NR	NR	20	NR
Iversen etal., 1990	C	30	90	NR	95	97	NR	NR
Davies etal., 1991	C	354						
		w/oaura	89	60	NR	NR	NR	NR
		w/aura	85	60	NR	NR	NR	NR
Rasmussen etal., 1991	P	740	82	50	83	86	NR	NR
Lipton etal., 1992	P	2479 (physician	74(F)	39(F)	72(F)	68(F)	56(F)	NR
		diagnosed)	66(M)	63(M)	63(M)	61(M)	45(M)	
		(non-physician	60(F)	18(F)	63(F)	65(F)	30(F)	
		diagnosed)	49(M)	18(M)	61(M)	63(M)	29(M)	
Rasmussen & Olesen, 1992	P	58	95	62	95	98	NR	NR
Russell etal., 1992	C	61 (clinical interview)						
		w/oaura	85	NR	98	82	NR	NR
		w/aura	100	NR	100	100	NR	NR
		61 (headachediary)						
		w/oaura	80	NR	82	75	NR	NR
		w/aura	53	NR	68	60	NR	NR

the fluid retention after the headache resolves. [50,51]

The prevalence of associated symptoms is higher in clinic-based than in population-based studies, probably because more effective interviewing techniques and more definitive criteria are used in the clinic. In addition, a selection bias toward patients with more severe headache may result in more symptoms being reported. [41] Studies that graded the severity of nausea, photophobia, and phonophobia improved the differentiation of migraine from TTH; by definition, these symptoms were more prevalent and more severe in migraineurs.[41]

Celentano et al., using a population-based telephone interview, estimated the prevalence of severe headaches in adolescents and young adults. Symptoms usually considered diagnostic of migraine (nausea and/or vomiting, visual disturbances, and photophobia) were significantly associated with prolonged duration and more severe pain; although these symptoms were reported relatively infrequently in the study population, they were associated with headaches that caused the greatest impairment [41]. Bigal et al. found similar results in a large population study.[52]

The prevalence of migraine-associated symptoms, particularly nausea and vomiting, has also been estimated by placebo-controlled drug studies. Forty-five percent to 100% of patients had nausea prior to treatment, which was similar to prevalence rates observed in other studies of adult migraineurs. The prevalence of vomiting was much lower, but varied dramatically from study to study, as might be anticipated, as a result of treatment of the acute migraine attack. Photophobia, when analyzed, occurred in 86%–97% of patients, while phonophobia was rarely analyzed.[41]

Silberstein performed a telephone interview survey of 500 self-reported migraine sufferers in 1994.[41] The most commonly reported symptoms associated with migraine, in addition to pain, were nausea, visual problems, and vomiting. Nausea occurred in more than 90% of all migraineurs; nearly one-third of these experienced nausea during every attack. Vomiting occurred in almost 70% of all migraineurs; nearly one-third of these vomited in the majority of attacks. Thirty and one-half percent of those who experienced nausea and 42.2% of those with vomiting indicated that the symptom interfered with their ability to take their oral migraine medication. Visual problems and vomiting were also reported to occur in most attacks by 70% and 32% of respondents, respectively. The only other symptom that occurred in more than 20% of respondents in a majority of attacks was sound sensitivity or auditory problems. Some symptoms that were reported by 10% or less of respondents (light sensitivity, dizziness, and neck pain) occurred in a high percentage of their attacks, suggesting that these symptoms may be specific but not sensitive indicators of migraine. Most of the commonly associated symptoms were most often rated as moderate to severe, consistent with the increased severity that would be expected with the more severe headaches in this study (as a result of selection criteria).[41]

Lipton et al. analyzed respondents to the 2009 US population sample (AMPP survey) who met criteria for episodic migraine (EM) and were identified using ICHD-2 criteria (< 15 headache days/month). Among 6,448 persons with EM and nausea symptom data, nearly half (49.5%) reported frequent nausea (≥ half the time) with headache, 29.1% reported nausea less than half the time, and 21.4% reported nausea never or rarely with their headaches. Frequent nausea was commoner in females (52.4%) versus males (39.2%, $p < .001$). Subjects with frequent nausea were more likely to be occupationally disabled or on medical leave than those with no or rare nausea (OR 2.13, CI 1.66–2.73, $p < 001$). Respondents with frequent versus no/ rare nausea more often reported that their headache medications interfered with work or school functioning (OR 1.66, CI 1.41–.94, $p < .0001$), the ability to perform household work (OR 1.49, CI 1.28–1.74, $p < .0001$), or family or social activities (OR 1.50, CI 1.29–1.75, $p < .0001$). Frequent headache-related nausea was associated with greater medication-related impairment at work or school, with household work, and in social and leisure activities. Less satisfaction with treatment was seen with increases in nausea frequency. Nausea appears to be a substantially debilitating feature of EM, leading to significantly worse outcomes in those who experience it and providing an important target for treatment.[53]

Nausea and/or vomiting, photophobia, and phonophobia are important criteria for migraine diagnosis, particularly if the headache is not accompanied by aura. Nausea and vomiting also interfere with medication ingestion and were among the principal reasons that patients discontinued a specific migraine medication. Gastric emptying can be delayed and oral drug absorption impaired during an attack of migraine, and vomiting may result in drug loss, thereby compromising the therapeutic effectiveness of orally administered drugs.[41]

Common Non-ICHD Symptoms

Recent studies indicate that atypical symptoms are common in migraine. These include neck pain/discomfort (59%–61%), as well as sinus pain/pressure (39%–44%).[54] Osmophobia and menstrual exacerbation can also be associated with migraine. The ICHD diagnostic criteria for migraine do not include autonomic nasal symptoms, such as congestion or rhinorrhea, or ocular symptoms, such as lacrimation, despite their frequent occurrence. Across studies, the frequency of nasal and ocular symptoms among patients with migraine ranges from 25% to 98%. [55–57] Conversely, the frequency of migraine meeting ICHD-1 or ICHD-2 diagnostic criteria is high among those with self-described or physician-diagnosed "sinus" headache. [58,59] In the Sinus, Allergy, and Migraine Study (SAMS), for example, more than half (52%) of 100 consecutively consulting patients who believed they had sinus headache were determined to have migraine with or without aura and 23% to have probable migraine.[58] Among those determined to have migraine, 62% experienced bilateral forehead and maxillary pain with their headaches; 56% experienced nasal congestion, 37% eyelid edema, 25% rhinorrhea, 22% conjunctival injection, and 19% lacrimation. In one clinic-based study (n = 47), 98% of patients with at least a 1-year history of self-described sinus headaches and no previous diagnosis of migraine or triptan use were determined, based on a detailed history, to have symptoms fulfilling ICHD criteria for migraine.[55] ICHD symptoms common among these patients included moderate/severe pain (98% of patients), photophobia (72%), and phonophobia (49%).[55] Nasal and ocular symptoms were at least as common or commoner than ICHD-defined symptoms in these patients: 74% reported stuffiness and 60% reported runny nose.[55] In another study (n = 2991), 88% of patients with a history of self-described or physician-diagnosed "sinus" headache and no previous diagnosis of migraine were determined by physician diagnosis to have migraine-type headache (80% with migraine with or without aura and 8% with migrainous disorder).[59] The authors concluded that the presence of nasal or ocular symptoms may be part of the migraine process in patients with recurrent headaches without fever or purulent discharge and that migraine should be included in the differential diagnosis of these patients. Results of these studies demonstrate that some patients' "sinus" headaches, often characterized by autonomic nasal and/or ocular symptoms, are actually migraine headaches (Figures 1.3 and 1.4).

Both headache and nasal/ocular symptoms respond to migraine-specific therapy with triptans. In the 47-patient clinic-based study described earlier,[55] patients were asked to treat two of their headaches with sumatriptan tablets (50 mg). Moderate or severe pre-dose pain was reduced to mild or no pain 2 hours post-dose in 66% of headaches (39/59) and to no pain in 34% of headaches (20/59). In the 3038-patient study described earlier,[59] patients diagnosed at the screening visit with migraine by ICHD-1 criteria entered a randomized, double-blind, parallel-group treatment phase, during which they treated a headache with either sumatriptan tablets (50 mg) or placebo. [60] Moderate or severe pre-dose pain was reduced to mild or no pain 2 hours post-dose in 69% of sumatriptan-treated patients compared with 43% of placebo-treated patients (p < 0.001). Likewise, more sumatriptan-treated patients than placebo-treated patients were free of sinus pain 2 hours post-dose (63% vs. 49%, p < 0.05).

The overlapping anatomy of primary sinonasal pain and migraine suggests a possible mechanism for autonomic nasal and ocular symptoms during migraine. Migraine headache is considered to be secondary to recurrent activation of the trigeminovascular system.[61,62] The trigeminal nerve contains three main divisions that carry pain information: the ophthalmic division (V1), the maxillary division (V2), and the mandibular division (V3). The trigeminal nerve thus innervates widespread areas of the head, face, and neck. The sensory trigeminal nerve network converges at the trigeminal nucleus caudalis, which relays pain signals to

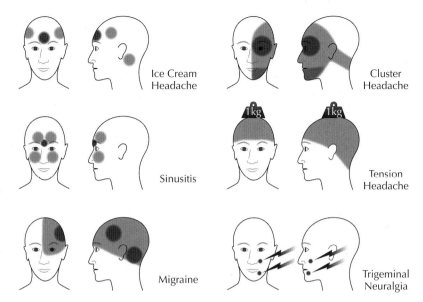

Figure 1.3. Location of typical headache types.

higher-order neurons in the thalamus and cortex. A branch of the cranial parasympathetic nerves, which to branch the sinus cavities and tears ducts, is contiguous with the maxillary branch of the trigeminal nerve along portions of its length. If one of these nerves is activated, it can activate the other; or both nerves may be activated simultaneously through a brainstem reflex between the trigeminal nucleus caudalis and the superior salivatory nucleus, the latter of which gives rise to cranial parasympathetic efferents that innervate the lacrimal gland and nasal/sinus mucosa. Activation of the cranial parasympathetic efferents can result in sinus-like symptoms, such as lacrimation, rhinorrhea, and nasal congestion. These connections possibly explain the occurrence of autonomic nasal and ocular symptoms in migraine. Circumstantial evidence supports this possibility,[63] but the anatomic and physiologic bases of nasal and ocular symptoms in migraine remain to be elucidated.

In two identical, randomized, multicenter, double-blind, placebo-controlled, multiple-attack, early intervention, crossover trials in 1266 adult migraineurs, the incidences of traditional migraine symptoms (nausea, vomiting, photophobia, phonophobia) and non-traditional symptoms associated with migraine (sinus pain/pressure and neck pain/discomfort) were determined before and after treatment with sumatriptan RT/naproxen sodium.

[54] The mean baseline incidence ranges for sinus pain/pressure (39%–44%) were greater than those for nausea (27%–33%) or vomiting (1%–3%), and the resolution of sinus pain/pressure after treatment with sumatriptan RT/naproxen sodium was significantly greater than placebo at all time points measured between 2 and 6 hours.

Patients having autonomic nasal and ocular symptoms or sinus pain/pressure with headaches and meeting ICHD criteria for migraine often mislabeled their headaches as "sinus" headaches or were misdiagnosed as having a non-migraine headache type. Adding autonomic symptoms to the diagnostic criteria for migraine may help to improve diagnostic clarity.

ICHD diagnostic criteria for migraine do not include neck pain despite its frequent occurrence in migraine. In a prospective study of 144 patients diagnosed with migraine according to ICHD-1 criteria, 75% indicated that their migraine episodes were accompanied by neck pain, most often described as tightness (69% of patients), stiffness (17% of patients), or throbbing (5% of patients).[64] The majority of patients (92%) indicated that neck pain occurred during the headache phase of a migraine attack; however, occurrence of neck pain during the prodrome (61% of patients) and the postdrome (41% of patients) was also common. In another study, which included 412 patients meeting ICHD-1 criteria for migraine, 51.2% described neck or shoulder stiffness or tightness in association with migraine attacks, and 36.7% described tenderness of the neck muscles.[65]

The location of pain often varies between attacks in the same individual and between patients with the same disorder. Headache and pain location may also help to distinguish between primary headache disorders (Figure 1.3). Neck pain associated with migraine attacks appears to respond to migraine-specific therapy with triptans. A subset of 30 patients from the 144-patient study described in the preceding paragraph used migraine-specific therapy with a triptan to treat 278 headaches, of which 231 (83%) were accompanied by neck pain.[64] Patients were instructed to treat at the onset of mild headache pain, with 83% of attacks associated with some neck pain. All patients were asked to treat with the most effective oral dose of their traditional triptan agent. The 2-hour pain-free rates for head and neck pain were nearly identical, with 68% (n = 278) head-pain free and 73% (n = 231) neck-pain free responses, respectively. Pain-free response 2 hours after treating mild, moderate, or severe headache pain was reported in 68% of attacks for head pain and in 73% of attacks for neck pain. In another study, of randomized,

double-blind, parallel-group design, patients self-reporting tension/stress headache and meeting ICHD-1 criteria for migraine treated moderate or severe headache pain with either sumatriptan tablets 100 mg (n = 130) or placebo (n = 123).[66] The majority of patients (84%) had neck pain at the time of dosing. Relief of neck pain/discomfort was reported in numerically (but not statistically significantly) more patients with sumatriptan than placebo 2 hours (44% vs. 42%) and 4 hours post-dose (60% vs. 55%). In another study of the effect of migraine-specific therapy on neck pain,[66] relief of neck pain was reported in significantly more patients treated with sumatriptan/naproxen sodium than placebo 2, 3, 4, and 6 hours post-dose in a randomized, double-blind, placebo-controlled, parallel-group study of the combination tablet sumatriptan/naproxen sodium taken as early intervention for mild pain for up to four migraine attacks by patients with ICHD-2-defined migraine. In this study, the mean baseline incidence of neck pain ranged from 59% to 61% across attacks. (The incidences of ICHD-defined migraine symptoms across attacks were 69%–74% for photophobia, 62%–69% for phonophobia, and 27%–33% for nausea.)

Calhoun et al. determined the prevalence of neck pain at the time of migraine treatment

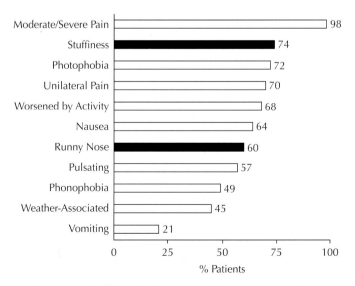

Figure 1.4. Percentage of patients with self-described "sinus" headache reporting specific symptoms. The headaches of nearly all of these patients (46 of 47) met ICHD-1 criteria for migraine. Many patients reported nasal symptoms with their migraine headaches.[55]

relative to the prevalence of nausea in a prospective, observational, cross-sectional study of 113 migraineurs, ranging in attack frequency from episodic to chronic migraine. Details of all migraines were recorded over the course of at least 1 month and until six qualifying migraines had been treated. Subjects recorded 2411 headache days, of which 786 were migraines. Most migraines were treated in the moderate pain stage. Regardless of the intensity of headache pain at time of treatment, neck pain was a more frequent accompaniment of migraine than was nausea ($p < .0001$). Neck pain and nausea occurred increasingly in mild (42.8 vs. 17.5), moderate (61.1 vs. 35.7), and severe (72.8 vs. 48.4) migraine attacks. Neck pain prevalence correlated with headache chronicity as attacks moved from episodic to chronic daily headache.[67]

The trigeminocervical nucleus, a spinal-cord region where descending sensory nerve fibers of the trigeminal nerve converge upon second-order neurons down to the level of C2, constitutes a possible substrate for the occurrence of neck pain in migraine. In addition to being a component of migraine, neck pain might also occur as a migraine trigger with myofascial and neurogenic underpinnings, or as a result of migraine and a manifestation of central sensitization.

Olfactory impairment is common in neurologic disorders. Many report changes in their sense of smell or osmophobia (aversion to odors) during migraine. Osmophobia is not included as a clinical feature of migraine in the ICHD-2 criteria. However, it is included as a symptom of migraine in the Canadian Headache Society migraine diagnostic guidelines,[68] which describe osmophobia as a highly sensitive and specific feature of migraine based on a 2000-case study published in 1954.[69] Osmophobia is also included in the ICHD-2 Appendix as a feature of migraine.[6] The ICHD-2 Appendix identifies novel entities that, consensus opinion suggests, may prove to be useful in diagnosis but have not been sufficiently validated for inclusion in ICHD-2 criteria.

Osmophobia is consistently and frequently reported as a migraine symptom in studies that include osmophobia in symptom checklists used to survey patients; studies that do not report osmophobia as a migraine symptom generally did not include it in symptom checklists. In one small study ($n = 50$), 50% of migraineurs experienced osmophobia or hyperosmia during migraine attacks. In a study of 1025 migraineurs consulting a headache center, 28% reported osmophobia as a migraine-associated symptom.[70] Other common symptoms included nausea (90.1%), vomiting (51.8%), photophobia (93.9%), phonophobia (91.4%), and dizziness (72.4%). The presence of osmophobia was correlated with both headache intensity and headache duration.

Migraine sufferers will occasionally report that an attack is provoked by exposure to certain odors. The triggers are usually of the intense variety, such as gasoline, acetone, or strong perfume.[12] Olfactory hallucinations, usually unpleasant, may occur as part of the aura, although this is rare, affecting only four of 551 migraineurs in one study.[12] In this series, osmophobia was a frequent complaint during the attack, involving more than one-quarter of the patients, most of whom were female.[71] Apart from precipitating migraine, smells may aggravate the headache, a finding that led to the suggestion that odors might be used to distinguish tension-type headache from migraine.[72]

Some data suggest that osmophobia is a specific migraine marker that differentiates migraine from other primary headache types and discriminates between migraine and secondary headaches.[73–76] In a clinic-based sample that included 477 migraineurs without aura, 92 migraineurs with aura, 135 patients with episodic tension-type headache, 44 with episodic cluster headache, and 25 with other primary headaches, osmophobia during headache attacks was reported by 43% of patients with migraine without aura, 39% of patients with migraine with aura, 7% of patients with episodic cluster headache, and 0% of patients with episodic tension-type headache or other primary headache disorders.[74] The authors concluded that osmophobia should be considered a candidate criterion for the diagnosis of migraine because of its specificity.[74] Osmophobia also was identified as a migraine marker in a review of medical records of 96 children consulting a headache clinic between December 2004 and March 2005.[75] Of the 96 children, 57% were classified as having migraine, 25% as having other primary headaches, and 18% as having secondary headaches. Osmophobia was present in 20% of migraineurs but was absent in patients with other primary headaches or secondary headaches.

Like osmophobia, olfactory triggers appear to be common in migraine. Migraine attacks were reported to be triggered by odors in 11 of 50 patients in one study.[77] Similarly, in a study of 74 patients with migraine and 30 non-migrainous control individuals, olfactory hypersensitivity was identified in 35.2% of patients with migraine and none of the controls.[76] The presence of olfactory hypersensitivity was associated with more frequent migraine attacks, more odor-triggered migraine attacks, and visual hypersensitivity. Whether osmophobia occurring during a migraine attack is phenomenologically related to olfactory hypersensitivity that can trigger migraine attacks is not known.

Migraineurs display hypersensitivity to sensory stimuli; however, olfactory acuity has not been well established. Hyperosmia is reported on rare occasions, and persists in some patients beyond the headache phase.[77] Interictal hyperosmia, as measured by thresholds to vanillin and acetone, was described in a group of 20 migraine sufferers.[78] This finding is in accord with reports that migraine sufferers are hypersensitive to sensory stimuli in general, including smell, taste, light, touch, and sound. In contrast to these observations, Hirsch[79] found elevated olfactory detection thresholds to pyridine in 12/67 (18%) migraineurs, compared with just 1% of the general population[79] and suggested that there was in fact an olfactory defect in migraine. These conflicting results indicate the need for further study, employing strict criteria for the diagnosis of headache and the timing of olfactory assessment in relation to the headache phase.[80]

Marmura and Anjum measured olfaction between, during, and after treated migraine compared with age- and sex-matched controls to determine if subjects could predict changes in olfaction during migraine. They used the University of Pennsylvania Smell Identification Test (UPSIT), a 40-item test to diagnose olfactory deficits. They recruited 50 subjects (13 men and 37 women, aged 19–60) with episodic migraine, excluding patients who had significant head injuries and sinus-nasal disease. They measured smell acuity by using UPSIT at three different intervals: between attacks, during acute migraine, and after successfully treated migraine. Age- and sex-matched controls with

no disabling headaches completed the UPSIT in the office on two separate occasions. In addition, they administered a questionnaire to determine odor sensitivity and perceived olfactory acuity during migraine. Subjectively, olfaction improved in six patients and worsened in six patients during migraine. Thirty-eight patients had no change. Using UPSIT, most subjects (43/50, mean 36.1) had normal olfactory acuity at baseline. The mean UPSIT was lower during acute migraine (34.8) and after treated attacks (35.6). Of six patients reporting subjectively improved olfaction, none had an improved UPSIT and four scored lower during migraine. Controls (mean = 36.8) had slightly higher UPSIT scores than subjects. There was a trend for more abnormal UPSIT scores (women < 35, men < 34) in acute migraine (11/35, p = 0.063), and after treated attacks (10/31, p = 0.090). The majority of subjects with migraine had normal baseline olfaction. Subjects claiming enhanced olfactory acuity with migraine were actually more likely to have a lower UPSIT score.[81]

Vertigo is not included in the ICHD classification for migraine with or without aura, but does appear to occur as a feature of migraine in some patients. An association between migraine and vertigo, defined as a symptom arising from the vestibular system rather than non-vestibular dizziness (e.g., lightheadedness, unsteadiness, impending faint), was documented more than 100 years ago.[82] Several studies[83,84] have demonstrated an excess prevalence of vestibular laboratory abnormalities and vertigo in migraine sufferers. Across studies, vestibular abnormalities were identified in approximately one-third of patients with migraine.[84] Conversely, an excess prevalence of migraine in individuals with vertigo has also been found.[83] More research on the phenomenology, epidemiology, pathophysiology, and response to therapy of migraine-associated vertigo is necessary before this clinical feature is considered as part of an expanded case definition of migraine.

Silberstein et al. investigated the efficacy and tolerability of a fixed-dose, single-tablet formulation of sumatriptan 85 mg, formulated with RT Technology, and naproxen sodium 500 mg (sumatriptan/naproxen) as early intervention acute therapy for migraine in two identically designed, randomized, double-blind, parallel-group, placebo-controlled studies. They not only evaluated the traditional migraine-associated symptoms (nausea, photophobia, and phonophobia) but non-traditional migraine-associated symptoms (neck pain/discomfort and sinus pain/pressure). The fixed-dose, single-tablet formulation of sumatriptan/naproxen was effective and well tolerated in an early intervention paradigm for the acute treatment of migraine, including traditional and non-traditional symptoms. Sinus pain and pressure were reported at baseline in 42% (study 1) and 52% (study 2) of patients. Neck pain and discomfort were reported in 58%–63% (study 1) and 63% (study 2) of patients. In the current studies, sinus pain/pressure and neck pain/discomfort at baseline were more common than vomiting (2%) and nausea (27%–30% [study 1] and 33%–34% [study 2]).[85]

During migraine attacks, more than 70% of patients exhibit cutaneous allodynia—that is, the perception of pain when ordinarily non-painful stimuli are applied to the skin. [86] Table 1.6 lists examples of signs of cutaneous allodynia. The allodynia can be either restricted (i.e., confined to the pain-referred area) or extended (i.e., experienced both within and outside the pain-referred area).[86] In patients who develop extended allodynia, cutaneous allodynia progresses during the course of a migraine attack from restricted allodynia to extended allodynia over a 1–2-hour period. This progression of allodynia as a migraine attack develops may reflect the sequential recruitment and sensitization of peripheral and central pain pathways.[86–89] The pathway

Table 1.6 Signs of Cutaneous Allodynia

During headache, skin pain or discomfort is worsened by
- Combing hair or pulling it back
- Wearing a hairband or hat
- Wearing glasses
- Wearing earrings
- Shaving
- Letting shower water hit the scalp
- Sleeping with head resting on the headache side
- Breathing cold air through the nose
- Wearing tight clothes, particularly turtleneck shirts
- Wearing a necklace
- Being hugged
- Wearing socks
- Wearing a bra

for trigeminal nociception involves afferent fibers of dural nociceptors with cell bodies in the trigeminal ganglion (first-order neurons), the spinal trigeminal nucleus (second-order neurons), the thalamus (third-order neurons), and the facial representation in the primary somatosensory cortex (fourth-order neurons). In the progression of allodynia, peripheral pain pathways originating from neurons with cell bodies in the trigeminal ganglion are recruited and sensitized first, and then the peripheral nerve activity contributes to the sensitization of central pain pathways originating from neurons with cell bodies in the dorsal horn of the spinal cord. Central sensitization can occur as early as 1 hour after the onset of migraine pain. It appears that, while initiation of central sensitization depends on input from sensitized peripheral pathways, central sensitization can be maintained independently of peripheral input.[86]

Changes in cutaneous allodynia may reflect changes in the extent of sensitization as a migraine attack progresses. Cutaneous allodynia may reflect the progression of neural sensitization during a migraine and, correspondingly, the progression of symptom severity. Typically during a migraine, pain progresses from mild to moderate or severe. The pain, often throbbing, associated with the onset of a migraine attack is thought to be caused by initial peripheral sensitization in the trigeminal nociceptive system. The moderate to severe pain that develops later in a full-blown migraine attack is associated with central sensitization involving second- and third-order neurons of the trigeminal nociceptive system. Central sensitization can occur as early as 1 hour after the onset of migraine pain. These observations have led to the suggestion that migraine therapy with triptans, which act peripherally on $5HT_{1B}$ receptors on the cranial vasculature and $5HT_{1D}$ receptors on meningeal pain fibers,[90] can be optimized by administering them immediately after the onset of mild pain to prevent sensitization of central pain pathways and the development of a full-blown migraine attack.[86] Clinical data support this practice of early intervention and its theoretical underpinnings by showing that therapeutic success is greater when migraine attacks are treated early, while pain is mild, rather than later, when pain has progressed to moderate or severe.[91–93] Furthermore, administering a triptan before the establishment of cutaneous allodynia during a migraine attack was substantially more likely to bring about a pain-free response than was treating after cutaneous allodynia was established.[88] In a study of 31 migraineurs treating 34 allodynia-associated migraine attacks and 27 attacks not associated with allodynia, patients were pain-free within 2 hours of dosing with a triptan in 93% of non-allodynic attacks compared with 15% of allodynic attacks.[87] In the presence of allodynia, triptan treatment was similarly ineffective for migraine attacks treated 1 hour *versus* 4 hours after the onset of pain. In the absence of allodynia, triptan treatment was similarly effective for migraine attacks treated 1 hour *versus* 4 hours after the onset of pain. The presence or absence of allodynia predicted the ability of a triptan to render a migraine attack pain-free with 90% accuracy. Consistent with these results, administration of sumatriptan at the same time that an inflammatory mixture was topically applied to the dura in an animal model (i.e., early intervention) prevented the development of central sensitization as measured by neuronal activity, whereas sumatriptan administered 2 hours after the inflammatory mixture was applied (i.e., late intervention) did not prevent central sensitization.[87]

In addition to reflecting the extent of trigeminal nociceptive sensitization within patients during a given migraine attack, differences in cutaneous allodynia may reflect differences *between* patients in the extent of trigeminal nociceptive sensitization.[94] The localized intracranial hypersensitivity (manifested as pain intensification triggered by bending over, sneezing, or coughing) that all patients experience with migraine is thought to be mediated by the sensitization of meningeal nociceptors on first-order neurons that arise from the trigeminal ganglion. For the minority of patients who do not progress to cutaneous allodynia during migraine, this sensitization of dural nociceptors may be the extent of sensitization occurring during an attack.[94] In allodynic patients, the progression from localized intracranial hypersensitivity to restricted/cephalic allodynia and then to extended/extracephalic allodynia may involve the subsequent sequential sensitization of second- and third-order neurons. Localized/cephalic allodynia may reflect sensitization of central trigeminal neurons (second-order neurons) in the brainstem,

and extended/extracephalic allodynia may reflect additional sensitization of third-order neurons that receive converging information from other body areas, such as the head and forearms.[94]

If differences in cutaneous allodynia reflect differences between patients in the extent of trigeminal nociceptive sensitization, then between-patient responsiveness to triptans, like responsiveness within a given migraine attack, may be predicted by degree of cutaneous allodynia. Those who never experience allodynia may respond to triptans equally as well when they are administered while pain is moderate or severe compared to early administration while pain is mild. (In the 31-patient study described earlier, patients who never developed allodynia were in fact highly likely to become pain-free after using a triptan, regardless of the time of triptan administration relative to the onset of pain.[87]) Those who develop allodynia during the later phase of the migraine attack may respond particularly well to triptans administered early in the course of the attack while pain is mild. Those who experience constant allodynia, both during and between migraine attacks, may constitute a group that never responds to triptans. These possibilities warrant evaluation in clinical studies.

Allodynia is prevalent in patients with migraine, and its presence is 90% accurate in predicting early pain-free efficacy of triptans.

Postdrome

Following the headache, the patient may have impaired concentration or may feel tired, washed out, irritable, and listless. Some people, however, feel unusually refreshed or euphoric after an attack. Muscle weakness and aching and anorexia or food cravings can occur.

Using a questionnaire, a Spanish study looked at the postdromal symptoms of 100 migraineurs who consulted their general physician. Postdromal symptoms were those experienced the day after the headache had started, but only if the symptoms had not been present on a questionnaire completed in a pain-free period. Postdromal symptoms were experienced by 80% of subjects for the first attack (mean and range 4.7 and 0–15). Asthenia (55%), tiredness (46%), somnolence (29%), concentration difficulties (28%), phonophobia (27%), photophobia (26%), unhappiness (26%), and yawning (24%) were the most common symptoms. As with premonitory symptoms, postdromal symptoms were more frequent in migraine-with-aura subjects. Headache severity was associated with a higher frequency of postdromal symptoms. Almost two-thirds of the symptoms were noticed in at least two of three attacks, while more than a quarter of the symptoms were repeated in three of three attacks.[15]

In the Griffin study,[11] the postdrome was defined as the time between the patient's regarding the headache as resolved and feeling completely back to normal. There was a return to normal within 6 hours of the end of the headache after 55% of migraines with a postdrome, with only 7% requiring more than 24 hours. Tiredness was the most common symptom in the postdrome (88%), with other symptoms similar to those expressed in the premonitory period. Nausea (23.5 vs. 14.8), photophobia (48.8 vs. 36), and phonophobia (38.4 vs. 31.8) were expressed at high percentages in the premonitory and postdrome phases.

Kelman documented the frequency, duration, and types of postdromal symptoms in 827 consecutive migraine patients who were evaluated at their first headache clinic visit. Sixty-eight percent reported postdrome (69.1% females, 56.8% males, < 0.007) with an average duration of 25.2 hours. Fifty-six percent had postdrome for ≤12 hours, 32% for 12–24 hours, 88% for 24 hours, and 12% for > 24 hours. The most common symptoms were tiredness (71.8%), head pain (33.1%), cognitive difficulties (11.7%), "hangover" (10.7%), gastrointestinal symptoms (8.4%), mood change (6.8%), and weakness (6.2%). Patients with postdrome had more characteristic and more frequent migraine features compared with those without postdrome. This study demonstrated postdrome in 68% of patients, duration ≤ 24 hours in most patients, more often associated with a full-blown migraine attack, commoner in females, and with commonest symptoms being tiredness and low-grade headache.[95]

Ng-Mak et al. interviewed migraine patients with postdrome symptoms as a prelude to developing a postdrome migraine questionnaire. Qualitative concept-elicitation focus groups were conducted with 34 patients in three geographically diverse US cities to elicit the symptoms and burden of migraine postdrome. Patients defined the onset of postdrome as the point at which they no longer experienced the migraine pain. Postdrome was often described as "[being] or [feeling] wiped out" and "headache hangover." The symptoms most frequently reported were tiredness, difficulty concentrating, weakness, dizziness, lightheadedness, and decreased energy. Patients also reported decreased activity levels as a result of postdrome symptoms. Postdrome symptoms impacted the ability to work, affected family interactions and social life, and caused cognitive impairment. A preliminary questionnaire measuring the severity and duration of symptoms and the severity of impacts of the post-migraine experience, with an 11-point (0 to 10) response scale, was developed. In this study, headache pain and nausea were excluded from the list of symptoms in the draft measure because they overlapped with primary symptoms of the headache phase.[96]

THE CLASSIFICATION OF MIGRAINE

In the ICHD-3 β, migraine is divided into two major categories: (1.1) migraine without aura (characterized by headache with specific features and associated symptoms); and (1.2) migraine with aura (characterized by the transient focal neurologic symptoms that usually precede or sometimes accompany the headache). Other major categories include chronic migraine (1.3), complications of migraine. (1.4), probable migraine (1.5), and episodic syndromes that may be associated with migraine (1.6).[8]

Migraine without Aura

The diagnostic criteria for migraine without aura (1.1) in ICHD-3 β, published in 2013, are little changed from those published in 1988 and 2004.[8] They require at least five lifetime attacks lasting 4–72 hours. In children, attacks may be shorter, 1–72 hours, and photophobia and phonophobia may be inferred from behavior, rather than reported, in young children.[6]

As before, criteria for migraine without aura are met by various combinations of features.

Table 1.7 ICHD-3 β Diagnostic Criteria for 1.1 Migraine Without Aura

A. At least 5 attacks fulfilling criteria B–D
B. Headache attacks lasting 4–72 hours (untreated or unsuccessfully treated)
C. Headache has at least two of the following characteristics:
   1. Unilateral location
   2. Pulsating quality
   3. Moderate or severe pain intensity
   4. Aggravation by or causing avoidance of routine physical activity (e.g., walking or climbing stairs)
D. During headache at least one of the following:
   1. Nausea and/or vomiting
   2. Photophobia and phonophobia
E. Not better accounted for by another ICHD-3 β diagnosis

Table 1.8 ICHD-3 β Diagnostic Criteria for 1.2 Migraine with Aura

A. At least 2 attacks fulfilling criteria B–C
B. One or more of the following fully reversible aura symptoms: visual, sensory, speech/language, motor, brainstem, or retinal symptoms
C. At least 2 of the following characteristics
   1. At least one aura symptom spreads gradually over 5 minutes or more and/or 2 or more symptoms occur in succession.
   2. Each single aura symptom lasts 5–60 min.
   3. At least one aura symptom is one-sided.
   4. The aura is accompanied or followed by headache. A possible lag phase lasts maximally 60 minutes.
D. Not better accounted for by another ICHD-3 β diagnosis.

Two of four features are required (Table 1.7). A typical unilateral, pulsating headache meets the criteria, but so does a bilateral, pressing headache if it is moderate or severe in intensity and aggravated by routine physical activity. Associated features include nausea with or without vomiting or both photophobia and phonophobia. In addition, neck pain, sinus pain, osmophobia, movement sensitivity, and menstrual exacerbation are part of migraine, although they are not ICHD-2 defining features.

Migraine with Aura

The ICHD-3 β criteria for migraine with aura (Table 1.8) are similar to the ICHD-2 criteria. [8] The typical aura of migraine is characterized by focal neurologic features that usually precede migrainous headache but may accompany it or occur in the absence of the headache. [97] Typical aura symptoms develop over ≥ 5 minutes and last no more than 60 minutes, and visual aura is overwhelmingly the most common symptom.[16] Typical visual auras have a hemianopic distribution. Scotomas (graying out of vision), photopsia or phosphenes, and other visual manifestations may occur. This mixing of positive and negative features is the hallmark of migraine aura. Visual distortions, such as metamorphopsia, micropsia and macropsia, are more common in children[12,17,98] (Table 1.9).

Auras are not always visual. Sensory symptoms occur in up to one-third of patients who have migraine with aura.[28] Sensory auras include numbness (negative symptom) and tingling or paresthesia (positive symptoms). The distribution may be cheiro-oral (face and hand). Word-finding difficulty, or dysphasia, may be part of typical aura. Motor weakness, symptoms of brainstem dysfunction, and changes in level of consciousness all occur,[27] usually signaling particular subtypes of migraine with aura (hemiplegic and basilar-type).

Typical migraine aura sometimes occurs with headache types other than migraine (i.e., headache not fulfilling the criteria of 1.1). Typical aura occurs with cluster headache, chronic paroxysmal hemicrania, and hemicrania continua. [99–101] These cases were classified based on the aura and the headache (*typical aura with non-migraine headache*). The ICHD-3 β now regards this as a migraine headache because of its relation to the aura.

Table 1.9 ICHD-3 β Diagnostic Criteria for 1.2.1 Typical Aura with Migraine Headache

1.2.1.1 *typical aura with headache*
Diagnostic criteria
A. Fulfills criteria for 1.2.1 *migraine with typical aura*
B. Headache, with or without migraine characteristics, accompanies or follows the aura within 60 minutes.

Migraine Aura Without Headache

When typical aura occurs in the absence of headache,[19,102,103] it is *typical aura without headache*, a disorder most often reported by middle-aged men (Table 1.10).[104] These periodic neurologic phenomena (scintillating scotomata, recurrent sensory, motor, and mental phenomena) must be differentiated from transient ischemic attacks (TIAs) and focal seizures, and are diagnosed as migraine only after full investigation and reasonable follow-up. Investigation is particularly needed when these phenomena first occur after age 40, when negative features (i.e., hemianopia) are predominant, or when the aura is of atypical duration[8,30] (Table 1.11).

Transient visual disturbances (TVDs), with flickering or scintillating phenomena, also occur with numerous other conditions, including blood cell diseases, retinal detachment, cluster headaches, trauma, and syncope, but are not generally associated with cerebrovascular embolic or thrombotic disease.[105] Headache occurring in association with aura symptoms will help confirm the diagnosis but does not exclude transient ischamia attack. Ziegler and Hassanein[19] reported that 44% of their patients who had headache with aura had aura without headache at some time.

Levy[106] found that 32% of Cornell neurologists had a history of transient neurologic loss, most commonly visual (field cuts, obscurations, scotomata) and less commonly nonvisual (hemiparesis, clumsiness, paresthesias, dysarthria) symptoms. Migraine was reported in 29%, occurring in 44% of those reporting and 22% of those not reporting transient CNS dysfunction. None developed any residual deficit or chronic neurologic disorder at 5-year followup, suggesting that these are benign migrainous accompaniments.

Table 1.10 ICHD-3 β Diagnostic Criteria for 1.2.3 Typical Aura Without Headache

A. Fulfills criteria for 1.2.1 *migraine with typical aura*

B. No headache accompanies or follows the aura within 60 minutes.

Table 1.11 Migraine Equivalents

Scintillating scotoma
Paresthesias
Aphasia
Dysarthria
Hemiplegia
Blindness
Blurring of vision
Hemianopia
Transient monocular blindness
Ophthalmoplegia
Oculosympathetic palsy
Mydriasis
Confusion-stupor
Cyclical vomiting
Seizures
Diplopia
Deafness
Recurrence stroke deficit
Chorea

Fisher[30] described transient neurologic phenomena characteristically not associated with headache (late life migrainous accompaniments or transient migrainous accompaniments) in 188 patients over the age of 40; 60% were men and 57% had a history of recurrent headache. The attacks of episodic neurologic dysfunction lasted from 1 minute to 72 hours and had variable recurrence rates (one attack 27%, 2–10 attacks 45%, and more than 10 attacks 28%). Scintillating scotoma was considered to be diagnostic of migraine even when it occurred in isolation, whereas other episodic neurologic symptoms (paresthesias, aphasia, and sensory and motor symptoms) needed more careful evaluation.

Wijman et al.[107] determined the frequency, characteristics, and stroke outcome of subjects with visual migrainous symptoms in the Framingham study. Visual symptoms occurred in 186 subjects. Visual symptoms that corresponded to the visual aura of migraine were reported by 26 of 186 subjects (14%), with a prevalence of 1.23% overall (1.33% in women and 1.08% in men). Their numbers ranged from 1 to 500 (10 or more in 69% of subjects) and lasted 15 to 60 minutes in 50% of subjects. The episodes were stereotypical in 65% of subjects. They began after the age of 50 in 77%. The pattern of visual manifestations varied widely among subjects. The episodes were never accompanied by headaches in 58%, and 42% had no headache history. In only 19%

of subjects did the migrainous visual episodes meet the IHS criteria for migraine aura, usually because one of the criteria ("at least one aura symptom develops gradually over more than four minutes") could not be reliably ascertained.

Three of 26 subjects (11.5%) had a stroke 1 or more years later; one had a subarachnoid hemorrhage 1 year later; one had a brainstem infarct 3 years later; and one had a cardioembolic stroke secondary to atrial fibrillation 27 years later. This stroke incidence rate of 11.5% was significantly lower than the stroke incidence rate of 33.3% in subjects with TIAs in the same cohort ($p = 0.030$). These usually occurred within 6 months and did not differ from the stroke incidence rate of 13.6% of those without migrainous phenomena or TIAs.

O'Connor and Tredici [108] described 61 cases of transient neurologic dysfunction in men seen during a 15-year period at the US Air Force School of Aerospace Medicine. These cases were derived from a selected group of highly trained young men whose profession required outstanding visual abilities. Age of onset was 12 to 44 years. Family history was present in 15 (24.6%) subjects, and a personal history of migraine was present only in two (3.3%). Eighteen subjects (29.5%) had nonvisual neurologic deficits during the episodes. One patient experienced permanent neurologic deficiency.

Cohen et al.[109] reported 31 cases of TVD attributed to migraine. Headache was present in 20 patients (64.5%). A family history of migraine was found in 61%, and 57% had a personal history of migraine. After approximately 2 years, one patient died of cardiac disease, none had a stroke, one developed amaurosis fugax, and one developed transient global amnesia.

Mattsson and Lundberg[105] estimated the prevalence and characteristics of TVD of possible migraine origin in both a clinical and a general population. One hundred consecutive women migraine patients 17–69 years of age and 245 women 40–75 years of age from the general population were interviewed. Lifetime prevalence was 37% in migraine patients and 13% in the general population. There were no differences in the TVD characteristics between the groups. Slightly less than half of each group had a gradual onset of 5 or more minutes (45% and 46% of the groups, respectively).

Headache following TVDs had more migrainous features in patients than in controls. The TVDs that did not fulfill the IHS criteria for migraine with aura probably represented abortive migraine phenomena.

In Alabama, a questionnaire survey of 1000 patients presenting for a comprehensive eye examination revealed that 6.5% reported experiencing visual sensations consistent with migraine aura without headache. The prevalence was 2.9% in males and 8.6% in females. A multivariate analysis revealed that female gender (odds ratio [OR] = 2.3), a history of migraine headaches (OR = 3.2), and a history of childhood motion sickness (OR = 2.7) were significantly related to migraine aura without headache.[110]

A Japanese study demonstrated that 35 of 1063 patients (3.2%; 1.1% males and 2.1% females) in general ophthalmologic clinics had typical aura without headache. The age of patients with typical aura without headache showed a biphasic distribution: 20–39 years and 60–69 years.[111]

Visual migrainous phenomena are not rare, since they occur in 1.33% of women and 1.08% of men in a general population sample and are usually benign. Transient migrainous accompaniments (scintillating scotomata, numbness, aphasia, dysarthria, and motor weakness) may occur for the first time after the age of 45 and can be easily confused with TIAs of cerebrovascular origin. Diagnosis is still by exclusion in all but the most classic cases.

Chronic Migraine

Chronic migraine (Table 1.12) was previously considered a complication of migraine. A diagnosis of chronic migraine requires that headaches occur on 15 or more days a month for more than 3 months. These headaches must be migraines on at least 8 days per month. A chronic migraine diagnosis excludes the diagnosis of tension-type headache because tension-type symptomatology is part of the diagnostic criteria for chronic migraine. It is impossible to distinguish the individual episodes of headache in patients with such frequent or continuous headaches; the characteristics often change, even within the same day. Chronic migraine is frequently associated with medication overuse. Patients with chronic

Table 1.12 ICHD-3 β Diagnostic Criteria for 1.2.3 Chronic Migraine

A. Headache (tension-type-like and/or migraine-like) on ≥ 15 days per month for at least 3 months
B. Occurring in a patient who has had at least five attacks fulfilling criteria for 1.1 *migraine without aura* and/or 1.2 *migraine with aura*
C. On ≥ 8 days per month for at least 3 months one or more of the following criteria were fulfilled[3]
   1. Criteria C and D for 1.1 *migraine without aura*
   2. Criteria B and C for 1.2 *migraine with aura*
   3. Headache considered by patient to be onset migraine and relieved by a triptan or an ergotamine derivative
D. Not better accounted for by another ICHD-3 β diagnosis.

migraine and medication overuse should have two diagnoses, chronic migraine and medication overuse headache (see Chapter 9 for more details).

Complications of Migraine

The ICHD-3 β criteria include a number of complications of migraine. Status migrainosus (1.5.2) (Table 1.13) refers to an attack of migraine with a headache phase that lasts > 72 hours.[112] The pain is severe (a diagnostic criterion) and debilitating. Status migrainosus may be caused by medication overuse. If chronic headache and medication overuse have been present, diagnoses are chronic migraine,

Table 1.13 ICHD-3 β Diagnostic Criteria for 1.4.1 Status Migrainosus

A. The present attack in a patient with 1.1 *migraine without aura* and/or 1.2 *migraine with aura* is typical of previous attacks except for its duration and severity.
B. All of the following features:
   1. Unremitting for > 72 hours
   2. Pain and/or other symptoms debilitate the patient
C. Not better accounted for by another ICHD-3 β diagnosis
   1. Remission for up to 12 hours due to medication or sleep is accepted.
   2. Milder cases are coded 1.5.1 *probable migraine.*

Table 1.14 ICHD-3 β Diagnostic Criteria for 1.4.2 Persistent Aura Without Infarction

A. The present attack in a patient with 1.2 *migraine with aura* is typical of previous attacks except that one or more aura symptoms persist for ≥ 1 week.
B. Not better accounted for by another ICHD-3 β diagnosis.

medication overuse headache, and status migrainosus. Non-debilitating attacks lasting > 72 hours but otherwise meeting these criteria are probable migraine without aura. If headache persists for 3 months or more, the diagnosis should be chronic migraine or new daily persistent headache.[8]

Persistent aura without infarction (Table 1.14) is diagnosed when aura symptoms, otherwise typical of past attacks, persist for > 1 week, and neuroimaging shows no evidence of infarction. It is an unusual but well-documented complication of migraine.[112] If aura symptoms last more than 1 hour (typical aura), but less than 1 week (persistent aura without infarction), the ICHD-3 β diagnosis is probable migraine with prolonged aura. Persisting aura symptoms are rare but well documented. They are often bilateral and may last for months or years. The 1-week cut-off is based on the opinion of experts and should be formally studied.[8]

Migrainous infarction (Table 1.15) is uncommon. One or more otherwise typical aura symptoms persist beyond 1 hour, and neuroimaging confirms ischemic infarction. Strictly applied, these criteria distinguish this disorder from other causes of stroke, which must be excluded.[113] The neurologic deficit develops during the course of an apparently typical attack of migraine with aura and exactly mimics the aura of previous attacks. Ischemic stroke in

Table 1.15 ICHD-3 β Diagnostic Criteria for 1.4.3 Migrainous Infarction

A. The present attack in a patient with 1.2 *migraine with aura* is typical of previous attacks except that one or more aura symptoms persists for > 60 minutes.
B. Neuroimaging demonstrates ischemic infarction in a relevant area
C. Not better accounted for by another ICHD-3 β diagnosis.

a migraine sufferer may be categorized as cerebral infarction of other cause coexisting with migraine, cerebral infarction of other cause presenting with symptoms resembling migraine with aura, or cerebral infarction occurring during the course of a typical migraine with aura attack. Only the last fulfills criteria for migrainous infarction. Migrainous infarction mostly occurs in the posterior circulation and in younger women. A twofold increased risk of ischemic stroke in migraine with aura patients has been demonstrated in several population-based studies. However, these infarctions are not migrainous infarctions. Most studies have shown a lack of association between migraine without aura and ischemic stroke.[8]

Migraine Aura-Triggered Seizure

Migraine and epilepsy are comorbid disorders. Headaches are common in the post-ictal period. Sometimes a seizure occurs during or following a migraine attack. A migraine aura-triggered seizure (Table 1.16) is a seizure fulfilling diagnostic criteria that occurs during or within 1 hour after a migraine aura.[8] This phenomenon, sometimes referred to as migralepsy, is rare. Evidence for association with migraine without aura is still lacking.

Episodic Syndromes That May Be Associated with Migraine

This group of disorders occurs in patients who have migraine with or without aura or have an increased likelihood of developing migraine with or without aura. Although they historically occur in childhood, they may also occur in adults. Additional conditions that these patients may have include episodes of motion sickness, and periodic sleep disorders including

Table 1.16 ICHD-3 β Diagnostic Criteria for 1.4.4 Migraine Aura-Triggered Seizure

A. Migraine fulfilling criteria for 1.2 *migraine with aura*
B. A seizure fulfilling diagnostic criteria for one type of epileptic attack occurs during or within 1 hour after a migraine with aura.

sleep walking, sleep talking, night terrors, and bruxism.[25]

Disorders classified under this heading include recurrent gastrointestinal disturbance, cyclic vomiting syndrome, abdominal migraine, benign paroxysmal vertigo, and benign paroxysmal torticollis.[8]

Recurrent episodic attacks of diffuse abdominal pain and/or discomfort include nausea and/or vomiting that may occur infrequently (episodic abdominal pain), chronically (chronic recurrent abdominal pain), with vomiting (recurrent vomiting syndrome), at predictable intervals (cyclic vomiting syndrome, or in association with migraine-like symptoms without headache (abdominal migraine).

Benign paroxysmal vertigo is characterized by recurrent, brief, episodic attacks of vertigo that occur without warning and resolve spontaneously in otherwise healthy children. One needs to rule out posterior fossa tumors, seizures, and vestibular disorders. Benign paroxysmal torticollis is defined as recurrent episodes of head-tilt to one side, often with slight rotation, that remit spontaneously. It occurs in infants and small children, with onset in the first year. It may evolve into benign paroxysmal vertigo or migraine with or without aura or remit without further symptoms. These disorders are discussed in Chapter 3.

Migraine Diagnosis Using ID Migraine™

Can the diagnosis of migraine be made with a simple screening test? Lipton et al. tried to establish the validity and reliability of a brief, self-administered migraine screener given in the primary care setting to patients with headache complaints. A total of 563 patients who presented for routine primary care appointments and reported headaches in the previous 3 months completed a self-administered migraine screener. All patients were then referred for an independent diagnostic evaluation by a headache expert, and 451 (80%) completed a full evaluation. A migraine diagnosis was assigned based on ICHD-2 criteria after a semi-structured diagnostic interview was completed. Of nine diagnostic screening questions (Table 1.17), a three-item subset of disability, nausea, and sensitivity to light provided optimum

Table 1.17 Sensitivity and Specificity of Individual Screener Items versus the Gold-Standard Migraine Diagnosis*

Item	Sensitivity	95% CI	Specificity	95% CI
1. Pain is worse on just one side	0.75	0.70–0.79	0.50	0.39–0.61
2. Pain is pounding, pulsing, or thobbing	0.87	0.83–0.90	0.22	0.14–0.33
3. Pain is moderate or severe	0.94	0.91–0.96	0.16	0.09–0.25
4. Pain is made worse by activities such as walking or climbing stairs.	0.67	0.62–0.72	0.57	0.46–0.68
5. You feel nauseated or sick to your stomach.	0.60	0.55–0.65	0.81	0.71–0.89
6. You see spots, stars, zigzags, lines, or gray areas for several minutes or more before or during your headaches (aura symptoms).	0.42	0.28–0.48	0.74	0.63–0.83
7. Light bothers you (a lot more than when you don't have headaches).	0.75	0.71–0.80	0.74	0.63–0.83
8. Sound bothers you (a lot more than when you don't have headaches).	0.83	0.78–0.86	0.56	0.45–0.67
9. Functional impairment due to headache in last 3 months.[†]	0.87	0.83–0.90	0.52	0.40–0.63

*Sample size ranged from 438 to 448 owing to occasional missing values.
[†]Scored positive if disability reported on any 1 day in the past 3 months.

information. Individuals who indicated that they had two of three of these features were said to screen positive for migraine, with a sensitivity of 0.81 (95% CI, 0.77–0.85), a specificity of 0.75 (95% CI, 0.64–0.84), and positive predictive value of 0.93 (95% CI, 89.9–95.8). Test-retest reliability was good, with a kappa of 0.68 (95% CI, 0.54–0.82). The sensitivity and specificity of the three-item migraine screener was similar regardless of sex, age, presence of other comorbid headaches, or previous diagnostic status. No additional gain in sensitivity or specificity was achieved with the longer nine-item version of the screener, whether using a quantitative scale or an algorithm based on IHS criteria. The presence of aura is the defining feature for one of the main clinical subtypes of migraine. In the current validation study, aura had good specificity but relatively low sensitivity (43%). The three-item Identification of Migraine (ID Migraine™) screener (Table 1.18) was found to be a valid and reliable screening instrument for migraine headaches. Its ease of use and operating characteristics suggest that it could significantly improve migraine recognition in primary care.[114]

Cousins et al. did a systematic review with meta-analysis to determine the diagnostic accuracy of the ID Migraine as a decision rule for identifying patients with migraine. A systematic literature search was conducted to identify all studies validating the ID Migraine, with the ICHD-2 criteria as the reference standard. Thirteen studies incorporating 5866 patients were included. The weighted prior probability of migraine across the 13 studies is 59%. The ID Migraine was useful for ruling out rather than ruling in migraine, with a greater pooled sensitivity estimate (0.84, 95% CI 0.75–0.90) than specificity (0.76, 95% CI 0.69–0.83). A negative ID Migraine score reduces the probability of migraine from 59% to 23%. The sensitivity analysis reveals similar results. This systematic review quantifies the diagnostic accuracy of the

Table 1.18 The ID Migraine

Do you have headaches that limit your ability to work, study or enjoy life?

Do you want to talk to your healthcare professional about your headaches?

Please answer these questions and give your answers to your healthcare professional.

During the last 3 months, did you have the following with your headaches:

You felt nauseated or sick to your stomach.

( ) Yes   ( ) No

Light bothered you (a lot more that when you don't have headaches).

( ) Yes   ( ) No

Your headaches limited your ability to work, study, or do what you needed to do for at least 1 day.

( ) Yes   ( ) No

ID Migraine as a brief, practical, and easy-to-use diagnostic tool. A positive score on the ID Migraine increases the pretest probability from 59% to 84%, whereas a negative ID Migraine score (less than two positive responses), reduces the probability to 23%.[114,115]

REFERENCES

1. Lipton RB, Stewart WF, Diamond S, Diamond ML, Reed M. Prevalence and burden of migraine in the United States: data from the American Migraine Study II. *Headache.* 2001;41:646–657.
2. Stewart WF, Lipton RB, Celentano DD, Reed ML. Prevalence of migraine headache in the United States: relation to age, income, race and other sociodemographic factors. *JAMA.* 1992;267:64–69.
3. Lipton RB, Stewart WF. Migraine in the United States: epidemiology and health care use. *Neurology.* 1993;43:S6–S10.
4. Silberstein SD, Lipton RB. Overview of diagnosis and treatment of migraine. *Neurology.* 1994;44:6–16.
5. Headache Classification Committee of the International Headache Society. Classification and diagnostic criteria for headache disorders, cranial neuralgia, and facial pain. *Cephalalgia.* 1988;8:1–96.
6. Headache Classification Committee. The International Classification of Headache Disorders, 2nd Edition. *Cephalalgia.* 2004;24:1–160.
7. Critchley M. *Migraine: from Cappadocia to Queen Square.* London: Heinemann, 1967.
8. Headache Classification Subcommittee of the International Headache Society: The International Classification of Headache Disorders, 3rd Edition, Beta Version. *Cephalalgia.* 2013;33(9):629–808.
9. Blau JN. Migraine prodromes separated from the aura: complete migraine. *Br Med J.* 1980;281:658–660.
10. Isler H. Frequency and time course of premonitory phenomena. In: Amery WK, Wauquier A, eds. *The prelude to the migraine attack.* London: Bailliere Tindall, 1986:44–53.
11. Giffin NJ, Ruggiero L, Lipton RB, et al. Premonitory symptoms in migraine: an electronic diary study. *Neurology.* 2003;60:935–940.
12. Kelman L. The premonitory symptoms (prodrome): a tertiary care study of 893 migraineurs. *Headache.* 2004;44:865–72.
13. Amery WK, Waelkens J, Caers I. Dopaminergic mechanisms in premonitory phenomena. In: Amery WK, Wauquier A, eds. *The prelude to the migraine attack.* London: Bailliere Tindall, 1986:64–77.
14. Amery WK, Waelkens J, Van den Bergh V. Migraine warnings. *Headache.* 1986;26:60–66.
15. Quintela E, Castillo J, Munoz P, Pascual J. Premonitory and resolution symptoms in migraine: a prospective study in 100 unselected patients. *Cephalalgia.* 2006;26:1051–1060.
16. Jensen K, Tfelt-Hansen P, Lauritzen M, Olesen J. Classic migraine, a prospective recording of symptoms. *Acta Neurol Scand.* 1986;73:359–362.
17. Silberstein SD, Young WB. Migraine aura and prodrome. *Seminars Neurol.* 1995;45:175–182.
18. Sacks O. *Migraine: understanding a common disorder.* Berkeley: University of California Press, 1985.
19. Ziegler DK, Hassanein RS. Specific headache phenomena: their frequency and coincidence. *Headache.* 1990;30:152–156.
20. Lance JW, Anthony M. Some clinical aspects of migraine: a prospective survey of 500 patients. *Arch Neurol.* 1966;15:356–361.
21. Wilkinson M. Clinical features of migraine. In: Rose FC, ed. *Handbook of clinical neurology.* Vol. 48. New York: Elsevier, 1986:117–133.
22. Hupp SL, Kline LB, Corbett JJ. Visual disturbances of migraine. *Surv Ophthalmol.* 1989;33:221–236.
23. Hachinski VC, Porchawka J, Steele JC. Visual symptoms in the migraine syndrome. *Neurology.* 1973;23:570–579.
24. Selby G, Lance JW. Observation on 500 cases of migraine and allied vascular headaches. *J Neurol Neurosurg Psychiatry.* 1960;23:23–32.
25. Hosking G. Special forms: variants of migraine in childhood. In: Hockaday JM, ed. *Migraine in childhood.* Boston: Butterworths, 1988:35–53.
26. Diamond S, Freitag FG, Prager J, Gandhi S. Olfactory aura in migraine. *N Eng J Med.* 1985;312:1390–1391.
27. Russell MB, Olesen J. A nosographic analysis of the migraine aura in a general population. *Brain.* 1996;119 (Pt 2):355–361.
28. Manzoni G, Farina S, Lanfranchi M, Solari A. Classic migraine-clinical findings in 164 patients. *Eur Neurol.* 1985;24:163–169.
29. Young WB, Gangal KS, Aponte RJ, Kaiser RS. Migraine with unilateral motor symptoms: a case-control study. *J Neurol Neurosurg Psychiatry.* 2007;78:600–604.
30. Fisher CM. Late life migraine accompaniments as a cause of unexplained transient ischemic attacks. *Can J Neurol Sci.* 1980;7:9–17.
31. Ashkenazi A, Sholtzow M, Shaw JW, Burstein R, Young WB. Identifying cutaneous allodynia in chronic migraine using a practical clinical method. *Cephalalgia.* 2007;27:111–117.
32. Stewart WF, Schechter A, Lipton RB. Migraine heterogeneity: disability, pain intensity, attack frequency, and duration. *Neurology.* 1994;44:S24–S39.
33. Drummond PD. Scalp tenderness and sensitivity to pain in migraine and tension headache. *Headache.* 1987;27:45–50.
34. Olesen J. Some clinical features of the acute migraine attack: an analysis of 750 patients. *Headache.* 1978;18:268–271.
35. Drummond PD, Lance JW. Clinical diagnosis and computer analysis of headache symptoms. *J Neurol Neurosurg Psychiatry.* 1984;47:128–133.
36. Silberstein SD. Chronic daily headache and tension-type headache. *Neurology.* 1993;43:1644–1649.
37. Cady RK, Gutterman D, Saiers JA, Beach ME. Responsiveness of nonIHS migraine and tension-type headache to sumatriptan. *Cephalalgia.* 1997;17:588–590.
38. Lipton RB, Cady RK, O'Quinn S, Hall CB, Stewart WF. Sumatriptan treats the full spectrum of headache in individuals with disabling IHS migraine. *Headache.* 1999;40:783–791.

39. Kelman L. Pain characteristics of the acute migraine attack. *Headache*. 2006;46:942–953.

40. Yoon MS, Mueller D, Hansen N, et al. Prevalence of facial pain in migraine: a population-based study. *Cephalalgia*. 2010;30:92–96.

41. Silberstein SD. Migraine symptoms: results of a survey of self-reported migraineurs. *Headache*. 1995;35:387–396.

42. Volans GN. Research review: migraine and drug absorption. *Pharmacokinetics*. 1978;3:313–318.

43. Saper JR. *Headache disorders: current concepts in treatment strategies*. Littleton, CO: Wright-PSG, 1983.

44. Boyle R, Behan PO, Sutton JA. A correlation between severity of migraine and delayed emptying measured by an epigastric impedance method. *Br J Clin Pharmacol*. 1990;30:405–409.

45. Russell MB, Rasmussen BK, Brennum J, Iversen HK, Jensen RA, Olesen J. Presentation of a new instrument: the diagnostic headache diary. *Cephalalgia*. 1992;12:369–374.

46. Anthony M, Rasmussen BK. Migraine without aura. In: Olesen J, Tfelt-Hansen P, Welch MA, eds. *The headaches*. New York: Raven Press, 1993:255–261.

47. Rasmussen BK, Jensen R, Olesen J. A population-based analysis of the diagnostic criteria of the international headache society. *Cephalalgia*. 1991;11:129–134.

48. Drummond PD. A quantitative assessment of photophobia in migraine and tension headache. *Headache*. 1986;26:465–469.

49. Kuritzky A, Ziegler KE, Hassanein R. Vertigo, motion sickness and migraine. Headache 1981;21:227–231.

50. Dalessio DJ. *Wolff's headache and other head pain*. 4th ed. Oxford: Oxford University Press, 1980.

51. Dalessio DJ. Migraine. In: Dalessio DJ, ed. *Wolff's headache and other head pain*. New York: Oxford University Press, 1980:56–130.

52. Bigal ME, Liberman JN, Lipton RB. Age-dependent prevalence and clinical features of migraine. *Neurology*. 2006;67:246–251.

53. Lipton RB, Reed ML, Fanning K, Buse DC. Relationship between high frequency nausea and treatment satisfaction in episodic migraine (EM): results of the American Migraine Prevalence and Prevention (AMPP) study. *Headache*. 2011;51:32(Abstract).

54. Dodick DW, Kaniecki R, Mathew N, Kori S, McDonald S, Nelsen A. Traditional and non-traditional migraine-associated symptoms: incidence and consistent responsiveness across 4 migraine attacks with sumatriptan 85 RT technology and naproxen sodium 500 mg (SumaRT/Nap). *Neurology*. 2007;68:A195(Abstract).

55. Cady RK, Schreiber CP. Sinus headache or migraine? Considerations in making a differential diagnosis. *Neurology*. 2002;58:S10–S14.

56. Wilson CWM, Kirker JG, Warnes H. The clinical features of migraine as a manifestation of allergic disease. *Postgrad Med J*. 1980;21:295(Abstract).

57. Barbanti P, Fabbrini G, Pesare M. Neurovascular symptoms during migraine attacks. *Cephalalgia*. 2001;21:295(Abstract).

58. Eross E, Dodick D, Eross M. The Sinus, Allergy and Migraine Study (SAMS). *Headache*. 2007;47:213–224.

59. Schreiber CP, Hutchinson S, Webster CJ, Ames M, Richardson MS, Powers C. Prevalence of migraine in patients with a history of self-reported or physician-diagnosed "sinus" headache. *Arch Intern Med*. 2004;164:1769–1772.

60. Ishkanian G, Blumenthal H, Webster CJ. Efficacy of sumatriptan tablets in migraineurs self-described or physician-diagnosed as having sinus headache: a randomized, double-blind, placebo-controlled study. *Clin Ther*. 2007;29:99–109.

61. Hargreaves RJ, Shepheard SL. Pathophysiology of migraine-new insights. *Can J Neurol*. 1999;26:S12–S19.

62. Goadsby PJ. Recent advances in understanding migraine mechanisms, molecules, and therapeutics. *Trends Mol Med*. 2007;13:39–44.

63. Bellamy JL, Cady RK, Durham PL. Salivary levels of CGRP and VIP in rhinosinusitis and migraine patients. *Headache*. 2006;46:24–33.

64. Kaniecki RG. Migraine and tension-type headache: an assessment of challenges in diagnosis. *Neurology*. 2002;58:S15–S20.

65. Smith T, Stoneman J, Smith C. Variability of presenting symptoms in a population of patients with IHS migraine with or without aura. *Headache*. 2003;43:417–18.(Abstract).

66. Kaniecki R, Ruoff G, Smith T. Prevalence of migraine and response to sumatriptan in patients self-reporting tension/stress headache. *Curr Med Res Opin*. 2006;22:1535–1544.

67. Calhoun AH, Ford S, Millen C, Finkel AG, Young T, Nie Y. The prevalence of neck pain in migraine. *Headache*. 2010;50:1273–1277.

68. Pryse-Phillips WEM, Dodick DW, Edmeads JG, et al. Guidelines for the diagnosis and management of migraine in clinical practice. *Can Med Assoc J*. 1997;156:1273–1287.

69. Friedman AP, Von Storch TJC, Merritt HH. Migraine and tension headaches. A clinical study: 2000 cases. *Neurology*. 1964;4:773.

70. Kelman L, Tanis D. The relationship between migraine pain and other associated symptoms. *Cephalalgia*. 2006;26:548–553.

71. Kelman L. Osmophobia and taste abnormality in migraineurs: a tertiary care study. *Headache*. 2004;44:1019–1023.

72. Spierings EL, Ranke AH, Honkoop PC. Precipitating and aggravating factors of migraine versus tension-type headache. *Headache*. 2001;41:554–558.

73. Merikangas KR, Dartigues JF, Whitaker A. Diagnostic criteria for migraine: a validity study. *Neurology*. 2004;44:S11–S16.

74. Zanchin G, Dainese F, Mainardi F. Osmophobia in primary headaches. *J Headache Pain*. 2005;6:213–215.

75. Raiele V, Pandolfi E, La Vecchia M. The prevalence of allodynia, osmophobia, and red ear syndrome in the juvenile headache: preliminary data. *J Headache Pain*. 2005;6:271.

76. Demarquay G, Royet JP, Giraud P. Rating of olfactory judgments in migraine patients. *Cephalalgia*. 2006;26:1123–1130.

77. Blau JN, Solomon F. Smell and other sensory disturbances in migraine. *J Neurol*. 1985;232:275–276.

78. Snyder RD, Drummond PD. Olfaction in migraine. *Cephalalgia*. 1997;17:729–732.

79. Hirsch AR. Olfaction in migraineurs. *Headache*. 1992;32:233–236.

80. Hawkes CH, Doty RL. General disorders of olfaction. In: Hawkes CH, Doty RL, eds. *The neurology of olfaction*. New York: Cambridge University Press, 2009:111–152.

81. Marmura MJ, Anjum M. Olfactory acuity in migraine during and between attacks: a case control study. *Neurology*. 2011;76:A198(Abstract).

82. Liveing E. *On megrim, sick headache, and some allied disorders: a contribution to the pathology of nerve-storms*. London: Churchill, 1873.

83. Eggers SD. Migraine-related vertigo: diagnosis and treatment. *Curr Pain Headache Rep*. 2007;11:217–226.

84. Furman JM, Marcus DA, Balaban CD. Migrainous vertigo: development of a pathogenetic model and structured diagnostic interview. *Curr Opin Neurol*. 2003;16:5–13.

85. Silberstein SD, Mannix LK, Goldstein J, et al. Multimechanistic (sumatriptan-naproxen) early intervention for the acute treatment of migraine. *Neurology*. 2008;71:114–121.

86. Burstein R, Yarnitsky D, Goor-Aryeh I, Ransil BJ, Bajwa ZH. An association between migraine and cutaneous allodynia. *Ann Neurol*. 2000;47:614–624.

87. Burstein R, Jakubowski M. Analgesic triptan action in an animal model of intracranial pain: a race against the development of central sensitization. *Ann Neurol*. 2004;55:27–36.

88. Burstein R, Collins B, Jakubowski M. Defeating migraine pain with triptans: a race against the development of cutaneous allodynia. *Ann Neurol*. 2004;55:19–26.

89. Yarnitsky D, Goor-Aryeh I, Bajwa Z, Ransail B, Cutrer M, Burstein R. Possible parasympathetic contributions to peripheral and central sensitization during migraine. *Headache*. 2003;43:(Abstract).

90. Goadsby PJ, Lipton RB, Ferrari MD. Migraine-current understanding and treatment. *N Engl J Med*. 2002;346:257–270.

91. Cady RK, Sheftell F, Lipton RB. Effect of early intervention with sumatriptan on migraine pain: retrospective analyses of data from three clinical trials. *Clin Therap*. 2000;22:1035–1048.

92. Winner P, Mannix LK, Putnam DG, et al. Pain-free results with sumatriptan taken at the first sign of migraine pain: 2 randomized, double-blind, placebo-controlled studies. *Mayo Clin Proc*. 2003;78:1214–1222.

93. Brandes JL, Kudrow D, Cady R, Tiseo PJ, Sun W, Sikes CR. Eletriptan in the early treatment of acute migraine: influence of pain intensity and time of dosing. *Cephalalgia*. 2005;25:735–742.

94. Borsook D, Burstein R, Becerra L. Functional imaging of the human trigeminal system: opportunities for new insights into pain processing in health and disease. *J Neurobiol*. 2004;61:107–125.

95. Kelman L. The postdrome of the acute migraine attack. *Cephalalgia*. 2006;26:214–220.

96. Ng-Mak DS, Fitzgerald KA, Norquist JM, et al. Key concepts of migraine postdrome: a qualitative study to develop a post-migraine questionnaire. *Headache*. 2011;51:105–117.

97. Olesen J, Friberg L, Skyhoj-Olsen T. Timing and topography of cerebral blood flow, aura and headache during migraine attacks. *Ann Neurol*. 1990;28:791–798.

98. Klee A, Willanger R. Disturbances of visual perception in migraine. *Acta Neurol Scand*. 1966;42:400–414.

99. Matharu MJ, Goadsby PJ. Post-traumatic chronic paroxysmal hemicrania (CPH) with aura. *Neurology*. 2001;56:273–275.

100. Peres MF, Siow HC, Rozen TD. Hemicrania continua with aura. *Cephalalgia*. 2002;22:246–248.

101. Silberstein SD, Niknam R, Rozen TD, Young WB. Cluster headache with aura. *Neurology*. 2000;54:219–221.

102. Whitty CWM. Migraine without headache. *Lancet*. 1967;ii:283–285.

103. Willey RG. The scintillating scotoma without headache. *Ann Ophthalmol*. 1979;11:581–585.

104. Staehelin-Jensen T. Familial hemiplegic migraine: a reappraisal and long-term follow-up study. *Cephalagia*. 1981;1:33–39.

105. Mattsson P, Lundberg PO. Characteristics and prevalence of transient visual disturbances indicative of migraine visual aura. *Cephalalgia*. 1999;19:479–484.

106. Levy DE. Transient CNS deficits: a common, benign syndrome in young adults. *Neurology*. 1988;38:831–836.

107. Wijman C, Wolf PA, Kase CS, Kelly-Hayes M, Beiser AS. Migrainous visual accompaniments are not rare in late life: the Framingham Study. *Stroke*. 1998;29:1539–1543.

108. O'Connor PS, Tredici TJ. Acephalgic migraine: fifteen years experience. *Ophthalmology*. 1981;88:999–1003.

109. Cohen GR, Harbison JW, Blair CJ, Ochs AL. Clinical significance of transient visual phenomena in the elderly. *Ophthalmology*. 1984;91:436–442.

110. Fleming JB, Amos AJ, Desmond RA. Migraine aura without headache: prevalence and risk factors in a primary eye care population. *Optometry*. 2000;71:381–389.

111. Aiba S, Tatsumoto M, Saisu A, et al. Prevalence of typical migraine aura without headache in Japanese ophthalmology clinics. *Cephalalgia*. 2010;30:962–967.

112. Bento MS, Esperanca P. Migraine with prolonged aura. *Headache*. 2000;40:52–53.

113. Rothrock J, North J, Madden K, Lyden P, Fleck P, Dittrich H. Migraine and migrainous stroke: risk factors and prognosis. *Neurology*. 1993;43:2473–2476.

114. Lipton RB, Kolodner K, Dodick D, et al. A self-administered screener for migraine in primary care: the ID Migraine Validation Study. *Headache*. 2003;43:(Abstract).

115. Cousins G, Hijazze S, Van de Laar FA, Fahey T. Diagnostic accuracy of the ID Migraine: a systematic review and meta-analysis. *Headache*. 2011;51:1140–1148.

Chapter 2

Migraine Genetics

INTRODUCTION

Significant progress in molecular genetics has advanced our understanding of the genetic basis of migraine. The fundamentals of molecular genetics, and the recent advances in the field, are important for clinicians to understand, as they provide a foundation for critical appraisal of the literature and unprecedented insights into the pathogenesis of the disorder, and reveal promising treatment targets for future drug development. This chapter first provides a primer of molecular genetics, followed by sections on the genetic advances in migraine, the methodology of genome-wide association studies, and the potential clinical implications.

In the past, it was believed that the gene was a unit of hereditary information aligned along a chromosome, each coding for one protein. Genetic information was believed to flow from DNA (deoxyribonucleic acid) to RNA (ribonucleic acid) to protein. But genes can code not only for protein but for functional RNA molecules. A coding gene was defined as a DNA sequence that encodes messenger RNA (mRNA) that is subsequently translated into protein. A non-coding gene was defined as a DNA sequence that codes for non-coding RNA (ncRNA) with intrinsic functional properties that do not require translation to protein. Examples include small nucleolar RNAs (snRNAs), microRNAs (miRNAs), ribosomal RNA (rRNA), and transfer RNA (tRNA).

The Encyclopedia of DNA Elements (ENCODE) project was created to delineate all functional elements encoded in the human genome.[1] A functional element is now defined by ENCODE as a discrete genome segment that encodes a defined product (for example, protein or non-coding RNA) or displays a reproducible biochemical signature (for example, protein binding or a specific chromatin structure). This greatly expands the traditional view of the functional elements from the exon (a region of a eukaryotic gene that codes for amino acids or RNA) to the intron (intervening sequence between exons). A strict dichotomy between protein-coding and non-coding RNA transcripts no longer exists. Some ncRNAs can be translated and, in addition to encoding proteins, bifunctional RNA transcripts participate in cellular regulatory and functional processes, rather than serving simply as intermediates for translation.

The genetic code resides in DNA because only it is passed to the next generation. Most DNA is located in the cell nucleus (nuclear DNA); some is found in the mitochondria (mitochondrial DNA or mtDNA). DNA (deoxyribonucleic acid) is a large polymer of alternating sugar (deoxyribose) attached to a nitrogenous base and phosphate residues (nucleotides). A nucleoside consists of deoxyribose attached to a nitrogenous base [adenine (A), cytosine (C), guanine (G) or thymine (T)] at the 1′ position. A nucleotide is a nucleoside with an attached phosphate group at the 5′ or 3′ position. RNA (ribonucleic acid) contains ribose as its sugar (instead of deoxyribose) and uracil (U) as its nitrogenous base (instead of thymine). RNA normally exists as single molecules. DNA is a double helix of two antiparallel DNA molecules (DNA strands) linked by weak hydrogen bonds from adenine (A) to thymine (T) [A–T] and cytosine (C) to guanine (G) [C–G].

During DNA replication, the two complimentary chromosomal DNA strands unwind. Each strand directs the synthesis of complimentary DNA to generate two daughter DNAs. DNA is synthesized by the enzyme DNA polymerase in the 5′ to 3′ direction by successively adding nucleotides to the free 3′ hydroxyl group of the growing strand.[2,3] DNA is the template for RNA synthesis. Transcription, the synthesis of messenger RNA (mRNA) from a sequence of DNA, is carried out by the DNA-dependent enzyme RNA polymerase. The RNA sequence determines the amino acid sequence. Translation (polypeptide synthesis from mRNA) occurs in ribosomes, which are large RNA-protein complexes.

THE GENOME

An organism's complete set of DNA is called its genome. The latest protein-coding gene count is about 20,687, accounting for about 3% of the human genome—less if one counts only their coding regions. The DNA sequence of these genes consists of exons and introns (Figure 2.1). An exon (from "expressed") is a region of a eukaryotic gene that codes for amino acids or RNA. An intron is the intervening sequence between the exons. It does not contribute to protein specification. Introns may contain regulatory information that is critical to appropriate gene expression. Intron sequences are transcribed into RNA and are spliced out from the RNA molecule before it can be translated into protein (intron splicing). Some genes contain a large number of introns that make up the bulk of the DNA sequence. Introns are also found in genes whose RNA is not translated (i.e., eukaryotic ribosomal RNA [rRNA] and transfer RNA [tRNA] genes). Epigenetic phenomena, such as methylation and histone modification, can alter the effect of a gene (see discussion later in this chapter). Another 11,224 DNA stretches are classified as pseudogenes, "dead" genes now known to be active in some cell types or individuals.[4] In contrast to what was previously believed, the vast majority of the human genome (80.4%) is transcribed into RNA and participates in at least one biochemical RNA and/or chromatin-associated event in at least one cell type. Much of the genome lies close to a regulatory event: 95% of the genome lies within 8 kilobases (kb) of a DNA–protein interaction, and 99% is within 1.7 kb of at least one of the biochemical events measured by ENCODE. There are approximately 399,124 regions with enhancer-like features (sequence of DNA that increases the rate of transcription of adjacent sequences). There are 70,292 regions with promoter-like features (DNA region, usually upstream to the coding sequence of a gene or operon, which binds RNA polymerase and directs the enzyme to the correct transcriptional start site), as well as hundreds of thousands of quiescent regions.

RNA transcription is tightly regulated. The primary RNA transcripts are synthesized in the nucleus and then processed to mRNA and other types of RNA. This includes the addition of a (5'-5'-linked 7-methylguanylate) "cap" at the 5' end and a sequence of adenylate groups at the 3' end (the poly-A tail), as well as the removal of any introns and exons splicing. Only about 10% of the primary RNA transcript leaves the nucleus. Processed mRNA is exported to the cytoplasm, where protein synthesis takes place. Alternative exon splicing (cutting out and combining different exons) of the primary RNA transcript produces different mRNAs.[2,5] Alternate splicing can result in the production of multiple proteins from the same exons; almost 100,000 proteins can be derived from the 20,687 protein-coding genes.

Genetic information is encoded in a linear sequence of three bases in the DNA strands (codon) (Figure 2.2). There are 64 possible codons for 20 different amino acids. Each amino acid is specified by approximately three different codons (Figure 2.3). In addition, there are three stop codons, UAA, UGA, and UAG (they stop protein synthesis). If the rate of variation at a specific point in DNA is greater than 1% it is called a *polymorphism*; if less than 1% it is a *mutation*. An allele is one of two or more alternative forms of a DNA sequence. A single nucleotide polymorphism (SNP) occurs when one base pair varies: AGC (Ser) versus AAC (Asn). There are approximately 10 million common SNPs; many are transmitted across generations in blocks. SNPs occur every 200 base pairs in humans, but just 1% result in alteration in protein coding.[2,3] A *haplotype* is a set of SNPs on a chromosome that are associated statistically. The identification of a few alleles of a haplotype sequence can frequently identify all other polymorphic sites in its region. These alleles, called *Tag SNPs* (an easily measured SNP that serves as a proxy for the blocks), can be used to capture most SNP variation within each block. A haplotype may be one locus, several loci, or an entire chromosome, depending on the number of recombination events that have occurred between a given set of loci.

THE CHROMOSOME

The term *chromosome* was coined by Waldeyer in 1888 from the Greek words for "colored" (*chroma*) and "body" (*soma*). It is an organized structure of one double-stranded DNA molecule combined with proteins, including

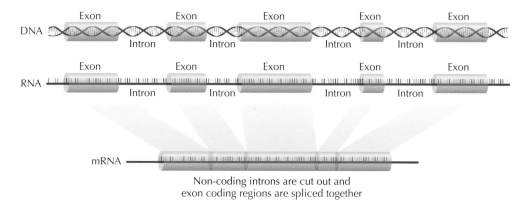

Non-coding introns are cut out and exon coding regions are spliced together

Figure 2.1. The DNA sequence of genes consist of exons and introns. An exon is a region that codes for amino acids or RNA. An intron is the intervening sequence between the exons.

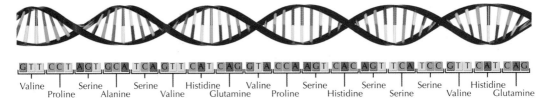

GTT	CCT	AGT	GCA	TCA	GTT	CAT	CAG	GTA	CCA	AGT	CAC	AGT	TCA	TCC	GTT	CAT	CAG
Valine		Serine		Serine		Histidine		Valine		Serine		Serine		Serine		Histidine	
	Proline		Alanine		Valine		Glutamine		Proline		Histidine		Serine		Valine		Glutamine

Figure 2.2. Genetic information is encoded in a linear sequence of three bases in the DNA strands.

histones (DNA + histones + regulatory proteins = chromatin) (Figure 2.4). Histones are highly conserved proteins grouped into five major classes (H1, H2A, H2B, H3, and H4).[6] Chromatin condenses during the metaphase stage of mitosis and becomes visible by light microscopy (Figure 2.1). There are 23 pairs of human chromosomes (22 pairs of autosomes and one pair of sex chromosomes), for a total of 46 per cell. The gene-dense areas contain mainly guanine (G) and cytosine C (light bands on chromosomes), the gene-poor areas mainly adenine (A) and thymine (T) (dark bands on chromosomes). Genes are concentrated in random areas, with vast expanses of non-protein-coding DNA between genes (up to 30,000 C/G repeats occur next to gene-rich areas). There are approximately 3 billion base pairs (adenine, cytosine, thymine, and guanine): 1% exons, 24% introns, and 75% intergenic DNA. The average gene has 30,000 bases, but there is great variation. The largest gene is dystrophin, with 2.4 million bases. Chromosome 1 has the most genes; the Y chromosome has the fewest.[7–9]. The most highly repeated DNA sequences are called "satellite DNA" because they can be easily separated from other DNA. They are found at the centromeres (or centers) and telomeres (ends) of chromosomes (Figure 2.2).

Within a chromosome, physical position is specified by the chromosome arm and in relation to specific banding patterns observed on the chromosome with Giemsa staining (also known as G-banding). The centromere, a constriction between the short and long arms of a chromosome, divides the chromosome into two arms: the short arm, "p" (from the French *petite*—small), and the long arm "q" (the letter following "p"). Giemsa staining results in distinct banding patterns, enabling division and subdivision of each chromosome arm into numbered segments. Gene positions can be described with reference to the chromosome number, arm, region, band, sub-band, and secondary sub-bands. The beta-globin gene (*HBB*) resides on chromosome 11q15.4 (read "eleven—q—one five point four," not "15 point four").

Telomeres are complexes comprising DNA and protein that cap and protect the ends of eukaryotic chromosomes. They are characterized by repetitive, single-strand DNA sequences that decrease in length with each cell division. When telomeres shorten to a critical length, cells become senescent. Some cells are protected by telomerase,

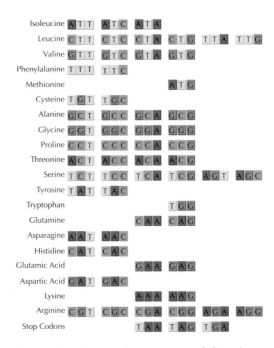

Figure 2.3. Genetic information is encoded in a linear sequence of three bases in the DNA strands (codon). There are 64 possible codons for 20 different amino acids. Each amino acid is specified by approximately three different codons. In addition, there are three stop codons, UAA, UGA, and UAG (they stop protein synthesis).

which adds telomeric DNA sequence repeats to the ends of chromosomes.[10] Telomerase may be a barometer of the organism's cumulative response to long-term endogenous and exogenous stressors. Older adults with chronic pain and high stress had significantly shorter leukocyte by telomerase activity than individuals reporting no chronic pain and low stress.[11]

EPIGENETICS

Epigenetic mechanisms modify DNA or chromatin without changing the DNA sequence (Figure 2.3). Epigenetics modulate gene expression and can have dramatic effects on protein expression. Epigenetic mechanisms include DNA methylation, histone methylation, repressive protein complexes, and RNA interference (RNAi).[12] During DNA methylation, a methyl group is attached to the 5' position of the cytosine found at C-G dinucleotides, catalyzed by DNA methyltransferase. This modifies the chemical structure of DNA and if it occurs in the promoter region can result in gene silencing. DNA methylation can result from environmental exposure, especially when it occurs during critical periods of development or with aging.[13]

Histone modification, another form of epigenetic regulation, results from acetylation, phosphorylation, and/or methylation of the histone proteins amino terminal tail. This modifies how tightly chromatin is packaged, thus controlling gene accessibility and expression. DNA methylation and histone modification work in concert to affect epigenetic regulation of gene expression.[14]

A third form of epigenetic regulation is through non-coding RNA molecules that regulate gene expression post-transcriptionally.[15] Epigenetic modification may underlie susceptibility to primary headache disorders.[16]

NON-CODING RNA (NCRNA)

RNA molecules that function as RNAs (rather than as templates for protein synthesis) in a regulatory, structural, or functional role are called non-coding RNAs (ncRNAs). Transfer RNA (tRNA) and ribosomal RNA are examples of ncRNAs. Transfer RNA

mediates the decoding process: each tRNA molecule binds a different amino acid and has a specific trinucleotide sequence, called the anticodon, that binds to mRNA. Ribosomal RNA is the catalytic component of the ribosomes: large, two-subunit RNA-protein complexes involved in the translation of RNA into protein. Other ncRNAs can target transcriptional activators or repressors and even DNA to regulate gene transcription and expression.

ENCODE defined 8800 small RNA molecules and 9600 long non-coding RNA molecules, each of which is at least 200 bases long. The RNAs can be subtyped into antisense RNAs (at least one transcript intersects any exon of a protein-coding locus on the opposite strand, or published evidence of antisense regulation of a coding gene); large intergenic non-coding RNA (LincRNA); sense overlapping (contains a coding gene within an intron on the same strand); sense intronic (within intron of a coding gene but does not intersect any exons on the same strand); and processed transcript (transcripts do not contain an open reading frame and cannot be placed in any of the other categories because of complexity in their structure).[17] DNA sequences that are present between start, or initiation, codons and stop, or termination, codons constitute an open reading frame. These sequences are translated into proteins.

Long non-coding RNAs (lncRNAs) are at least 200 nucleotides in length (but are often much longer) and are transcribed from intergenic regions, from gene regulatory regions, and from specific chromosomal regions (telomeres22). lncRNAs are also derived from the mitochondrial genome. lncRNAs can enhance gene expression or repress genomic regions or even entire chromosomes. In mammals, several classes of genes are expressed from only one allele per cell. Two examples are X-chromosome inactivation and genomic imprinting. Only one copy of each X-linked gene is active in female cells (XX). In genomic imprinting, genes within a discrete domain are coordinately regulated and expressed according to parent of origin; lncRNAs may be the master regulator of this phenomena. lncRNAs have been proposed to serve as recruiting tools for chromatin-modifying complexes.[18] lncRNAs have a role in transcriptional and epigenetic mechanisms via the recruitment of

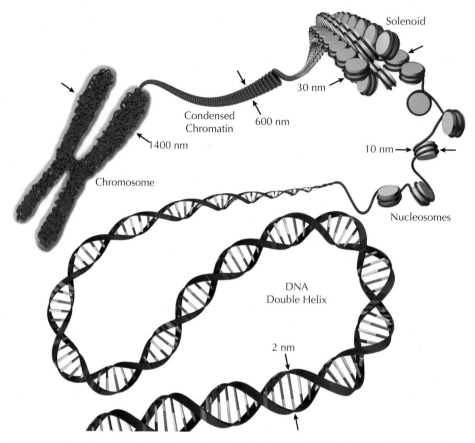

Figure 2.4. DNA (deoxyribonucleic acid) packaging. DNA packaging is regulated by histones. They create histone-DNA complexes, called nucleosomes, which are folded into higher-order chromatin structures.

transcription factors and chromatin-modifying complexes that would in turn silence or activate genes residing within the allelically regulated clusters.

lncRNAs can also affect alternative splicing and other post-transcriptional RNA modifications through the assembly of nuclear domains containing RNA-processing factors, nuclear-cytoplasmic shuttling, and translational control. lncRNAs act as signals for integrating temporal, spatial, developmental, and stimulus-specific cellular information—decoys with the ability to sequester RNA and protein molecules, thereby inhibiting their functions; as guides for genomic site-specific and more widespread recruitment of transcriptional and epigenetic regulatory factors; and as scaffolds for macromolecular assemblies with varied functions.[19] lncRNAs can also act as precursors for small ncRNAs.

Small ncRNAs are involved in post-transcriptional regulation of target RNAs via RNA interference (RNAi). Small ncRNAs include miRNAs, endogenous small interfering RNAs (endosiRNAs), and PIWI-interacting RNAs (piRNAs). Some miRNAs and siRNAs can cause genes they target to be methylated, modulating their transcription. Mature miRNAs are 20–23 nucleotide, single-stranded RNAs (ssRNAs), derived from longer primary transcripts (pri-miRNA). They are integrated and associated with Argonaute proteins, the catalytic components of the RNA-induced silencing complex (RISC). RISCs are responsible for the gene-silencing phenomenon known as RNA interference (RNAi).[20] Argonaute proteins bind different classes of small non-coding RNAs, including microRNAs (miRNAs), small interfering RNAs (siRNAs), and Piwi-interacting RNAs (piRNAs).[21] Small RNAs guide Argonaute proteins to their specific targets through sequence complementarity; they block mRNA from being translated, or accelerate its degradation. An individual miRNA can regulate hundreds of different mRNAs and multiple miRNAs and can also target a single mRNA.[6] miRNAs can also target and repress other ncRNAs.

Endogenous small interfering RNAs (endo-siRNAs) are 21–26 nucleotide double-stranded RNAs (dsRNAs) that are cleaved from longer dsRNA intermediates and incorporated into RNA-induced silencing complexes (RISCs), in which they function as single-stranded entities. Endo-siRNAs are involved in gene regulation and genome defense via silencing of mRNAs and transposon-derived ncRNAs. In contrast to miRNAs, endo-siRNAs act on RNA molecules containing perfectly complementary sequences.[6]

A *transposable element* (TE) is a DNA sequence that can change its position within the genome, sometimes creating mutations and altering the cell's genome size Transposable genetic elements (TEs) can move to new sites in genomes either directly, by a cut-and-paste mechanism (transposons) or indirectly, through an RNA intermediate (retrotransposons). Retrotransposons copy themselves in two stages, first from DNA to RNA by transcription, then from RNA back to DNA by reverse transcription. The DNA copy is then inserted into the genome in a new position. Retrotransposons behave very similarly to retroviruses, such as HIV. DNA transposons use a cut-and-paste transposition mechanism that does not involve an RNA intermediate. The transpositions are catalyzed by various types of transposase enzymes. The duplications at the target site can result in gene duplication. TEs constitute more than half of the DNA in many higher eukaryotes.[12]

PIWI-interacting RNAs are small ncRNAs (26–30 nucleotides) associated with the PIWI subclass of Argonaute proteins and are involved in silencing mRNAs and transposons. Those derived from transposon elements regulate transposon activity; piRNAs derived from piRNA clusters modulate gene expression. piRNAs were initially found in germ cells; recent studies have established that piRNAs are expressed in somatic cells, including neurons.[6]

Small nucleolar RNAs are derived from intronic regions with roles in promoting RNA modifications, including pseudouridylation and methylation, as well as pre-mRNA processing. They can also guide RNA-modifying enzyme complexes to other RNA molecules (such as rRNAs) in the nucleolus. This is mediated by the formation of duplexes between snoRNAs and RNAs with complementary sequences.[6]

IMPLICATIONS FOR MIGRAINE RESEARCH

Several strategies have been employed to identify genes for migraine. The most successful approach has been the identification of gene mutations in families with familial hemiplegic migraine, a rare monogenic subtype of migraine. This has been done by using positional cloning techniques, mutation analysis, and traditional linkage analysis, which requires testing several hundreds or thousands of genetic markers across the genome and selecting those chromosomal regions that most closely segregate with the disease. A second linkage analysis strategy that is often used in complex traits is affected sib-pair analysis in which chromosomal regions shared by affected siblings that occur with a probability higher than by chance alone are identified. This is then followed by case-control association studies testing single nucleotide polymorphisms (SNPs) in candidate genes in the shared regions. The goal is to identify SNPs, and thus gene alleles, that statistically differ in frequency between cases and controls and that cause increased susceptibility to the disease. A third, hypothesis-driven approach is direct testing of candidate genes in case-control association studies. A promising extension of this approach is the possibility of testing for genome-wide association by scanning hundreds of thousands of SNPs in large and clinically homogenous populations. Genome-wide association studies (GWAS) use SNP chip genotyping in large populations. It is based on the fact that long segments of chromosomes are transmitted in blocks from parents to children. GWAS look for a statistically significant association between SNPs and a specific trait or disease. Individuals are distinguished by unique SNP alleles combinations called haplotypes ("tag SNPs"), which are the accumulation of SNP variants that have been inherited intact over many generations. In many regions of the genome, 95% or more of the existing diversity is defined by just 5 to 10 alternative haplotypes. A haplotype, containing dozens or hundreds of SNP alleles, can be identified by tag SNPs that serve as a proxy for the entire haplotype. A nearly complete whole-genome profile can be obtained with the use of a DNA microarray that distinguishes genotypes at just 500,000 tag SNPs.[22]

GWAS normally compare the DNA of cases to controls using tagged haplotypes. If one variant is more frequent in cases, the SNP is said to be "associated" with the disease. GWAS alone cannot specify which genes are causal, but they can lead to the identification of the precise DNA sequence that is responsible.[22,23]

GWAS have so far linked 3800 SNPs to 427 diseases and traits.[24] Only 12% of SNPs associated with traits are located in, or occur in, protein-coding regions of genes. Most SNPs reside in regions that are outside protein-coding genes; approximately 40% are in intergenic regions, and another 40% are located in non-coding introns. Disease phenotypes can be associated with a specific cell type or transcription factor. Maurano et al. examined 349 types of cells.[25] Each cell type had about 200,000 accessible locations and at least 3.9 million regions where transcription factors can bind in the genome. These functional regions overlap with specific DNA bases linked to higher or lower risks of various diseases, suggesting that gene regulation might account for variations in risk.[24] In fact, 12% of these SNPs collocate with transcription factor binding sites, and 34% are in open chromatin. It has recently been demonstrated that these variants are concentrated in regulatory DNA marked by deoxyribonuclease I (DNase I) hypersensitive sites (DHSs) and suggest pervasive involvement of regulatory DNA variation in common human disease and provide pathogenic insights into diverse disorders.[25] This method, called DNAseseq, cuts DNA wherever chromatin has unwound enough to let regulatory proteins bind to it.

Stamatoyannopoulos has cataloged such gene regulatory sites in 130 human cell types and developmental stages, including fetal tissues, adult organ tissues, and cancer cell lines. Different cell types have different subsets of hypersensitive sites, depending on their gene expression profiles. He found 2.1 million of these sites, taking up well more than 11% of the genome. Some 7500 were identified in all cell types, while about 450,000 were found in just one cell type, suggesting that those latter sites are involved in regulating genes for specific kinds of cells. Stamatoyannopoulos found that about 53% were located at the hypersensitive sites; only about 7% of the SNPs fall in the DNA sequences that actually encode proteins.

Disease-associated SNP variants perturb transcription factor recognition sequences, alter allelic chromatin states, and form regulatory networks. Maurano et al. found tissue-selective enrichment of more weakly disease-associated variants within DHSs and the de novo identification of pathogenic cell types for Crohn's disease, multiple sclerosis, and an electrocardiogram trait, without prior knowledge of physiological mechanisms. Human regulatory DNA encompasses a variety of cis-regulatory elements, within which the cooperative binding of transcription factors creates focal alterations in chromatin structure. A cis-regulatory element, or cis-element, is a region of DNA or RNA that regulates the expression of genes located on that same molecule of DNA (often a chromosome). DNase I mapping has been instrumental in the discovery and census of human cis-regulatory elements.[25,26] These results suggest pervasive involvement of regulatory DNA variation in common human disease and provide pathogenic insights into diverse disorders.

MIGRAINE GENETICS

In the first of section of this chapter, the fundamentals of molecular genetics and the recent advances that are important for understanding the genetics of migraine were reviewed. This section provides an update on the genetic advances in migraine and insights into the pathogenesis that these advances have provided.

Migraine is recognized to cluster in families and has long been considered to be a strongly heritable disorder. Migraine, with aura (MA) or without aura (MO), has a substantial risk of familial occurrence, and genetic epidemiologic studies suggest that MO and MA have distinct and unique heritability; first-degree relatives of

MO probands have 1.9 times the risk of MO and 1.4 times the risk of MA, whereas first-degree relatives of MA probands have nearly four times the risk of MA and no increased risk of MO[27]. Concordance rates for migraine are higher among monozygotic (MZ) than dizygotic (DZ) twins; heritability estimates are around 52% in female twin pairs raised together or apart since infancy. In MZ Danish twin pairs, liability to MO resulted from additive genetic effects (61%) and from individual-specific environmental effects (39%), while in MA, correlation in liability was 0.68 in MZ and 0.22 in DZ, with heritability estimated at 0.65. Twin studies reveal that approximately one-half of the variation in migraine is attributable to additive genes, while the remainder is caused by unshared rather than shared environmental factors between twins.[28,29]

Complex segregation analyses have demonstrated that a multifactorial heredity model, wherein multiple genetic susceptibility factors interact with multiple environmental factors and render an individual susceptible to recurrent attacks, is most compatible with the mode of inheritance of migraine.[30] Migraine, like many complex multifactorial inherited diseases, is co-transmitted with other disorders. Migraine, anxiety, and depression are comorbid and share common genetic traits.[31]

As reviewed in the first section of this chapter, identifying genes for multifactorial disorders like migraine is challenging, since multiple genes, most with low penetrance, contribute to susceptibility of the disorder.[32] Moreover, the resulting phenotype is influenced by both endogenous and exogenous non-genetic factors. Case ascertainment can be a serious confounder that influences the validity of genetic analysis, particularly with migraine, in which there is no biomarker to aid in diagnosis. Thus for large population-based studies, questionnaires, which are less reliable than the gold-standard specialist interview, are relied upon not only for case ascertainment, but for control ascertainment as well.

Familial Hemiplegic Migraine: A Monogenic Migraine Subtype

Hemiplegic migraine (HM) is a rare subtype of migraine with aura that may occur as a familial or a sporadic condition. Familial hemiplegic migraine (FHM) is an autosomal dominant disorder associated with attacks of MA and MO and hemiparesis. The headache and aura features, apart from the hemiparesis, are identical to MA,[33] and two-thirds of the FHM patients, in addition to attacks of FHM, also have attacks of common non-hemiplegic migraine.[34]

Three genes have been identified in families with FHM. The first FHM gene that was identified is *CACNA1A* (*FHM1*), which is located on chromosome 19p13.[35,36] *CACNA1A* encodes the α_1-subunit of a voltage dependent P/Q Ca^{2+} channel,[37] which is widely expressed throughout the central nervous system (CNS). The defect is due to at least 21 different mis-sense mutations in the *CACNA1A* gene. The same gene is associated with episodic ataxia with cerebellar vermal atrophy[35] and epilepsy, during severe FHM attacks or independent of FHM attacks. The phenotype in *FHM1 S218L* mutation carriers can be very severe, even lethal, after mild head trauma. [38,39] P-type neuronal Ca^{2+} channels mediate 5-HT and excitatory neurotransmitter release. Dysfunction may impair 5-HT release and may predispose patients to migraine attacks or impair their self-aborting mechanism. Voltage-gated P/Q-type calcium channels mediate glutamate release, are involved in cortical spreading depression (CSD), and may be integral in initiating the migraine aura.[40] Spontaneously occurring or engineered mutations within the *CACNA1A* gene modulate CSD threshold. Mutant mice expressing human FHM type 1 mutations in the *CACNA1A* gene (*R192Q* or *S218L*) show increased CSD susceptibility [41] and facilitated subcortical propagation of CSD. Female mice expressing the *R192Q* or *S218L* mutation exhibited a significantly higher susceptibility than male mice toward CSD; this was eliminated by ovariectomy.[42]

A second gene, *FHM2*, has been mapped to chromosome 1 q 21-23. The defect is a new mutation in the alpha 2 subunit of the Na/K pump (*ATP1A2*).[43] This mutation results in reduced activity or decreased affinity for K+ of Na+/K+ pump, leading to impaired clearance of K+ and glutamate from the extracellular space. More than 30 *FHM2* mutations have been identified; most are amino acid changes, but there are also small deletions and a mutation affecting the stop codon, which causes an extension of the *ATP1A2* protein by 27 amino acid residues. Most of the *ATP1A2* mutations are associated with pure FHM; some are associated with FHM and cerebellar problems, childhood convulsions, epilepsy, and permanent mental retardation. Some *ATP1A2* mutations are associated with non-hemiplegic migraine phenotypes, such as basilar migraine [44] and even common migraine.[39] A third gene (*FHM3*) has been linked to chromosome 2q24. It is due to a mis-sense mutation in gene *SCN1A* (*Gln1489Lys*), which encodes an α1 subunit of a neuronal voltage-gated Na+ channel (Na$_v$1.1). This results in charge-altering AA exchange in hinged-lid domain of the protein, which is critical for fast inactivation of the channel. The mutation induces two- to fourfold accelerated recovery from fast inactivation. Excessive firing of neurons due to mutant Na$_v$1.1 channels could facilitate CSD by several mechanisms. High-frequency firing might lead to a rise in extracellular K+ concentration and thus further depolarization. In addition, repetitive firing might enhance the release of the excitatory neurotransmitter glutamate. This mutation might have effects similar to those of *CACNA1A* mutations in *FHM1*, which enhance neurotransmitter release and facilitate CSD. This is also similar to the effects of the *ATP1A2* mutations in *FHM2*.[45]

SCN1A is a well-known epilepsy gene with over 100 truncating and mis-sense mutations that are associated with childhood epilepsy (i.e., severe myoclonic epilepsy of infancy or generalized epilepsy with febrile seizures). [46,47] *SCN1A* encodes the pore-forming subunit of neuronal Nav1.1 channels. Only five *FHM3* mutations that change amino acid residues have been identified.[45,48,49,50] Mis-sense mutations *Q1489K* and *L1649Q* were identified in large families and are associated with pure FHM.[45,48] Notably, three of five FHM carriers of the *L263V* mutation had generalized tonic-clonic epileptic attacks, occurring independently from their HM attacks.[49] Two novel *FHM3 SCN1A* mutations (*Q1489H* and *F1499L*) were reported. [50] Four of five carriers of the *FHM3 Q1489H* mutation, in addition to having HM, also suffered from elicited repetitive transient daily blindness that was not associated with headache or other neurologic symptoms. [51] New clinical data support cosegregation of FHM and the new-eye phenotype of elicited repetitive daily blindness and two novel *SCN1A* mutations as the underlying genetic defect in two unrelated families (c.4495T_C/ p.Phe1499Leu and c.4467G_C/p. Gln1489His mis-sense substitutions [in exons 24 and 23, respectively]). This remarkably stereotyped new-eye phenotype has clinical characteristics of abnormal propagation of the retinal electrical signal that may be a retinal spreading depression.[50]

A mutation in *SLC1A3*, encoding the glial glutamate transporter EAAT1, which removes glutamate from the synaptic cleft, has been identified in a boy with pure hemiplegic migraine,[52] and a homozygous deletion in *SLC4A4*, encoding the electrogenic sodium bicarbonate (Na+−HCO3−) cotransporter NBCe1, was associated with FHM in two sisters who were also affected by renal tubular acidosis and ocular abnormalities.[53] *SLC1A3* and *SLC4A4* might be the fourth and fifth genes to be implicated in FHM.

The proline-rich transmembrane protein (PRRT2) has been recently implicated as the fourth FHM gene.[53a] The finding of similar or identical PRRT2 truncating deletions in several hundred non-migraine patients with migraine infantile convulsion choreoathetosis, paroxysmal kinesigenic dyskinesia, and benign familial infantile convulsions has questioned the relevance of this gene in FHM.[53b] The increasing availability of exome and genome data will facilitate the correlation between clinical phenotype with genetic variants in multiple loci and determine the true relevance of the PRRT2 gene in FHM.

Sporadic hemiplegic migraine (SHM) exhibits clinical symptoms that are similar to HM. Screening of FHM genes in previous series of patients with SHM detected a very low proportion of mutated patients. Riant et al. screened 25 patients.[54] Sequencing of *ATP1A2* and *CACNA1A* was conducted in each proband, and all identified variants were looked for in both parents. Twenty-three different amino acid variants were identified in 23 of the 25 patients. The variants occurred de novo in 19 patients (76%), strongly in favor of their causal role. *SCN1A* analysis did not show any mutation. Among the 19 patients with a de novo mutation, 5 had a pure HM and 14 had associated neurologic signs, such as ataxia, epilepsy, or intellectual disabilities. Thus, FHM genes are involved in early-onset SHM, particularly when associated with neurologic signs. Molecular analysis identified 14 novel de novo mutations.[54] The fact that not all FHM families are linked to one of the three known FHM loci implies that there are additional FHM genes. There are no obvious clinical differences between the three FHM types, although patients with *FHM1* mutations more often exhibit cerebellar ataxia or trauma-triggered attacks.[37,55,55] All three FHM types have associated epilepsy.[56]

Genes for Common Migraine Subtypes

GENOME-WIDE ASSOCIATION STUDIES

Genome-wide association studies (GWAS) depend on the ability to map the patterns of inheritance for the most common form of genomic variation, the single nucleotide polymorphism (SNP). There are approximately 10 million common SNPs; those with a minor-allele frequency of at least 5% are transmitted across generations in blocks, allowing a few particular, or tag, SNPs to capture the great majority of SNP variation within each block. (A tag SNPs is readily measured SNP that is in strong linkage disequilibrium with multiple other SNPs, so that it can serve as a proxy for these SNPs on large-scale genotyping platforms.) GWAS compare DNA from individuals with a disease (cases) and similar individuals without the disease (controls). The genome from each individual is read using SNP arrays containing large numbers of genetic variants. If one type of variant is more frequent in individuals with the disease, the SNP (often a tag SNP) is said to be "associated" with the disease. The associated SNPs are then considered to mark a region of the human genome that influences the risk of disease. As noted earlier, GWAS identify SNPs and other variants in DNA that are associated with a disease, but cannot on their own specify which genes are causal. SNPs associated with disease by GWAS are enriched within non-coding functional elements, with a majority residing in or near ENCODE-defined regions that are outside of protein-coding genes (see first section of this chapter).[1]

While GWAS appear to show great promise, it is important to understand that common DNA sequence variations, as identified in GWAS, do not directly lead to changes in disease-related phenotypes, but instead lead to changes in molecular phenotypes, which then affect molecular and cellular processes that lead to changes in physiological states. Understanding the extent to which and under what conditions this DNA is accessible to proteins that control expression will help to elucidate the functional consequences of these SNPs.

GWAS have identified many non-coding variants associated with common diseases and traits, like migraine. These variants are concentrated in regulatory DNA marked by deoxyribonuclease I (DNase I) hypersensitive sites (DHSs), which suggests pervasive involvement of regulatory DNA variation in common human disease and provides pathogenic insights into diverse disorders.[25] For example, the connection of numerous DHSs harboring GWAS SNPs with promoters of distant genes amplifies the genetic basis of disease and trait associations, provides a wealth of plausible causal genes to explain associations, and unifies seemingly unconnected variants associated with related diseases by way of convergent perturbation of common transcription factor networks.[33]

MIGRAINE GENOME-WIDE ASSOCIATION STUDIES

A meta-analysis of GWAS on migraine evaluated six population-based European migraine cohorts with a total sample size of 10,980 individuals (2446 cases and 8534 controls from six Dutch and Icelandic samples).[57] For replication, three population-based samples (two of Dutch and one of Australian origin) were tested. A total of 32 SNPs showed marginal evidence for association ($p < 10^{-5}$). The best result was obtained for SNP rs9908234, located in the nerve growth factor receptor gene ($p = 8 \times 10^{-8}$). This SNP did not replicate in three cohorts from the Netherlands or Australia. In addition, none of the additional 18 additional leading SNPs that were tested in two replication cohorts could be replicated successfully. A possible explanation for the negative results could be reduced power to detect an association based on diagnostic inaccuracy, since diagnoses were rendered based on questionnaires, rather than the gold standard of direct specialist-patient interviews. Another explanation offered by the authors is the heterogeneity of the population-based sample, with a less severe phenotype and consequently a lower genetic risk compared with patients seen in clinical practice.

The authors of this study also investigated SNP rs1835740, located on 8q21 between the metadherin (MTDH) and PGCP genes, which was found to be significantly associated with migraine with aura in the first GWA study of clinic-based populations.[57,58] The SNP was not associated with migraine, but a gene-based analysis identified a modest gene-based significant association with migraine. The MTDH gene down-regulates SLC1A2 (also known as EAAT2 and GLT-1), the gene encoding the major glutamate transporter in the brain, providing a possible link between this variant and glutamate regulation, a neurotransmitter long considered to play a role in migraine pathogenesis. Down-regulation of EAAT2 could result in excess glutamate at the neuronal synapse, and this accumulation could account for the electrophysiological and imaging evidence of cortical excitability and provide a substrate for CSD, the presumed biological substrate of migraine aura, and central sensitization, postulated to be the underlying mechanism of allodynia during a migraine attack. These results also support the hypothesis that complementary pathways, such as the glutamate system, may link the Mendelian channelopathies with the pathogenic mechanisms of more common forms of episodic neurologic disorders, such as migraine.

Another GWA study that was conducted involved a large population-based cohort of 23,230 women (5122 migraineurs and 18,108 non-migraineurs), with complete genotype and phenotype information and verified European ancestry from the Women's Genome Health Study (WGHS).[59] This study identified three SNPs with genome-wide significant association for common migraine at the population level: rs2651899 (1p36.32, PRDM16), rs10166942 (2q37.1, TRPM8), and rs11172113 (12q13.3, LRP1). These SNPs were significant in a meta-analysis among three replication cohorts and met genome-wide significance in a meta-analysis combining the discovery and replication cohorts. Two of the SNPs (rs2651899 and rs10166942) were specific for migraine compared to those without migraine, though none of the SNP associations was preferential for MA or MO, nor were any associations specific for individual migraine features.

The SNP rs10166942 was also found to be stronger among women (this may relate to the higher prevalence of migraine in women). The LRP1 locus, a member of the lipoprotein receptor family that serves as a sensor of the extracellular environment, is involved in the proliferation of vascular smooth muscle cells and modulates synaptic transmission.[60] The LRP1 protein and glutamate (NMDA) receptors are co-localized on neurons. This finding provides a further link between genetic associations and altered glutamate homeostasis in the pathogenesis of migraine. Importantly, however, this study also identified a new locus, TRPM8, which encodes a sensor for cold and cold-induced burning pain and is primarily expressed in sensory neurons, and is a target in animal models of neuropathic pain.[61–63] This new locus could be a pathophysiological link between migraine and other pain syndromes. This study also suggests a shared pathophysiology between MA and MO.

The first GWA clinic-based study of MO recently replicated associations at the TRPM8 and LRP1 loci, and reported several additional associated loci.[64] In this study, GWA data from 2,326 clinic-based German and Dutch individuals with MO and 4,580 population-matched controls was analyzed. SNPs at two of 12 loci demonstrated convincing replication at 1q22 (MEF2D) and 3p24 (TGFBR2). The MEF2D protein is a transcription factor that is highly expressed in the brain, regulates neuronal differentiation, and restricts the number of excitatory synapses when activated.[65,66] MEF2D dysregulation may affect neuronal excitatory neurotransmission in individuals with MO. In support of this hypothesis, MEF transcriptional targets have been associated with other neurologic disorders, including epilepsy.[66] The TGFBR2 protein is involved in the regulation of cell proliferation and differentiation, as well as in extracellular matrix production.[65] Missense mutations in TGFBR2 have been shown to cause monogenic familial aortic dissection as well as migrainous headaches in 11/14 mutation carriers in a large multigenerational family.[67] This locus is, therefore, an attractive candidate gene for migraine, especially since migraine sufferers are known to have increased risk of carotid dissection.

In this important study, SNPs at the PHACTR1 and ASTN2 loci also showed suggestive evidence of replication. The PHACTR1 locus encodes a protein (a member of the PHACTR/scapinin family) that controls synaptic activity and synaptic morphology and has been implicated in endothelial cell function and susceptibility to early-onset myocardial infarction.[68–71] The link between PHACTR and migraine pathogenesis could, therefore, either be neuronal, through aberrant synaptic transmission, or vascular, since endothelial dysfunction, cardiovascular disease, and myocardial infarction have all been linked to migraine.[72]

Variants within the *ASTN2* locus, a member of the astroactin gene family, have a role in glial guided migration and appear important for the development of the laminar architecture of cortical regions of the brain.[73] It is unclear how this links to the pathophysiology of migraine.

As illustrated in a recent state-of-the-art review,[73a] the findings from a large population-based GWAS study[73b] and a meta-analysis of 29 cohorts[59] have resulted in the identification of 12 susceptibility loci. The genes assigned to these loci seem to mainly affect neuronal pathways (MTDH, LRP1, PRDM16, MEF2D, ASTN2, PHACTR1, FHL5, MMP16), metalloproteinases (in case of MMP16, TSPAN2, AJAP1), and vascular pathways (in case of PHACTR1, TGFBR2, C7orf10). While the genetic association between these loci and migraine are robust based on the replication in independent cohorts, disease risk ascertainment and the functional consequences of these findings are difficult given the low odds ratios and the finding of GWAS hits outside coding regions. However, their association identifies potentially new pathogenetic mechanisms and treatment targets and are expected to ultimately have translational relevance to patients with migraine.

Other Migraine Genes

Migraine is comorbid with numerous other disorders, and it is likely that an underlying shared biology between two comorbid disorders is driven, in part, by a similar genetic substrate. Recently, two distinct mis-sense mutations in two independent families with MA and familial advanced sleep phase syndrome was identified in the gene encoding CKIδ.[74] The CKIδ protein is pivotal in the function of the biological clock that influences the circadian rhythm. The resulting alterations (T44A and H46R) occurred in the conserved catalytic domain of CKIδ, where they caused reduced enzyme activity. Mice engineered to carry the CKId-T44A allele demonstrated significantly lowered mechanical and thermal sensory thresholds after infusion with nitroglycerin, a prototypic migraine trigger, and a significant increase in cFOS-positive neurons was demonstrated in the trigeminal-cervical complex. Also, consistent with the premise that migraine is characterized by neuronal hyperexcitability and that CSD of neuronal and glial membranes is responsible for the migraine aura, CKId-T44A mice demonstrated a reduced threshold for CSD after the application of potassium chloride to exposed cerebral cortex, and increased spontaneous and evoked calcium signaling in astrocytes. These in vitro and in vivo data suggest that CKIδ activity may contribute to the pathogenesis of migraine and may potentially uncover protein targets of CKIδ as new targets for drug discovery.

The two-pore domain (K2P) potassium channel, TWIK-related spinal cord potassium channel (TRESK, encoded by *KCNK18*), has been implicated in the regulation pain pathways.[75] K2P channels are important in the control of neuronal resting membrane potential and neuronal excitability and are distributed throughout the CNS.[76] The TRESK K2P channel is activated by calcineurin after G$_q$ α receptor stimulation and a subsequent rise in intracellular calcium.[77,78] It is, therefore, a potential target of pain mediators that exert their action via these pathways, and a role has recently been suggested for TRESK in the calcineurin inhibitor–induced pain syndrome.[78,79] TRESK is also activated by volatile anesthetics, such as halothane,[80] which have been shown to inhibit CSD.

Lafreniere et al. examined the potential role of TRESK in typical MA.[81] They sequenced the entire coding region of the *KCNK18* gene in a panel and examined whether TRESK is involved in migraine by screening the *KCNK18* gene in subjects diagnosed with migraine. They reported a frame-shift mutation, F139WfsX24, which segregates perfectly with typical migraine with aura in a large pedigree. They also identified prominent TRESK expression in migraine-salient areas, such as the trigeminal ganglion. Functional characterization of this mutation demonstrates that it causes a complete loss of TRESK function and that the mutant subunit suppresses wild-type channel function through a dominant-negative effect, thus explaining the dominant penetrance of this allele. These results support a role for TRESK in the pathogenesis of typical migraine with aura and further support the role of this channel as a potential therapeutic target.[81]

This finding has potential therapeutic implications. Since TRESK is an ion channel expressed at the surface of the neuron, highly selective and potent small molecule agonist compounds could be developed and evaluated pre-clinically for acute and preventive efficacy in animal models of migraine. Because the gene is expressed in a very limited set of neurons, and since the trigeminal ganglion also lies outside the blood–brain barrier, modulating its activity should have minimal off-target or central nervous system toxicity. Any such agonists however would have to avoid anesthetic or immune system side effects.[82]

The possibility of migraine as an X-linked disorder is suggested by the female preponderance and evidence that a high proportion of affected males have a greater number of affected first-degree relatives.[83] In a linkage analysis of six migraine pedigrees and a case-control cohort study that evaluated 11 candidate genes, two distinct susceptibility variants were identified at Xq27 (marked by DXS8043—DXS297) and Xq28 (DXS8061—XqTer).[84] Since these susceptibility regions were also associated in the case-control population, the possibility was raised that these loci are not pedigree-specific and may be contributing to migraine in the general population.

Migraine and Genetic Vasculopathies

Migraine, particularly MA, is associated with several hereditary and acquired cerebrovascular disorders, including arterial dissection, ischemic stroke, and cardiovascular disease. It has been speculated that migraine and stroke may both be triggered by hypoperfusion and could therefore exist on a continuum of vascular complications in a subset of patients who have these hereditary or acquired comorbid vascular conditions.[85] Indeed, evidence suggests that certain migraine mutations may increase the vulnerability for stroke by facilitating ischemic depolarizations.[86]. FHM type 1 (FHM1) mutant mice, with mutations in CaV2.1 voltage-gated calcium channels, develop earlier onset of anoxic depolarization and more frequent peri-infarct depolarizations, resulting in more extensive cerebral infarctions and worse neurological outcomes. Enhanced susceptibility to ischemia-induced CSD may predispose migraine sufferers to infarction during mild ischemic events and that this in part may account for the higher stroke risk in migraineurs.

The mechanism underlying the frequent association between migraine and genetic small vessel arteriopathies is unclear, but a common underlying factor may be the propensity for transient cerebral ischemia or hypoperfusion to trigger an underlying cascade of events that culminate in a migraine attack.(63) Indeed, recent experimental data have indicated that focal, mild, and transient hypoperfusion (cerebral ischemia without infarction) can trigger CSD.[87] MA and MO have been associated as a common trait in several genetic small vessel vasculopathies, as illustrated in the following sections.

CEREBRAL AUTOSOMAL DOMINANT ARTERIOPATHY WITH SUBCORTICAL INFARCTS AND LEUKOENCEPHALOPATHY

The clinical observation of an association between migraine and several genetic vasculopathies supports the concept that transient hypoperfusion or ischemic depolarization increase the susceptibility to migraine. One such genetic vasculopathy is cerebral autosomal dominant arteriopathy with subcortical infarcts and leukoencephalopathy (CADASIL). CADASIL is a systemic, nonamyloid, nonatherosclerotic vasculopathy and is the most common monogenic-inherited form of adult-onset stroke and vascular dementia, linked to mutations in the Notch 3 gene (located on chromosome 19p13.2-p13.1), which encodes a cell surface receptor that, in human adult tissue, is solely expressed on vascular smooth muscle cells.[88] The Notch3 protein is part of a signal transduction pathway, critical for aspects of vascular development, homeostasis, and vascular smooth muscle cell differentiation. Most mutations in CADASIL are mis-sense mutations and involve the loss or gain of a cysteine residue in the Notch3 protein (specifically the extracellular epidermal-growth-factor-like repeat).[88,89] The Notch3 transgenic mouse model demonstrates that degeneration of vascular smooth muscle cells (VSMCs) precedes the deposition of granular osmiophilic material (GOM) in the basement membrane and extracellular matrix of VSMCs and mutations in the *NOTCH3* gene have a gain-of-function effect on the protein, and that dysfunctional anchoring of vascular smooth muscle cells to the extracellular matrix and adjacent cells triggers VSMC degeneration.[90] The variable disease course of CADASIL, ranging from relatively mild to very severe, might be an indication for the involvement of other genetic and environmental modifying factors.[91,92]

The incidence of MA, typically the first disease symptom of CADASIL, is five times greater compared to the general population.[87,93,94] Visual and sensory auras are most common in CADASIL, although 50% of the patients also experience atypical attacks with basilar, hemiplegic, or prolonged aura, and even coma. [95,96] The explanation for the predilection for MA attacks in patients with CADASIL was recently demonstrated in a study that showed that CSD, the electrophysiological substrate of migraine aura, is enhanced in mice expressing a vascular Notch 3 CADASIL mutation (R90C) or a Notch 3 knockout mutation.[97] The phenotype was stronger in Notch 3 knockout mice, implicating both loss of function and neomorphic mutations in its pathogenesis. The mechanism underlying CSD increased susceptibility in CADASIL is unclear, but dysfunctional communication within the neurovascular unit has been raised as a possibility.[97,98] Abnormal Notch 3 signaling may disrupt normal astrocyte-smooth muscle communication and may result in impaired neurovascular coupling, or Notch 3 mutations expressed in neural progenitor cells and transiently in newly born neurons may lead to enhanced CSD susceptibility phenotype later in life. [99]

RETINAL VASCULOPATHY WITH CEREBRAL LEUKODYSTROPHY (RVCL)

Retinal vasculopathy with cerebral leukodystrophy (RVCL) is a neurovascular syndrome (formerly referred to in three separate families and publications as cerebroretinal vasculopathy (CRV),[100] hereditary vascular retinopathy (HVR),[101] and hereditary endotheliopathy, retinopathy, nephropathy and stroke (HERNS),[102]) characterized by vascular retinopathy, cognitive impairment, depression, migraine (mainly without aura), focal neurologic symptoms, and, in later disease stages, characteristic contrast-enhancing intracerebral mass lesions. Several systemic symptoms can be present as well, including renal and liver dysfunction, Raynaud's phenomenon, and gastrointestinal bleeding. Although reported independently, the discovery of the gene defect, carboxyl-terminal truncations causing frame-shifts in the *TREX1* gene encoding the 3'-5' DNA-specific exonuclease *TREX1*(3p21.1-p21.3), showed that they are different phenotypic variants of the same genetic disorder.[103]

It is unclear how the carboxyl truncating mutations in *TREX1* lead to the phenotype or pathogenesis of RVCL. Functional studies with mutant TREX1 suggest that forms lacking their native carboxyl-termini cannot localize to their usual perinuclear site within the cell and freely diffuse throughout the cytoplasm, thereby rendering the gene product unable to perform its physiological function.[104]

HEREDITARY SYSTEMIC ANGIOPATHY

Hereditary systemic angiopathy (HSA) manifests with cerebral calcifications, retinopathy, progressive nephropathy and hepatopathy, and appears to be a variant of RVCL. Small and medium-sized subcortical white matter lesions are seen on magnetic resonance imaging—a finding consistent with a vasculopathy of small and medium-sized cerebral vessels. Subjects usually present in the fourth decade of life with visual impairment, migraine-like headaches, skin rash, seizures, motor weakness, and cognitive impairment. In the later stages, patients may develop liver sclerosis, with progressive hepatic impairment and renal microangiopathy leading to organ failure and chronic anemia.[105] HSA has several similarities with RVCL; the cerebral calcification, perivascular inflammatory response and progressive hepatic and renal failure are unique to this disorder.[82]

COL4A1-RELATED DISORDER

Autosomal dominant *COL4A1* gene-related disorders are described in at least 12 white European families with 100% penetrance of disease.[106] Thus far, 12 different missense mutations have been described in the *COL4A1* gene. Mutations in the *COL4A1* gene, located on chromosome 13q34, are associated with several unique phenotypes with overlapping features, including a condition exhibiting perinatal hemorrhage with porencephaly in survivors;[107–110] a small vessel disease with hemorrhage of adult onset or with infantile hemiparesis;[111] and hereditary angiopathy, nephropathy, aneurysms and muscle cramps (HANAC syndrome).[108,112] Along with hemorrhagic strokes, *COL4A1* mutations may cause variable degrees of retinal arteriolar tortuosity, cataracts, glaucoma, and anterior segment dysgenesis of the eye.

Neurologic symptoms in *COL4A1* mutation carriers may vary in degree of severity, even within families. Depending on the age of onset, affected individuals present with infantile hemiparesis, seizures, visual loss, dystonia, strokes, migraine, mental retardation, cognitive impairment, and dementia. Single or recurrent intracranial hemorrhages may occur in non-hypertensive adults less than 50 years of age. These hemorrhages can occur spontaneously, subsequent to trauma, or as a result of anticoagulant use. Stroke often occurs as the first presentation of the disease, with a mean age of onset of 36 years.[106] MRI generally demonstrates typical features of other small vessel diseases, including diffuse leukoencephalopathy with deep white matter involvement of posterior periventricular areas, subcortical infarctions, microhemorrhages, and dilated perivascular spaces.

The association with migraine in individuals with *COL4A1* mutations is unclear, and may either be coincidental or mutation specific. Migraine with aura was described in one family with hereditary porencephaly secondary to a *COL4A1* mutation, while in two other patients the migraine subtype was not specified.[108] However, as in six other families with hereditary porencephaly, migraine was not described.

REFERENCES

1. The ENCODE Project Consortium. An integrated encyclopedia of DNA. *Nature*. 2012;480:57–74.
2. Strachan T, Read AP. *Human molecular genetics*. 2nd ed. New York: Wiley-Liss, 1999.
3. Guttmacher AE, Collins FS. Genomic medicine: a primer. *N Engl J Med*. 2002;347:1512–1520.
4. Pennisi E. Genomics. ENCODE project writes eulogy for junk DNA. *Science*. 2012;337:1159, 1161.
5. Spurbeck JL, Adams SA, Stupca PJ, Dewald GW. Primer on medical genomics. Part XI: Visualizing human chromosomes. *Mayo Clin Proc*. 2004;79:58–75.
6. Qureshi IA, Mehler MF. Emerging roles of non-coding RNAs in brain evolution, development, plasticity and disease. *Nat Rev Neurosci*. 2012;13:528–541.
7. Ensenauer RE, Reinke SS, Ackerman MJ, Tester DJ, Whiteman DA, Tefferi A. Primer on medical genomics. Part VIII: Essentials of medical genetics for the practicing physician. *Mayo Clin Proc*. 2003;78:846–857.
8. Ansell SM, Ackerman MJ, Black JL, Roberts LR, Tefferi A. Primer on medical genomics. Part VI: Genomics and molecular genetics in clinical practice. *Mayo Clin Proc*. 2003;78:307–317.
9. Tefferi A, Wieben ED, Dewald GW, Whiteman DA, Bernard ME, Spelsberg TC. Primer on medical genomics part II: Background principles and methods in molecular genetics. *Mayo Clin Proc*. 2002;77:785–808.
10. Chan SR, Blackburn EH. Telomeres and telomerase. *Philos Trans R Soc Lond B Biol Sci*. 2004;359:109–121.
11. Sibille KT, Langaee T, Burkley B, et al. Chronic pain, perceived stress, and cellular aging: an exploratory study. *Mol Pain*. 2012;8:12.
12. Fedoroff NV. Presidential address. Transposable elements, epigenetics, and genome evolution. *Science*. 2012;338:758–767.
13. Mathews HL, Janusek LW. Epigenetics and psychoneuroimmunology: mechanisms and models. *Brain Behav Immun*. 2011;25:25–39.
14. Kouzarides T. Chromatin modifications and their function. *Cell*. 2007;128:693–705.
15. Sato F, Tsuchiya S, Meltzer SJ, Shimizu K. MicroRNAs and epigenetics. *FEBS J*. 2011;278:1598–1609.
16. Montagna P. The primary headaches: genetics, epigenetics and a behavioural genetic model. *J Headache Pain*. 2008;9:57–69.

17. Harrow J, Frankish A, Gonzalez JM, et al. GENCODE: the reference human genome annotation for The ENCODE Project. *Genome Res.* 2012;22:1760–1774.

18. Lee JT, Bartolomei MS. X-inactivation, imprinting, and long noncoding RNAs in health and disease. *Cell.* 2013;152:1308–1323.

19. Wang KC, Chang HY. Molecular mechanisms of long noncoding RNAs. *Mol Cell.* 2011;43:904–914.

20. Cenik ES, Zamore PD. Argonaute proteins. *Curr Biol.* 2011;21:R446–R449.

21. Ghildiyal M, Zamore PD. Small silencing RNAs: an expanding universe. *Nat Rev Genet.* 2009;10:94–108.

22. Hartwell LH, Hood L, Goldberg ML, Reynolds AE, Silvre LM. *Genetics: from genes to genomes.* 4th ed. New York: McGraw Hill, 2011.

23. Manolio TA. Genomewide association studies and assessment of the risk of disease. *N Engl J Med.* 2010;363:166–176.

24. Pennisi E. Disease risk links to gene regulation. *Science.* 2011;332:1031.

25. Maurano MT, Humbert R, Rynes E, et al. Systematic localization of common disease-associated variation in regulatory DNA. *Science.* 2012;337:1190–1195.

26. Gross DS, Garrard WT. Nuclease hypersensitive sites in chromatin. *Annu Rev Biochem.* 1988;57:159–197.

27. Russell MB, Iselius L, Olesen J. Migraine without aura and migraine with aura are inherited disorders. *Cephalalgia.* 1996;16:305–309.

28. Ulrich V, Gervil M, Kyvik KO, Olesen J, Russell MB. The inheritance of migraine with aura estimated by means of structural equation modelling. *J Med Genet.* 1999;36:225–227.

29. Russell MB, Ulrich V, Gervil M, Olesen J. Migraine without aura and migraine with aura are distinct disorders: a population-based twin survey. *Headache.* 2002;42:332–336.

30. Russell MB, Andersson PG, Thomsen LL, Iselius L. Cluster headache is an autosomal dominantly inherited disorder in some families: a complex segregation analysis. *J Med Genet.* 1995;32:954–956.

31. Merikangas KR, Merikangas JR, Angst J. Headache syndromes and psychiatric disorders: associations and familial transmission. *J Psychiatric Res.* 1993;27:197–210.

32. Ferrari MD, Dichgans M. Genetics of primary headache. In: Silberstein SD, Lipton RB, Dodick DW, eds. *Wolff's headache and other head pain.* 8th ed. New York: Oxford University Press, 2007:133–149.

33. Thomsen LL, Eriksen MK, Roemer SF, Anderson I, Olesen J, Russell MB. A population-based study of familial hemiplegic migraine suggests revised diagnostic criteria. *Brain.* 2002;125:1379–1399.

34. Russell MB, Ducros A. Sporadic and familial hemiplegic migraine: pathophysiological mechanisms, clinical characteristics, diagnosis, and management. *Lancet Neurol.* 2011;10:457–470.

35. Ophoff RA, Terwindt GM, Vergouwe MN. Familial hemiplegic migraine and episodic ataxia type-2 are caused by mutations in the Ca2+ channel gene CACNLA4. *Cell Tiss Res.* 1996;87:543–552.

36. Joutel A, Bousser MG, Biousse V. A gene for familial hemiplegic migraine maps to chromosome 19. *Nature Genetics.* 1993;5:40–45.

37. Ducros A, Deiner C, Joutel A, et al. The clinical spectrum of familial hemiplegic migraine associated with mutations in a neuronal calcium channel. *N Eng J Med.* 2001;345:17–24.

38. Chan YC, Burgunder JM, Wilder-Smith E, et al. Electroencephalographic changes and seizures in familial hemiplegic migraine patients with the CACNA1A gene S218L mutation. *J Clin Neurosci.* 2008;15:891–894.

39. de Vries B, Frants RR, Ferrari MD, van den Maagdenberg AM. Molecular genetics of migraine. *Hum Genet.* 2009;126:115–132.

40. Ferrari MD, Haan J. Genetics of headache. In: Silberstein SD, Lipton RB, Dalessio DJ, eds. *Wolff's headache and other head pain.* 7th ed. New York: Oxford University Press, 2001:73–84.

41. Eikermann-Haerter K, Dilekoz E, Kudo C. Genetic and hormonal factors modulate spreading depression and transient hemiparesis in mouse models of familial hemiplegic migraine type I. *J Clin Invest.* 2009;119:99–109.

42. Eikermann-Haerter K, Ayata C. Cortical spreading depression and migraine. Curr *Neurol Neurosci Rep.* 2010;10:167–173.

43. De Fusco M, Marconi R, Silvestri L, et al. Haploinsufficiency of ATP1A2 encoding the Na(+)/K(+) pump alpha2 subunit associated with familial hemiplegic migraine type 2. *Nat Genet.* 2003;33:192–196.

44. Ambrosini A, D'Onofrio M, Grieco GS, et al. Familial basilar migraine associated with a new mutation in the ATP1A2 gene. *Neurology.* 2005;65:1826–1828.

45. Dichgans M, Freilinger T, Eckstein G, et al. Mutation in the neuronal voltage-gated sodium channel SCN1A in familial hemiplegic migraine. *Lancet.* 2005;366:371–377.

46. Meisler MH, Kearney JA. Sodium channel mutations in epilepsy and other neurological disorders. *J Clin Invest.* 2005;115:2010–2017.

47. Mulley JC, ScheVer IE, Petrou S, Dibbens LA, Berkovic SF, Harkin LA. SCN1A mutations and epilepsy. *Hum Mutat.* 2005;25:535–542.

48. Vanmolkot KR, Babini E, de VB, et al. The novel p.L1649Q mutation in the SCN1A epilepsy gene is associated with familial hemiplegic migraine: genetic and functional studies. Mutation in brief #957. Online. *Hum Mutat.* 2007;28:522.

49. Castro MJ, Stam AH, Lemos C, et al. First mutation in the voltage-gated Nav1.1 subunit gene SCN1A with co-occurring familial hemiplegic migraine and epilepsy. *Cephalalgia.* 2009;29:308–313.

50. Vahedi K, Depienne C, Le FD, et al. Elicited repetitive daily blindness: a new phenotype associated with hemiplegic migraine and SCN1A mutations. *Neurology.* 2009;72:1178–1183.

51. Le FD, Safran AB, Picard F, Bouchardy I, Morris MA. Elicited repetitive daily blindness: a new familial disorder related to migraine and epilepsy. *Neurology.* 2004;63:348–350.

52. Freilinger T, Koch J, Dichgans M, et.al. A novel mutation in SLC1A3 associated with pure hemiplegic migraine. *J Headache Pain.* 2010;11(Suppl 1):90.

53. Suzuki M, Van Paesschen ESI, et al. Defective membrane expression of the Na(+)-HCO(3)(-) cotranssporter NBCel1 is associated with familial migraine. *Proc Natl Acad Sci USA*. 2010;107:15963–15968.

53a. Riant F, Roze E, Barbance C, Méneret A, Guyant-Maréchal L, Lucas C, Sabouraud P, Trébuchon A, Depienne C, Tournier-Lasserve E. PRRT2 mutations cause hemiplegic migraine. *Neurology*. 2012;79:2122–2124.

53b. Pelzer N, de Vries B, Kamphorst JT, Vijfhuizen LS, Ferrari MD, Haan J, van den Maagdenberg AM, Terwindt GM. PRRT2 and hemiplegic migraine: a complex association. *Neurology*. 2014;83:288–290.

54. Riant F, Ducros A, Ploton C, Barbance C, Depienne C, Tournier-Lasserve E. De novo mutations in ATP1A2 and CACNA1A are frequent in early-onset sporadic hemiplegic migraine. *Neurology*. 2010;75:967–972.

55. van den Maagdenberg AM, Haan J, Terwindt GM, Ferrari MD. Migraine: gene mutations and functional consequences. *Curr Opin Neurol*. 2007;20:299–305.

56. Haan J, Terwindt GM, van den Maagdenberg AM, Stam AH, Ferrari MD. A review of the genetic relation between migraine and epilepsy. *Cephalalgia*. 2008;28:105–113.

57. Litthart L, de Vries B, Smith AV, et.al. Meta-analysis of genome-wide association for migraine in six population-based European cohorts. *Eur J Human Genet*. 2011;19:901–907.

58. Anttila V, Stefansson H, Kallela M, et al. Genome-wide association study of migraine implicates a common susceptibility variant on 8q22.1. *Nat Genet*. 2010;42:869–873.

59. Chasman D, Schurks M, Antilla V, et.al. Genome-wide association study reveals three susceptibility loci for common migraine in the general populaton. *Nature Genetics*. 2011;43:695–698.

60. Lillis AP, VanDuyn LB, Murphy-Ullrich JE, Stickland DK. LDL receptor-related protein 1: unique tissue-specific functions revealed by selective gene knock-out studies. *Physiol Rev*. 2008;88:887–918.

61. Proudfoot CJ, et.al. Analgesia medicated by the TRPM8 cold receptor in chronic neuropathic pain. *Curr Biol*. 2006;16:1591–1605.

62. Peier AM, et al. A TRP channel that senses cold stimuli and menthol. *Cell*. 2002;108:705–715.

63. Dray A. Neuropathic pain: emerging treatments. *Br J Anaesth*. 2008;101:48–58.

64. Freilinger T, Antilla V, de Vries B, et.al. Genome-wide Association analysis identifies susceptibility loci for migraine without aura. *Nature Genetics*. 2012;44:777–782.

65. Lin X, Shah S, Bulleit RF. The expression of MEF2 genes is implicated in CNS neuronal differentiation. *Brain Res Mol Brain Res*. 1996;42:307–316.

66. Flavell SW. Genome-wide analysis of MEF2 transcriptional program reveals synaptic target genes and neuronal activity-dependent polyadenylation site selection. *Neuron*. 208;60:1022–1038.

67. Law C, et al. Clinical features in a family with an R460H mutation in transforming growth factor a receptor 2 gene. *J Med Genet*. 2006;43:908–916.

68. AnonymousPhactrs 1–4: a family of protein phosphatise 1 and actin regulatory proteins. *Proc Natl Acad Sci USA*. 2004;101:7187–7192.

69. Greengard P, Allen PB, Nairn AC. Beyond the dopamine receptor: the DARPP-32 protein phosphatase-1 cascade. *Neuron*. 1999;23:435–447.

70. Jarray R, et al. Depletion of the novel protein PHACTR-1 from human endothelial cells abolishes tube formation and induces cell death receptor apoptosis. *Biochimie*. 2011;93:1668–1675.

71. Myocardial Infarction Genetics Consortium. Genome-wide association of early-onset myocardial infarction with single nucleotide polymorphisms and copy number variants. *Nat Genet*. 2009;41:334–341.

72. Tietjen GE. Migraine as a systemic vasculopathy. *Cephalalgia*. 2009;29:987–996.

73. Wilson PM, Fryerk RH, Fang Y, Hatten ME. Astn2, a novel member of the astrotactin gene family, regulates the trafficking of ASTN1 during glial-guided neuronal migraion. *J Neurosci*. 2010;30:8529–8540.

73a. Tolner EA, Houben T, Terwindt GM, de Vries Bb, Ferrari MD, van den Maagdenberg AMJM. From migraine genes to mechanisms. *Pain*. 2015;156:S64–S74.

73b. Anttila V, Winsvold BS,Gormley P, Kurth T, Bettella F, McMahonG, et al. Genome-wide meta-analysis identifies new susceptibility loci for migraine. *Nat Genet*. 2013;45:912–917.

74. Brennan KC, Bates EA, Shapiro RE, et al. Casein kinase idelta mutations in familial migraine and advanced sleep phase. *Sci Transl Med*. 2013;5:183ra56,1–11.

75. Huang DY, Yu BW, Fan QW. Roles of TRESK, a novel two-pore domain K+ channel, in pain pathway and general anesthesia. *Neurosci Bull*. 2008;24:166–172.

76. Enyedi P, Czirjak G. Molecular background of leak K+ currents: two-pore domain potassium channels. *Physiol Rev*. 2010;90:559–605.

77. Czirjak G, Toth ZE, Enyedi P. The two-pore domain K+ channel, TRESK, is activated by the cytoplasmic calcium signal through calcineurin. *J Biol Chem*. 2004;279:18550–18558.

78. Mathie A. Neuronal two-pore-domain potassium channels and their regulation by G protein-coupled receptors. *J Physiol*. 2007;578:377–385.

79. Smith HS. Calcineurin as a nociceptor modulator. *Pain Physician*. 2009;12:E309–E318.

80. Liu C, Au JD, Zou HL, Cotten JF, Yost CS. Potent activation of the human tandem pore domain K channel TRESK with clinical concentrations of volatile anesthetics. *Anesth Analg*. 2004;99:1715–22, table.

81. Lafreniere RG, Cader MZ, Poulin JF, et al. A dominant-negative mutation in the TRESK potassium channel is linked to familial migraine with aura. *Nat Med*. 2010;16:1157–1160.

82. Lafreiniere RG, Rouleau GA. Migraine: role of the TRESK two-port potassium channel. *Int J Biochem Cell Biol*. 2011;43:1533–1536.

83. Stewart WF, Bigal ME, Kolodner K, Dowson F, Liberman FN, Lipton RB. Familial risk of migraine: variation by proband age at onset and headache severity. *Neurology*. 2006;66:344–348.

84. Maher BH, Kerr M, Cox HC, et al. Confirmation that Xq27 and Xq28 are susceptibility loci for migraine in independent pedigrees and a case-control cohort. *Neurogenetics*. 2012;13:97–101.

85. Dalkara T, Nozari A, Moskowitz MA. Migraine aura pathophysiology: the role of blood vessels and microembolism. *Neurology.* 2012;9:309–317.

86. Eikermann-Haerter K, Lee JH, Yuzawa I, et al. Migraine mutations increase stroke vulnerability by facilitating ischemic depolarizations. *Circulation.* 2012;125:335–345.

87. Nozari A, Dilekoz E, Sukhotinsky I, et al. Microemboli may link spreading depression, migraine aura, and patent foramen ovale. *Ann Neurol.* 2010;67:221–229.

88. Chabriat H, Joutel A, Dichgans M, et.al. CADASIL. *Lancet Neurol.* 2009;8:643–653.

89. Morrow D, Guha S, Sweeney C, Birney Y, Walshe TOC, et.al. Notch and vascular smooth muscle cell phenotype. *Circ Res.* 2008;103:70–82.

90. Monet M, Domenga V, Lemaire B, et al. The archetypal R90C CADASIL-NOTCH3 mutation retains NOTCH3 function in vivo. *Hum Mol Genet.* 2007;16:982–992.

91. Opherk C, Peters N, Herzog J, Leudtke R, Dichgans M. Longterm prognosis and causes of death in CADASIL: a retrospective study in 411 patients. *Brain.* 2004;127:2533–2539.

92. Opherk C, Peters N, Holtmanspotter M, Gschwendtner A, Muller-Myshok B, Dichgans M. Heritability of MRI lesion volume in CADASIL: evidence for genetic modifiers. *Stroke.* 2006;37:2684–2689.

93. Chabriat H, Vahedi K, Iba-Zizen MT, et al. Clinical spectrum of CADASIL: a study of seven families. *Lancet.* 1995;346:934–939.

94. Vahedi K, Chabriat H, Levy C, et.al. Migraine with aura and brain magnetic resonance imaging abnormalities in patients with CADASIL. *Arch Neurol.* 2002;61:1237–1240.

95. Feuerhake F, Volk V, Ostertag CB, et.al. Reversible coma with raised intracranial pressure: an unusual clinical manifestation of CADASIL. *Acta Neuropathol.* 2002;103:188–192.

96. Schon F, Martin RJ, Prevett M, et.al. "CADASIL coma": an underdiagnosed acute encephalopathy. *J Neurol Neurosurg Psychiatry.* 2003;74:249–252.

97. Eikermann-Haerter K, Yuzawa I, Dilekoz E, et.al. Cerebral autosomal dominant arteriopathy with subcortical infarcts and leukoencephalopathy syndrome mutations increase susceptibility to spreading depression. *Ann Neurol.* 2011;69:413–418.

98. Joutel A, Monet-Lepretre M, Gosele C, et.al. Cerebrovascular dysfunction and microcirculation rare fraction precede white matter lesions in a mouse genetic model of cerebral ischemic small vessel disease. *J Clin Invest.* 2010;120:433–445.

99. Arboleda-Velasquez JF, Zhou Z, Shin HK, et.al. Linking Notch signaling to ischemic stroke. *Proc Natl Acad Sci USA.* 2008;105:4856–4861.

100. Grand MG, Kaine J, Fulling K, et al. Cerebroretinal vasculopathy: a new hereditary syndrome. *Ophthalmology.* 1988;95:649–659.

101. Terwindt GM, Haan J, Ophoff RA, et al. Clinical and genetic analysis of a large Dutch family with autosomal dominant vascular retinopathy, migraine and Raynaud's phenomenon. *Brain.* 1988;121:303–316.

102. Jen J, Cohen AH, Yue Q, et al. Heridtary endotheliopathy with retinopathy, nephropathy, and stroke (HERNS). *Neurology.* 1997;49:1322–1330.

103. Richard A, Van den Maagdengerg AM, Jen JC, et al. Truncations in the carboxyl-terminus of human 3'-5' DNA exonuclease TREX1 cause retinal vasculopathy with cerebral leukodystrophy. *Nat Genet.* 2007;39:1068–1070.

104. Chowdhury D, Beresford PJ, Zhu P, et al. The exonuclease TREX1 is in the SET complex and acts in concert with NM23H1 to degrade DNA during granzyme A-mediated cell death. *Mol Cell.* 2006;23:133–142.

105. Winkler DT, Lyrer P, Probst A, et al. Hereditary systemic angiopathy (HSA) with cerebral alcifications, retinopathy, progressive nephropathy, and hepatopathy. *J Neurol.* 2008;255:77–88.

106. Lanfranconi S, Markus HS. COL4A1 mutations as a monogenic cause of cerebral small vessel disease: a systemic review. *Stroke.* 2010;41:e513–518.

107. Gould DB, Phalan FC, Breedveld GJ, et al. Mutations in COL4A1 cause perinatal cerebral hemorrhage and porencephaly. *Science.* 2005;308:1167–1171.

108. Breedveld G, de Coo IF, Lequin MH, et al. Novel mutations in three families confirm a major role of COL4A1 in hereditary porencephaly. *J Med Genet.* 2006;43:490–495.

109. van der Knaap MS, Smit LM, Barkhof F, et al. Neonatal porencephaly and adult stroke related to mutations in collagen IV A1. *Ann Neurol.* 2006;59:504–511.

110. de Vries LS, Koopman C, Groenendall F, et al. COL4A1 mutation in two preterm siblings with antenatal onset of parenchymal hemorrhage. *Ann Neurol.* 2009;12–18.

111. Vahedi K, Kubis N, Boukobza M, et al. COL4A1 mutation in a patient with sporadic, recurrent intrcerebral hemorrhage. *Stroke.* 2007;38:1461–1464.

112. Plaisier E, Gribouval O, Alamowitch S, et al. COL4A1 mutation and hereditary antiopathy, nephropathy, aneurysms, and muscle cramps. *N Engl J Med.* 2007;357:2687–2695.

Chapter 3

Less Common Migraine Subtypes

PROBABLE MIGRAINE

HEMIPLEGIC MIGRAINE

MIGRAINE WITH BRAINSTEM AURA

RETINAL MIGRAINE

VISUAL SNOW

VESTIBULAR MIGRAINE

EPILEPSY AND MIGRAINE

REFERENCES

Migraine and its common subtypes have been described in Chapter 1. In this chapter, we will review less common ICHD-3 β migraine subtypes, including probable migraine, hemiplegic migraine, migraine with brainstem aura, retinal migraine, visual snow, vestibular migraine, and postictal headache.

PROBABLE MIGRAINE

Probable migraine (1.5), a frequent primary headache disorder, has replaced the previous term, migrainous disorder, in the ICHD-2.[1] Between 10% and 45% of those who suffer from headache with features of migraine fail to fully meet the ICHD criteria for migraine with or without aura.[2] Most meet criteria for probable migraine, a migraine subtype fulfilling all criteria but one for migraine with or without aura (as long as the full set of criteria for another disorder are not met) (Table 3.1). There are two probable migraine

subtypes: probable migraine without aura (1.5.1) and probable migraine with aura (1.5.2). Probable migraine is common and is associated with temporary disability and reduction in the health-related quality of life. [3] In a large epidemiologic study conducted in the United States in which 162,576 individuals aged 12 years or older were interviewed, the 1-year period prevalence of probable migraine among those with severe headaches was 4.5% (3.9% in men and 5.1% in women). Prevalence was higher in women and men between the ages of 30 and 59 years. Prevalence was significantly higher in African Americans than in whites (female 7.4% vs. 4.8%; male 4.8% vs. 3.7%) and was inversely related to household income. During their headaches, most sufferers (48.2%) had at least some impairment, while 22.1% were severely disabled. Only 21% of those with probable migraine ever received a medical diagnosis of migraine. Sinus headache (34.9%), tension-type headache (25.2%), and stress headache

Table 3.1 ICHD-3 β Criteria for 1.5 Probable Migraine (Previously Migrainous Disorder)

Diagnostic criteria

A. Attacks fulfilling all but one of criteria for 1.1 *migraine without aura* or 1.2 *migraine with aura*
B. Not fulfilling criteria for a recognized headache disorder
C. Not better accounted for by another ICHD-3 β diagnosis.

1.5.1 *Probable migraine without aura*

Diagnostic criteria

A. Attacks fulfilling all but one of criteria A–D for 1.1 *migraine without aura*
B. Not better accounted for by another ICHD-3 β diagnosis.

1.5.2 *Probable migraine with aura*

Diagnostic criteria

A. Attacks fulfilling all but one of criteria A–C for 1.2 *migraine with aura* or any of its subforms
B. Not better accounted for by another ICHD-3 β diagnosis.

(22%) were more common medical diagnoses than probable migraine.[4] This study concluded that probable migraine is a frequent, underdiagnosed, undertreated, and sometimes disabling disorder. Its epidemiologic profile is similar to that of migraine.

Patel et al. found that in a health plan the prevalence of probable migraine was 14.5% (19.6% in women, 13.1% in men).[5] This study used a telephone interview instead of a mailed questionnaire and did not screen for severe headache. Lanteri-Minet conducted a population study in France: 10,532 subjects were assessed using validated questionnaires that followed the ICHD-2 criteria (Framig 3 study). In the Framig 3 study, which also did not exclude less than severe migraine, the prevalence of probable migraine was 10.1%. In this study, 12.3% of probable migraine sufferers had moderate or severe disability,[6] which is comparable to the Silberstein et al. study.[4]

At times the diagnosis of probable migraine overlaps with and is misdiagnosed as tension-type headache. We believe the default should be probable migraine, as the clinical, demographic, and impairment profiles and the treatment response to migraine-specific drugs more closely resemble migraine. In fact, the Spectrum study demonstrated that a clinical diagnosis of migraine is usually correct in patients with disabling episodic headache. A clinical diagnosis of episodic tension-type headache in patients with disabling headache proves to be incorrect in one-third of patients when a headache diary is used.[7]

HEMIPLEGIC MIGRAINE

The typical aura of migraine is characterized by focal neurologic features that usually precede the headache, but may accompany it or occur in the absence of the headache. Hemiplegic migraine is a rare form of migraine with aura that involves motor aura (weakness)[8,9] (Tables 3.2 and 3.3).

The ICHD-3 β[1] subdivides hemiplegic migraine into familial and sporadic forms. (Tables 3.4 and 3.5). Diagnostic criteria are similar, except for familiarity—that is, no affected relatives in the sporadic form versus affected first-degree or second-degree relative(s) in the familial form. The criteria for hemiplegic

Table 3.2 ICHD-3 β Diagnostic Criteria for 1.2. Migraine With Aura

A. At least 2 attacks fulfilling criteria B–C
B. One or more of the following fully reversible aura symptoms: visual, sensory, speech/language, motor, brainstem or retinal symptoms
C. At least 2 of the following characteristics
   1. At least one aura symptom spreads gradually over 5 minutes or more and/or 2 or more symptoms occur in succession.
   2. Each single aura symptom lasts 5–60 minutes.
   3. At least one aura symptom is one-sided.
   4. The aura is accompanied or followed by headache. A possible lag phase lasts maximally 60 minutes.
D. Not better accounted for by another ICHD-3 β diagnosis.

Table 3.3 ICHD-3 β Diagnostic Criteria for 1.2.3 Hemiplegic Migraine

A. At least 2 attacks fulfilling criteria B–C
B. Fully reversible motor weakness and one or more of the following fully reversible aura symptoms: visual, sensory, or speech symptoms
C. At least 2 of the following 4 characteristics
1. At least one aura symptom spreads gradually over 5 minutes or more, or, 2 or more symptoms occur in succession.
2. Each non-motor aura symptom lasts 5–60 minutes and motor symptoms < 72 hours.
3. At least one aura symptom is one-sided.
4. The aura is accompanied or followed by headache. A possible lag phase lasts maximally 60 minutes.
D. Not better accounted for by another ICHD-3 β diagnosis.

migraine[10] are the same as those for *Migraine with aura* (1.2), except that the aura includes some degree of motor weakness (hemiparesis) and the motor symptoms often last longer than 60 minutes. (They can last up to 24 hours and even weeks.) In addition to weakness, one or more fully reversible visual, sensory, or speech aura symptoms must be present. (This can also be basilar-type migraine aura.) At least one aura symptom must be one-sided. (Aphasia is always a one-sided symptom, but dysarthria is not.) When weakness lasts for weeks, it may be difficult to distinguish it from sensory loss with give-way weakness (which defines migraine with unilateral motor symptoms [MUMS]). MUMS motor symptoms begin with the onset of the headache or worsen as the headache pain intensifies. Motor symptoms are usually accompanied by sensory symptoms. MUMS weakness always has a give-way character and often persists between attacks. Except for the distinction between true and give-way weakness, many patients with MUMS fulfill the ICHD criteria for hemiplegic migraine. As patients do not report the difference between true weakness and give-way weakness, and as distinguishing give-way and true weakness on examination may be difficult,[11,12] reports of sporadic hemiplegic migraine may include patients with MUMS.[13] The differential diagnosis of hemiplegic migraine also includes focal seizures, conversion disorder, stroke, homocystinuria, CADASIL, and MELAS syndrome.[9,14]

Table 3.4 Familial Hemiplegic Migraine

Migraine with aura including motor weakness and at least one first- or second-degree relative has migraine aura including motor weakness.

Diagnostic criteria

A. Fulfills criteria for 1.2.3 *hemiplegic migraine*
B. At least one first- or second-degree relative has had attacks fulfilling criteria for 1.2.3 *hemiplegic migraine*.

1.2.3.1.1 *Familial hemiplegic migraine 1 (FHM1)*

Diagnostic criteria

A. Fulfills criteria for 1.2.3.1 *familial hemiplegic migraine*
B. A causative mutation on the *CACNA1A* gene has been demonstrated.

1.2.3.1.4 *Familial hemiplegic migraine (FHM) other loci*

Diagnostic criteria

A. Fulfills criteria for 1.2.3.1 *familial hemiplegic migraine*
B. No mutation on the *CACNA1A, ATP1A2*, or *SCN1A* gene has been demonstrated

1.2.3.1.2 *Familial hemiplegic migraine 2 (FHM2)*

Diagnostic criteria

A. Fulfills criteria for 1.2.3.1 *familial hemiplegic migraine*
B. A causative mutation on the ATP1A2 gene has been demonstrated

1.2.3.1.3 *Familial hemiplegic migraine 3 (FHM3)*

Diagnostic criteria

A. Fulfills criteria for 1.2.3.1 *familial hemiplegic migraine*
B. A causative mutation on the *SCN1A* gene has been demonstrated

1.2.3.1.4 *Familial hemiplegic migraine (FHM) other loci*

Diagnostic criteria

A. Fulfills criteria for 1.2.3.1 *familial hemiplegic migraine*
B. No mutation on the *CACNA1A, ATP1A2*, or *SCN1A* gene has been demonstrated.

Table 3.5 1.2.3.2 Sporadic Hemiplegic Migraine

Diagnostic criteria

A. Fulfills criteria for 1.2.3 hemiplegic migraine
B. No first-degree or second-degree relative fulfills criteria for 1.2.3 *hemiplegic migraine.*

Hemiplegic migraine attacks usually start in the first two decades of life and include gradually progressing visual, sensory, motor, aphasic, and often basilar-type symptoms accompanied by headaches. Most patients have attacks of migraine with typical aura without weakness. Sporadic and familial hemiplegic migraine varies in its manifestation, from hemiparesis alone to severe early-onset forms with recurrent coma and cerebral edema, permanent cerebellar ataxia, and, rarely, epilepsy-elicited repetitive transient blindness or mental retardation.[9] In a population-based Danish epidemiological survey of hemiplegic migraine, the prevalence of the sporadic form was 0.002% and the familial form was 0.003%. [15,16]

Familial hemiplegic migraine (FHM), in addition to requiring migraine with aura and motor weakness, requires that at least one first- or second-degree relative has had similar attacks, including motor weakness[10] (Table 3.4). FHM is the first migraine syndrome to be linked to a specific set of genetic polymorphisms.[17,18] The onset of weakness may be abrupt, but it usually lasts less than 1 hour [19]. All of Bradshaw and Parsons's patients had associated paresthesias; 88% had visual auras and 44% had speech disturbances. Weakness lasted less than 1 hour in 58% of patients; however, it lasted 1–3 hours in 14% of patients, 3–24 hours in 12%, and between 1 day and 1 week in 16% of patients.[20] The syndrome can change over an affected individual's lifetime. A person who has FHM in adolescence may develop migraine with aura as an adult and migraine without aura later in life.[21]

The three known loci for FHM are on chromosomes 1, 2, and 19, but some families do not link to any of these, indicating that there is at least one additional locus.[22,23] Patients who otherwise meet these criteria but have no family history of this disorder are classified as *sporadic hemiplegic migraine* (SHM, 1.2.3.2) [15] (Table 3.5).

Specific genetic subtypes of FHM have been identified: in FHM1 there are mutations in the *CACNA1A* gene (coding for a calcium channel) on chromosome 19; in FHM2 there are mutations in the *ATP1A2* gene (coding for a K/Na-ATPase) on chromosome 1; and in FHM3 there are mutations in the *SCN1A* gene (coding for a sodium channel) on chromosome 2. If genetic testing is done, the genetic subtype

should be specified at the fifth digit. It has been shown that FHM often has basilar-type symptoms, in addition to the typical aura symptoms, and that headache is almost always present. Rarely, during FHM attacks, disturbances of consciousness (sometimes including coma), fever, CSF pleocytosis, and confusion can occur. FHM attacks can be triggered by (mild) head trauma. In approximately 50% of FHM families (usually FHM1), chronic progressive cerebellar ataxia occurs independent of the migraine attacks. FHM may be mistaken for epilepsy and (unsuccessfully) treated as such. See Chapter 2 for more details on FHM.

Sporadic and familial hemiplegic migraine attacks are similar, but they vary among patients. Onset is usually during youth, with a low but variable attack frequency (about three attacks per year). The frequency and severity of attacks usually deceases in adulthood. Trigger factors include minor head trauma, exertion, and emotional stress.[9] FHM subjects are not hypersensitive to calcitonin gene-related peptide and nitric oxide, in contrast to subjects with migraine with or without aura.[24,25]

MIGRAINE WITH BRAINSTEM AURA

In the ICHD-1, migraine with brainstem aura (MWBA; 1.2.2) was called basilar artery migraine (Table 3.6). To remove the implication that the basilar artery is involved, "basilar-type migraine" replaced the term "basilar migraine" in the ICHD-2. The ICHD-3 β then replaced "basilar-type migraine" with the term "MWBA." Bickerstaff was the first to propose the concept of "basilar artery migraine."[26] He found two patients with identical symptoms that could only be explained by an abnormality of the basilar artery circulation.[27] One patient was a 14-year-old whose symptoms lasted a few hours and recurred on numerous occasions. The other was an elderly man whose symptoms progressed rapidly to coma and death: thrombotic occlusion of the basilar artery with infarction in the brainstem and occipital cortex was demonstrated at autopsy. So it was by clinical analogy with the structural lesion in the basilar artery and the symptoms of basilar artery territory ischemia that the syndrome "basilar artery migraine" was first described.

Table 3.6 **ICHD-3 β Criteria for 1.2.2 Migraine with Brainstem Aura**

Previously used terms: Basilar artery migraine, basilar migraine, basilar-type migraine

Diagnostic criteria

A. At least 2 attacks fulfilling criteria B–D
B. One or more of the following fully reversible aura symptoms: visual, sensory, or speech/language but no motor symptoms
C. At least two of the following brainstem symptoms: dysarthria, vertigo, tinnitus, hypacusis, diplopia, ataxia, decreased level of consciousness
D. At least 2 of the following 4 characteristics
  1. At least one aura symptom spreads gradually over 5 minutes or more, and/or, 2 or more symptoms occur in succession
  2. Each single aura symptom lasts 5–60 minutes.
  3. At least one aura symptom is one-sided.
  4. The aura is accompanied or followed by headache. A possible lag phase lasts maximally 60 minutes.
E. Not better accounted for by another ICHD-3 β diagnosis.

The distinguishing feature of MWBA is a symptom profile that suggests brainstem involvement.[28] The ICHD-3 β requires at least two of the following aura symptoms, all fully reversible: visual, sensory, or speech/language symptoms, but no motor symptoms. In addition, at least two of the following brainstem symptoms are required: dysarthria, vertigo, tinnitus, hyperacusis, diplopia, ataxia, and/or decreased level of consciousness. Because 60% of patients with FHM have brainstem symptoms, MWBA should be diagnosed only when weakness is absent.

More than one-third of subjects have their first attack of MWBA in the second decade of life. It occurs frequently in children[29] and may present for the first time after age 50, although in this age group, a very thorough investigation for alternative diagnoses, especially transient ischemic attack, is essential. MWBA may occur in combination with other types of migraine, and remains the dominant form in more than 75% of cases.[30] At first, Bickerstaff noted a predominance of teenage girls in his basilar artery migraine population, but subsequent experience revealed a female incidence similar to that of other types of migraine [26]. Precipitating factors were identified by 71% of subjects in one series[30]. Emotions, stress, menstruation, and weather change were among the predominant triggers, although head injury, food, and contraceptive drugs were also common.

The aura lasts from 5 to 60 minutes in most cases, but it can last long as3 days. Visual symptoms usually occur first, and the visual disturbance may consist of blurred vision, teichopsia, scintillating scotoma, and graying or total loss of vision. The visual disturbance may start in one visual field and then spread to become bilateral. Hallucinations of body magnification, especially that of the head and hands corresponding to the dominance of these regions in the sensory cerebral cortex, are also seen.[31]. Bickerstaff pointed out that when vision is not completely obscured, diplopia might occur, usually as a sixth nerve palsy.[32] Some form of diplopia may appear in as many as 16% of cases.[30]

Vertigo is the next most common symptom, occurring in up to 63% of patients.[30,33] Ataxia and tinnitus may accompany vertigo or may occur independently. Dysarthria is as frequent as vertigo.

Tingling and numbness occur in more than 60% of cases, in the typical cheiro-oral spreading pattern that is seen in migraine with aura. It is usually bilateral and symmetrical, but it may alternate sides. Impairment of consciousness is common.[30] Patients may enter a state of impaired consciousness that resembles sleep; they may be easily aroused by stimulation, only to return to the same state.[34]. Rarely, this progresses to stupor and prolonged coma.[35,36] Seizures have been observed in association with MWBA.[27,37]

Headache is usually located in the occipital region; it is throbbing and accompanied by severe nausea and vomiting. It is unusual for the headache to be unilateral or localized to the more anterior head. Photophobia and phonophobia occur in one-third to one-half of patients. As with other forms of migraine, the symptoms may occur without headache, but this is seen in less than 4% of cases.[30]

Is MWBA just a variant of migraine with aura? Kirchmann et al. studied the clinical features of 38 patients with what was then called basilar-type migraine.[33] The median duration of aura was 60 minutes (range 2 minutes to 72 hours), and symptoms included vertigo (61%), dysarthria (53%), tinnitus (45%), diplopia (45%), bilateral visual symptoms (40%), bilateral paresthesias (24%), decreased level of consciousness (21%), hyperacusis (21%), and ataxia (5%). All patients described visual aura symptoms during the attacks of MWBA: 61% had a unilateral or bilateral sensory aura, and 40% had an aphasic aura. Overall, 95% of the patients with MWBA (36 of 38) also reported attacks of migraine with typical aura at other times. The study concluded that there was no firm evidence to establish MWBA as an independent disease.

RETINAL MIGRAINE

Retinal migraine (Table 3.7) is a rare disorder characterized by at least two attacks of monocular visual disturbances associated with migraine headache. Carroll introduced the term "retinal migraine" to describe patients with episodes of transient and permanent monocular visual loss, specifically in the absence of migraine headache.[38] The term "retinal migraine" is now used when monocular visual impairment is temporally associated with attacks of migraine headache. However, unilateral visual loss is not restricted just to the retina, and the term "anterior visual pathway migraine" or "ocular migraine" may be more accurate.[39]

Recurrent monocular visual disturbances is a strictly unilateral disorder. Most patients do not experience side shift, although some experience side-alternating attacks. Visual disturbances may include scintillations, scotomata, or blindness (blurring, "gray-outs," and "black-outs") that affect only one eye and are accompanied or followed within 1 hour by migraine headache. Positive visual phenomena include flashing rays of light, zigzag lightning, and other teichopsia, whereas perceptions of bright-colored streaks, halos, or diagonal lines are less common.[40,41] Visual field defects can be altitudinal, quadrantic, central, or arcuate. Complex monocular visual impairment ("black paint dripping down from the upper corner of my left eye," the coalescence of peripherally located spots, and tunnel vision)

Table 3.7 1.2.4 Retinal Migraine

Diagnostic criteria

A. At least 2 attacks fulfilling criterion B–D
B. Fully reversible monocular positive and/or negative visual phenomena (e.g., scintillations, scotomata, or blindness) confirmed by examination during attack or by the patients drawing of a monocular field defect (after proper instruction) during attack
C. At least 2 of the following 3 characteristics
    1. The aura spreads gradually over 5 minutes or more.
    2. The aura symptoms last 5–60 minutes.
    3. The aura is accompanied or followed by headache. A possible lag phase lasts maximally 60 minutes.
D. Not better accounted for by another ICHD-3 β diagnosis.

can rarely occur.[39,42] Rare cases of transient monocular visual loss have also been reported with cluster headache, idiopathic stabbing headache, chronic daily headache, cerebral autosomal dominant arteriopathy with subcortical infarcts and leukoencephalopathy, and an unspecified headache type.[43–46]

Other causes of monocular visual loss, including transient ischemic attack, optic neuropathy, and retinal detachment, must be ruled out by appropriate investigation.[47] Although the ICHD-3 β criteria require the visual features to be fully reversible, a recent review suggests that patients with monocular "aura" experience retinal infarction of migrainous origin.[48] These patients should be diagnosed with migrainous infarction.[40]

The migraine headache is usually ipsilateral to the visual loss. In contrast to the current ICHD-2 criteria for retinal migraine, nearly 50% of patients with monocular visual loss had a history of migraine with typical visual aura. The onset of visual loss usually precedes (by definition within 1 hour of headache onset) or accompanies the headache; less often, the visual loss follows the headache. The duration of transient monocular visual loss varies widely between and within patients. The duration ranges from a few seconds to 1 hour. Prolonged, fully reversible monocular visual loss can rarely occur (days to weeks). Nearly half of reported cases had permanent monocular visual defects, but no consistent pattern of visual field loss was noted.

Elicited repetitive daily blindness is a recently described syndrome that appears to segregate as a monogenic, autosomal dominant condition in which affected individuals experience multiple daily episodes of transient visual loss.[49] The episodes are commonly bilateral and may occur daily (up to 10 times per day). The episodes are usually short-lasting (10 seconds), manifested as rapid and complete visual loss, beginning and recovering from the peripheral to the central visual field. During attacks, individuals may have fully dilated pupils with absent direct and indirect pupillary reflexes. These transient visual symptoms may occur spontaneously or may be triggered by eye rubbing, sudden changes of light, sudden direct eye illumination, or sudden standing. Rubbing on one eye triggers a unilateral and ipsilateral transient blindness, sometimes followed within less than 2 seconds by a contralateral transient blindness. Rubbing both eyes triggers simultaneous bilateral transient blindness. There is no associated headache or any other neurologic symptoms before, during, or after the transient blindness episodes. The disorder appears to be part of the FHM spectrum and recently two novel *SCN1A* mutations in a family with the syndrome were identified.[50]

VISUAL SNOW

Patients with visual snow have a persistent positive disturbance in their entire visual field, resembling the "static" or "snow" of a badly tuned television. The disturbance consists of white and black dots in the entire visual field and can persist for years. Additional visual phenomena include palinopsia (trailing and after-images), entoptic phenomena (floaters, spontaneous photopsia, blue field entoptic phenomenon, self-light of the eye), photophobia, and nyctalopia (impaired night vision). It has a major impact on patients' quality of life. Visual snow is often confused with persistent visual aura in migraine. The symptoms are generally very poorly responsive to all treatment attempts with numerous modalities (see Figure 3.1).

Schankin et al. did a retrospective survey of patients with visual snow. They found 120 patients (female: male ratio = 1:2.2) with a mean age of onset of 16.8±10.9 years. Most

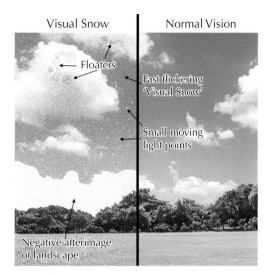

Figure 3.1. Visual snow.

(88%) had visual snow during the daytime and almost all (98%) at night. Additional visual symptoms were floaters (73%), persistent after-images (63%), "hard time seeing at night" (58%), "little cells that travel on a wiggly path" (57%), photophobia (54%), "moving objects leave trails" (48%), flashes (44%), and "swirls with eyes closed" (41%). Most disturbing were visual snow, floaters, and "hard time seeing at night." Ninety-two percent of patients had no response to medication.[51]

Their preliminary clinical criteria for "visual snow" were (A) persistent, dynamic, black and white visual disturbance in the entire visual field; (B) at least one of the following: moving objects leave trails, persistent after-images, floaters, bright flashes, "little cells that travel on a wiggly path," "swirls, clouds or waves with eyes closed," "hard time seeing at night," photophobias; (C) absence of the pattern of typical migraine aura; (D) not attributed to another disorder. They tested these criteria prospectively in 68 patients with self-reported visual snow. Thirty (44%) met criterion A. Symptoms had been present since childhood in 19. Age of onset (mean±SD) in the remaining 17 patients was 21±9 years. Additional visual symptoms were floaters (83%), persistent after-images (83%), "hard time seeing at night" (83%), "little cells that travel on a wiggly path" (83%), photophobia (70%), "moving objects leave trails" (60%), "swirls, clouds, or waves with eyes closed" (60%), and bright flashes (57%).

Criteria C and D were fulfilled in all patients. Requiring at least one, two, or three elements of criterion B reduced the sensitivity by 0%, 0%, and 7%, respectively. In patients with late-onset visual snow, seven (41% of 17) recalled having headache within 1 week of onset; five met ICHD-2 criteria for migraine. In three patients, a visual aura (followed by headache in two) preceded the onset. A history of migraine was seen in 22 (73%) patients; 16 (53%) had migraine with aura. None had used illicit drugs in the week prior to the onset of visual snow. Retinal tear was found in two patients, papilledema in one, and crowded optical disc in one. Otherwise, all ophthalmology tests were normal. Schankin et al. concluded that visual snow is almost always associated with at least three other visual symptoms (criterion B). Visual snow is a visual clinical syndrome distinct from migraine with aura. The onset of visual snow is frequently associated with headache. There is susceptibility in patients with migraine and especially migraine with aura. Rarely there is a secondary ophthalmological cause.[52]

Jäger et al. studied four patients with visual snow using MR perfusion and MR diffusion imaging.[53] Two patients had typical visual aura and two had a primary persistent visual disturbance that involved large areas, if not the entire visual field. Patients reported bright spots and sometimes colorful change or haziness, and often compared their vision to that of a poorly tuned television. The authors were not able to detect any significant changes in cerebral water diffusion and perfusion in patients with either migraine with persistent aura or primary persistent visual disturbance. Schankin et al. believe that visual snow is a unique, often disabling visual disturbance distinct from migraine aura. While a significant proportion of such patients have a history of migraine with or without aura, the standard acute and preventive migraine treatments are often unhelpful.

VESTIBULAR MIGRAINE

An association between migraine and vertigo, defined as a symptom arising from the vestibular system rather than non-vestibular dizziness (e.g., lightheadedness, unsteadiness, impending faint), was documented more than 100 years ago.[54] Studies[55,56] have demonstrated an excess prevalence of vestibular laboratory abnormalities and vertigo in migraine sufferers. Vestibular abnormalities occur in approximately one-third of patients with migraine[56] and excess migraine prevalence is found in patients with vertigo.[55] The differential diagnosis includes Ménière's disease and benign paroxysmal positional vertigo, and differentiation is difficult because of symptom overlap.[57,58] In the absence of specific neurotologic findings, the diagnosis of vestibular migraine is often based on a history of recurrent episodes of vertigo unexplained by other central or otological disease in patients with migraine. Only a minority of patients with vertigo and migraine meet criteria for MWBA, [59–62] and the link with migraine may be obscured when vertigo is dissociated temporarily from headache.[59,60,63–66] The study of migraine-associated vertigo is complicated by heterogeneity in the nature, duration, and frequency of vertigo.[55]

Vertigo has not appeared in the ICHD classification until recently. However, based on emerging evidence, it has been included in the appendix of ICHD-3 β. According to the ICHD-3 β, in addition to a diagnosis of migraine with aura or migraine without aura, at least 50% of attacks must be associated with at least one of the following: headache criteria for migraine, photophobia and phonophobia, or visual aura. The duration of the vertigo attacks does not generally correspond to a typical migraine aura.[59,63]. The proportion of patients who have attacks lasting minutes, hours, or days is split equally by roughly one-third each. A small proportion have vertigo symptoms that last only seconds and often occur repeatedly during head motion or visual stimulation or after changes of head position. In these patients, episode duration is defined as the total period during which short attacks recur. While the majority of episodes do not last longer than 72 hours, some patients may not recover fully until 1 month has passed.

Vestibular symptoms, as defined by the Bárány Society's Classification of Vestibular Symptoms and qualifying for a diagnosis of A1.6.5 *vestibular migraine*, include the following:

a. spontaneous vertigo:
   i. internal vertigo (a false sensation of self-motion);

   ii. external vertigo (a false sensation that the visual surround is spinning or flowing);

b. positional vertigo, occurring after a change of head position;

c. visually induced vertigo, triggered by a complex or large moving visual stimulus;

d. head motion–induced vertigo, occurring during head motion;

e. head motion–induced dizziness with nausea (dizziness is characterized by a sensation of disturbed spatial orientation; other forms of dizziness are currently not included in the classification of vestibular migraine).

In a systematic epidemiologic study, Neuhauser et al. found that the lifetime prevalence of migraine-associated vertigo was 0.98% in a representative sample of the adult German population.[62] Their diagnostic criteria for migraine-associated vertigo included (1) recurrent vestibular vertigo; (2) ICHD-defined migraine; (3) migrainous symptoms (i.e., headache, photophobia, phonophobia, or aura) during at least two vertiginous attacks; and (4) vertigo not attributed to another disorder. Among patients with migraine-associated vertigo, 67% reported spontaneous rotational vertigo and 24% reported positional vertigo. The patients with migraine-associated vertigo had impaired health-related quality of life compared with vertigo-free controls as measured with the Short Form-8 Health Survey. The study of migraine-associated vertigo is complicated by heterogeneity in the nature, duration, and frequency of vertigo.[55] For example, although vertigo can occur during headache in patients with ICHD-defined migraine, it commonly occurs during headache-free periods or during the migraine prodrome. In the Neuhauser et al. study,[62] only a minority of patients (24%) always experienced headaches with their vertigo. Headaches were also not consistently associated with vertigo in a study of 40 patients with benign recurrent vertigo whose headache episodes met ICHD criteria for migraine.[67] Vertigo occurred concurrently with headache in only half of the cases.

The response of migraine-associated vertigo to migraine-specific therapy has not been assessed in a controlled fashion, with the exception of one small (*n* = 10) study with inconclusive results.[68] In a survey of 53 migraineurs who identified dizziness or vertigo as symptoms of their headache episodes, the reported efficacy of anti-migraine medications for headache was directly correlated with efficacy at alleviating dizziness or vertigo.[69] Additional research to determine the responsiveness of migraine-associated vertigo to migraine-specific therapy is needed. Anatomic and physiologic links involving the vestibular nuclei, the trigeminal system, and the thalamocortical processing centers have been proposed to explain the occurrence of vertigo in association with migraine.[56] Central sensitization has been suggested as a potentially important mechanism for migraine-related vestibular symptoms, including vertigo. Emerging evidence demonstrates altered ictal and interictal functional brain activity in individuals with vestibular migraine. Using F-fluorodeoxy glucose (FDG) positron-emission tomography (PET), Shin and colleagues demonstrated ictal activation (increased metabolism) in two patients in the bilateral cerebellum, frontal cortices, temporal cortex, posterior insula, and thalami and decreased metabolism in the occipital cortex. [70] The authors proposed that these findings may represent reciprocal inhibition between the visual and vestibular systems. In another functional imaging study of 17 patients with vestibular migraine compared to 17 controls, Obermann and colleagues demonstrated widespread gray matter volume reduction in pain and vestibular processing areas, including bilateral thalamus and cingulate cortex, that correlated with increasing disease duration. [71] They also showed significant frontal and insula cortical volume decrease that correlated with headache severity, indicating a strong affective component in vestibular migraine. The observed changes, which reflected multisensory vestibular processing and central vestibular compensation, similar to what is seen after a peripheral vestibular injury, were considered to reflect adaptation related to cortical plasticity in patients with vestibular migraine.

Radtke et al.[65] have reformulated their diagnostic criteria[62] for vestibular migraine and provide criteria for definite vestibular migraine (dVM) and probable vestibular migraine (pVM) for those who may not exhibit all the typical features of dVM. (Table 3.8) This differed from their previous proposed criteria in which response to anti-migrainous medication or migraine precipitants of vertigo were not included in the definition of pVM.[64] They then reassessed 75 patients (67 women, aged

Table 3.8 **Vestibular Migraine**

Definite Vestibular Migraine
1. ≥ 2 attacks of vestibular vertigo (rotational vertigo, other illusory self or object motion, positional vertigo, head motion intolerance, i.e., sensation of imbalance or illusory self or object motion that is provoked by head motion)
2. Migraine according to ICHD
3. Concomitant migrainous symptoms during ≥ 2 vertigo attacks
4. No evidence of other central or otological causes of vertigo.

Possible Vestibular Migraine

1. ≥ 2 attacks of vestibular vertigo
2. At least one of the following:
   a. Migraine according to ICHD
   b. At least one migrainous symptom during ≥ 2 vertigo attacks:
      (i) Migrainous headaches
      (ii) Photophobia
      (iii) Phonophobia
      (iv) Visual or other auras
3. No evidence of other central or otological causes of vertigo.

A1.6.5 Vestibular Migraine

Previously used terms:
Migraine-associated vertigo/dizziness; migraine-related vestibulopathy; migrainous vertigo.

Diagnostic criteria
A. At least five episodes fulfilling criteria C and D
B. A current or past history of *1.1 migraine without aura* or *1.2 migraine with aura*
C. Vestibular symptoms of moderate or severe intensity, lasting between 5 minutes and 72 hours
D. At least 50% of episodes are associated with at least one of the following three migrainous features:
   1. Headache with at least two of the following four characteristics:
      a. Unilateral location
      b. Pulsating quality
      c. Moderate or severe intensity
      d. Aggravation by routine physical activity
   2. Photophobia and phonophobia
   3. Visual aura
E. Not better accounted for by another ICHD-3 β diagnosis or by another vestibular disorder.

24–76) with dVM ($n = 47$) or pVM ($n = 28$) after a mean follow-up of 8.75±1.3 years. Assessment included a comprehensive neurotological clinical examination, pure-tone audiometry, and caloric testing. dVM was confirmed in 40 of 47 patients with a prior diagnosis of dVM (85%). Fourteen of 28 patients initially classified as pVM met criteria for dVM (50%) and nine met criteria for pVM (32%). Six additional patients with dVM and two with pVM had developed mild sensorineural hearing loss, formally fulfilling criteria for bilateral Ménière's disease, but had clinical features atypical of Ménière's disease. Seven of these also met criteria for dVM at follow-up. The initial diagnosis was completely revised for four patients.

Although probable migraine diagnosis lacks a gold standard for evaluation of diagnostic criteria, repeated comprehensive neurotological evaluation after a long follow-up period indicates not only high reliability but also high validity of the clinical criteria (positive predictive value 85%). Half of patients with pVM evolve to meet criteria for dVM. However, in a subgroup of vestibular migraine patients with hearing loss, criteria for dVM and Ménière's disease are not sufficiently discriminative. Radtke et al.[72] assessed the evolution of clinical symptoms and vestibulocochlear function in 61 patients (54 women, 7 men, aged 24–76) with dVM according to validated diagnostic criteria after a median follow-up time of 9 years (range: 5.5–11). Assessment consisted of a clinical interview and neurotologic examination, including pure-tone audiometry and caloric testing. Most patients (87%) had recurrent vertigo at follow-up; frequency was reduced in 56%, increased in 29%, and unchanged in 16%. Mild persistent unsteadiness was reported in 18% of patients. Interictal ocular motor abnormalities had increased from 16% to 41%. The most frequent finding was positional nystagmus in 28% of patients, including definite central-type positional nystagmus in 18%. Concomitant cochlear symptoms with vertigo had increased from 15% to 49%. Eleven patients (18%) developed mild bilateral sensorineural hearing loss in the low-frequency range. They concluded that the majority of patients continue to have recurrent vertigo, the impact of which could be severe. Vestibulo-cochlear dysfunction progressed slowly in some patients with dVM. Interictal central-type positional nystagmus may help distinguish vestibular migraine from peripheral vestibular disorders such as Ménière's disease. While the data suggest an association between migraine and vertigo, the prevalence of vertigo in migraine remains poorly defined, and its responsiveness to migraine-specific therapy is unknown. Furthermore, the variable temporal association of vertigo with headaches in patients with ICHD-defined migraine makes identifying migrainous vertigo difficult.

EPILEPSY AND MIGRAINE

"Migralepsy" is an old term deriving from "migra(ine)" and "(epi)lepsy," introduced by Lennox and Lennox to describe a condition in which "ophthalmic migraine with perhaps nausea and vomiting was followed by symptoms characteristic of epilepsy."[73] After the first report, the term "migralepsy" was reintroduced by Marks and Ehrenberg.[74] Migraine followed by epilepsy (migralepsy) could be a seizure starting with an ictal epileptic headache, followed by a sensorimotor partial or generalized seizure. Headache may be the sole manifestation of epilepsy.[75]

Headache can occur prior to (pre-ictal headache), during (ictal headache), or after (post-ictal headache [PIH]) a seizure. Pre-ictal headache was evaluated in a small study of 11 patients with intractable focal epilepsy. Headache was frontotemporal, ipsilateral to the focus, in nine patients with temporal lobe epilepsy and contralateral in one patient with temporal lobe epilepsy and one with frontal lobe epilepsy.[76]

The ICHD-3 β has criteria for two types of headache associated with epileptic seizures: hemicrania epileptica (migrainous headache occurring during an epileptic seizure and ipsilateral to its focus) and PIH.[1] Hemicrania epileptica is an ipsilateral headache with migrainous features occurring as an ictal manifestation of the seizure discharge. In the first report, Isler et al. found that hemicranial attacks of pain coincided with seizure activity and lasted for seconds to minutes (i.e. hemicrania epileptica). Two exceptions were noted: (1) a case of complex status in which headache lasted for hours, and (2) a case in which the headache lasted most of the 20 minutes of a recorded seizure.[77] Belcastro et al. found five potential hemicrania epileptica patients in the literature. In all these patients, migraine/headache lasted longer than "seconds to minutes" and it appeared to be the sole manifestation of a non-convulsive status epilepticus. These patients did not meet ICHD-3 β criteria for hemicrania epileptica (Table 3.9). Four patients showed partial status epilepticus in the occipital lobes and one showed absence status. These observations suggest that headache/migraine could be the sole symptom not only of a partial but also of a generalized non-convulsive status epilepticus, and headache could be ipsilateral or contralateral to the ictal epileptiform discharge.[75]

PIH (Table 3.10) is defined as a headache of any type in a patient with a partial or generalized epileptic seizure if the headache has occurred or worsened in temporal relation (< 3 hours) to the termination of the partial or generalized epileptic seizure and has improved in temporal relation (< 72 hours) to the termination of the

Table 3.9 ICHD-3 β Criteria for 7.6.1 Hemicrania epileptica

Diagnostic criteria:
A. Headache of any type
B. The patient is having a partial epileptic seizure.
C. Evidence of causation shown by at least two of the following:
   1. Headache occurs simultaneous with onset of partial seizure.
   2. Headache is ipsilateral to the ictal discharge.
   3. Headache improves immediately after the partial seizure has terminated.
D. The headache is not better accounted for by another headache diagnosis.

Table 3.10 ICHD-3 β Diagnostic Criteria for 7.6.2 Post-ictal Headache

A. Headache of any type
B. The patient had a partial or generalized epileptic seizure.
C. Evidence of causation shown by both of the following:
 1. Headache has occurred or worsened in temporal relation (< 3 hours) to the termination of the partial or generalized epileptic seizure.
 2. Headache has improved in temporal relation (< 72 hours) to the termination of the partial or generalized epileptic seizure.
D. The headache is not better accounted for by another headache diagnosis

partial or generalized epileptic seizure. PIH occurs in over 40% of patients with either temporal or frontal lobe epilepsy and in up to 59% of patients with occipital lobe epilepsy. Patients with generalized tonic-clonic seizure have PIH more frequently than those without generalized tonic-clonic seizure.

The prevalence of PIH ranges between 12% and 52%.[78] PIH is often neglected because of the dramatic manifestation of the seizure and the fact that approved therapies for PIH are nonexistent. One study assessed the delay to the appearance of PIH and found that the headache began within 5 minutes after seizure termination in 92% of 36 children with PIH, and only rarely was it delayed up to one hour. [78–80] Other studies have defined PIH as a headache that begins after or immediately after a seizure. Other durations (30 minutes, 1 hour, and 3 hours [ICHD-3 β]) following the seizure have also been used. Migraine features of PIH were described in 34%–48% of cases in different studies of adult patients.[81–84] Other authors have reported migraine features in 55.7% of 115 patients with epilepsy and seizure-associated headaches (97% had PIH),[78] 27% of 71 patients with peri-ictal headaches (86% had PIH),[72] and 48% of another group of 56 people with epilepsy and seizure-related headaches (82% had PIH).[85,86]

Schön and Blau reported 100 epileptic patients, 51 of whom had PIH.[87] PIH was more commonly associated with generalized tonic-clonic seizures than with focal seizures; 9% of those with PIH had independent migraine attacks. PIH were either bilateral or unilateral; were associated with phonophobia and photophobia, throbbing pain, vomiting, nausea, and visual aura; and lasted 6–72 hours. Epileptic migraineurs recognized these headaches as being similar to their migraine.

Botha et al. described the clinical characteristics and associations of PIH in generalized epilepsy in a tertiary neurology clinic. Two hundred consecutive adults with generalized epilepsy underwent semi-structured interviews, dividing them into study (with PIH) and control (no PIH) patients. PIH occurred in 104/200 (52%) of patients; 63% had headache after every seizure. Pain duration was 4–24 hours in 43% of patients, and pain intensity was severe in 55%. ICHD-2 migraine was found in 47% of patients, tension-type headache in 38%, and 15% were unclassified (13% had probable migraine). Self-medication occurred in 81% of patients and interictal headache was significantly associated with PIH (present in 64% of study patients versus 5% of controls). They concluded that PIH occurs commonly in generalized epilepsy, mostly as migraine headache, with interictal headache a specific risk factor.[88] PIHs are prevalent, moderate to severe in intensity, last many hours, and frequently have characteristics of migraine. Although PIH is estimated to have a significant impact on the quality of life of people with epilepsy, it is frequently undertreated. Simple analgesics may prove beneficial.[78].

People at the highest risk of having PIH are young adults, both women and men, with relatively severe and long-standing epilepsy who have generalized tonic-clonic seizures and a personal history of interictal headaches. An occipital epileptogenic focus may be an additional risk factor. The high risk of having PIH, especially after generalized tonic-clonic seizures, may help differentiate epileptic from clinically similar non-epileptic psychogenic spells, especially when taken together with fatigue, as suggested by Ettinger et al.,[89] who found that only one patient of 23 documented cases of non-epileptic seizures mentioned headache as a post-ictal symptom, whereas 38% of 16 patients with epilepsy complained of PIH.

REFERENCES

1. Headache Classification Subcommittee of the International Headache Society. The International Classification of Headache Disorders, 3rd Edition, Beta Version. *Cephalalgia*. 2013;33(9):629–808.

2. Rains JC, Penzien DB, Lipchik GL, Ramadan NM. Diagnosis of migraine: empirical analysis of a large clinical sample of atypical migraine (IHS 1.7) patients and proposed revision of the IHS criteria. *Cephalalgia*. 2001;21:584–595.

3. Lipton, R, Patel N, Bigal ME, Kolodner K, Leotta C, Lafatta J, Lipton RB. Disability and health-related quality of life in strict migraine vs probable migraine (migrainous headache) and control subjects within a health plan. In Cephalalgia (Vol. 23, No. 7, pp. 593-593). Oxon, England: Blackwell Publishing Ltd. 2003;3:593.

4. Silberstein SD, Loder E, Diamond S, Bigal ME, Lipton RB. Probable migraine in the United States: results of the American Migraine Prevalence and Prevention (AMPP) study. *Cephalalgia*. 2007;27:220–234.

5. Patel NV, Bigal ME, Kolodner KB, Leotta C, Lafata JE, Lipton RB. Prevalence and impact of migraine and probable migraine in a health plan. *Neurology*. 2004;63:1432–1438.

6. Lanteri-Minet M, Valade D, Geraud G, Chautard MH, Lucas C. Migraine and probable migraine: results of FRAMIG 3, a French nationwide survey carried out according to the 2004 IHS classification. *Cephalalgia*. 2005;25:1146–1158.

7. Lipton RB, Cady RK, Stewart WF, Wilks K, Hall C. Diagnostic lessions from the spectrum study. *Neurology*. 2002;58:S27–S31.

8. Olesen J, Friberg L, Skyhoj-Olsen T. Timing and topography of cerebral blood flow, aura and headache during migraine attacks. *Ann Neurol*. 1990;28:791–798.

9. Russell MB, Ducros A. Sporadic and familial hemiplegic migraine: pathophysiological mechanisms, clinical characteristics, diagnosis, and management. *Lancet Neurol*. 2011;10:457–470.

10. Klee A, Willanger R. Disturbances of visual perception in migraine. *Acta Neurol Scand*. 1966;42:400–414.

11. Young WB, Gangal KS, Aponte RJ, Kaiser RS. Migraine with unilateral motor symptoms: a case-control study. *J Neurol Neurosurg Psychiatry*. 2007;78:600–604.

12. Fisher CM. Late life migraine accompaniments as a cause of unexplained transient ischemic attacks. *Can J Neurol Sci*. 1980;7:9–17.

13. Ashkenazi A, Sholtzow M, Shaw JW, Burstein R, Young WB. Identifying cutaneous allodynia in chronic migraine using a practical clinical method. *Cephalalgia*. 2007;27:111–117.

14. Hosking G. Special forms: variants of migraine in childhood. In: Hockaday JM, ed. *Migraine in childhood*. Boston: Butterworths, 1988:35–53.

15. Thomsen LL, Eriksen MK, Roemer SF, Anderson I, Olesen J, Russell MB. A population-based study of familial hemiplegic migraine suggests revised diagnostic criteria. *Brain*. 2002;125:1379–1399.

16. Thomsen LL, Ostergaard E, Olesen J, Russell MB. Evidence for a separate type of migraine with aura: sporadic hemiplegic migraine. *Neurology*. 2003;60:595–601.

17. De Fusco M, Marconi R, Silvestri L, et al. Haploinsufficiency of ATP1A2 encoding the Na(+)/K(+) pump alpha2 subunit associated with familial hemiplegic migraine type 2. *Nat Genet*. 2003;33:192–196.

18. Ducros A, Deiner C, Joutel A, et al. The clinical spectrum of familial hemiplegic migraine associated with mutations in a neuronal calcium channel. *N Eng J Med*. 2001;345:17–24.

19. Staehelin-Jensen T. Familial hemiplegic migraine: a reappraisal and long-term follow-up study. *Cephalagia*. 1981;1:33–39.

20. Bradshaw P, Parsons M. Hemiplegic migraine, a clinical study. *Q J Med*. 1965;34:65–85.

21. Stewart WF, Shechter A, Rasmussen RK. Migraine prevalence: a review of population-based studies. *Neurology*. 1994;44:S17–S23.

22. Ophoff RA, Terwindt GM, Vergouwe MN. Familial hemiplegic migraine and episodic ataxia type-2 are caused by mutations in the Ca2+ channel gene CACNLA4. *Cell Tiss Res*. 1996;87:543–552.

23. Ophoff RA, Terwindt GM, Vergouwe MN. Involvement of a Ca2+ channel gene in familial hemiplegic migraine and migraine with and without aura. Wolff Award 1997. Dutch Migraine Genetics Research Group. *Headache*. 1997;37:479–485.

24. Hansen JM, Thomsen LL, Marconi R, Casari G, Olesen J, Ashina M. Familial hemiplegic migraine type 2 does not share hypersensitivity to nitric oxide with common types of migraine. *Cephalalgia*. 2008;28:367–375.

25. Hansen JM, Thomsen LL, Olesen J, Ashina M. Calcitonin gene-related peptide does not cause the familial hemiplegic migraine phenotype. *Neurology*. 2008;71:841–847.

26. Bickerstaff ER. Basilar artery migraine. *Lancet*. 1961;1:15–17.

27. Bickerstaff ER. The basilar artery and the migraine-epilepsy syndrome. *Proc R Soc Med*. 1962;55:167–169.

28. Kuhn WF, Kuhn SC, Daylida L. Basilar migraine. *Eur J Emerg Med*. 1997;4:33–38.

29. Hockaday JM. Basilar migraine in childhood. *Dev Med Child Neurol*. 1979;21:455–463.

30. Sturzenegger MH, Meienberg O. Basilar artery migraine: a follow-up study of 82 cases. *Headache*. 1985;25:408–415.

31. Podoll K, Ebel H. Hallucinations of body magnification in migraine. *Fortschr Neurol Psychiatr*. 1998;66:259–270.

32. Bickerstaff ER. Basilar artery migraine. In: Rose C, ed. *Handbook of clinical neurology*. Amsterdam: Elsevier Science, 1986:135–140.

33. Kirchmann M, Thomsen LL, Olesen J. Basilar-type migraine: clinical, epidemiologic, and genetic features. *Neurology*. 2006;66:880–886.

34. Bickerstaff ER. Impairment of consciousness in migraine. *Lancet*. 1961;2:1057–1059.

35. Lawall JS, Oommen JK. Basilar artery migraine presenting as conversion hysteria. *J Nerv Men Dis*. 1978;166:809–811.

36. Ferguson KS, Robinson SS. Life-threatening migraine. *Arch Neurol*. 1982;39:374–376.

37. Basser LS. The relation of migraine and epilepsy. *Brain*. 1969;92:285–300.

38. Carroll D. Retinal migraine. *Headache*. 1970;9–13.

39. Corbett JJ. Neuro-ophthalmic complications of migraine and cluster headaches. *Neurol Clin*. 1983;1:973–995.

40. Grosberg BM, Solomon S, Friedman DI, Lipton RB. Retinal migraine reappraised. *Cephalalgia*. 2006;26:1275–1276.

41. Hachinski VC, Porchawka J, Steele JC. Visual symptoms in the migraine syndrome. *Neurology*. 1973;23:570–579.

42. Grosberg BM, Solomon S. Retinal migraine: two cases of prolonged but reversible monocular visual defects. *Cephalalgia*. 2006;26:75757.

43. Fisher CM. Cerebral ischemia: less familiar types. *Clin Neurosurg*. 1971;18:267–336.

44. Ammache Z, Graber M, Davis P. Idiopathic stabbing headache associated with monocular visual loss. *Arch Neurol*. 2000;57:745–746.

45. Evans RW, Daroff RB. Monocular visual aura with headache: retinal migraine? *Headache*. 2000;40:603–604.

46. Ravaglia S, Costa A, Santorelli FM, Nappi G, Moglia A. Retinal migraine as unusual feature of cerebral autosomal dominant arteriopathy with subcortical infarcts with leukoencephalopathy (CADASIL). *Cephalalgia*. 2004;24:74–77.

47. Troost BT, Zagami AS. Ophthalmoplegic migraine and retinal migraine. In: Olesen J, Tfelt-Hansen P, Welch KMA, eds. *The headaches*. Philadelphia: Lippincott Williams & Wilkins, 2000:511–516.

48. Grosberg BM, Solomon S, Lipton RB. Retinal migraine. *Curr Pain Headache Rep*. 2005;9:268–271.

49. Le FD, Safran AB, Picard F, Bouchardy I, Morris MA. Elicited repetitive daily blindness: a new familial disorder related to migraine and epilepsy. *Neurology*. 2004;63:348–350.

50. Vahedi K, Depienne C, Le FD, et al. Elicited repetitive daily blindness: a new phenotype associated with hemiplegic migraine and SCN1A mutations. *Neurology*. 2009;72:1178–1183.

51. Schankin C, Maniyar F, Hoffmann J, Chou D, Goadsby P: Visual snow: a new disease entity distinct from migraine aura. *Neurology*. 2012;78(suppl 1):PO1.227(Abstract).

52. Schankin C, Maniyar F, Goadsby P: Testing the criteria for visual snow (positive persistent visual disturbance). *Headache*. 2012;52:898(Abstract).

53. Jager HR, Giffin NJ, Goadsby PJ. Diffusion- and perfusion-weighted MR imaging in persistent migrainous visual disturbances. *Cephalalgia*. 2005;25:323–332.

54. Liveing E. *On megrim, sick headache, and some allied disorders: a contribution to the pathology of nervestorms*. London: Churchill, 1873.

55. Eggers SD. Migraine-related vertigo: diagnosis and treatment. *Curr Pain Headache Rep*. 2007;11:217–226.

56. Furman JM, marcus DA, Balaban CD. Migrainous vertigo: development of a pathogenetic model and structured diagnostic interview. *Curr Opin Neurol*. 2003;16:5–13.

57. Radtke A, Lempert T, Gresty MA, Brookes GB, Bronstein AM, Neuhauser H. Migraine and Meniere's disease: is there a link? *Neurology*. 2002;59:1700–1704.

58. von Brevern, M, Radtke A, Clarke AH, Lempert T. Migrainous vertigo presenting as episodic positional vertigo. *Neurology*. 2004;62:469–472.

59. Dieterich M, Brandt T. Episodic vertigo related to migraine (90 cases): vestibular migraine? *J Neurol*. 1999;246:883–892.

60. Kayan A, Hood JD. Neuro-otological manifestations of migraine. *Brain*. 1984;107 (Pt 4):1123–1142.

61. Cha YH, Lee H, Santell LS, Baloh RW. Association of benign recurrent vertigo and migraine in 208 patients. *Cephalalgia*. 2009;29:550–555.

62. Neuhauser HK, Radtke A, van Brevern M. Migrainous vertigo: prevalence and impact on quality of life. *Neurology*. 2006;67:1028–1033.

63. Cutrer FM, Baloh RW. Migraine-associated dizziness. *Headache*. 1992;32:300–304.

64. Neuhauser H, Leopold M, von Brevern M, Arnold G, Lempert T. The interrelations of migraine, vertigo, and migrainous vertigo. *Neurology*. 2001;56:436–441.

65. Radtke A, Neuhauser H, von Brevern M, Hottenrott T, Lempert T. Vestibular migraine: validity of clinical diagnostic criteria. *Cephalalgia*. 2011;31:906–913.

66. Cass SP, Furman JM, Ankerstjerne K, Balaban C, Yetiser S, Aydogan B. Migraine-related vestibulopathy. *Ann Otol Rhinol Laryngol*. 1997;106:182–189.

67. Brantberg K, Trees N, Baloh RW. Migraine-associated vertigo. *Acta Otolaryngol*. 2005;125:276–279.

68. Neuhauser H, Radtke A, von Brevern M. Zolmitriptan for treatment of migrainous vertigo: a pilot randomized placebo-controlled trial. *Neurology*. 2003;60:882–883.

69. Bikhazi P, Jackson C, Ruckenstein MJ. Efficacy of antimigrainous therapy in the treatment of migraine-associated dizziness. *Am J Otol*. 1997;18:350–354.

70. Shin JH, Kim YK, Hyo-Jung K, Kim J-S. Altered brain metabolism in vestibular migraine: Comparison of interictal and ictal findings. *Cephalalgia*. 2014;34:58–67.

71. Obermann M, Wurthmann S, Schulte-Steinberg B, Theyson N, Diener H-D, Naegal S. Central vestibular system modulation in vestibular migraine. *Cephalalgia*. 2014;34(13):1053–1061.

72. Radtke A, von Brevern M, Neuhauser H, Hottenrott T, Lempert T. Vestibular migraine: long-term follow-up of clinical symptoms and vestibulo-cochlear findings. *Neurology*. 2012;79:1607–1614.

73. Lennox WG, Lenox MA. *Epilepsy and related disorders*. Boston: Little,Brown, 1960.

74. Marks DA, Ehrenberg BL. Migraine related seizures in adults with epilepsy, with EEG correlation. *Neurology*. 1993;43:2476–2483.

75. Belcastro V, Striano P, Kasteleijn-Nolst Trenite DG, Villa MP, Parisi P. Migralepsy, hemicrania epileptica, post-ictal headache and "ictal epileptic headache": a proposal for terminology and classification revision. *J Headache Pain*. 2011;12:289–294.

76. Karaali-Savrun F, Goksan B, Yeni SN, Ertan S, Uzun N. Seizure-related headache in patients with epilepsy. *Seizure*. 2002;11:67–69.

77. Isler H, Wirsen ML, Elli N. Hemicrania epileptica: synchronous ipsilateral ictal headache with migraine features. In: Andermann F, Lugaresi E, eds. *Migraine and epilepsy*. Boston: Butterworths, 1987:246–263.

78. Ekstein D, Schachter SC. Postictal headache. *Epilepsy Behav*. 2010;19:151–155.

79. Cai S, Hamiwka LD, Wirrell EC. Peri-ictal headache in children: prevalence and character. *Pediatr Neurol*. 2008;39:91–96.

80. Leniger T, Isbruch K, von den DS, Diener HC, Hufnagel A. Seizure-associated headache in epilepsy. *Epilepsia*. 2001;42:1176–1179.

81. Syvertsen M, Helde G, Stovner LJ, Brodtkorb E. Headaches add to the burden of epilepsy. *J Headache Pain*. 2007;8:224–230.

82. Yankovsky AE, Andermann F, Bernasconi A. Characteristics of headache associated with intractable partial epilepsy. *Epilepsia*. 2005;46:1241–1245.

83. Forderreuther S, Henkel A, Noachtar S, Straube A. Headache associated with epileptic seizures: epidemiology and clinical characteristics. *Headache*. 2002;42:649–655.

84. HELP Study Group. Multi-center study on migraine and seizure-related headache in patients with epilepsy. *Yonsei Med J*. 2010;51:219–224.

85. Wawrzyniak B, Ghaeni L, Matzen J, Holtkamp M. Peri- and interictal headache in epilepsy: frequency, characteristics and predictors. *Epilepsia*. 2009;50(Suppl 6):37.

86. Doneva A, Cvetkovska E. Headache associated with epileptic seizures. *Epilepsia*. 2009;50(Suppl 4):166.

87. Schon F, Blau JN. Postepileptic headache and migraine. *J Neurol Neurosurg Psychiatry*. 1987;50:1148–1152.

88. Botha SS, Schutte CM, Olorunju S, Kakaza M. Postictal headache in South African adult patients with generalised epilepsy in a tertiary care setting: a cross-sectional study. *Cephalalgia*. 2010;30:1495–1501.

89. Ettinger AB, Weisbrot DM, Nolan E, Devinsky O. Postictal symptoms help distinguish patients with epileptic seizures from those with non-epileptic seizures. *Seizure*. 1999;8:149–151.

Chapter 4

Migraine Comorbidity

MIGRAINE, CARDIOVASCULAR, AND CEREBROVASCULAR DISEASE

CORONARY HEART DISEASE

CONGENITAL HEART DEFECTS

EPILEPSY

PSYCHIATRIC COMORBIDITY

PAIN

OBESITY

ALLERGY

ASSOCIATION BETWEEN RESTLESS LEGS SYNDROME AND MIGRAINE

MIGRAINE, RAYNAUD'S SYNDROME, AND OTHER RHEUMATOLOGIC DISORDERS

REFERENCES

Comorbidity indicates an association between two disorders that is more than coincidental. In contrast, coexistent (concomitant) illnesses occur together in the same person at a rate that would be expected by chance. Migraine is a common condition that is present in approximately 12% of the general population and thus is associated with a number of both comorbid and concomitant illnesses.[1,2]

Understanding the comorbidity of migraine is important for a number of reasons. Coexisting diseases can complicate diagnosis, as a high degree of symptomatic overlap occurs among the conditions associated with migraine. Migraine is comorbid with other disorders that share overlapping features. Both stroke and migraine, for example, can cause focal neurologic deficits associated with headache. Both migraine and depression can cause changes in mood or behavior associated with pain. Both migraine and epilepsy can cause transient alterations of consciousness, as well as headache.

The problem with comorbidity is not limited to differential diagnosis. When comorbid diseases occur, the challenge is to recognize that more than one disease may be present. As several of the conditions that are comorbid with migraine produce episodic manifestations, clinicians must be sensitive to reports of more than one kind of attack. The presence of migraine should increase, not reduce, the suspicion that other disorders may be present.

The study of comorbidity may provide epidemiological, biological, or genetic clues that provide a better understanding of the pathophysiology of migraine. Studies of migraine comorbidity require the consistent application

63

Table 4.1 **Risk-Ratio of comorbid mental disorders in migraine.**

Comorbid Disorder	Risk-Ratio and Confidence Interval				
Reference	Merikangas et al., 1990	Breslau et al., 1991	Swartz et al., 2000	Jette et al., 2008	Saunders et al., 2008
Major depressive disorder	2.2 (1.1–4.8)	4.3 (3.0–6.9)	3.2 (2.0–4.8)	2.3 (1.9–2.8)	3.5 (2.6–4.6)
Bipolar I and II	2.9 (1.1–8.6)	NS	7.3 (2.2–24.6)	3.7 (2.7–5.0)	3.9 (2.3–6.5)
Obsessive-compulsive disorder	1.0 NS	5.1 (2.3–11.2)	NS	—	—
Generalized anxiety disorder	3.3	5.7 (2.7–12.1)	NS		2.5 (1.6–4.0)
Panic disorder	5.3			2.8 (2.2–3.6)	3.6 (2.4–5.2)
Social phobia	3.4 (1.1–10.9)	2.6 (1.5–3.3)	1.6 (1.3–2.2)	2.3 (1.9–2.9)	2.4 (1.8–2.3)
Nicotine dependence	—	2.2 (1.5–3.3)	—	—	4.6 (1.4–11.1)
Substance-related disorders	—	2.2 (1.5–3.3)	NS	1.0 (NS)	1.6 (0.9–2.9) NS
Any mental disorder	**3.3 (0.8–13.8)**	**6.6 (3.2–13.9)**	**5.1 (2.6–9.8)**	**3.1 (2.4–4.1)**	**3.7 (2.2–6.2)**

of reliable and valid case definitions for both migraine and the other disorders being studied in representative samples. Studies must be adequately powered and free of bias. Reciprocal incidence studies, wherein persons with migraine, free of comorbidity, are followed to estimate rates of onset of the comorbidity, and similarly, individuals with the comorbidity are followed to estimate the rate of migraine onset, are ideal. Reciprocal incidence studies have been conducted for depression and anxiety disorders and, to some degree, for epilepsy.

The common illnesses that are associated with migraine and that influence its management include several comorbid conditions, such as depression, anxiety disorders, epilepsy, and stroke, and some concomitant illnesses, such as hypertension and obesity (Table 4.1). Both comorbid and concomitant medical conditions impact migraine treatment decisions. In practice, patients presenting with migraine must undergo a systematic diagnostic evaluation to ensure the accurate detection of coexisting illnesses or comorbid conditions so that both can be considered when designing treatment plans. How coexisting and comorbid disorders influence treatment is covered in Chapters 7 and 8, which deal with acute and preventive treatment.

In addition to diagnostic and therapeutic implications, the study of comorbidity may provide clues to the pathophysiology of migraine. When two conditions appear linked or associated with the other, several kinds of causal explanations should be considered (Figure 4.1). First, the disorders may not be associated. The method of subject ascertainment may result in apparent associations. For example, if patients with migraine and

1. Commorbidity may arise by coincidence or selection bias (spurious association).

2. One condition may cause the other (unidirectional causak models).

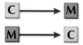

3. The conditions may related due to shared environmental or genetic risk factors.

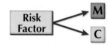

4. Environmental or genetic risk factors may produce a brain state that gives rise to both conditions.

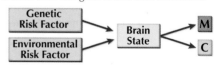

M = Migraine, C = comorbid condition

Figure 4.1. Possible causal explanations for comorbid conditions.

depression are more difficult to treat and are more likely to be referred to a headache specialist, the association between migraine and depression will be overestimated in studies conducted in headache specialty clinics (Berkson's bias).[3]

A second kind of causal model states that comorbid conditions may be associated because one condition causes the other. A third kind of causal model states that shared environmental or genetic risk factors might account for the co-occurrence of two disorders. Finally, independent genetic or environmental risk factors may produce a brain state that gives rise to migraine and a comorbid condition.[4]

MIGRAINE, CARDIOVASCULAR, AND CEREBROVASCULAR DISEASE

The association between migraine and ischemic stroke is well known and has been demonstrated in case-control, cohort, and observational studies. Overall, three meta-analyses of observational studies have demonstrated that individuals with migraine have a twofold increased risk of ischemic stroke.[7–9] The evidence is strongest for stroke in young women, particularly for migraine with aura and even more so for women who smoke or use oral contraceptives.[8,10–16] The combination of smoking and oral contraceptives in young women with migraine with aura increases the ischemic stroke risk by approximately ninefold compared to women without migraine. [8,17] The risk also appears to increase with increasing migraine attack frequency.[18] The association between migraine with aura and ischemic stroke appears to be independent of conventional cardiovascular risk factors,[7–9] even though migraine has been associated with elevated cardiovascular Framingham risk factors.[19,20]

A prospective analysis by Kurth and colleagues from the Women's Health Study extended findings to women over the age of 45.[5] Almost 30,000 female health professionals aged 45 and older were followed for an average of 10 years. Diagnosis of migraine and aura were based on self-report. In this population, migraine with aura was associated with incident ischemic stroke (HR 1.70 [1.1–2.6]). Ischemic stroke risk was most evident for those < 55 years of age at baseline (HR 2.25 [1.3–3.9]). Migraine with aura was also a risk factor for other forms of vascular disease, including myocardial infarction, coronary revascularization, and death due to cardiovascular disease. These results have been extended to studies in men over 45.[6]

Migraine has also been associated with white matter abnormalities, although there have been some inconsistencies. A meta-analysis by Swartz et al. summarized results from seven case-control studies.[21] The pooled risk of white matter abnormalities associated with migraine was increased fourfold (3.9 [2.3–6.7]), with the OR similar for studies that included (OR 3.6 [1.5–8.4]) or excluded (OR 4.1 [2.1–8.4]) individuals with cerebrovascular disease risk factors.

Several population-based studies have reported on the association between migraine, white matter hyperintense lesions, and silent infarctions. In an important population-based study known as the Cerebral Abnormalities in Migraine, an Epidemiological Risk Analysis (CAMERA), Kruit et al. found that some migraineurs are at increased risk for subclinical stroke, apparent on MRI.[22] A cohort of migraineurs with and without aura and a gender- and age-matched comparison group received an MRI and standard neurologic examination. No participant had an abnormal neurologic examination or reported a history of stroke or TIA. Migraine subjects and controls were recruited from the general population. MRI evaluations were performed by neuroradiologists blinded to migraine case status, and migraine aura classification was performed by expert headache clinicians. There was no difference overall in the prevalence of clinically relevant infarcts between migraineurs and controls. However, the migraineurs, particularly those with aura, had an increased likelihood of subclinical infarcts in the cerebellar region of the posterior circulation. The highest risk was found in those with migraine with aura and more than one attack per month (OR 15.8 [1.8–140]). Women with migraine were roughly twice as likely to have deep white matter lesions as the non-migraineurs (OR 2.1 [1.0–4.1]), although the risk was similar in women with and without aura. Consistent with the earlier studies on clinical stroke and white matter abnormalities, these findings were independent of measured cardiovascular risk factors. This study also demonstrated an increased prevalence of infratentorial (predominantly pontine) hyperintensities and posterior circulation-territory infarct-like lesions in those with migraine with aura (OR 13.7, 95% CI [1.7–112]), especially in those with at least one attack per month (OR 15.8, 95% CI [1.8–140]).[23] Another population-based study confirmed the association between migraine with aura and infarct-like lesions (OR 12.4, 95% CI [1.6–99.4], p for trend .005), but the lesions were not confined to the vascular territory of the posterior circulation.[24] In a population-based prospective study in Iceland, adults with midlife (mean age, 51 years) migraine with aura had an increased risk of late-life cerebellar infarct-like lesions (OR 1.4, 95% CI [1.1–1.8]) that was stronger in women (OR 1.9, 95% CI [1.4–2.6]).[25] There was no increased risk of migraine with aura and subcortical white matter hyperintensities, and there was no change in risk after adjustment for cardiovascular risk factors or history of cardiovascular diseases. Visual aura was associated with a higher risk of cerebellar infarcts (OR 2.2, 95% CI [2.5–3.1]) than sensory aura (OR 1.3, 95% CI [0.6–2.8]).

Palm-Meinders and colleagues reported on the 9-year follow-up of the Dutch population-based cohort (CAMERA-2 study).[26] They examined 203 of 295 participants with migraine and 83 of 140 age- and sex-matched control adults from the original CAMERA-1 study and determined the number and volumetric change of deep white matter hyperintensities, intratentorial hyperintensities, and posterior circulation territory infarct-like lesions. Progression of deep white matter hyperintensities was greatest in women with migraine without aura (OR 2.1, 95% CI [1.0–4.1], p = .04). Progression of white matter hyperintensity was not associated with the frequency of migraine episodes, duration, type of attacks, migraine therapy, or systemic hypertension. Lesions at baseline persisted but did not increase in size. New white matter hyperintense lesions accounted for the progression, but the overall volume of lesion burden was low (0.09 mL) at follow-up. Infratentorial hyperintensities progressed at the same rate in both the migraine and control groups. Patients with migraine were not at higher risk than controls for developing new posterior circulation territory infarct-like lesions. White matter hyperintense lesions were not associated with an increased risk of cognitive decline in migraine patients. The CAMERA-2 study demonstrated no increased risk of clinically manifest stroke or decline in fine motor skills or cognition measured by memory, concentration, attention, executive function, psychomotor and processing speed, organization, fluid intelligence, and visuospatial skills. This finding is consistent with results from a French population-based study.[24]

Given the previously demonstrated association of migraine with aura and ischemic stroke, it is somewhat surprising that the risk of progression of deep white matter hyperintensities was greatest in participants who had migraine without aura. It remains uncertain whether preventive migraine therapy reduces either progression of white matter hyperintensity or the risk of stroke, for less than 5% of participants with migraine in CAMERA-2 were taking preventive therapy. In addition, there is no evidence that triptans and ergots increase the risk of white matter hyperintense lesions. However, they were used in less than 15% of participants with migraine in CAMERA-2 and were not specifically analyzed. Because triptans have not been associated with incident ischemic stroke and triptans and ergotamine derivatives are not contraindicated in the setting of white matter hyperintense lesions, the results of this study should reassure clinicians who may be concerned about their use in patients with migraine.

PREGNANCY-RELATED HYPERTENSION

While the majority of studies have not confirmed a comorbid relationship between migraine and hypertension, there is substantial evidence of an association between migraine and pregnancy-related hypertension. In three case-control studies in the United States,[27] Canada,[28] and Peru,[29] individuals with migraine had, respectively, a 1.8- (95% CI [1.1–2.7]), 2.4- (95% CI [1.4–4.2]), and 4.0-fold (95% CI [1.9–8.2]) increased risk of preeclampsia compared to women without migraine. In a prospective cohort study of 702 normotensive women in Italy, migraine, diagnosed according to ICHD-2 criteria, was associated with incident hypertensive disorders in pregnancy (OR 2.9, 95% CI [1.4–5.8]).[30] Williams et al.

evaluated the influence of physician-diagnosed migraine on blood pressure levels and the risk of hypertensive disorders of pregnancy in a clinic-based prospective cohort study of 3373 healthy pregnant women.[31] Migraine was associated with elevated blood pressures, particularly mean third-trimester blood pressures. Adjusted mean third-trimester SBP, DBP, and MAP were 4.08, 2.39, and 2.95 mmHg, respectively, higher for individuals with migraine compared to those with migraine. Individuals with migraine had a 1.53-fold increased odds of preeclampsia (95% CI [1.09–2.16]). Overweight or obese individuals with migraine, compared with non-obese women without migraine, had a 6.10-fold increased odds of preeclampsia (95% CI [3.82–9.75]). The comorbid relationship between gestational hypertension and migraine may be related to the well-documented abnormality in endothelial function, platelet aggregation, and increased vascular resistance in individuals with migraine, which, combined with the dramatic and adaptive hemodynamic and hemostatic changes during pregnancy, may represent the biological substrate of this comorbid relationship.

In addition to hypertension, a US population-based study evaluated the association between migraine and all cardiovascular disease from 18,345,538 pregnancy-related discharges from 2000 to 2003.[32] Diagnoses that were associated with migraine codes during pregnancy (excluding preeclampsia) were stroke (OR 15.05, 95% CI [8.26–27.4]), myocardial infarction/heart disease (OR 2.11, 95% CI [1.76–2.54]), pulmonary embolus/venous thromboembolism (OR 3.23, 95% CI [2.06–7.07]), and hypertension (OR 8.61, 95% CI [6.43–11.54]), as well as preeclampsia/gestational hypertension (OR 2.29, 95% CI [2.13–2.46]), smoking (OR 2.85, 95% CI [2.53–3.21]), and diabetes (OR 1.96, 95% CI [1.64–2.35]).

CORONARY HEART DISEASE

Data on the association of migraine and coronary heart disease (CHD) have been inconsistent. Most studies have been positive for an association between migraine and angina and negative for an association with myocardial infarction. Early negative findings emerged from the Physicians Health Study, the Women's

Health Study, the ARIC study,[33] a study based on a managed care cohort by Sternfeld et al.,[34] and an earlier study by Waters. [35] All of these studies were either based on middle-aged or older adults or did not present risk separately for migraine with and without aura. Female migraineurs in the Cook study had a notably negative CHD risk profile compared to the non-headache controls based on traditional coronary risk factors.[36]

Recent population studies contradict these earlier findings. Kurth and coworkers from the Women's Health Study found that migraine with aura was a risk factor for all cardiovascular disease (CVD), including myocardial infarction. [5] In this very large prospective cohort, active migraine with aura in women was associated with increased risk of major CVD, myocardial infarction, ischemic stroke, and death due to ischemic CVD, as well as with coronary revascularization and angina. Active migraine without aura was not associated with increased risk of any CVD event. The results were meticulously controlled for many risk factors for coronary artery disease. Another population study by Scher et al.[19] compared the CHD risk profile of migraineurs with and without aura to the non-migraine population. They found that, compared to a control population, migraineurs were more likely to smoke (OR 1.43 [1.1–1.8]), less likely to consume alcohol (OR 0.58 [0.5–0.7]), and more likely to report a parental history of early myocardial infarction. Migraineurs with aura were more likely to have an unfavorable cholesterol profile (TC > or = 240 mg/dL [OR 1.43 (0.97–2.1)], TC:HDL ratio > 5.0 [OR 1.64 (1.1–2.4)]), to have elevated BP (systolic BP > 140 mm Hg or diastolic BP > 90 mm Hg [OR 1.76 (1.04–3.0)]), and to report a history of early onset CHD or stroke (OR 3.96 [1.1–14.3]); female migraineurs with aura were more likely to be using oral contraceptives (OR 2.06 [1.05–4.0]). The odds of having an elevated Framingham risk score for CHD were approximately doubled for the migraineurs with aura. Elevated blood pressure was found only in the migraineurs who had not consulted physicians for their headaches. The authors suggest that migraineurs who had consulted physicians may have received headache-specific treatment that lowered their blood pressure or may have been diagnosed with high blood pressure. This study also found that the women with migraine were more likely to have been diagnosed with gestational hypertension; this was after taking into account age and number of pregnancies.

CONGENITAL HEART DEFECTS

Patent foramen ovale (PFO) is a common, often incidental finding, occurring in approximately 25% of the general population.[37] PFO is believed to play a role in cryptogenic stroke, particularly in younger adults, via presumed paradoxical embolism through a right-to-left shunt. Several clinic-based case-control studies and a meta-analysis have suggested that PFO is more common among individuals with migraine with aura and that migraine with aura is more common among individuals with PFO. [38–41] This has led to the hypothesis that PFO might be causally linked with migraine with aura, the increased risk of ischemic stroke, and white matter hyperintense lesions in individuals with migraine with aura. Specifically, it has been suggested that the right-to-left shunt may serve as a conduit for the passage of particulate or humoral factors from the venous to arterial circulation, which then, in a predisposed individual with migraine, could serve to trigger migraine aura and the ensuing migraine attack. [42] Indeed, in a mouse model, microemboli triggered CSD, often without causing micro-infarction, and the authors speculated that paradoxical embolization may link cardiac and extracardiac right-to-left shunts to migraine aura, and if translatable to humans, a subset of migraine auras may belong to a spectrum of hypoperfusion disorders, along with transient ischemic attacks and silent infarcts.[42]

Conflicting evidence exists regarding the association between migraine and PFO.[43] In a multiethnic, elderly, population-based cohort from the prospective ongoing Northern Manhattan Study (NOMAS) project, PFO detected with transthoracic echocardiography and agitated saline was not associated with self-reported migraine among 1101 stroke-free subjects. The prevalence of PFO was not significantly different between subjects who had migraine (26/178, or 14.6%) and those who did not (138/923, or 15.0%; $p = 0.9$). In an adjusted multivariate logistic-regression model, the presence of PFO was not associated with increased migraine prevalence (odds ratio 1.01, 95% CI [0.63–1.61]). Not surprisingly, increasing age was associated with lower prevalence of migraine in subjects both with (odds ratio 0.94, 95% CI [0.90 to 0.99 per year]) and without PFO (odds ratio 0.97, 95% CI [0.95–0.99 per year]). The observed lack of association between PFO and migraine (with or without aura) was not modified by diabetes mellitus, hypertension, cigarette smoking, or dyslipidemia. The authors concluded that the causal relationship between PFO and migraine remains uncertain, and the role of PFO closure among unselected patients with migraine remains questionable, despite the limitations of this study, which included self-reported migraine history, recall bias with regard to migraine aura (given its high prevalence in this study), and a population that was significantly older (mean 69 years) than previous studies that did show a relationship between migraine with aura and the presence of a PFO.

The potential relationship between PFO and migraine led to several open-label, non-randomized, observational studies indicating that PFO closure leads to reduction or elimination of migraine.[44–51] However, the first controlled study evaluating the safety and efficacy of PFO closure in migraine with aura subjects failed to meet its primary and all secondary endpoints.[52] The Migraine Intervention with STARFlex© Technology (MIST) trial randomized 147 patients to either closure or sham-closure. No significant difference was observed in the primary end-point of migraine headache cessation between implant and sham groups (3 of 74 versus 3 of 73, respectively; $p = 0.51$). As expected, the implant arm experienced more serious procedural adverse events. In this study, 163 of 432 patients (38%) had a moderate or large right-to-left shunt. The authors stated that this trial confirmed the high prevalence of right-to-left shunts in patients with migraine with aura but failed to demonstrate a benefit with regard to reducing the impact of migraine in those undergoing closure. In a recently presented (American Headache Society, Washington DC, June 2015) but unpublished report of a second randomized sham-controlled trial of PFO closure in migraine patients (PREMIUM), the study also failed to achieve its primary endpoint (50% responder rate). However, the study did meet one of its main secondary endpoints (reduction in migraine days). Whether a small subgroup of patients exists for which PFO closure may lead to a significant reduction in attack frequency remains unclear.

Evidence from a clinic-based family study by Wilmshurst et al.[53] supports the notion that atrial shunts (PFO and atrial septal defects) segregate with familial migraine with aura. Probands (19 families) had a large atrial right-to-left shunt on contrast echocardiography or, in one family, a large ASD detected by transesophageal echocardiography. Most probands (13/20) also had migraine with aura. Seventy-one relatives had transthoracic contrast echocardiography. Excluding the probands, 47% of the family members had large shunts, 14% had small or medium shunts, and 39% had no shunt. The prevalence of migraine with aura in the relatives with large, medium and small, and no shunts was, respectively, 64%, 40%, and 30% ($p < 0.05$ for trend).

In light of abundant but conflicting evidence, the weight of evidence favors an association between migraine with aura and PFO. However, there is no evidence from controlled clinical trials that PFO closure alters the course of migraine. Therefore, in the absence of compelling factors such as transient ischemic attack or ischemic stroke, young patients with migraine should not undergo routine screening or PFO closure for the purpose of migraine prevention. If available, physicians should refer eligible patients with migraine for closure only within the context of a sham-controlled clinical trial.

EPILEPSY

Migraine and epilepsy are chronic neurologic disorders with paroxysmal attacks that may include alteration of consciousness, visual, sensory, or motor manifestations, and pain, as well as autonomic, gastrointestinal, and psychological features. In addition to overlapping clinical features, migraine and epilepsy also share genetic risk factors, an underlying pathophysiology, and medication treatment options. Migraine and epilepsy are comorbid. The 1-year period prevalence of epilepsy is 0.5% in the general population, but in individuals with migraine, the prevalence of epilepsy ranges from 1% to 17%, with a median of 5.9%. [54,55] Similarly, 14%–20% of individuals with epilepsy have been found to have ICHD-defined migraine.[56,57]

Ottman and Lipton examined the association between migraine and epilepsy[58,59] using data from the Epilepsy Family Study of Columbia University. Among probands with epilepsy, the prevalence of migraine was 24%. In their relatives with epilepsy, migraine prevalence was 26%. Only 14.5% of relatives without epilepsy had migraine. The incidence of migraine in persons with epilepsy was 2.4 times higher than in persons without epilepsy. Migraine risk was elevated in every subgroup of epilepsy defined by seizure type, age of onset, and etiology. The age of onset of epilepsy did not influence the risk of migraine. Migraine with aura may have an even greater comorbidity with epilepsy than migraine without aura. In two recent studies, the prevalence of epilepsy in children with migraine with aura was 30%, and the incidence of new-onset seizures was increased in pediatric patients with migraine with aura as compared to those with migraine without aura.[60,61]

The pathophysiological mechanisms that link migraine and epilepsy are complex. There is little evidence to support a unidirectional causal mechanism. While ictal and post-ictal migraine-like headaches have been well described, headache in these settings would be considered secondary.[62] Though seizures may occur immediately after or within 60 minutes of a migraine aura, a phenomenon known as *migralepsy*, this is rare in the migraine population without epilepsy. However, in individuals with both migraine and epilepsy, migralepsy has been reported to occur with a frequency range of 1.7%–16%.[56,57]

Shared environmental risk factors contribute little to the comorbidity of the two disorders. Of the well-known environmental and genetic risk factors for epilepsy evaluated in the Epilepsy Family Study (including head injury, meningitis, stroke, and structural brain disease), only head injury was associated with an increase in migraine, but it accounted for only a small proportion of the observed comorbidity.[50,63] However, specific genetic polymorphisms may contribute to the association between migraine and epilepsy. The three major loci thus far identified as being responsible for up to 70% of families with familial hemiplegic migraine (FHM) have also been associated with epilepsy (see Chapter 2). The neuronal P/Q type calcium channel (CACN1A), Na+/K+ ATPase (ATP1A2), and the voltage-gated neuronal sodium channel (SCN1A) have each of these genes that have also been identified in various forms of epilepsy.[64] The *CACNA1A* gene on chromosome 19, which codes for the main subunit of the CaV2.1 P/Q neuronal calcium channel, contains at least seven mutations that are also associated with epilepsy; these include localization-related seizures, generalized seizures, and seizures associated with fatal coma.[64] Like FHM itself, the epilepsy phenotypes associated with the *CACNA1A* and other *FHM* genes are highly variable among carriers with the same mutation and within the same family.[65–67] The mechanism of seizures in *FHM1* mutations likely relates to the shift in channel opening toward more negative membrane potentials, delayed channel inactivation, and channels that open with smaller depolarization and stay open longer. These physiological shifts allow more Ca^{2+} to enter presynaptic terminals, resulting in enhanced glutamate release. Genetically engineered mice with knock-in mutations of selective mutations that are involved in FHM1 demonstrate enhanced excitatory neurotransmission and increased susceptibility to cortical and subcortical spreading depression. Indeed, with specific types of mutations, spreading depression may propagate between cortex, basal ganglia, diencephalon, and hippocampus in genetically susceptible brains, which could explain the prolonged hemiplegia, coma, and seizure phenotype in this variant of migraine with aura.[68]

At least 10 mutations in the *FHM2* gene, which is found on the long arm of chromosome 1 in the 1q23 region and codes for the alpha1 subunit of a Na+/K+ ATPase, have been associated with multiple seizure types, including benign familial infantile convulsions and partial and generalized seizures.[64,69,70] A loss of function of the Na+/K+ase pumps lead to an increase in extracellular potassium and impaired clearance of glutamate from the synaptic cleft, both of which increase neuronal excitability and can cause both cortical spreading depression and the rapid synchronous depolarization on neurons that is characteristic of seizures. Mutations in the *SCN1A* gene, responsible for FHM3 and found on chromosome 2q24, encoding the neuronal voltage-gated sodium channel gene, has been well established as an important cause of a number of epilepsy syndromes. This gene is associated with a spectrum of epilepsy severity, ranging from generalized epilepsy with febrile seizures plus type 2 (GEFS+2), typically a mild form of epilepsy, to severe myoclonic epilepsy of infancy (SMEI).[71–73] Electrophysiological studies of the *SCN1A* mutations responsible for GEFS+2 revealed impaired sodium channel inactivation and excitability based on a reduced threshold for repetitive action potential generation and neuronal firing.[74] This mutation has also been shown to impair inactivation of sodium channels and is thought to play a role in the enhanced neuronal excitability leading to CSD.[75]

These data underscore the shared genetics and neurobiology of a subtype of migraine (FHM) and epilepsy. These mutations result in neuronal excitability by altering the flux of ions across the neuronal or glial cell membrane, altering membrane potential and the function of membrane voltage-gated ion channels and membrane pumps, lowering the threshold for neuronal firing, and altering the homeostasis of the extracellular space, particularly with regard the clearance of glutamate. The relevance of these mutations and the biological overlap between FHM and epilepsy to more common subtypes of migraine are not yet clear. The mutations thus far found to be responsible for a large percentage of families with FHM have not been found in individuals with migraine with or without aura. However, emerging results from genome-wide association studies have implicated a number of genetic variants associated with migraine with and without aura and which regulate excitatory neurotransmission (see Chapter 2).

PSYCHIATRIC COMORBIDITY

Numerous studies have reported the cross-sectional associations and bi-directional associations between migraine and a variety of psychiatric and somatic conditions. Depression is the most extensively studied psychiatric that is comorbid with migraine. Individuals with migraine are two- to fourfold more likely to experience a mood disorder.[76–83] Based on this extensive evidence base, the odds of depression in those with migraine range from

2.0 to 4.0. Breslau et al. measured the bidirectional associations of migraine, severe non-migraine headache, and depression in a 2-year, longitudinal, population-based cohort from the Detroit metropolitan area.[70] They examined the relationship between migraine and incident depression, as well as depression and incident migraine. The study also assessed the specificity of this association for migraine versus other severe headache. Over a 2-year period, having baseline depression increased the risk of incident migraine (RR 3.4 [1.4–8.7]) but did not increase the risk of other severe headache. In addition, the risk of incident depression was higher in those with baseline migraine (RR 5.8 [2.7–12.3]) and (marginally) of severe headache (RR 2.7 [0.9–8.1]).

Stewart et al.[84] studied the relationship of migraine to panic disorder and panic attacks in a population-based telephone interview survey of 10,000 residents of Washington County, Maryland, who were between the ages of 12 and 29. The highest rates of migraine headaches occurring in the preceding week were reported by men and women with a history of panic disorder. The relative risk of migraine headache occurring during the previous week and associated with a history of panic disorder was 6.96 in men and 3.70 in women.

In a follow-up analysis of the same sample, Stewart et al.[85] found that 14.2% of women and 5.8% of men who had experienced headache in the previous 12 months had consulted a physician for the problem. An unexpectedly high proportion of those who had consulted a physician for headache had a history of panic disorder. Of those who had recently seen a physician, 15% of women and 12.8% of men between 24 and 29 years of age had a panic disorder. This suggests that comorbid psychiatric disease is associated with seeking care for headache disorders.

Breslau et al.[76] studied the association of IHS-defined migraine with specific psychiatric disorders in a sample of 1007 young adults between 21 and 30 years of age in southeast Michigan. Persons with a history of migraine (n = 128) had significantly higher lifetime rates of affective disorder, anxiety disorder, illicit drug use disorder, and nicotine dependence. The sex-adjusted ORs were 4.5 for major depression (95% CI [3.0–6.9]), 6.0 (95% CI [2.0–18.0]) for manic episode, 3.2 (95% CI [2.2–4.6]) disorder for any anxiety, and 6.6

(95% CI [3.2–13.9]) for panic disorder.[77] The psychiatric comorbidity odds associated with migraine with aura were generally higher than those associated with migraine without aura. [76] Migraine with aura was associated with an increased lifetime prevalence of both suicidal ideation and suicide attempts, after the factors of sex, major depression, and other concurring psychiatric disorders were controlled for.[86]

Using follow-up data gathered 3.5 years after baseline, Breslau et al.[78] reported on the prospective relationship between migraine and major depression in a cohort of young adults. The relative risk for the first onset of major depression during the follow-up period in persons with prior migraine versus no prior migraine was 4.1 (95% CI [2.2–7.4]). The relative risk for the first onset of migraine during the follow-up period in persons with prior major depression vs no history of major depression was 3.3 (95% CI [1.6–6.6]).

In summary, recent epidemiologic studies support the association between migraine and major depression previously reported in clinic-based studies. The prospective data indicate that the observed cross-sectional or lifetime association between migraine and major depression could result from a bidirectional influence, from migraine to subsequent onset of major depression and from major depression to first migraine attack. Furthermore, these epidemiologic studies indicate that persons with migraine have increased prevalence of bipolar disorder, panic disorder, and one or more anxiety disorders [78,87–89]

A cross-sectional study of over 50,000 adults aged 20 and older by Zwart et al. (the Nord-Trøndelag Health Study) measured the co-occurrence of headache and depression or anxiety disorders.[83] Measurements included headache diagnosis, a medical examination, and administration of the Hospital Anxiety and Depression scale. Overall, individuals with migraine headache were more likely to have depression (OR 2.7 [2.3–3.2]) or anxiety disorders (OR 3.2 [2.8–3.6]) than non-headache controls. Similar associations were seen for non-migraine headache and depression (OR 2.2 [2.0–2.5]) or anxiety disorders (OR 2.7 [2.4–3.0]). There was a linear trend associated with headache frequency. Thus, for migraine headache < 7 days per month, 7–14 days/month, and 15+ days/month, respectively, the association with depression was OR 2.0 (1.6–2.5),

OR 4.2 (3.2–5.6), and OR 6.4 (4.4–9.3). A similar trend was seen for anxiety disorders and for non-migraine headache with depression or anxiety disorders.

This high degree of comorbidity appears to be even higher in specialty clinics, where up to 50% of migraine patients have elevated depression scores.[90,91] Migraine has also been associated with a greater risk of suicide, even after controlling for the presence of depression.[86,92] The association between migraine and the bipolar subtype of depression is greater than that for major depressive disorder alone; however, the lower prevalence of the bipolar subtype in many studies diminishes the power to discriminate differences across mood disorder subtypes.[93–97] In a large population-based study, individuals with bipolar disorder had a significantly higher prevalence of migraine compared to the general population (24.8% vs. 10.3%, $p < .05$).[82] The sex-specific prevalence of comorbid migraine in bipolar disorder was 14.9% for males and 34.7% for females, and males with bipolar disorder and migraine were more likely to live in a low-income household ($p < .05$), receive welfare and social assistance ($p < .05$), report an earlier age of onset of bipolar disorder ($p < .05$), and have a higher lifetime prevalence of comorbid anxiety disorders ($p < .05$). Bipolar females with comorbid migraine had, in addition, more comorbid medical disorders ($p < .05$). The authors concluded that screening for psychiatric comorbidity, including bipolar disorder, may be warranted in individuals presenting to tertiary care practice with migraine.

Migraine is also associated with anxiety disorders. There is a strong association between migraine and panic disorder, phobic disorders, and generalized anxiety disorder. There is a two- to sixfold increased risk for anxiety disorders in those with migraine compared to controls, and the occurrence of both anxiety and depression in those with migraine has been observed in population-based studies. [76,77,80,81,83,89,96–101]. While the onset of anxiety in individuals with migraine often occurs in childhood and adolescence, there is no evidence in population-based studies that anxiety occurs earlier among those with migraine. The fear and anxiety that occur in anticipation of the next attack may lead to avoidance behaviors and compulsive use (and overuse) of acute medications in an effort to reduce the likelihood of the next attack. McWilliams et al. examined the difference between migraine and other chronic pain disorders and their association with depression and anxiety.[99] Data from an adult US population (the Midlife Development in the United States Survey) were used to examine the cross-sectional associations between three pain conditions (migraine, arthritis, back pain) and three psychiatric disorders (depression, generalized anxiety disorder, panic attacks). The associations between the three psychiatric disorders were generally similar for the three pain conditions (i.e., the association between migraine and depression was roughly similar to the association between back pain and depression). However, the association between pain and anxiety was stronger than the association between pain and depression.

A comorbid relationship between attention deficit hyperactivity disorder (ADHD) and migraine has been implied from a case control sample of 572 adult patients with a diagnosis of ADHD and community controls ($n = 675$), who responded to questionnaires rating past and present symptoms of ADHD and comorbid conditions, including migraine diagnosis, treatment history and work status.[102] Migraine prevalence was significantly higher in the patient group compared to the controls (28.3% vs. 19.2%, $p < 0.001$, OR 1.67, CI 1.28–2.17). The difference from controls was especially notable for men (22.5% vs. 10.7%, $p < 0.001$, OR 2.43, CI 1.51–3.90) but was also significant for women (34.4% vs. 24.9%, $p = 0.008$, OR 1.58, CI 1.13–2.21). Migraine was associated with symptoms of mood and anxiety disorders in both patients and controls.

PAIN

Migraine is comorbid with other chronic pain conditions in children, adolescents, and adults. In one large prospective study, 1756 third- and fifth-grade schoolchildren in Finland were evaluated and followed for the presence of non-traumatic musculoskeletal pain symptoms.[103] They were re-evaluated after 1 and 4 years to determine factors related to the prognosis of musculoskeletal pain. Children with comorbid headache were more likely to have persistent musculoskeletal pain at follow-up compared to the children without comorbid headache.

In another study of 1290 Finnish children aged 8 to 9 years, otalgia, shoulder/neck pain, back pain, and abdominal pain were commoner in those with migraine compared to those with non-migraine headache.[104] In the same country, there was a high degree of comorbidity between headache and abdominal (OR 2.3, 95% CI [1.6–3.5]) and other pain (OR 3.8, 95% CI [2.7–5.8]) among almost 2000 8-year-old children.[105] A study of 793 Swedish adolescents found that two-thirds of those with frequent headache also complained of frequent pain involving muscles, back, abdomen, ears, and teeth.[106] In Germany, a study of 5474 children aged 7–14 [107] found an association between frequent headache and back and stomach pain. A prospective study among children in Scotland identified headache as a risk factor for persistent musculoskeletal pain 1 and 4 years later. [108] In a cross-sectional study involving more than 9000 Danish adolescents, Hestbaek et al. found that headache (not characterized by type) was associated with both moderate LBP (< = 30 days per year; OR 2.1 [1.8–2.5]) and with high frequency LBP (> 30 days per year; OR 3.4 [2.3–5.0]).[109]

The Norwegian HUNT studies, which comprise large numbers of health-related questionnaire and biometric data from a population of over 50,000, have provided considerable information on the comorbid relationship between headache and other pain disorders.[110] The prevalence of chronic musculoskeletal pain (lasting greater than 3 months) was almost twice as high among those with either migraine or non-migraine headache. While the elevated risk was similar in those with non-migraine (OR 1.8 [1.8–1.9]) and migraine (OR 1.9 [1.8–2.0]) headaches, headache frequency was a strong predictor of comorbid musculoskeletal symptoms, such that with headache present on less than 7 days per month, 7–14 days per month, more than 15 days per month, respectively, the association with musculoskeletal symptoms was OR 1.5 (1.4–1.6), OR 3.2 (2.9–3.5), OR 5.3 (4.4–6.5) for women, and OR 1.7 (1.6–1.8), OR 3.2 (2.8–3.8), OR 3.6 (2.9–4.5) for men. The age distribution for chronic musculoskeletal pain and headache differed, with the peak prevalence of headache reached in the forties,

while musculoskeletal pain increased gradually until the sixth decade of life.

In a population-based study from the National Comorbidity Survey Replication (NCS-R), a nationally representative face-to-face household survey of adults 18 years of age and older, the comorbidity of chronic spinal pain with other physical and mental disorders was analyzed.[111] Chronic spinal pain was defined as self-reported "chronic back or neck problems." Comorbid mental disorders were based on *DSM-IV* criteria, and included mood disorders, anxiety disorders, and substance use disorders. Chronic spinal pain was associated with mood disorders (OR 2.5 [1.9 = 3.2]), anxiety disorders (OR 2.3 [1.9–2.7]), and substance use disorders (primarily alcohol abuse or dependence) (OR 1.6 [1.2–2.2]). In addition, chronic spinal pain was associated with other chronic pain (OR 4.8 [3.9–5.8]), which included arthritis (OR 3.9 [3.2–4.7]), migraine (OR 5.2 (4.1–6.4)), other headache (OR 4.0 [2.9–5.3]), and other chronic pain (OR 3.7 [2.9–4.7]).

A population-based study among more than 30,000 US adults found that self-reported severe headache or migraine was commonly associated with facial jaw pain (OR women 7.6, OR men 5.4), low back pain (OR 4.2 and 3.9) or neck pain (OR 6.6 and 2.5).[112] In an adult population of 8000 Swedes aged 20 to 84 years, headache was highly comorbid with shoulder pain and painful conditions such as ulcer and dyspepsia.[113]

Fibromyalgia appears to be comorbid with primary headache disorders, but the association has mainly been demonstrated in clinical samples from tertiary referral centers and not from population-based studies. In a clinical sample of patients presenting to a tertiary center, the prevalence of fibromyalgia in a group of patients with frequent (transformed) migraine was 35.6%,[114] while in a study comprising 92 consecutive individuals with episodic migraine, the prevalence of fibromyalgia was 22%.[115] In a consecutive sample of 1123 patients screened at a tertiary referral pain center in Italy, fibromyalgia was most common in patients with episodic tension-type headache (35%, $p < 0.0001$) and chronic tension-type headache (44.3%, $p < 0.0001$).[116] Patients presenting with chronic migraine and chronic tension-type headache had a higher probability of sharing the fibromyalgia profile, especially when associated with frequent headache, anxiety, pericranial tenderness, poor sleep quality, and physical disability.

OBESITY

Evaluation for obesity is an important factor in the evaluation and management of patients with migraine, especially since weight gain is a frequent adverse event of several preventive medications used to treat migraine. Both obesity and migraine are risk factors for ischemic stroke, and obesity is a risk factor for the progression of migraine from episodic to chronic.

In the first of four population-based studies, Scher and colleagues demonstrated a fivefold increased risk of chronic daily headache in patients with episodic migraine who has a body mass index (BMI) > 30 and were followed for 1 year.[117] There appeared to be a graded effect such that those who were overweight (BMI 25–29.9) had a threefold increased risk. Subjects in this study were not classified as having chronic migraine or chronic tension-type headache. Obesity (BMI > 30) was found to be associated with chronic daily headache (CDH) associated with migraine features after adjustment for other risk factors and demographic variables.

In a subsequent population-based study, 3791 individuals were identified as having episodic migraine out of a total of 30,215 who were interviewed.[118,119] BMI was not associated with the prevalence of migraine, after adjusting for multiple covariates (age, sex, marital status, income, medical treatment, depressive symptoms, medication use), but was associated with the frequency of headache attacks, again in a *dose-dependent* fashion. In the severely obese group, 20.7% (OR 5.7, 95% CI [3.6–8.8]) had high-frequency episodic migraine (10–14 days per month) compared to 13.6% (OR 2.9, 95% CI [1.9–4.4]) in the obese group, 5.8% of the overweight group (OR 1.3, 95% CI [0.6–2.8]), and 4.4% in the normal body weight group.

A third population-based study evaluated the relationship between obesity and chronic headache, and participants with CM and CTTH were identified.[119] The study confirmed that obesity and CDH are comorbid but showed little to no relationship between obesity and

CTTH except in the severely obese group. The study also confirmed the suggestion from the previous population-based episodic migraine study that obesity is a risk factor not only for increased frequency of attacks, but for progression to chronic migraine. The prevalence of CM was 0.9% in the normal weight group, 1.2% of the overweight group (OR 1.4, 95% CI [1.1–1.8]), 1.6% of the obese group (OR 1.7, 95% CI [1.2–2.43]), and 2.5% of the severely obese group (OR 2.2, 95% CI [1.5–3.2]). Adjusted analyses demonstrated that obesity was associated with CDH and CM, but not CTTH.

In the American Migraine Prevalence and Prevention Study (AMPP), a validated questionnaire was mailed to 120,000 households selected to be representative of the US population; headaches were classified according to the International Classification of Headache Disorders, 2nd edition (ICHD-2) Headache Society criteria.[120] The prevalence of high-frequency episodic migraine was found to be significantly higher in the obese (8.2%, $p < 0.001$) and morbidly obese group (10.4%, $p < 0.0001$) compared to the normal body weight group (6.5%). Disability was also significantly higher in the overweight, obese, and morbidly obese groups. Obesity was not associated with frequency of tension-type or probable migraine headache in this study.

In contrast, investigators in Sweden conducted a population-based study in 684 women aged 40 to 74 who were attending a population-based mammography screening program.[121] The prevalence of obesity did not differ between women with active migraine, women with a history of migraine currently in remission, or women who had no prior history of migraine ($p = 0.96$). Obesity was not associated with the frequency, intensity, or duration of attacks.

Finally, in a recent prospective cohort study among 19,162 participants followed for 12.9 years in the Women's Health Study, 7916 incident overweight and 730 incident obesity cases occurred.[122] Through self-report using standardized questionnaires, 3,483 (18.2%) had migraine and the multivariable-adjusted Hazard Ratios (95% CI) among the migraine subjects was 1.11 (1.05–1.17) for becoming overweight and 1.00 (0.83–1.19) for becoming obese. This large prospective study of middle-aged women indicated that neither migraine itself nor the frequency of attacks is a risk factor for incident obesity.

Obesity is associated with increased frequency of attacks in episodic migraine and progression of episodic to chronic migraine, but there is no evidence that migraine sufferers with obesity are more treatment resistant to acute or preventive medications than those who are not obese.[123] Nevertheless, the use of preventive medications that are weight-neutral should be strongly considered in obese or morbidly obese patients with migraine who require preventive treatment. In a randomized, double-blind comparator study evaluating topiramate 100 mg and amitriptyline 100 mg in 331 subjects, 52 (16%) experienced major weight gain (> 5% total body weight) and 56 (17%) experienced major weight loss (> 5% of total body weight).[124] Those participants who gained weight were found to have elevations in mean diastolic blood pressure (+2.5 vs. –1.2 mmHg), heart rate (+7.6 vs. –1.3 b.p.m.), glycosylated hemoglobin (+0.09% vs. –0.04%), total cholesterol (+6.4 vs. –6.3 mg/dL), low-density lipoprotein cholesterol (+7.0 vs. –4.4 mg/dL), and triglycerides (+15.3 vs. –10.4 mg/dL), and an increase in high sensitivity C-reactive protein (+1.8 vs. –1.9 mg/L). These cardiovascular risk factors may further augment the cardiovascular risk already elevated in those with migraine and obesity.

The influence of bariatric surgery and weight loss on the clinical course of migraine has been evaluated. In one prospective observational study among 24 morbidly obese patients who had had bariatric surgery,[18] there was a reduction in headache days from 11.1±10.3 days preoperatively to 6.7±8.2 days postoperatively ($p < 0.05$).[125] In another prospective study of 29 women between 18 and 50 years of age who underwent bariatric surgery, the 6-month outcomes showed a lower frequency ($p < 0.001$) and shorter duration of the migraine attacks ($p < 0.02$); lower medication use during the attack ($p < 0.005$); and a reduction in migraine-related disability as measured by the Migraine Disability Assessment (MIDAS) questionnaire and Headache Impact Test (HIT-6).[126] There was a linear and significant decrease in BMI in this cohort over the course of 6 months. There was a reduction in mean monthly migraine frequency in both episodic (from 4 to 1 episodes per month) and chronic (from 16.8 to 8.5 episodes per month)

migraine patients. The absence of a control group, small sample sizes, and non-blinded nature of these studies are limitations, and conclusions regarding the association between weight loss from bariatric surgery and improvements in migraine must await larger controlled studies.

ALLERGY

Mixed evidence suggests a comorbid relationship between migraine and allergic disorders. Population-based and clinic-based studies have shown a weak association between migraine and asthma during childhood and adulthood [127–129] as well as with hay fever, rhinitis, and eczema.[130,131] In a large-scale, population-based, cross-sectional study involving 51,383 patients who completed headache and respiratory disease questionnaires as part of a Norwegian health study, those with current asthma, asthma-related symptoms, hay fever, and chronic bronchitis were approximately 1.5 times more likely to have migraine or non-migraine headache than those without allergy disorders. For both headache types, the association increased with increasing headache frequency, but the magnitude of the increase was similar for both.[132] In a US study involving 10,198 children ages 4 to 18 years, of whom 17.1% reported frequent or severe headaches (including migraine), the children were more likely to have asthma, hay fever, and ear infections.[133]

In a study involving more than 35,000 Norwegian patients who were 8 to 29 years of age and on active asthma treatments, increased migraine prevalence was found in asthmatics as compared with a non-asthmatic control group.[134] However, in a study involving more than 51,000 individuals with migraine in the UK General Practice Research Database, a thorough case-control analysis demonstrated a non-significant adjusted OR of 1.17 for developing asthma.[135]

The relationship between allergic symptoms and migraine is complicated by the fact that trigeminal autonomic symptoms, including lacrimation, rhinorrhea, and nasal stuffiness, are common during migraine attacks, and are therefore often mistakenly diagnosed as allergic rhinitis, headaches triggered by allergy, or sinus-related headaches.[136]

A recent study evaluated the association of migraine and asthma and estimated the risk of hypertensive disorders of pregnancy in relation to maternal comorbid migraine and asthma in a cohort of 3,731 women who were interviewed during early pregnancy.[137] Individuals with migraine had a 1.38-fold (95% CI [1.09–1.38]) increased odds of asthma as compared with individuals without migraine. The odds of pregnancy-related hypertensive disorders, including pregnancy-induced hypertension, preeclampsia, and both disorders combined, were 2.53 (95% CI [1.39–4.61]), 3.53 (95% CI [1.51–8.24]), and 2.64 (95% CI [1.56–4.47]), respectively, among those with comorbid migraine and asthma compared to those with neither disorder.

Allergic rhinitis and hay fever (seasonal allergic rhinitis) have also been reported to be associated with migraine. Migraine was found to be significantly more prevalent in individuals with allergic rhinitis (34%) compared with non-atopic, non-rhinitis controls (2%).[138] Hay fever has also been associated with migraine, especially as migraine frequency increases. [132] The relative odds of migraine in those with rhinitis were 1.5 for when attack frequency was less than 7 days per month, 1.9 for attacks 7–14 days per month, and 2.6 for attacks occurring on 15 or more days per month. In addition, persons with chronic rhinosinusitis (i.e., >15 headache days per month) are three times more likely to experience chronic headaches. [139] In the American Migraine Prevalence and Prevention Study, mixed rhinitis was present in 67% of 5849 individuals with migraine in the general population.[140] Those with rhinitis of any type were approximately one-third more likely to be in higher headache frequency and disability categories. The underlying mechanism that links migraine and rhinitis is not known, but may be biological and related to cranial autonomic activation during migraine attacks, mast cell degranulation, or shared genetic factors.

ASSOCIATION BETWEEN RESTLESS LEGS SYNDROME AND MIGRAINE

Migraine is now known to be comorbid with restless legs syndrome (RLS). Restless legs syndrome is a disorder of motor restlessness associated with paresthesia/dysesthesia in the arms or legs that affects up to 10%–15% of the population.[141] Symptoms are relieved with activity and exacerbated by rest.[142] It is most commonly idiopathic, but can be secondary to other neurologic disorders.[143] While no comprehensive explanation of the pathophysiology of RLS exists,[144] evidence suggests that it may be secondary to a central hypo-dopaminergic state. Direct dopamine stimulation with either carbidopa/levodopa or dopamine agonists is effective in relieving the symptoms of both idiopathic and secondary RLS.[145–152] In addition, both PET[153] and SPECT(154) studies implicate diminished striatal dopamine binding in RLS and periodic limb movements of sleep. Some RLS patients have low ferritin levels and may benefit from iron therapy. The D_2 receptor contains iron, perhaps linking the dopaminergic hypothesis of RLS with low iron levels.[155,156] RLS has been correlated with depressed moods and reduced libido, and morning (OR 4.7) and daytime (OR 2.8) headache.[157] Clinic-based studies have suggested that migraineurs have an increased prevalence of fibromyalgia[114] and fibromyalgia, in turn, has been correlated with RLS (OR 25.8).[158–160]

In 2003, Young et al. characterized RLS in a headache population and correlated treatment-induced risks with dopamine blockers.[161] They enrolled 50 patients with severe headaches admitted to an outpatient infusion center. The diagnosis of RLS was established using the International Restless Legs Syndrome Study Group criteria.[142] Patients were screened for baseline akathisia using the Barnes's akathisia scale[162] and were re-examined for akathisia after receiving intravenous infusion with one of four dopamine receptor-blocking agents as treatment for their headaches. Forty-one patients (82%) had episodic or chronic migraine. The rest had new daily persistent headache, cluster headache, or post-traumatic headache. Seventeen subjects (34%) met the criteria for RLS. Nineteen subjects (38%) developed drug-induced akathisia. Thirteen of the subjects with RLS (76.5%) developed akathisia, compared with only six of the 33 (18.2%) without RLS ($p < 0.0001$). The prevalence of RLS in this cohort was quite high (34%) compared with published population reports.[141,163] They proposed that RLS should be added to the list of disorders comorbidly associated with migraine. Headache patients with RLS are at a greatly increased risk of developing drug-induced akathisia when treated with intravenous dopamine receptor-blocking agents. Young's study had several limitations. Small sample sizes limited the ability to adequately assess subgroups, particularly headache diagnosis and concomitant medication use. The study was observational and was neither blinded nor controlled.

Rhode subsequently performed a case-control study on the comorbidity of RLS (International Restless Legs Syndrome Study Group) and migraine.[164] Patients with ICHD migraine (n = 411) and 411 sex- and age-matched control subjects were included. RLS frequency was significantly higher in migraine patients than in control subjects (17.3% vs. 5.6%, $p < 0.001$, OR 3.5, CI 2.2,5.8). There was no significant association between migraine and depression as defined by the Beck Depression Inventory score (9.6% in migraine vs. 4.0% in control subjects, $p = 0.190$). Depression was more frequent in migraine patients with (13.6%) than without (8.7%) RLS. They found an association between RLS and migraine and, in addition, a co-association with depression.

D'Onofrio et al. performed an observational study on the occurrence of RLS in patients affected by primary headaches.[165] Two hundred headache patients and 120 sex- and age-matched control subjects were included. RLS frequency was significantly higher in headache patients than in control subjects (22.4% vs. 8.3, $p = 0.002$) independent of gender, although with a female preponderance (84%) in both groups. More than 60% (n = 27) of RLS patients were affected by migraine without aura and 30% (n = 13) by a combination of two headache types ($p \geq 0.001$). RLS frequency for the other types of headaches was very low. In both headache and control groups, depression and anxiety were more frequent in subjects with RLS compared with those without RLS. Headache patients with RLS reported sleep disturbances more frequently than those without RLS (50.0% vs. 32.7%, $p < 0.0001$) and showed a normal or underweight body mass index. This data confirms the existence of an association between RLS and primary headaches, particularly migraine. These studies all suggested an association between RLS and migraine.

Chun et al. investigated the frequency of RLS in different primary headache disorders and its impact and clinical correlates in migraine patients.[166] Consecutive patients with migraine, tension-type headache, and cluster headache were recruited in their headache clinic in Taiwan. Each patient completed the MIDAS questionnaire, Hospital Anxiety and Depression Scale, Pittsburgh Sleep Quality Index, and the International RLS Study Group Rating Scale. A total of 1041 patients (migraine 772, TTH 218, CH 51) completed the study. RLS was more common in patients with migraine (11.4%) than those with TTH (4.6%) or CH (2.0%) ($p = 0.002$). In migraine patients, RLS was associated with higher frequencies of photophobia, phonophobia, exacerbation due to physical activities, vertigo, dizziness, tinnitus, and neck pain and higher mean scores of Migraine Disability Assessment and Hospital Anxiety and Depression Scale. Migraine patients with RLS had poorer sleep than those without RLS. RLS frequency increased with the number of migrainous symptoms. This study again demonstrated an association between migraine and RLS. Comorbid RLS worsened sleep quality in migraine patients. Treatment of RLS may improve sleep quality, but it is unknown if treatment of RLS in patients with migraine can improve their sleep quality and benefit migraine control.

Recent population-based studies have confirmed the comorbidity between RLS and migraine. In a cohort study of 31,370 women participating in the Women's Health Study, at baseline or during follow-up 6857 (21.9%) women reported any migraine.[167] These women had an increased risk for RLS (multivariable-adjusted OR 1.22, 95% CI [1.13–1.32]). A similar association was found for migraine with aura (multivariable-adjusted OR 1.27, 95% CI [1.10–1.48]), migraine without aura (multivariable adjusted OR 1.24, 95% CI [1.09–1.40]), and new reports of migraine during the follow-up period (multivariable-adjusted OR 1.30, 95% CI [1.10–1.54]). A similar finding in men was found in a cross-sectional study among 22,926 participants in the Physicians' Health Study. In this population, 2816 (12.3%) reported migraine and 1717 (7.5%) reported a diagnosis of RLS. The magnitude of the association in men was similar to that found in women, where migraine was associated with an increased multivariable-adjusted odds ratio (OR1.20, 95% CI [1.04–1.38]) for having RLS.[168]

An association between migraine and RLS was also demonstrated in a pediatric population. A case-control study involving 111 consecutive patients with migraine presenting to a tertiary care headache center was compared to 73 headache-free controls for the presence of RLS using a semi-structured interview. The frequency of RLS in migraine patients was significantly higher than in controls (22% vs. 5% [$p < 0.001$] and 8% [$p < 0.001$]).[169]

Why is RLS comorbid with migraine? RLS may be related to a dopaminergic system dysfunction.[145] The A11 dopaminergic nucleus of the dorsal-posterior hypothalamus is hypothesized to be involved in the pathophysiology of RLS in an animal model.[171,172] Animal studies have shown that lesioning the A11 nucleus facilitates trigeminovascular nociception.[173] Therefore, a shared dopaminergic dysfunction in A11 nucleus may be the neuroanatomical substrate linking migraine and RLS. As Chen et al. stated, this can explain the higher frequencies of migraine features and accompanying symptoms, as well as a higher headache disability in migraine patients with RLS.

MIGRAINE, RAYNAUD'S SYNDROME, AND OTHER RHEUMATOLOGIC DISORDERS

There is increased prevalence of migraine in individuals who have rheumatologic disorders, including Sjogren's syndrome[174] and systemic lupus erythematosus.[175] Several case series[174–181] have suggested that migraine is comorbid with Raynaud's phenomenon (RP). Zahavi et al.[181] found an increased prevalence of RP in migraineurs. O'Keeffe et al.[178] found an increased prevalence of migraine and chest pain in a sample of patients with primary RP. In a follow-up study, O'Keeffe et al.[178] found an increased prevalence of migraine in a group of patients with RP compared with controls. Miller et al.[176] found an increased prevalence of both migraine and RP in patients with variant angina. Leppert et al.[180] found a high prevalence of recurrent headaches in a population of women with RP. Recently, Terwindt et al.[182] found a genetic link between migraine and RP and vascular retinopathy in one extended Dutch family. Finding a gene for this family may help to elucidate the genetic background of migraine and other vascular disorders indicating RP.[183]

REFERENCES

1. Lipton RB, Diamond S, Reed M, Diamond ML, Stewart WF. Migraine diagnosis and treatment: results from the American Migraine Study II. *Headache*. 2001;41:638–645.
2. Lipton RB, Stewart WF, Diamond S, Diamond ML, Reed M. Prevalence and burden of migraine in the United States: data from the American Migraine Study II. *Headache*. 2001;41:646–657.
3. Berkson J. Limitations of the application of fourfold table analysis to hospital data. *Biometries Bulletin*. 1946;2:47–53.
4. Lipton RB, Silberstein SD. Why study the comorbidity of migraine? *Neurology*. 1994;44(17):4–5.
5. Kurth T, Gaziano JM, Cook NR, Logroscino G, Diener HC, Buring JE. Migraine and risk of cardiovascular disease in women. *JAMA*. 2006 Jul 19;296(3):283–291.
6. Kurth T, Gaziano JM, Cook NR, Bubes V, Logroscino G, Diener HC, et al. Migraine and risk of cardiovascular disease in men. *Arch Intern Med*. 2007 Apr 23;167(8):795–801.
7. Etminan M, Takkouche B, Isoma FC, Samii A. Risk of ischaemic stroke in people with migraine: systematic review and meta-analysis of observational studies. *BMJ*. 2005;330(7482):63.
8. Schurks M, Rist PM, Bigal ME, Buring JE, Lipton RB, Kurth T. Migraine and cardiovascular disease: systematic review and meta-analysis. *BMJ*. 2009;339:b3914.
9. Spector JT, Kahn SR, Jones MR, Jayakumar M, Dalal D, Nazarian S. Migraine headache and ischemic stroke risk: an updated meta-analysis. *Am J Med*. 2010;123:612–624.
10. Henrich JB, Horowitz RI. A contolled study of ischemic stroke risk in migraine patients. *J Clin Epidemiol*. 1989;42:773–780.
11. Chang CL, Donaghy M, Poulter N. Migraine and stroke in young women: case-control study. The World Health Organization Collaborative Study of Cardiovascular Disease and Steroid Hormone Contraception. *Br Med J*. 1999;318(7175):13–18.
12. Chang CL, Donaghy M, Poulter N. WHO Collaborative Study of Cardiovascular Disease and Steroid Hormone Contraception. Migraine and stroke in young women: case control study. *Br Med J*. 1999;318:13–18.
13. Tzourio C, Iglesias S, Tehindrazanarivelo A, Chedru F, Bousser MG, The AICSJ Group. Migraine and ischemic stroke in young women. *Stroke*. 1994;25:15(Abstract).
14. Tzourio C, Tehindrazanarivelo A, Iglesias S. Case-control study of migraine and risk of ischemic stroke in young women. *Br Med J*. 1995;310:830–833.
15. Tzourio C, Iglesias S, Hubert JB. Migraine and risk of ischemic stroke: a case-control study. *Br Med J*. 1993;307:289–292.

16. Kurth T, Slomke MA, Kase CS, Cook NR, Lee IM, Gaziano JM, et al. Migraine, headache, and the risk of stroke in women: a prospective study. *Neurology*. 2005 Mar 22;64(6):1020–1026.

17. MacClellan LR, Cole J, Wozniak MA, Stern B, Mitchell B, et.al. Probable migraine with visual aura and risk of ischemic stroke: the Stroke Prevention in Young Women Study. *Stroke*. 2013;38:2438–2445.

18. Kurth T, Schurks M, Logroscino G, Buring JE. Migraine frequency and risk of cardiovascular disease in women. *Neurology*. 2009;73:581–588.

19. Scher AI, Terwindt GM, Picavet HS, Verschuren WM, Ferrari MD, Launer LJ. Cardiovascular risk factors and migraine: the GEM population-based study. *Neurology*. 2005 Feb 22;64(4):614–620.

20. Bigal ME, Golden W, Buse D, Chen YT, Lipton RB. Triptan use as a function of cardiovascular risk: a population-based study. *Headache*. 2010;50:256–263.

21. Swartz RH, Kern RZ. Migraine is associated with magnetic resonance imaging white matter abnormalities: a meta-analysis. *Arch Neurol*. 2004;61:1366–1368.

22. Kruit MC, vanBuchem MA, Hofman PA, Bakkers JT, Terwindt GM, Ferrari MD, et al. Migraine as a risk factor for subclinical brain lesions. *JAMA*. 2004;921:427–434.

23. Kruit MC, Launer LJ, Ferrari MD, van Buchem MA. Brain stem and cerebellar hyperintense lesions in migraine. *Stroke*. 2006 Apr;37(4):1109–1112.

24. Kurth T, Mohamed S, Maillard P, et.al. Headache, migraine, and structural brain lesions and function: population based Epidemiology of Vascular Ageing-MRI study. *BMJ*. 2011;342:c7357.

25. Scher AI, Gudmundsson LS, Sigurdsson S, et.al. Migraine headache in middle age and late-life brain infarcts. *JAMA*. 2013;301(24):2563–2570.

26. Palm-Meinders IH, Koppen H, Terwindt GM, et.al. Structural brain changes in migraine. *JAMA*. 2013;308(18):1889–1897.

27. Adeney KL, Williams MA, Miller RS, Frederick IO, Sorenson TK, Luthy DA. Risk of preeclampsia in relation to maternal history of migraine headaches. *J Matern Fetal Neonatal Med*. 2005;18:167–172.

28. Marcoux S, Berube S, Brisson J, Fabia J. History of migraine and risk of pregnancy-induced hypertension. *Epidemiology*. 1992;3:53–56.

29. Sanchez SE, Qui C, Williams MA, Lam N, Sorensen TK. Headaches and migraines are associated with an increased risk of preeclampsia in Peruvian women. *Am J Hypertens*. 2008;21:360–364.

30. Facchinetti F, Allais G, Nappi RE, D'Amico R, Marozio L, Bertozzi L, et al. Migraine is a risk factor for hypertensive disorders in pregnancy: a prospective cohort study. *Cephalalgia*. 2009 Mar;29(3):286–292.

31. Williams MA, Peterlin BL, Gelaye B, Enquobahrie DA, Miller RS, Aurora SK. Trimester-specific blood pressure levels and hypertensive disorders among pregnant migraineur. *Headache*. 2011;51(10):1468–1482.

32. Bushnell CD, Jamison M, James AH. Migraines during pregnancy linked to stroke and vascular diseases: US population based case-control study. *BMJ*. 2009;338:b664.

33. Carson AP, Rose KM, Sanford CP, et.al. Lifetime prevalence of migraine and other headaches lasting 4 or more hours: the Atherosclerosis Risk in Communities (ARIC) study. *Headache*. 2004;44:20–28.

34. Sternfeld B, Stang P, Sidney S. Relationship of migraine headaches to experience of chest pain and subsequent risk for myocardial infarction. *Neurology*. 1995;45(2):2135–2142.

35. Waters WE. Headache and blood pressure in the community. *Br Med J*. 1971;1:142–143.

36. Cook NR, Bensenor IM, Lotufo PA, et.al. Migraine and coronary heart disease in women and men. *Headache*. 2002;42:715–727.

37. Hagen PT, Scholz DG, Edwards WD. Incidence and size of patent foramen ovale during the first 10 decades of life: an autopsy study of 965 normal hearts. *Mayo Clin Proc*. 1984;59(1):17–20.

38. Schwerzmann M, Nedeltchev K, Lagger F, Mattle HP, Windecker S, Meier B. Prevalence and size of directly detected patent foramen ovale in migraine with aura. *Neurology*. 2005;65(9):1415–1418.

39. Anzola GP, Magoni M, Guindani M, Rozzini L, Dalla VG. Potential source of cerebral embolism in migraine with aura: a transcranial Doppler study. *Neurology*. 1999 May 12;52(8):1622–1625.

40. Schwedt TJ, Demaerschalk BM, Dodick DW. Patent foramen ovale and migraine: a quantitative systematic review. *Cephalalgia*. 2008 May;28(5):531–540.

41. Dalla Volta G, Guindani M, Zavarise P, Griffini S, Pezzini A, Padovani A. Prevalence of patent foramen ovale in a large series of patients with migraine with aura, migraine without aura and cluster headache, and relationship with clinical phenotype. *J Headache Pain*. 2005;6(4):328–330.

42. Nozari A, Dilekoz E, Sukhotinsky I, Stein T, Eikermann-Haerter K, Liu C, et al. Microemboli may link spreading depression, migraine aura, and patent foramen ovale. *Ann Neurol*. 2010 Feb;67(2):221–229.

43. Rundek T, Elkind MS, Di Tullio MR, et.al. Patent foramen ovale and migraine: a cross-sectional study from the Northern Manhattan Study (NOMAS). *Circulation*. 2008;1181419:1419–1424.

44. Schwerzmann M, Wiher S, Nedeltchev K, Mattle HP, Wahl A, Seiler C, et al. Percutaneous closure of patent foramen ovale reduces the frequency of migraine attacks. *Neurology*. 2004;62:1399–1401.

45. Morandi E, Anzola GP, Angeli S, Melzi G, Onorato E. Transcatheter closure of patent foramen ovale: a new migraine treatment? *J Interv Cardiol*. 2003; 16(1):39–42.

46. Post MC, Thijs V, Herroelen L, Budts WI. Closure of a patent foramen ovale is associated with a decrease in prevalence of migraine. *Neurology*. 2004;62:1439–1448.

47. Post MC, Van Deyk K, Budts W. Percutaneous closure of a patent foramen ovale: Single-centre experience using different types of devices and mid-term outcome. *Acta Cardiologica* 2005;60(5):515–519.

48. Reisman M, Christofferson RD, Jesurum J, Olsen JV, Spencer MP, Krabill KA. Migraine headache relief after transcatheter closure of patent foramen ovale. *J Am Coll Cardiol*. 2005;45(4):493–495.

49. Kimmelstiel C, Gange C, Thaler D. Is patent foramen ovale closure effective in reducing migraine symptoms? A controlled study. *Catheter Cardio Interv*. 2007;69(5):740–746.

50. Rigatelli G, Cardaioli P, Braggion G, Giordan M, Fabio D, Aggio S. Resolution of migraine by transcatheter patent foramen ovale closure with premere occlusion system in a preliminary series of patients with

previous cerebral ischemia. . *Catheter Cardio Interv*. 2007;70(3):429–433.

51. Wilmshurst PT, Nightingale S, Walsh KP, Morrison WL. Effect on migraine of closure of cardiac right-to-left shunts to prevent recurrence of decompression illness or stroke or for haemodynamic reasons. *Lancet*. 2000;356:1648–1651.

52. Dowson A, Mullen MJ, Peatfield R, Muir K, Khan AA, Wells C, et al. Migraine Intervention With STARFlex Technology (MIST) trial: a prospective, multicenter, double-blind, sham-controlled trial to evaluate the effectiveness of patent foramen ovale closure with STARFlex septal repair implant to resolve refractory migraine headache. *Circulation*. 2008 Mar 18;117(11):1397–404.

53. Wilmshurst PT, Pearson MJ, Nightingale S, Walsh KP, Morrison WL. Inheritance of persistent foramen ovale and atrial septal defects and the relation to familial migraine with aura. *Heart*. 2004;90:1315–1320.

54. Andermann F. Migraine and epilepsy: an overview. In: Andermann F, Lugaresi E, editors. *Migraine and epilepsy*. Boston: Butterworths, 1987:405–421.

55. Andermann E, Andermann FA. Migraine-epilepsy relationships: epidemiological and genetic aspects. In: Andermann FA, Lugaresi E, editors. *Migraine and epilepsy*. Boston: Butterworths, 1987:281–291.

56. Marks DA, Ehrenberg BL. Migraine related seizures in adults with epilepsy, with EEG correlation. *Neurology*. 1993;43:2476–2483.

57. Velioglu SK, Ozmenoglu M. Migraine-related seizures in an epileptic population. *Cephalalgia*. 1999;19(797):801.

58. Ottman R, Lipton RB. Comorbidity of migraine and epilepsy. *Neurology*. 1994;44:2105–2110.

59. Lipton RB, Ottman R, Ehrenberg BL, Hauser WA. Comorbidity of migraine: the connection between migraine and epilepsy. *Neurology*. 1994;44(Suppl 7):28–32.

60. Piccinelli P, Borgatti R, Nicoli F, Calcagno P, Bassi MT, Quadrelli M, et al. Relationship between migraine and epilepsy in pediatric age. *Headache*. 2006 Mar;46(3):413–421.

61. Ludvigsson P, Hesdorffer D, Olafsson E, Kjartansson O, Hauser WA. Migraine with aura is a risk factor for unprovoked seizures in children. *AnnNeurol*. 2006;59:210–213.

62. Haut S, Bigal ME, Lipton RB. Chronic disorders with episodic manifestations: focus on epilepsy and migraine. *Lancet Neurol*. 2006;5:148–157.

63. Ottman R, Lipton RB. Is the comorbidity of epilepsy and migraine due to a shared genetic susceptibility? *Neurology*. 1996;47:918–924.

64. Haan J, Terwindt GM, van den Maagdenberg AM, Stam AH, Ferrari MD. A review of the genetic relation between migraine and epilepsy. *Cephalalgia*. 2008 Feb;28(2):105–113.

65. Ophoff RA, van Eijk R, Sandkuijl LA, et al. Genetic heterogeneity of familial hemiplegic migraine. *Genomics*. 1994;22:21–26.

66. Kors EE, Melberg A, Vanmolkot KR, et.al. Childhood epilepsy, familial hemiplegic migraine, cerebellar ataxia, and a new CACNA1A mutation. *Neurology*. 2004;63:1136–1137.

67. Beauvais K, Cave-Riant F, De Barace C, Tardieu M, Tournier-Lasserve E, Furby A. New CACNA1A gene mutation in a case of familial hemiplegic migraine with status epilepticus. *Eur J Neurol*. 2004;52:58–61.

68. Eikermann-Haerter K, Yuzawa I, Qin T, Wang Y, Baek K Kim YR, Hoffman uDE, et al. Enhanced subcortical spreading depression in familial hemiplegic migraine type 1 mutant mice. *J Neurosci*. 2011;31(15):5755–5763.

69. Lebas A, Guyant-Marechal L, Hannequin D, Riant F, Tournier-Lasserve E, Parain D. Severe attacks of familial hemiplegic migraine, childhood epilepsy and ATP1A2 mutation. *Cephalalgia*. 2008 Jul;28(7):774–777.

70. Kaate R, Kors E.E., Hottenga J, et.al. Novel mutationsin the Na/K ATPase pump gene ATP1A2 associated with familial hemiplegic migraine and benign infantile convulsions. *Ann Neurol*. 2003;54:360–366.

71. Claes L, Del-Favero J, Ceulemans B, Lagae L, Van Broeckhoven C, De Jonghe P. De novo mutations in the sodium-channel gene SCN1A cause severe myoclonic epilepsy of infancy. *Am J Hum Genet*. 2001;68:1327–1332.

72. Ceulemans BP, Claes LR, Lagae LG. Clinical correlations of mutations in the SCN1A gene: from febrile seizures to severe myoclonic epilepsy in infancy. *Ped Neu*. 2004;30:234–243.

73. Escayg A, MacDonald BT, Meisler MH, et.al. Mutations of SCN1A, encoding a neuronal sodium channel, in two families with GEFS+2. *Nature Genetics*. 2013;24:343–345.

74. Lossin CWDW, Rhodes TH, Vanoye CG, George AL. Molecular basis of an inherited epilepsy. *Neuron*. 2002;34:877–884.

75. Dichgans M, Freilinger T, Eckstein G, Babini E, Lorenz-Depiereux B, Biskup S, et al. Mutation in the neuronal voltage-gated sodium channel SCN1A in familial hemiplegic migraine. *Lancet*. 2005 Jul 30;366(9483):371–377.

76. Breslau N, Davis GC, Andreski P. Migraine, psychiatric disorders and suicide attempts: an epidemiological study of young adults. *Psychiatry Res*. 1991;37:11–23.

77. Breslau N, Davis GC. Migraine, physical health and psychiatric disorders: a prospective epidemiologic study of young adults. *J Psychiatr Res*. 1993;27(2):211–221.

78. Breslau N, Davis GC, Schultz LR, Peterson EL. Migraine and major depression: a longitudinal study. *Headache*. 1994;7:387–393.

79. Breslau N, Schultz LR, Stewart WF, Lipton RB, Lucia VC, Welch KM. Headache and major depression: is the association specific to migraine? *Neurology*. 2000;54(2):308–313.

80. Merikangas KR, Merikangas JR, Angst J. Headache syndromes and psychiatric disorders: associations and familial transmission. *J Psychiatric Res*. 1993;27:197–210.

81. Lipton RB, Hamelsky S, Kolodner KB, Steiner TJ, Stewart WF. Migraine, quality of life, and depression: a population-based case-control study. *Neurology*. 2000;55(5):629–635.

82. Breslau N, Lipton RB, Stewart WF, Schultz LR, Welch KM. Comorbidity of migraine and depression: investigating potential etiology and prognosis. *Neurology*. 2003 Apr 22;60(8):1308–1312.

83. Zwart JA, Dyb G, Hagen K, Odegard KJ, Dahl AA, Bovim G, et al. Depression and anxiety disorders associated with headache frequency. The Nord-Trondelag Health Study. *Eur J Neurol*. 2003 Mar;10(2):147–152.

84. Stewart WF, Linet MS, Celentano DD. Migraine headaches and panic attacks. *Psychosom Med.* 1989;51:559–569.

85. Stewart WF, Shechter A, Liberman J. Physician consultation for headache pain and history of panic: results from a population-based study. *Am J Med.* 1992;92:35S–40S.

86. Breslau N. Migraine, suicidal ideation, and suicide attempts. *Neurology.* 1992;42:392–395.

87. Silberstein SD, Lipton RB, Breslau N. Migraine: Association with personality characteristics and psychopathology. *Cephalalgia.* 1995;15:337–369.

88. Breslau N, Davis GC. Migraine, major depression and panic disorder: a prospective epidemiologic study of young adults. *Cephalalgia.* 1992;12:85–89.

89. Breslau N, Merikangas K, Bowden CL. Comorbidity of migraine and major affective disorders. *Neurology.* 1994;44(Suppl 7):17–22.

90. Marazziti D, Toni C, Pedri S, Bonuccelli U, Pavese N, Nuti A, et al. Headache, panic disorder and depression: comorbidity or a spectrum? *Neuropsychobiology.* 1995;31(3):125–129.

91. Juang KD, Wang SJ, Fuh JL, Lu SR, Su TP. Comorbidity of depressive and anxiety disorders in chronic daily headache and its subtypes. *Headache.* 2000 Nov;40(10):818–823.

92. Wang SJ. Migraine and suicide. *Expert Rev Neurotherapeutics.* 2007;7:1069–1071.

93. Mahmood T, Romans S, Silverstone T. Prevalence of migraine in bipolar disorder. *J Affect Disord.* 1999 Jan;52(1–3):239–241.

94. Oedegaard KJ, Neckelmann D, Mykletun A, Dahl AA, Zwart JA, Hagen K, et al. Migraine with and without aura: association with depression and anxiety disorder in a population-based study. The HUNT Study. *Cephalalgia.* 2006 Jan;26(1):1–6.

95. McIntyre RS, Konarski JZ, Wilkins K, Bouffard B, Soczynska JK, Kennedy SH. The prevalence and impact of migraine headache in bipolar disorder: results from the Canadian Community Health Survey. *Headache.* 2006 Jun;46(6):973–982.

96. Jette N, Patten S, Williams J, Becker W, Wiebe S. Comorbidity of migraine and psychiatric disorders: a national population-based study. *Headache.* 2008 Apr;48(4):501–516.

97. Swartz KL, Pratt LA, Armenian HK, Lee LC, Eaton WW. Mental disorders and the incidence of migraine headaches in a community sample: results from the Baltimore Epidemiologic Catchment area follow-up study. *Arch Gen Psychiatr.* 2000;57(10):945–950.

98. Devlen J. Anxiety and depression in migraine. *J R Soc Med.* 1994 Jun;87(6):338–341.

99. McWilliams LA, Goodwin RD, Cox BJ. Depression and anxiety associated with three pain conditions: results from a nationally representative sample. *Pain.* 2004;111:77–83.

100. Saunders K, Merikangas K, Low NC, Von Korff M, Kessler C. Impact of comorbidity on headache-related disability. *Neurology.* 2008;70:538–547.

101. Breslau N, Schultz LR, Stewart WF, Lipton R, Welch KM. Headache types and panic disorder: directionality and specificity. *Neurology.* 2001 Feb 13;56(3):350–354.

102. Fasmer OB, Halmoy A, Oedegaard KJ, Haavik J. Adult attention deficit hyperactivity disorder is associated with migraine headaches. *Eur Arch Psychiatr Clin Neurosci.* 2011;261:595–602.

103. Mikkelsson M, El-Metwally A, Kautiainen H, Auvinen A, Macfarlane GJ, Salminen JJ. Onset, prognosis and risk factors for widespread pain in schoolchildren: a prospective 4-year follow-up study. *Pain.* 2008 Sep 15;138(3):681–687.

104. Anttila P, Metsahonkala L, Mikkelsson M, Helenius H, Sillanpaa M. Comorbidity of other pains in schoolchildren with migraine or nonmigrainous headache. *J Pediatr.* 2001;138(2):176–180.

105. Santalahti P, Aromaa M, Sourander A, Helenius H, Pija J. Have there been changes in children's psychosomatic symptoms? A 10-year comparison from Finland. *Pediatrics.* 2005;115:e434–e442.

106. Fichtel A, Larsson B. Psychosocial impact of headache and comorbidity with other pains among Swedish school adolescents. *Headache.* 2002;42:766–775.

107. Kroner-Herwig B, Heinrich M, Morris L. Headache in German children and adolescents: a population-based epidemiological study. *Cephalalgia.* 2007 Jun;27(6):519–527.

108. El-Metwally A, Halder S, Thompson D, Macfarlane GJ, Jones GT. Predictors of abdominal pain in schoolchildren: a 4-year population-based prospective study. *Arch Dis Child.* 2007;92:1094–1098.

109. Hestbaek L, Leboeuf-Yde C, Kyvik KO, et.al. Comorbidity with low back pain: a cross-sectional population-based survey of 12- to 22-year-olds. *Spine.* 2004;29:1483–1491.

110. Hagen K, Einarsen C, Zwart JA, Svebak S, Bovim G. The co-occurrence of headache and musculoskeletal symptoms amongst 51 050 adults in Norway. *Eur J Neurol.* 2002 Sep;9(5):527–533.

111. Von KM, Crane P, Lane M, Miglioretti DL, Simon G, Saunders K, et al. Chronic spinal pain and physical-mental comorbidity in the United States: results from the national comorbidity survey replication. *Pain.* 2005 Feb;113(3):331–339.

112. Strine TW, Chapman DP, Balluz LS. Population-based U.S. study of severe headaches in adults: psychological distress and comorbidities. *Headache.* 2006 Feb;46(2):223–232.

113. Bingefors K, Isacson D. Epidemiology, comorbidity, and impact on health-related quality of life of self-reported headache and musculoskeletal pain: a gender perspective. *Eur J Pain.* 2004;8:435–450.

114. Peres MF, Young WB, Kaup AO, Zukerman E, Silberstein SD. Fibromyalgia is common in patients with transformed migraine. *Neurology.* 2001;57(7):1326–1328.

115. Ifergane G, Buskila D, Simiseshvely N, Zeev K, Cohen H. Prevalence of fibromyalgia syndrome in migraine patients. *Cephalalgia.* 2006 Apr;26(4):451–456.

116. de Tommaso M, Federico A, Serpino C, Vecchio E, Franco G, Sardaro M, et al. Clinical features of headache patients with fibromyalgia comorbidity. *J Headache Pain.* 2011;12(6):629–638.

117. Scher AI, Stewart WF, Ricci JA, Lipton RB. Factors associated with the onset and remission of chronic daily headache in a population-based study. *Pain.* 2003;106 (81):89.

118. Bigal ME, Liberman JN, Lipton RB. Obesity and migraine: a population study. *Neurology.* 2006;66:545–550.

119. Bigal ME, Lipton RB. Obesity is a risk factor for transformed migraine but not chronic tension-type headache. *Neurology*. 2006 Jul 25;67(2):252–257.

120. Bigal ME, Tsang A, Loder E, Serrano D, Reed ML, Lipton RB. Body mass index and episodic headaches: a population-based study. *ArchIntern Med*. 2007;167:1964–1970.

121. Mattsson P. Migraine headache and obesity in women aged 40–74 years: a population-based study. *Cephalalgia*. 2007 Aug;27(8):877–80.

122. Winter AC, Wang L, Buring JE, et al. Migraine, weight gain and the risk of becoming overweight and obese: a prospective cohort study. *Cephalagia*. 2012;32(13):963–971.

123. Bigal ME, Gironda M, Tepper SJ, Feleppa M, Rapoport AM, Sheftell FD, et al. Headache prevention outcome and body mass index. *Cephalalgia*. 2006 Apr;26(4):445–450.

124. Dodick DW, Freitag F, Banks J, Saper J, Xiang J, Rupnow, et al. Topiramate versus amitriptyline in migraine prevention: a 26-week, multicenter, randomized, double-blind, parallel-group non-inferiority trial in adult migraineurs. *Clin Ther*. 2009;31(3):542–559.

125. Bond DS, Vithiananthan S, Nash JM, Thomas JG, Wing RR. Improvement of migraine headaches in severely obese patientss after bariatric surgery. *Neurology*. 2010;76(13):1135–1138.

126. Novack V, Fuchs L, Lantsberg L, Kama S, Lahoud U, Horev A, et al. Changes in headache frequency in premenopausal obese women with migraine after bariatric surgery: a case series. *Cephalalgia*. 2011;31:1336–1342.

127. Chen TC, Leviton A. Asthma and eczema in children born to women with migraine. *Arch Neurol*. 1990;47:1227–1230.

128. Strachnan DP, Butland BK, Anderson HR. Incidence and prognosis of asthma and wheezing illness from early childhood to age 33 in a national British cohort. *BMJ*. 1996;312:1195–1199.

129. Von Behren J, Kreutzer R, Hermandez A. Self-reported asthma prevalence in adults in California. *J Asthma*. 2002;39:429–440.

130. Mortimer MJ, Kay J, Gawkrodger DJ, Jaron A, Barker DC. The prevalence of headache and migraine in atropic children: an epidemiological study in general practice. *Headache*. 1993;33:427–431.

131. Davey G, Sedgwick P, Maier W, Visick G, Strachnan DP, Anderson HR. Association between migraine and asthma: matched case-control study. *Br J Gen Pract*. 2002;52:723–727.

132. Aamodt AH, Stovner LJ, Langhammer A, Hagen K, Zwart J-A. Is headache related to asthma, hay fever, and chronic bronchitis? The Head-HUNT Study. *Headache*. 2007;47:204–212.

133. Lateef TM, Merikangas KR, He J, et.al. Headache in a national sample of American children: prevalence and comorbidity. *J Child Neurol*. 2009;24(5):536–543.

134. Karlstad O, Nafstad P, Tverdal A, Skurtveit S, Furu K. Comorbidities in an asthma population 8–29 years old: a study from the Norwegian prescription database. *Pharmacoepidem Dr S*. 2012;21:1045–1052.

135. Becker C, Brobert GP, Almqvist PM, Johansson S, Jick SS, Meier CR. The risk of newly diagnosed asthma in migraineurs with or without previous triptan prescriptions. *Headache*. 2008 Apr;48(4):606–610.

136. Barbanti P, Fabbrini G, Pesare M, Vanacore N, Cerbo R. Unilateral cranial autonomic symptoms in migraine. *Cephalalgia*. 2002 May;22(4):256–259.

137. Czerwinski S, Gollero J, Qui C, Sorenson TK, Williams M. Migraine-asthma comorbidity and risk of hypertensive disorders of pregnancy. *J Pregnancy*. 2012; 2012: 858097.

138. Ku M, Silverman B, Prifti N, Ying W, Persaud Y, Schneider A. Prevalence of migraine headaches in patients with allergic rhinitis. *Ann Allergy Asthma Immunol*. 2006;97:226–230.

139. Aaseth K, Grande RB, Kvaerner K, Lundqvist C, Russell MB. Chronic rhinosinusitis gives a ninefold increased risk of chronic headache. The Akershus study of chronic headache. *Cephalalgia*. 2010 Feb;30(2):152–160.

140. Martin VT, Fanning KM, Serrano D, Buse DC, Reed ML, Bernstein JA, et al. Chronic rhinitis and its association with headache frequency and disability in persons with migraine: results of the American Migraine Prevalence and Prevention (AMPP) Study. *Cephalalgia*. 2014;34:336–348.

141. Lavigne GJ, Montplaisir JY. Restless legs syndrome and sleep bruxism: prevalence and association among Canadians. *Sleep*. 1994;17:739–743.

142. Walters AS. Toward a better definition of the restless legs syndrome. *Move Disor*. 1995;10:634–642.

143. Ondo W, Jankovic J. Restless legs syndrome: clinicoetiologic correlates. *Neurology*. 1996;47:1435–1441.

144. Chokroverty S. Sleep disorders. In: Bradley WG, Daroff RB, Fenichel GM, Marsden CD, editors. *Neurology in clinical practice*. 3rd ed. Boston: Butterworth-Heinemann; 2000:1781–1727.

145. Brodeur C, Montplaisir J, Godbout R, Marinier R. Treatment of restless legs syndrome and periodic movements during sleep with L-dopa: a double-blind, controlled study. *Neurology*. 1988 Dec;38(12):1845–1848.

146. Walters AS, Hening JW, Kavey N, Chokroverty S, Frank SG. A double-blind randomized crossover trial of bromocriptine and placebo in restless legs syndrome. *Ann Neurol*. 1988;24:455–458.

147. Trenkwalder C, Stiasny K, Pollmacher T, Wetter T, Schwarz J, Kohnen R. L-dopa therapy of uremic and idiopathic restless legs syndrome: a double-blind, crossover trail. *Sleep*. 1995;18:681–688.

148. Wetter TC, Stiasny K, Winkelmann J, Buhlinger A, Brandenburg U, Penzel t. A randomized controlled study of pergolide in patients with restless legs syndrome. *Neurology*. 1999;52:944–950.

149. Montplaisir J, Nicolas A, Denesle R, Mancilla BG. Restless legs syndrome improved by pramipexole: a double-blind randomized trail. *Neurology*. 1999;52:938–943.

150. Reuter I, Ellis CM, Chaudhuri KR. Nocturnal subcutaneous apomorphien infusion in Parkinson's disease and restless legs syndrome. *Acta Neurol Scand*. 1999;100:163–7.

151. Ondo W. Ropinirole for restless legs syndrome. *Movement Disord*. 1999;14:138–140.

152. Inoue Y, Mitani H, Nanba K, Kawahara R. Treatment of periodic leg movements disorder and restless legs

syndrome with talipexole. *Psychiatr Clin Neurosci.* 1999;53:283–285.

153. Turjanski N, Lees AJ, Brooks DJ. Striatal dopaminergic function in restless legs syndrome: 18F-dopa and 11C-raclopride PET studies. *Neurology.* 1999;52:932–937.

154. Staedt J, Stoppe G, Kogler A, Riemann H, Hajak G, Munz DL. Nocturnal myoclonus syndrome (periodic movements in sleep) related to central dopamine D2 receptor alteration. *Eur Arch Psychiatr Clin Neurosci.* 1995;245:8–10.

155. O'keeffe ST, Gavin K, Lavan JN. Iron status and restless legs syndrome in the elderly. *Age Aging.* 1994;23:200–203.

156. Sachdev P. The neuropsychiatry of brain iron. *J Neuropsychiatr Clin Neurosci.* 1993;5:18–29.

157. Ulfberg J, Nystrom B, Carter N, Edling C. Restless legs syndrome among working-aged women. *Eur Neurol.* 2001;46:17–19.

158. Yunus MB. Psychological aspects of fibromyalgia syndrome: a component of the dysfunctional spectrum syndrome. *Baillieres Clin Rheumatol.* 1994;8:811–837.

159. Yunus MB. Central sensitivity syndromes: a unified concept for fibromyalgia and other similar maladies. *J Indian Rheum Assoc.* 2000;8:27–33.

160. Yunus MB. A comprehensive medical evaluation of patients with fibromyalgia syndrome. *Rheumatic Dis Clin N Amer.* 2002;28:201–217.

161. Young WB, Piovesan E, Biglan KM. Restless legs syndrome and drug-induced akathesia in headache patients. *CNS Spectr.* 2003 Aug 6;6:450–456.

162. Barnes TR. A rating scale for drug-induced akathisia. *Br J Psychiatr.* 1989;154:672–676.

163. Ekbom KA. Restless legs syndrome. *Neurology.* 1960;10:868–873.

164. Rhode AM, H"sing VG, Happe S. Comorbidity of migraine and restless legs syndrome: a case control study. *Cephalagia.* 2007;27:1255–1260.

165. d'Onofrio F, Bussone G, Cologno D, Petretta V, Buzzi MG, Tedeschi G, et al. Restless legs syndrome and primary headaches: a clinical study. *Neurol Sci.* 2008 May;29 Suppl 1:S169–S172.

166. Chen P-K, Fuh J-L, Chen S-P, et al. Association between restless legs syndrome and migraine. *J Neurol Neurosurg Psychiatr.* 2010;81:524e8.

167. Schurks M, Winter AC, Berger K, Buring JE, Kurth T. Migraine and restless legs syndrome in women. *Cephalalgia.* 2012;32:382–389.

168. Winter AC, Schurks M, Berger K, Buring JE, Gaziano JM, Kurth T. Migraine and restless legs syndrome in men. *Cephalalgia.* 2012;33:130–135.

169. Seidel S, Bock A, Schlegel W, Kilic A, Wagner G, Gelbmann G, et al. Increased RLS prevalence in children and adolescents with migraine: a case-control study. *Cephalalgia.* 2012;32:693–699.

170. Silberstein SD, Lipton RB. Overview of diagnosis and treatment of migraine. *Neurology.* 1994;44(suppl 7):6–16.

171. Ondo WG, He Y, Rajasekaran S, et al. Clinical correlates of 6-hydroxydopamine injections into A11 dopaminergic neurons in rats: a possible model for restless legs syndrome. *Movement Disord.* 2009;(15):154–158.

172. Clemens S, Rye D, Hochman S. Restless legs syndrome: revisiting the dopamine hypothesis from the spinal cord perspective. *Neurology.* 2006 Jul 11;67(1):125–30.

173. Charbit A, Holland PR, Goadsby PJ. Stimulation or lesioning of dopaminergic A11 cell group affects neuronal firing in the trigeminal nucleus caudalis. *Cephalagia.* 2007;27:605(Abstract).

174. Pal B, Gibson C, Passmore J, Griffiths ID, Dick WC. A study of headaches and migraine in Sjogren's syndrome and other rheumatic disorders. *Ann Rheum Dis.* 1989;48:312–316.

175. Isenberg DA, Thomas DM, Snaith ML, Mckeran RO, Royston JP. A study of migraine in systemic lupus erythematosis. *Ann Rheum Dis.* 1982;41:30–32.

176. Miller D, Waters DD, Warnica W, Szlachcic J, Kreeft J, Theroux P. Is variant angina the coronary manifestation of a generalized vasospastic disorder? *N Eng J Med.* 1981;304(13):763–766.

177. Atkinson RA, Appenzeller O. Hemicrania and Raynaud's phenomenon; manifestations of the same disease? *U NM Headache Rounds.* 1976 March; 1–3.

178. O'Keeffe ST, Tsapatsaris NP, Beetham WP. Increased prevalence of migraine and chest pain in patients with primary Raynaud disease. *Ann Int Med.* 1992;116(12, Part 1):985–989.

179. O'Keeffe ST, Tsapatsaris NP, Beetham WP. Association between Raynaud's phenomenon and migraine in a random population of hospital employees. *J Rheum.* 1993;20(7):1187–1188.

180. Leppert J, Aberg H, Ringqvist I, Sorensson S. Raynaud's phenomenon in a female population: prevalence and association with other conditions. *J Vas Dis.* 1987;38(12):871–877.

181. Zahavi A. Prevalence of Raynaud's phenomenon in patients with migraine. *Arch Int Med.* 1984;144:742–744.

182. Terwindt GM, Haan J, Ophoff RA, Groenen SM, Storimans CW, Lanser JB, et al. Clinical and genetic analysis of a large Dutch family with autosomal dominant vascular retinopathy, migraine, and Raynaud's phenomenon. *Brain.* 2000;121(Part 2):303–316.

183. Shechter AL, Rozen TD, Silberstein SD, Stewart WF, Lipton RB. Raynaud's phenomenon and migraine: are they comorbid? *Neurology.* 1998;50, 435(Abstract).

Chapter 5

Migraine Pathogenesis

INTRODUCTION

Migraine is a primary brain disorder resulting from altered modulation of normal sensory stimuli and dysfunction of the trigeminal nerve and its central connections. Migraine starts in the brain; the premonitory symptoms and typical migraine triggers (stress, sleep deprivation, oversleeping, hunger, and prolonged sensory stimulation) can only be accounted for by a central process.[1,2] Migraineurs show interictal hypersensitivity to sensory stimuli and abnormal processing of sensory information, characterized by increased amplitudes and reduced habituation of evoked and event-related potentials.[3]

Migraine headache is a neurovascular event with dilation of blood vessels, neuronal activation, and pain. Migraine most likely results from a dysfunction of the trigeminal nerve and its central connections that normally modulate sensory input. The following components are believed to be involved: (1) the cranial blood vessels and meninges; (2) the trigeminal innervation of the vessels and meninges; (3) the reflex connections of the trigeminal system with cranial parasympathetic pathways; and (4) local and descending pain modulation.

The key pain pathways are the afferent peripheral and ascending central trigeminal sensory pathways. Brain imaging studies suggest that important modulation of the trigeminal sensory transmission involves the dorsal raphe nucleus, locus ceruleus, and nucleus raphe magnus.[4]

PATHOPHYSIOLOGY

Anatomy of Cephalic Pain

The classic studies of Ray and Wolff [5] and Penfield [6] demonstrated that the brain itself is largely insensitive to pain, but the dura mater, the intracranial segments of the trigeminal, vagus, and glossopharyngeal nerves, and the proximal portions of the large intracranial vessels, including the basilar, vertebral, and carotid branches, are pain-sensitive (Figure 5.1). Surrounding the large cerebral vessels, the pial vessels, the large venous sinuses, and the dura mater is a plexus of largely unmyelinated fibers that arise from the ophthalmic division of the trigeminal nerve and the upper cervical dorsal roots.[7] The central convergence of the ophthalmic division of the trigeminal nerve and the branches of C2 nerve roots explain the typical distribution of migraine pain over the frontal and temporal regions and the referral of pain to the parietal, occipital, and high cervical regions.[4]

The dura is innervated by sensory, sympathetic, and parasympathetic nerve fibers. A single neurite emerges from the cell bodies of the sensory neurons in the trigeminal ganglion; it bifurcates and projects out to the periphery and into the medullary dorsal horn (trigeminal nucleus caudalis [TNC]). Sympathetic fibers arise from the ipsilateral superior cervical ganglion.[8] Parasympathetic fibers arise from the sphenopalatine and otic ganglia and in ganglia associated with the internal carotid artery. Nerve fibers differ in their peptidergic content.

Most meningeal sensory fibers are unmyelinated C-units or thinly myelinated Aδ-units; some Aδ fibers are also present.[9] Sensory fibers can be activated by mechanical, thermal, and chemical stimuli. Applying an inflammatory soup (bradykinin, PGE2, serotonin, and histamine) to the dura produces not only activation but also sensitization of meningeal nociceptors. [10] Meningeal sensory nerve fibers contain calcitonin-gene-related peptide (CGRP), substance P (SP), and neurokinin A (NKA).[11] Neuropeptide Y (NPY) is a marker for sympathetic neurons, vasoactive intestinal polypeptide (VIP) for parasympathetic neurons.[9] Trigeminal nociceptive fibers innervating cerebral vessels contain glutamate as well as SP and

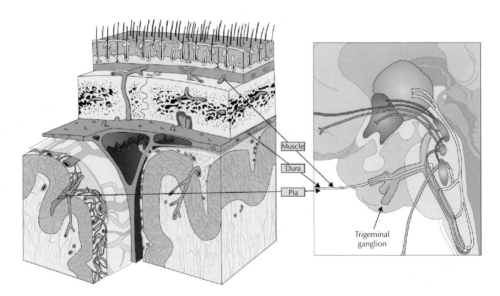

Muscle

Dura

Pia

Trigeminal ganglion

Figure 5.1. Extracranial and intracranial pain-sensitive structures.

CGRP, which are released when the trigeminal ganglion is stimulated.

The trigeminal nerve has three divisions: ophthalmic, mandibular, and maxillary. Anterior pain-producing structures are innervated by the ophthalmic (first) division. Posterior regions are subserved by the upper cervical nerves. Afferent fibers of the trigeminal nerve converge to form the sensory root of the trigeminal nerve, which enters the brainstem at the pontine level and terminates in the trigeminal brainstem nuclear complex (TBNC), the major relay nucleus for head and face pain. It receives nociceptive input from cephalic blood vessels and pericranial muscles (via the trigeminal and upper cervical nerves), as well as inhibitory and facilitory suprasegmental input. The TBNC is composed of the principal trigeminal nuclei (Vp) and the spinal trigeminal nuclei (Vsp) (subdivided into three regions: the rostral subnucleus nucleus oralis, the middle subnucleus interpolaris, [Vi], and the caudal subnucleus nucleus caudalis [Vc] (also called TNC).[12] In the Vc, the rostrocaudal axis of the face is represented from rostral to caudal.[13] Vc is primarily responsible for processing nociceptive and temperature information from the face and head, whereas Vp is involved in processing tactile information. Nociceptive input from the cervical nerves also activates the neurons in the TNC, which extends to the C2 spinal segment.

The TBNC is analogous to the dorsal horn of the spinal canal, the first synapse in the central nervous system. The primary afferents terminate in lamina I and II and, to a lesser extent, the deeper lamina III–V. Second-order neurons in Vc and C1–2 consist of low-threshold mechanoreceptive neurons, innocuous thermoreceptive wide-dynamic-range (WDR) neurons, and nociceptive-specific neurons, which respond solely to noxious stimuli. WDR neurons are more responsive to noxious than to innocuous stimuli. WDR and nociceptive-specific neurons receive primary afferent input from slowly conducting fibers (Aδ alone or Aδ plus C); WDR neurons also receive input from Aβ fibers, accounting for their tactile sensitivity. Nociceptive neurons in Vc and C1–2 also respond to stimulation of muscles, temporomandibular joint, intranasal mucosa, cornea, tooth pulp, and blood vessels of the intracranial dura. The convergence of afferent input from superficial and deep tissues has been postulated as the basis for the clinical phenomenon of referred pain of deep or visceral origin.

Depolarization of the small caliber pseudounipolar neurons projecting from the trigeminal ganglion, which invest these meningeal structures and cerebral vessels, results in activation of second-order neurons within the brainstem areas of the medullary TBNC and the dorsal horn of the upper cervical spinal cord segments. Second-order neurons in the TBNC and cervical dorsal horn are modulated by projections from the nucleus raphe magnus, periaqueductal gray (PAG),[14] rostral trigeminal nuclei,[15] and descending cortical inhibitory systems.[16] Second-order neurons from the TBNC form the trigeminothalamic tract and project to other brainstem nuclei,[17,18] such as the PAG, as well as to the contralateral dorsomedial and ventroposteromedial nuclei of the thalamus[19] and hypothalamus. The trigeminothalamic tract is analogous to the spinothalamic tract. Most spinothalamic and trigeminothalamic tract neurons that originate from the dorsal horn and project to ventroposterior lateral and ventroposterior medial nuclei have WDR characteristics.[20] The major thalamic pain and temperature projection arises from neurons in Vc that reach the thalamus via a crossed pathway that joins the contralateral spinothalamic tract. Ventroposterior medial neurons (VPN) project mainly to the primary sensory cortex. Most VPN, some with wide-dynamic-range characteristics, respond to low-threshold stimuli.[21] PO neurons project to the primary sensory cortex and granular insular cortex. TBNC neurons also project to a number of diencephalic and brainstem areas involved in the regulation of autonomic, endocrine, affective, and motor functions. All TBNC subnuclei project directly to the hypothalamus.[9]

Trigeminal nociceptive fibers that innervate the meninges also give rise to collateral branches that cross the calvarial sutures and innervate the periosteum and pericranial muscles.[22] Bidirectional action potential propagation through antidromic activation of meningeal nociceptors by extracranial pathology (e.g., head trauma, pericranial muscle inflammation) or antidromic activation of extracranial sensory fibers from intracranial pathology (e.g., aura) provides a mechanism by which extracranial pathology can triggers migraine attacks in susceptible individuals and pericranial muscle tenderness can result from a migraine attack triggered by an intracranial process (e.g., cortical spreading depression).

The existence of nociceptive pathways that bypass the thalamus and project directly and indirectly to cortical areas such as the amygdala and orbitofrontal cortex suggests that some aspects of pain sensation could arise without relay in the thalamus.[9]

Trigeminal pain is associated with activation in several cortical areas, including the insular cortex, the anterior cingulate cortex, and the somatosensory cortex.[23] In the primary somatosensory cortex, painful trigeminal stimulation results in a laminar configuration similar to that observed within the brainstem trigeminal nuclei, with V1 more caudal, V2 more rostral, and V3 medial, abutting the area of activation observed after stimulating the thumb.[24] The cortex is involved in processing and modulating pain perception. The primary sensory cortex is involved in sensory discrimination aspects of pain perception; the granular insular cortex is involved primarily in affective and perhaps autonomic responses to pain.[9]

PREMONITORY PHASE

Premonitory symptoms occur in the majority of migraine sufferers and precede the development of aura and/or headache. In a prospective electronic diary study in subjects with a historically consistent premonitory phase, premonitory symptoms were followed more than half the time by a migraine headache within 72 hours.[1] Fatigue, neck stiffness, and concentration difficulties were the most common symptoms, while yawning, emotional changes, and difficulty with reading and writing were the most predictive for a migraine headache.

A clear understanding of the anatomical and physiological basis of the premonitory phase would undoubtedly provide important insights into the origin of a migraine attack as well as identify potential targets for acute pre-headache phase treatment or more effective preventive therapies.

A lack of stimulus-induced habituation of cortical responses that increase progressively during the premonitory phase, and normalize with the onset of headache, have been reproducibly demonstrated.[25] More recently, Maniyar and colleagues used nitroglycerin to trigger premonitory symptoms and migraine

headache in subjects with episodic migraine without aura who habitually experienced premonitory symptoms during spontaneous attacks.[26] They performed positron emission tomography scans with H_2O^{15} at baseline, in the premonitory phase prior to the onset of headache pain, and during migraine headache in eight patients. They demonstrated activations in the posterolateral hypothalamus, midbrain tegmental area, periaqueductal gray, dorsal pons, and various cortical areas including the occipital, temporal, and prefrontal cortex. Hypothalamic involvement may explain many of the premonitory symptoms and may provide some insight into why migraine is commonly triggered by a change in homeostasis, while brainstem activation in the regions of the PAG, locus ceruleus, and dorsal raphe may explain the abnormal processing of sensory stimuli (photophobia and phonophobia) and the generation of headache that are the seminal features of migraine attacks. This is supported by the finding that hypothalamic and brainstem activations in the premonitory phase were exclusively right-sided, and patients developed purely or predominantly right-sided headache during the migraine headache phase, suggesting that ipsilateral involvement of these structures before the onset of headache may be involved in headache generation. As the authors suggested, these data are not only the most robust imaging data seen during the premonitory phase of migraine attacks, but highlight potential neurotransmitter systems, such as dopamine and orexin, as future targets for novel therapeutics.

AURA

It was previously believed that the migraine aura was caused by cerebral vasoconstriction and that the headache was associated with cerebral or meningeal reactive vasodilation.[5,6,27] This explained the headache's throbbing quality and its relief by ergots. It is now believed that the migraine aura is due to neuronal dysfunction, not ischemia; ischemia rarely, if ever, occurs. Headache often begins while cortical blood flow (CBF) is reduced (cerebral oligemia);[28–30] thus headache is not due to simple reflex vasodilation.[31,32] Woods et al.[33] reported a PET study of a migraine patient that showed propagated hypoperfusion during the pain phase of a migraine attack; Denuelle et al.

[34] investigated migraine patients using PET and also found cortical hypoperfusion during the pain phase of migraine. These findings are not consistent with vasodilation as a primary trigger for pain; to the contrary, they suggest that headache is associated with and may be triggered by hypoperfusion.

The fortification spectrum of the visual aura corresponds to an event moving across the cortex at 2–3 mm/min.[35] Noxious stimulation of the rodent cerebral cortex produced a spreading decrease in electrical activity that moved at 2–3 mm/min.[36] Cortical spreading depression (CSD), originally described by Leão (36), is an intense depolarization of neuronal and glial membranes accompanied by a massive disruption of ionic gradients and loss of membrane resistance. CSD is characterized by shifts in cortical steady state potential, cessation of spontaneous or evoked synaptic activity, transient massive glutamate, and K+ release, causing extracellular K+ concentrations ($[K^+]_e$) to rise above 50 mM increases, increases in nitric oxide, and transient increases, followed by sustained decreases, in CBF.[28] Elevated extracellular K+ promotes the contiguous spread of a depolarization wave across neural tissue. Large unregulated release of excitatory amino acids, like glutamate, and direct intercellular transfer of ions and small molecules through gap junctions facilitate the spread (Figure 5.2).

CSD in the cerebral cortex is associated with characteristic blood flow fluctuations: an initial, small, brief, species-dependent reduction in cerebral blood flow is followed by a profound hyperemia, reaching up to 200% of baseline, and then by a longer lasting oligemia (60%–90% of baseline) that usually lasts up to 1 hour, but can last as long as 3 days.[37] CSD has multiple additional effects on blood vessel tone: by

inducing changes in second messenger cascades, immediate early genes, growth factors, neurotransmitter and neuromodulatory systems, as well as inflammatory mediators such as interleukin-1β or tumor necrosis factor-α. CSD does not cause injury or cell death in the normal brain. Evidence supporting CSD in the human brain in situ has been obtained using functional MRI (fMRI)[31] (epidural electrophysiological recordings)[38] and intracortical multiparametric electrodes.[39] However, under conditions of energy compromise (e.g., stroke), anoxic depolarization and peri-infarct spreading depolarizations are associated with a reduction in tissue ATP, oxygen, and pH.[40]

CSD has been implicated in progressive neuronal injury after stroke and head trauma. Takano et al.[41] used two-photon microscopic nicotinamide adenine dinucleotide (NADH) imaging and oxygen sensor microelectrodes in live mouse cortex. They found that CSD is linked to severe hypoxia and marked neuronal swelling that can last up to several minutes. Changes in dendritic structures and loss of spines during CSD are comparable to those that occur during anoxic depolarization. Increasing O_2 availability shortens the duration of CSD and improves local redox state. Their results indicate that tissue hypoxia associated with CSD is caused by a transient increase in O_2 demand exceeding vascular O_2 supply and can produce hypoxia.

Glutamate plays a pivotal role in CSD. After depolarization, glutamate is released into the synaptic cleft regulated by Cav2.1 gating calcium influx. Synaptic activity is terminated in part by astrocytic uptake of glutamate via transporters driven by sodium gradients. Na gradients are maintained by activity of Na, K-ATPase removing sodium from inside cells.

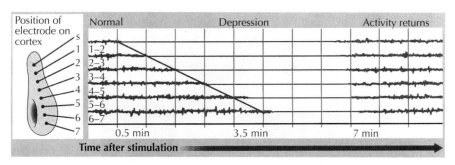

Figure 5.2. Cortical spreading depression (CSD).

Energy is required and achieved by glucose utilization after uptake from blood vessels. Susceptibility to CSD is enhanced by gain of function mutation in Cav2.1 and increased synaptic release of glutamate from neurons. Loss of function mutation in Na, K-ATPase expressed by astrocytes raises extracellular glutamate and potassium. Excessive firing of neurons due to mutant Nav1.1 channels can also enhance glutamate release.

The migraine aura is associated with an initial hyperemic phase, followed by reduced CBF, which moves across the cortex (spreading oligemia).[42] (Figure 5.3) Olesen and Lauritzen[42,43] found 17%–35% reductions in posterior CBF, which spread anteriorly at 2–3 mm/min. It crossed brain areas supplied by separate vessels and thus is not due to segmental vasoconstriction.[43] Reduced CBF persisted from 30 minutes to 6 hours, then slowly returned to baseline or even increased. Milner[44] pointed out the similarity between the velocity of CSD propagation and the march of the visual aura reported by Lashley. [35] The rates of progression of spreading oligemia are similar to those of fortification spectra and CSD, suggesting that they are related. [32,36,44]

Additional studies[29,33,45–47] support the hypothesis that CSD produces the aura.[28] During visual auras, CBF decreased 15%–53%, cerebral blood volume decreased 6%–33%, and mean transit time increased 10%–54% in the occipital cortex contralateral to the aura. The perfusion defect moved anteriorly.[47] The absence of diffusion abnormalities suggests that ischemia does not occur during the aura.[30]

The first PET study performed from the start of a migraine attack was done when a subject who was participating in a visual activation paradigm developed a migraine attack. [33] The patient was scanned with 12 successive measurements of regional CBF (rCBF). After the sixth scan, the patient developed an occipital headache, with nausea, photophobia, vertigo, anorexia, visual blurring, and difficulty in focusing on the images presented. The first decrease in rCBF was found bilaterally in the visual association cortex. The decrease in rCBF spread across the cortical surface toward the parietal and occipitotemporal areas at a constant rate, sparing the cerebellum, the basal ganglia, and the thalamus. The changes were short-lasting, with recovery by the time of the next measurement (12–15 minutes later). Since the visual disturbance did not fulfil ICHD-2 criteria for a visual aura, the attack was classified as migraine without aura.

Blood oxygenation level-dependent (BOLD) functional MRI reflects the relative concentration of deoxyhemoglobin in venous blood. Visual stimulation was used to trigger headache in six patients with migraine with aura and two patients with migraine without aura.[46] Their typical headache with ($n = 2$) or without visual change was visually triggered at 7.3 minutes (mean time) after visual stimulation began. In five patients, the onset of headache or visual change, or both, was preceded by suppression of initial activation (mean onset time, 4.3

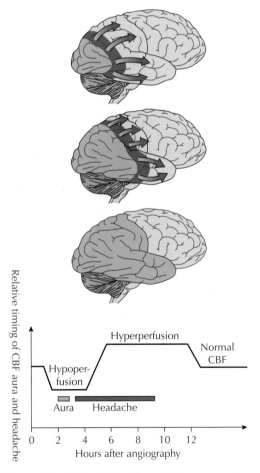

Figure 5.3. CSD and blood flow. CSD causes migraine aura. It is a wave of cortical excitation and depression associated with changes in blood flow.

minutes; p = .001) The suppression slowly propagated into contiguous occipital cortex at a rate ranging from 3 to 6 mm/min. This neuronal suppression was accompanied by baseline contrast intensity increases that indicated vasodilatation and tissue hyperoxygenation. Utilizing fMRI BOLD, a focal increase in blood flow during migraine visual aura was detected. The BOLD signal spread within occipital cortex at a rate of 3.5 mm/min and was retinotopically congruent with the patient's aura. This initial increased BOLD signal was followed minutes later by a decrease, suggesting a rise and then a fall in CBF.[31] Magnetoencephalography (MEG) demonstrates changes in migraineurs, but not controls, consistent with CSD.[48,49]

CORTICAL EXCITABILITY

Cortical responsiveness is abnormal in episodic migraine between migraine attacks.[1,12] There is a deficit of habituation (or adaptation) in visual-evoked cortical response; that is, the amplitude of the cortical potential does not decrease over successive blocks of 50–100 averaged responses in migraine patients, as in healthy subjects. The first block of averaged responses is smaller in migraineurs than in healthy controls.[2] Habituation, deficient outside of an attack, normalizes just before and during the migraine attack, and the amplitude of the first block of responses increases. [3] The cortical responsivity abnormality fluctuates in relation to the migraine attack; it is most pronounced during the days immediately preceding the attack and normalizes during the attack.[7]

Chen et al.[50] recorded visual evoked magnetic fields (VEF) using MEG in 25 CM patients and 38 episodic migraineurs (29 interictally, 9 ictally) and 32 healthy controls. CM patients were recorded in a pain-free interval. Grand average P100m amplitudes as well as the first block amplitude were significantly larger in CM patients and ictal episodic migraine patients compared to interictal episodic migraine subjects. On stimulus repetition, P100m amplitude habituated equally in CM patients, ictal episodic migraine patients, and control subjects, whereas a habituation deficit was found interictally in episodic migraineurs. Evoked-potential amplitude to low numbers of stimuli is a marker of sensitization, while amplitude reduction over large numbers of stimuli reflects habituation. In CM and interictal episodic migraine, the P100m parameters did not correlate with any clinical variable.[51] The normal ictal-like pattern is independent of the presence or intensity of headache at the time of recording and is not a non-specific consequence of the pain.[52] Normal VEF habituation in CM (n = 18) was confirmed by Chen et al. in another study: they found, on the contrary, that the VEF potentiates in patients with persistent visual aura (n = 6).[53] Chen et al. have shown that the response pattern of the visual cortex in CM is similar to that found during a migraine attack in patients with EM, that is, both normal with regard to habituation and abnormal regarding amplitude of the evoked response after a low number of stimuli. In CM, and during EM attacks, the brain becomes more sensitive to stimuli but tends to adapt normally to repeated stimuli.

Transcranial magnetic stimulation (TMS) applies magnetic fields of increasing intensity to evaluate cerebral cortical excitability. Several,[54,55] but not all[56] studies have demonstrated that phosphenes are generated in migraineurs at lower thresholds than in controls, and that it is easier to visually trigger headache in those with lower thresholds.

In another paradigm, cortical excitability at baseline with phosphene thresholds (PTs) and magnetic suppression of perceptual accuracy profiles has been measured.[57] Five episodic migraine patients, five CM patients, and five normal controls participated. Visual target stimuli consisted of low-contrast letter trigrams presented centrally within a frame. The letters were presented in upper case Arial 48-point font, followed at variable intervals by a single TMS pulse over the occipital area. They measured the effect of TMS to suppress the recall of these trigrams. Lack of suppression indicated cortical excitability. Both PTs and magnetic suppression of perceptual accuracy measures were consistent, indicating a continuum of excitability across the three groups: chronic migraine patients had the highest excitability, followed by episodic migraine, then controls. Aurora et al.[57] also used the magnetic suppression of perceptual accuracy (MSPA) paradigm to study cortical inhibition in 25 CM patients (with or without medication overuse) compared to episodic migraine patients and healthy controls. CM patients had the lowest subjective phosphene threshold and the smallest suppression index; healthy controls had the highest threshold and the largest suppression; and episodic migraineurs fell in between them.[58] Ten of these 25 CM patients had 18 Fludeoxyglucose PET scans, which showed increased metabolism in the pons and the right temporal cortex, and decreased metabolism in bilateral medial frontal, parietal, and somatosensory areas and caudate nuclei.[58]

TMS has been used to examine cortical excitability between migraine attacks in children. In 10 children suffering from migraine without aura and 10 healthy age-matched controls, TMS was employed to study regional excitability of the occipital (PT and suppression of visual perception) and motor (resting motor threshold and cortical silent period) cortex. Patients were studied 1–2 days before and after a migraine attack, as well as during the interictal period. Migraineurs had lower PTs compared with healthy participants at each time-point, indicating increased occipital excitability. This increase in occipital excitability was attenuated 1–2 days before a migraine attack, as indicated by a relative increase in PTs. The increase in PTs before the next attack was associated with a stronger TMS-induced suppression of visual perception and a prolongation of the motion aftereffect. Motor cortex excitability was not altered in patients and did not change during the migraine cycle. These findings show that pediatric migraine without aura is associated with a systematic shift in occipital excitability preceding the migraine attack. Similar systematic fluctuations in cortical excitability might be present in adult migraineurs and may reflect either a protective mechanism or an abnormal decrease in cortical excitability that predisposes an individual to a migraine attack.[59]

Other evidence of increased CNS excitability comes from studies using evoked and event-related potentials (such as visual,[60] auditory,[61] somato-sensory,[62] nociceptive,[63] and olfactory[64] stimuli, and brainstem reflexes[65]). The most consistent finding is that repetitive stimulation led to attenuated responses, pointing to habituation behavior in healthy subjects, while migraine patients showed an unchanged or even increased response.[3,66–68] A few studies found no difference between migraineurs and unaffected controls.[66,69] It is crucial to note that the altered habituation pattern in migraineurs was only found interictally; amplitudes seem to normalize just before and during the headache attack.[52,70]

Somatosensory evoked potentials (SSEPs) show lack of both habituation and sensitization in migraine patients between attacks.[71] When MOH patients were studied in a pain-free state or with mild headaches, the amplitude of the most prominent SSEP component, N20-P25, was initially (1st block) greater in MOH patients and in episodic migraineurs without aura studied ictally than in the subgroup studied interictally and in healthy controls.[72] In control subjects and migraineurs without aura studied ictally, N20-P25 habituation was normal; it was reduced in MOH and in migraine without aura patients interictally. The increased MOH SSEP amplitude was proportional to the duration of headache chronification, reflecting central sensitization.[72] NSAIDs overuse induced SSEP sensitization that persisted over time, while triptans reduced both sensitization and habituation.[72] Triptans and NSAIDs, when overused, influence excitability of the somatosensory and the motor cortices differently. While NSAID overuse promotes sensitization in the sensory system, triptan overuse does not, but reduces inhibitory mechanisms in the motor cortex in proportion to the degree of overconsumption.[73]

Contingent negative variation (CNV) is the surface negative slow wave potential elicited in expectancy conditions. It represents the excitability of cortical pyramidal neurons; CNV consists of a negative wave generated in a reaction-time paradigm. Its early component (related to the warning stimulus) represents the level of expectation, and it is modulated by the noradrenergic system. The late component is related to motor readiness under dopaminergic control.[20] Migraine patients have enhanced negativity and reduced habituation compared with non-migraine controls. Siniatchkin et al.[43] studied CNV amplitude and habituation in a group of 15 CDH patients with MOH compared to 15 episodic migraineurs and 15 healthy controls. Amplitude of total CNV and its early component was greater in episodic migraine patients than in CDH patients or controls. In CDH patients there was a smaller late CNV component and an enhanced post-imperative negative variation (PINV). The early component did not habituate in either episodic migraine or CDH, but was of significantly lower amplitude in CDH. CDH patients may have lost the compensatory mechanism that is present in episodic patients, leading to chronification and lower negativity of the slow wave.

Lack of habituation is not specific for migraine and may be mainly based on nonspecific processes, such as the chronicity of the disease. The same findings have been reported in chronic low back pain patients [74–76] and may be related to the duration and severity of the disorder. Long-lasting and/or repetitive pain sensations can lead to profound functional[77] as well as structural[78] changes in the brain. The lack of habituation may not be specific for pain as such. This phenomenon was also shown in patients with tinnitus,[79] schizophrenia,[80] and Parkinson's disease.[81]

Is migraine due to neuronal hyperexcitability, perhaps due to cortical disinhibition?[52] It has been postulated that the pre-activation level in migraine patients may not be a predisposing factor to develop migraine.[52] Instead, the pivotal pathogenic process may be an imbalance in the cortical excitability level, which can be affected by intrinsic and external aspects. A disturbance of the balance of these intracortical neurons may lead to an oscillatory effect of the excitability level: the cortical preactivation level changes between high and low excitability. If the system is particularly vulnerable, external factors such as stress, visual stimuli, hormonal changes, hypoglycemia, or sleep deprivation may trigger an attack. In other words, abnormal modulation of excitability rather than general hyper- or hypo-excitability may be the crucial underlying factor responsible for the genesis of migraine attacks.

Headache

Pain has three spatiotemporal characteristics: (1) as pain intensity increases, the area in which it is experienced may enlarge (radiation); (2) the pain may outlast the evoking stimulus; and (3) repeated nociceptive stimuli may increase the perceived pain intensity, even without increased input (sensitization).[82] Pain has both sensory and affective dimensions. In addition to being physically unpleasant, pain is associated with negative emotional feelings shaped by anticipation, attitudes, and context.[20] Pain unpleasantness is in series with pain sensation intensity.

There are two prevailing concepts regarding the generation of headache in migraine. The central hypothesis states that migraine pain originates in the brain. The peripheral or afferent hypothesis argues that migraine headache results from the activation of meningeal and blood vessel nociceptors combined with a change in central pain modulation. In this model, nociception may originate from pial, dural, or extracranial periarterial sensory afferents alone or in combination.[83,84]

A sterile meningeal inflammatory process (neurogenic inflammation [NI]) may underlie the sustained activation and sensitization of perivascular meningeal afferents during migraine attacks (Figure 5.4). Trigeminal sensory neurons contain the neuropeptides SP, CGRP, and neurokinin A NKA and glutamate. [85] In animal models, activation of meningeal nociceptors leads to release of vasoactive proinflammatory peptides such as CGRP substance P (SP), and neurokinin A from the peripheral nerve terminals (NI). These mediators produce vasodilation of meningeal blood vessels (CGRP), plasma protein extravasation (PPE) (extravasation of fluid into the perivascular space around the dural blood vessels), mast cell activation, platelet activation, and sensitization of the nerve terminals.[86] SP and CGRP further amplify the trigeminal terminal sensitivity by stimulating the release of bradykinin and other inflammatory mediators from non-neuronal (glial) cells.[87,88] Inflammatory mediators increase the responsiveness of and turn on silent, or sleeping, nociceptors. Intense neuronal stimulation causes induction of c-fos (an immediate early gene product) in the TNC of the brainstem. Neurotropins, such as nerve growth factor (NGF), are synthesized locally and can also activate mast cells and sensitive nerve terminals.[89] Bradykinin and kallidin, both acting through the B1 and B2 receptors, can activate primary afferent nociceptors.[90] Prostaglandins and nitric oxide (a diffusible gas that acts as a neurotransmitter)[91] are endogenous mediators that can be produced locally and can sensitize nociceptors.

After meningeal irritation, c-fos expression (a marker for neuronal activation) occurs in the TNC[92] and in the dorsal horn at the C_1 and C_2 levels.[93,94] C-fos may also be a signal for the nervous system's adaptive responses to insult. [95] This may produce long-lasting neuronal sensitization with increased activation of the

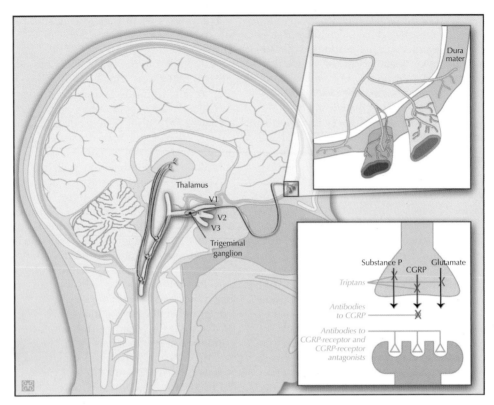

Figure 5.4. Central and peripheral connections of the trigeminal nerve and sites of action of triptans, antibodies to CGRP, and antibodies to CGRP receptor and CGRP-receptor antagonists.CGRP = calcitonin gene-related peptide.

trigeminal vascular system.[96] Reflex connections to the cranial parasympathetics form the trigeminoautonomic reflex. Activation results in VIP release and vasodilation.[32] SP and NKA mainly cause PPE, while CGRP is a powerful vasodilator of intracranial arteries[97,98] and an effective mast cell degranulator in the cranial dura mater.[99] PPE in the guinea pig dura mater, induced by antidromic stimulation of the trigeminal ganglion, was quantified as a measure for the extent of NI and for the effectiveness of anti-migraine drugs, such as the triptans, which reduce PPE.[100] One study suggests that NI occurs in humans.[101] The NI model had been used as an assay to predict probable anti-migraine efficacy. Several highly effective compounds in animal models, however, failed to relieve migraine in clinical trials. NK1 receptor antagonists are not effective in the acute treatment of migraine. Neither is the endothelin receptor antagonist bosentan[102] or the sumatriptan analogue CP-122,288. [103,104] Cortical spreading depression (the

cause of the aura) can activate the trigeminal system. Repeated episodes of neurogenic inflammation may chronically sensitize the pain pathways and may contribute to the development of daily headache.

Superior sagittal sinus stimulation results in CGRP, but not SP, release.[105] This is important: CGRP, not SP, is elevated in external jugular venous blood during migraine.[106] Sumatriptan reduced elevated CGRP levels in a migraine attack and in experimental animals during trigeminal ganglion stimulation. [107,108] Intracisternal inflammatory soup also leads to a significant release of CGRP into the external jugular vein and cerebrospinal fluid (CSF). Neonatal capsaicin treatment destroys primary trigeminal afferents. Hoffmann et al. found that inflammatory soup–induced CGRP release was significantly reduced after neonatal capsaicin treatment, but inhibition was more pronounced in jugular vein blood than in CSF. Baseline CGRP levels were not affected by neonatal capsaicin treatment. Following neonatal capsaicin treatment, CGRP mRNA was significantly reduced in the trigeminal ganglion, but not in the brainstem. These results suggest that resting-state CGRP levels can be maintained after trigeminal denervation of the meninges. However, for functional purposes, primary trigeminal afferents are mandatory, as they are the major source for stimulus-induced CGRP release.[109]

CGRP appears to play a pivotal role in the generation of migraine headache.[110,111] The first potent specific selective small molecule CGRP antagonist, BIBN-4096BS,was shown to be effective in acute migraine treatment.[112] Its development was stopped since it could only be administered intravenously. Gepants is now the class name for CGRP antagonists. Four additional chemically unrelated CGRP receptor antagonists (olcegepant, telcagepant, MK-3207, and BI 44370TA) have been shown to be effective in the acute treatment of migraine.[112–117]

Astrocytes and microglia play a vital role in this process. They are involved in the initiation and maintenance of pathological pain. Astrocytes remove neurotransmitters such as glutamate, gamma-aminobutyric acid (GABA), norepinephrine, dopamine, serotonin, and acetylcholine from the synaptic cleft.[118] Neurotransmitters are converted into metabolites that are utilized for alternative functions or secreted into the extracellular space. Glutamate released in the synaptic cleft is taken up by astrocytes through Na+-dependent excitatory amino acid transporters EAAT1 and EAAT2. Astrocytes produce many trophic factors including brain-derived neurotrophic factors, glial-derived neurotrophic factor, NGF, neurotrophins, and insulin-like growth factor I. They are coupled to each other via gap junctions, mainly connexins 30 and 43.[119] Gap junctions are clusters of closely packed hemichannels, which align between neighboring cells head to head to form channels. They provide direct cytoplasmic passage of ions and small molecules. Ca2+-mediated intercellular signaling works by releasing ATP, which activates purinergic receptors on neighboring astrocytes. This is a mechanism by which astrocytes communicate with each other and modulate the activity of adjacent cells, including neurons, oligodendrocytes and microglia.[120] Through ATP release, astrocytes mediate the neuroinflammatory

response of microglia. After a given stimulus, microglia remain "primed," that is, they overrespond to subsequent stimuli and exaggerate pain.[121–123] Glial activation (astrocytes and/or microglia) increases production of pro-inflammatory cytokines (e.g. interleukin-1b [IL-1b], interleukin-6 [IL-6], tumor necrosis factor-a [TNFa],[124] chemokines,[125] arachidonic acid and prostaglandins, excitatory amino acids, ATP, reactive oxygen species, nitric oxide, and NGF)[124] and increases neuronal excitability.[124]

Neurotransmitters released in the synaptic cleft can stimulate astrocytes to release neuroactive substances (gliotransmitters) that can feed back onto presynaptic terminals or directly stimulate postsynaptic neurons. Activation of spinal microglia and astrocytes has been demonstrated in animal models of trigeminal pain models.[126] Glia-to-neuron signaling via toll-like receptor 4 (TLR-4) may play a role in the initiation and maintenance of pathological pain.[127–130] The TLRs, primarily expressed on microglia, are a family of innate immune pattern recognition receptors that contribute to their activation.[131,132]

Opioid-induced glial activation, by TLR-4 activation, opposes opioid analgesia and enhances opioid adverse effects.[133,134] Opioids produce analgesia via neuronal μ-opioid receptor agonism, but glial cells activation occurs via TLR-4, resulting in the production of neuroexcitatory mediators.[135] Prolonged opioid administration increases glial activation and pain facilitation, producing opioid tolerance and hyperalgesia.[136] Ibudilast, a non-selective phosphodiesterase inhibitor,[137] has glial-attenuating properties, including the ability to inhibit TLR-4 signaling. [135] A trial of ibudilast in MOH treatment in patients who overuse opioids is under way (clinicaltrials.gov identifier NCT01317992). (+)-naltrexone, the enantiomer of the selective μ-receptor antagonist (-)-naltrexone, has no m-receptor antagonism but is a potent TLR-4 antagonist. (+)-naltrexone potentiates acute morphine analgesia, blocks opioid reward,[138] decreases analgesic tolerance and hyperalgesia,[135] and reverses allodynia.[129] Pre-clinical evidence suggests that opioids cause hyperalgesia through activation of glial cells via TLR-4 stimulation. Furthermore, evidence is emerging that in humans, chronic pain is associated with increased TLR-4 sensitivity.

Sarchielli et al.[139] measured CSF levels of NGF, CGRP, and SP in patients with TM both with and without medication overuse. Higher NGF, CGRP, and SP levels were found in CSF in both groups of patients compared with controls. A correlation was found between NGF and SP levels. All levels correlated with the duration of the disorder. This study suggests the involvement of NGF and chronic activation of the trigeminal vascular system in TM. NGF production could arise from peripheral trigeminal nerve terminals as well as the TNC and pain facilitating pathways. Ashina et al.[140] compared interictal plasma levels of CGRP of patients with chronic TTH and healthy control subjects. Patients whose usual headache quality was throbbing had a higher interictal plasma CGRP level than control subjects ($p = 0.002$), whereas plasma CGRP level was normal in 22 patients with pressing headaches ($p = 0.36$). This strongly suggests that the patients with an elevated CGRP level had TM and that the trigeminal vascular system is activated as part of the process of TM.

The peripheral or afferent hypothesis argues that headache results from the activation of meningeal and blood vessel nociceptors, combined with a change in central pain modulation.[83] Lambert argues this is still speculative as (1) no one has found convincing, significant, and consistent pathology in migraine; and (2) no one has demonstrated in migraineurs any increase in traffic in the trigeminal sensory fibers that ought to relay the pain signals generated out in the sensory field.[141]

Does Migraine Headache Result from Vasodilation?

Vasodilating medications, such as nitroglycerin and phosphodiesterase inhibitors, can trigger migraine. This was used as an argument that cerebral blood vessel dilation is a cause of migraine pain. This has been challenged by imaging studies, which demonstrate that these medication-evoked migraine-like headaches begin after the cerebral vessels are no longer dilated.[142,143] In addition, some cerebral vasodilation-inducing agents (e.g., VIP) do not evoke headache.[144,145] In another study using 3T MRA, Schoonman et al.[143] measured blood flow in the basilar artery and internal carotid artery and diameters of the middle meningeal, external carotid, internal carotid, middle cerebral, basilar, and posterior cerebral arteries. During nitroglycerine (but not placebo) infusion, there was a transient 6.7%–30.3% vasodilation ($p < 0.01$) of all blood vessels, but no change in blood flow. During migraine, there was no vasodilation or change in blood flow.

These results are in conflict with a recent study. Asghar et al.[146] examined the diameter of extra- and intracranial vessels in patients with migraine without aura using high-resolution direct magnetic resonance angiography imaging to measure the arterial circumference of the extracranial middle meningeal artery (MMA) and the intracranial middle cerebral artery (MCA). They induced an attack of migraine without aura by infusing CGRP. Dilation of both the MMA and the MCA occurred during the induced migraine attack. In unilateral migraine attacks, there was dilation of the MMA and MCA on the headache side but no dilation on the non-headache side. In bilateral headache, there was bilateral dilation of both the MMA and MCA. Sumatriptan administration caused amelioration of headache and contraction of the MMA but not the MCA.

These data suggest that migraine without aura is associated with dilation of extra- and intracerebral arteries and that the headache location is associated with the location of the vasodilation. In contrast, Schoonman et al.[143] found that nitroglycerin-provoked migraine attacks were not associated with dilation of the MMA and the MCA. Both studies used the same MRI, head coil, and vessel-wall software. The major differences were that Ashgar et al. applied predefined pain intensity criteria (VRS ≥ 4) before a migraine attack qualified for MRA scans, and they calculated the artery circumference, not the average diameter. Thus, the Schoonman et al. study might have been unable to detect the subvoxel size dilation of the MMA and MCA observed by Ashgar et al.

Could the modest 9%–12% dilation be sufficient to activate normal sensory afferents in the perivascular space, or could it have an effect only on sensitized nociceptors? Ashgar et al. suggest the latter, because arterial diameters may dilate markedly, during hypotension, and pulsation may increase during physical exercise without accompanying head pain. In the Ashgar et al. study, subcutaneous sumatriptan reversed dilation and even contracted MMA (but not MCA) during migraine attacks. This is the strongest evidence that sumatriptan blocks dilation in the major dural artery during the migraine attack. In another animal model of migraine, triptans exerted their anti-migraine action through presynaptic 5-HT1B/1D receptors in the nucleus caudalis, blocking synaptic transmission between axon terminals of the peripheral trigeminovascular neurons and cell bodies of their central counterparts. [147] Sumatriptan may exert its anti-migraine effect by a combined constriction of extracerebral arteries and inhibition of nociceptive input from these arteries.

What, if any, is the role of vasodilation? There is considerable evidence against intracranial vasodilatation as the triggering mechanism of migraine headache. But Levy et al. suggest the possibility of a distinct non-vasodilatory peripheral headache generator. According to them, a given triggering factor might activate the migraine pain pathway by acting locally within the intracranial meningeal milieu. It might affect meningeal nociceptors directly or indirectly by acting on other meningeal constituents. Factors capable of interacting with meningeal vascular cells or local immune cells could potentially promote local release of mediators capable of activating meningeal nociceptors.[148]

SENSITIZATION IN MIGRAINE

Most migraineurs exhibit cutaneous allodynia inside and outside their pain-referred areas during migraine attacks. Selby and Lance observed that, during migraine attacks, patients complain of increased pain with stimuli that would ordinarily be non-nociceptive. [149] These stimuli include hair-brushing, wearing a hat, and resting the head on a pillow. This phenomenon of pain being produced by non-painful stimuli is referred to as allodynia. In a series of now classic experiments, Burstein et al.[150] explored allodynia development in patients with migraine.

They measured pain thresholds for hot, cold, and pressure stimuli, both within the region of spontaneous pain and outside it. As an attack progressed in a selected group of migraine sufferers, cutaneous allodynia developed in the region of pain and then outside it (extra-cephalic locations). He found that 33 of 42 patients (79%) developed allodynia. Allodynia began over the first half of the attack in those in whom it eventually developed.

Many patients had periorbital cutaneous allodynia ipsilateral to the headache. Patients with allodynia were significantly older than those without cutaneous allodynia, suggesting a possible correlation between age and sensitization. Triptans can prevent, but not reverse, cutaneous allodynia.[151] Cutaneous allodynia can be used to predict triptans' effectiveness. [152] Without allodynia, triptans completely relieved the headache and blocked the development of allodynia. In 90% of attacks with established allodynia, triptans provided little or no headache relief and did not suppress allodynia. However, late triptan therapy eliminated peripheral sensitization (throbbing pain aggravated by movement), even when pain relief was incomplete and allodynia was not suppressed. [152] Early intervention may work by preventing cutaneous allodynia and CS.

Peripheral Sensitization

Sensitization of nociceptors results in increased spontaneous neuronal discharge rate (Figure 5.5). Neurons show increased responsiveness to both painful and non-painful stimuli. The receptive fields expand and, as a result, pain is felt over a greater part of the dermatome. This results in hyperalgesia (increased sensitivity to pain) and cutaneous allodynia. An example of this is sunburn, with increased sensitivity to temperature (i.e., a warm shower feels painfully hot).

How does sensitization occur? Tissue injury and inflammation result in the release of inflammatory mediators, such as prostaglandin E2, bradykinin, and NGF. These substances act on G-protein-coupled receptors or tyrosine kinase receptors expressed on nociceptor terminals. This activates intracellular signaling pathways, resulting in phosphorylation of receptors and ion channels. Phosphorylation changes the threshold and kinetics of the nociceptor terminals, producing increased sensitivity and excitability that result in peripheral sensitization.[153] Transcriptional or translational regulation can also contribute to peripheral sensitization.

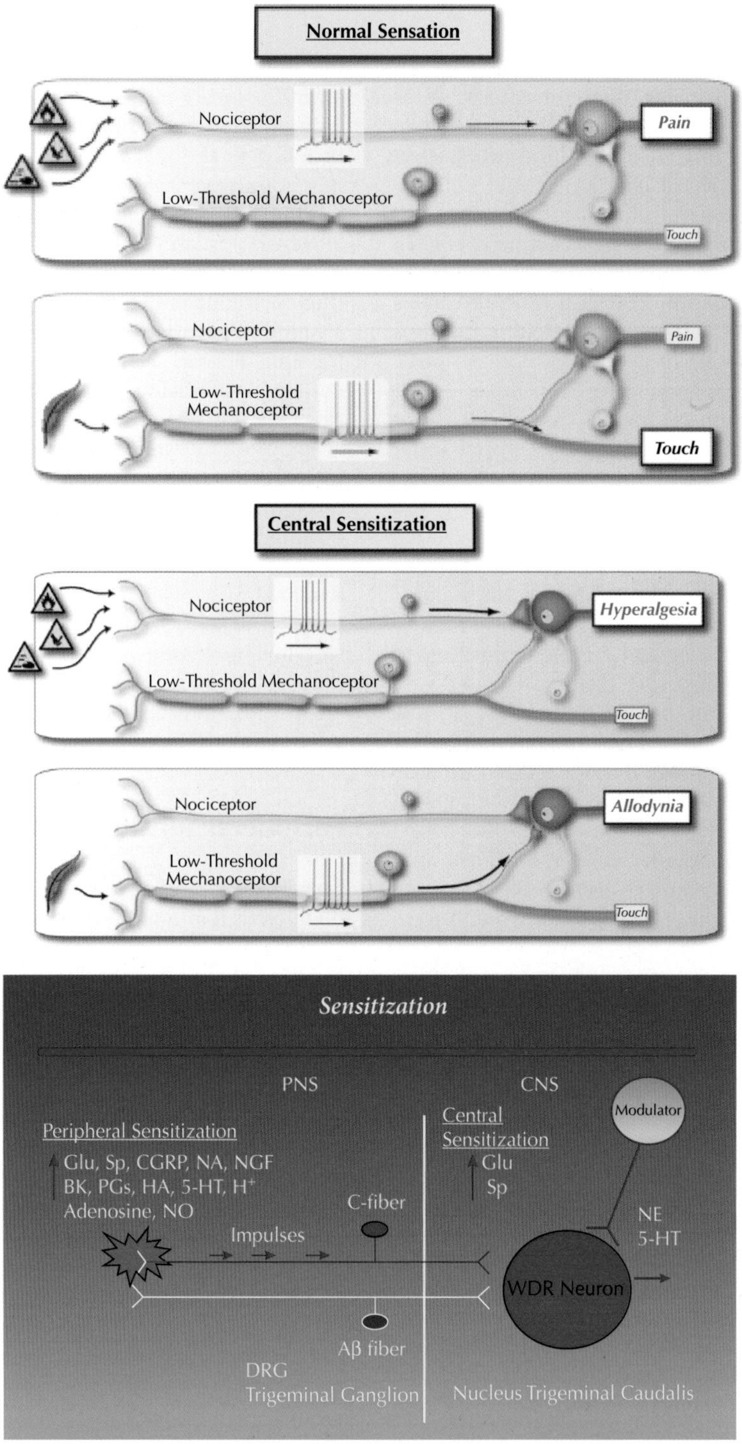

Figure 5.5. Sensitization.
Normal sensation. The somatosensory system is organized such that the highly specialized primary sensory neurons that encode low-intensity stimuli only activate those central pathways that lead to innocuous sensations, while high-intensity stimuli that activate nociceptors only activate the central pathways that lead to pain, and the two parallel pathways do not functionally inter-sect. This is mediated by the strong synaptic inputs between the particular sensory inputs and pathways and inhibitory neurons that focus activity to these dedicated circuits.Central sensitization. With the induction of central sensitization in somatosensory pathways with increases in synaptic efficacy and reductions in inhibition, a central amplification occurs, enhancing the pain response to noxious stimuli in amplitude, duration, and spatial extent, while the strengthening of normally ineffective synapses recruits subliminal inputs such that inputs in low-threshold sensory inputs can now activate the pain circuit.

NGF-induced activation of p38 mitogen-activated protein kinase in primary sensory neurons after peripheral inflammation increases the expression and peripheral transport of TRPV1 (a member of the transient receptor potential [TRP] family), exacerbating heat hyperalgesia.[154] (The TRP superfamily consists of cation channels related to the product of the *Drosophila trp* [for transient receptor potential] gene. The vanilloid receptor 1 [VR1] forms a distinct subgroup of the TRP family of ion channels. Members of the vanilloid receptor family [TRPV] are activated by a diverse range of stimuli, including heat, protons, lipids, phorbols, phosphorylation, changes in extracellular osmolarity and/or pressure, and depletion of intracellular $Ca2+$ stores. However, VR1 remains the only channel activated by vanilloids such as capsaicin.)

Brief chemical irritation of the dura with an inflammatory soup of four inflammatory mediators (histamine, serotonin, bradykinin, and prostaglandin E2) made meningeal perivascular neurons pain-sensitive for a period of 1–2 hours.[155] This peripheral sensitization can explain the intracranial hypersensitivity (i.e., the worsening pain during coughing, bending over, or any head movement).[156]

Can NI in the meninges and dura with dural peripheral sensitization[155] account for the pain of migraine?[157] Despite the fact that the throbbing quality of migraine pain is often attributed to the periodic activation of trigeminovascular sensory afferents triggered by the distension of cranial arteries during systole, little direct evidence for this model exists. Ahn studied patients with throbbing migrainous pain and asked them to signal in real time the occurrences of their subjective experience of pulsating pain, during which time their arterial pulse was independently monitored. Overall, the throbbing pain rate was substantially slower than the arterial pulse rate, and among the few individuals in whom the rates were the same, the occurrences of throbbing and arterial pulsations fell in and out of phase with each other. The lack of a simple correspondence between the subjective experience of throbbing pain and the arterial pulse requires refinement of the view that the subjective experience of throbbing migraine pain is directly related to the distension of cranial arteries and the activation of associated sensory afferents.[158] Burstein believes the throbbing pain is due to

CSF pulsations that produce the rhythmic pulsation of the meninges. With the increase in intracranial neuronal sensitivity that migraine patients experience, the normal rhythmic pulsation is interpreted as painful.

Central Sensitization

Central sensitization needs to be differentiated from windup, which is an immediate activity-dependent plasticity characterized by a progressive increase in action potential output from dorsal horn neurons during a conditioning train of repeated low-frequency C-fiber nociceptor stimuli.[159] It results in increased synaptic efficacy, that is, enhanced responses in the conditioning nociceptor pathway (homosynaptic potentiation).[159] C-fiber activation elicits slow synaptic potentials that last several hundred milliseconds.[160,161] Windup results from the summation of these slow synaptic potentials at relatively low-afferent input frequencies.

Windup is accompanied by calcium entry via N-methyl-D-aspartate (NMDA) channels. The increased intracellular calcium induces translocation (from cytosolic to membrane-bound form) and activation of protein kinase C and phosphorylation of the NMDA channel, which relieves the $Mg+2$ block on the ion channel.[162] The increased calcium may also be responsible for the induction of the two early gene products, c-fos and c-jun, which can alter other peptides, proteins, and receptors.[162] This results in increased glutamate sensitivity; the action potential progressively increases in response to each stimulus in a train of inputs.[163] NGF and inflammatory cytokines may change the phenotype of sensory neurons, making them more sensitive to nociception.[164] NGF increases the synthesis, transport, and neuronal content of SP and CGRP. It also regulates two ion channels in sensory neurons: the capsaicin receptor ion channel and the tetrodotoxin-resistant Na+ channel.[165] Neurons that exhibit windup are less sensitive to opioids than are neurons that do not exhibit this phenomenon.166] Morphine pretreatment and NMDA receptor antagonists block windup, mediated by NMDA and tachykinin receptors.

Central sensitization, in contrast, refers to an activity- or use-dependent increase in the excitability of nociceptive neurons as a result of, and outlasting, a short barrage of nociceptor input. This activity-dependent central sensitization is normally initiated only by nociceptor sensory inflow and can take up to 60 minutes to develop. Sensitization results from the activation of multiple intracellular signaling pathways in dorsal horn neurons by the neurotransmitter (glutamate) and neuromodulators (SP, brain-derived neurotrophic factor, and ephrin-B ligands). Central sensitization is characterized by an increased spontaneous discharge rate, reductions in threshold, increased responsiveness to both noxious and nonnoxious peripheral stimuli, and expanded receptive fields of CNS nociceptive neurons.[167–169] Most dorsal horn neuronal input is sub-threshold—the synaptic strength is too weak to evoke an action potential output.[170] After induction of central sensitization, by a brief intense nociceptor-conditioning stimulus, this normally subliminal input can activate dorsal horn neurons as a result of increases in synaptic efficacy.[171] A striking feature of the increased synaptic efficacy of activity-dependent central sensitization is that, in addition to including nociceptor central terminal synapses activated by the conditioning stimulus (a form of homosynaptic facilitation), it is also associated with synapses made by low-threshold mechanosensitive Ab fibers on dorsal horn neurons. Because Ab fibers are not activated by the nociceptive conditioning stimuli necessary to induce central sensitization, this is an example of heterosynaptic facilitation (i.e., the synapses activated by the conditioning and test inputs are different). As a result of central sensitization, low-threshold sensory fibers activated by innocuous stimuli, such as light touch, can activate normally high-threshold nociceptive secondary sensory neurons in the dorsal horn. The increased excitability of CNS neurons results in a reduction in pain threshold (tactile allodynia). Cutaneous allodynic pain is referred to the periphery, but it arises from within the CNS. This activity-dependent central facilitation manifests within seconds of an appropriate nociceptive conditioning stimulus and can outlast the stimulus for several hours.[168] If the stimulus is maintained, central sensitization persists.[168] Clinically, central sensitization contributes to pain hypersensitivity in the skin, muscle, joints, and viscera.[172]

Does Sensitization Play a Role in Headache?

Brief dural chemical irritation of the dura may result first in peripheral, then in central sensitization, with changes in the central trigeminal neurons that receive convergent input from the dura and the skin. Their threshold decreases and their excitability increases in response to brushing and heating of the periorbital skin—stimuli to which they showed only minimal or no response prior to chemical stimulation.[173] In addition, the threshold of cardiovascular responses to facial and intracranial stimuli decreased.[174] Applying an inflammatory soup to the dura sensitizes second-order trigeminovascular neurons (increased spontaneous activity and response to mechanical and thermal skin stimulation). [155] Triptans administered early prevented CS: dural and facial receptive fields did not expand, and spontaneous activity and mechanical and thermal sensitivity did not increase. Late triptan intervention did not reverse CS, but shrunk the expanded dural receptive fields and normalized intracranial mechanosensitivity. CS may play a key role in maintaining the headache.[151,152]

Central sensitization results in muscle tenderness and cutaneous allodynia in migraineurs. Bendtsen et al.[175] has also found evidence for sensitization in patients with chronic tension-type headache. Pericranial myofascial tenderness, evaluated by manual palpation, was considerably higher in patients than in controls ($p < 0.00001$). The stimulus-response function from highly tender muscle was qualitatively different than from normal muscle, suggesting that myofascial pain may be mediated by low-threshold mechanosensitive afferents projecting to sensitized dorsal horn neurons.

Gallai et al.[176] found elevated CSF levels of glutamate and nitrite (a nitric oxide [NO] metabolite) in TM patients with and without medication overuse. The increase in CSF nitrite, a marker for NO production, was accompanied by an increase in cGMP. CGRP, SP, and, to a lesser extent, neurokinin A were also elevated in patients compared with controls. NO plays a crucial role in animal models of sensitization. Its formation is triggered by glutamate receptor activation.

Increased headache frequency, expansion of the headache area, and cutaneous allodynia suggest sensitization of the trigeminal nociceptive neurons. In MOH, facilitation of pain processing has been established. Perrotta et al. found the threshold and temporal summation threshold of the nociceptive withdrawal reflex to be markedly reduced in patients with MOH. There was enhanced pain perception following single and repeated stimulation in MOH patients as compared to episodic migraineurs. Withdrawal of the overused medication was associated with an improvement in these findings.[177] These findings provide a neural basis for the pathophysiology of migraine pain and suggest a basis for continued head pain.

PAIN MODULATION

The mammalian nervous system contains networks that modulate nociceptive transmission. The TBNC receives monoaminergic, enkephalinergic, and peptidergic projections from regions known to be important in the modulation of nociceptive systems. A descending inhibitory neuronal network extends from the frontal cortex and hypothalamus through the ventrolateral periaqueductal gray (PAG) to the rostral ventromedial medulla (RVM). The RVM, in turn, can either inhibit or facilitate pain transmission through direct projections to the spinal and medullary dorsal horn.[178] The RVM includes the nucleus raphe magnum and the adjacent reticular formation and projects to the outer laminae of the spinal and medullary dorsal horn. Electrical stimulation or injection of opioids into the PAG reduces nociceptive-responsive neuron activity of medullary dorsal horn neurons. The PAG receives projections from the insular cortex and the amygdala.[21] Stimulation of the RVM, a relay in descending modulation of nociception, can result in inhibition and/or facilitation of nociceptive and non-nociceptive input.

Anti-nociception can be measured by nociceptive reflex inhibition.[179] RVM stimulation at relatively high current intensities results in anti-nociception (in the tail-flick test) and is responsible for decreased responses of dorsal horn neurons. By contrast, lower current intensity stimulation is pro-nociceptive (facilitatory).[180–182] Excitatory neurotransmitters (e.g., glutamate, neurotensin) microinjected into the RVM replicated the effects of stimulation, facilitating and inhibiting spinal nociception at lower and higher doses, respectively. [181–184] Microinjection of NMDA into the RVM facilitated the tail-flick reflex in a dose-dependent manner, an effect blocked by an NMDA receptor antagonist.[185]

In the RVM and PAG, three classes of neurons have been identified.[186] "Off-cells" pause immediately before the nociceptive reflex, whereas "on-cells" are activated. Neutral cells show no consistent changes in activation. [21] On-cells and off-cells fire in a reciprocating pattern: tail-flick latency was longer during periods of increased off-cell activity and was shorter when on-cells were active.

Acute opioid administration activates off-cells and inhibits on-cells; nociceptive reflexes are inhibited. Naloxone-precipitated opioid withdrawal increases on-cell activity,[187,188] which is abolished by intra-RVM lidocaine injection.[189,190] Thus, off-cell activity suppresses nociception, whereas on-cell activity enhances the response to noxious stimuli. On- and off-cell activity is modulated by 5-HT_1 receptor agonists.[21] Off- and on-cells (descending inhibitory and facilitatory pathways) project from the RVM through both dorsal and ventral parts of the spinal cord to the spinal dorsal horn.[179]

Paradoxically, more prolonged exposure to opioids can induce pain and decrease tolerance to nociception, in part enhancing the influence of pain facilitating "on" cells.[191] This may also be similar mechanistically to the abnormal pain that follows peripheral nerve injury. Both are less responsive to the anti-nociceptive effects of morphine and are reversed by NMDA antagonists.[192] Both activate the RVM descending pain facilitation pathways. Increased RVM facilitation may be mediated by the pro-nociceptive peptide cholecystokinin (CCK), which is present throughout the brain and spinal cord, including the PAG and RVM. CCK can contribute to RVM neuron excitability. Intra-RVM CCK produces reversible thermal and tactile hypersensitivity[193] and prevents both the activation of off-cells and the anti-nociception produced by systemic morphine.[194] Conversely, microinjection of a CCK antagonist into the RVM blocks thermal and tactile hypersensitivity in rats with peripheral nerve injury.[193] CCK antagonists also enhance morphine-induced anti-nociception and reverse morphine tolerance.[195] In addition, the RVM produces descending facilitation by elevating spinal dynorphin expression.[196] Dynorphin acts as an endogenous pronociceptor mediator, resulting in enhanced release of CGRP and SP.[197–199] Lesions in the RVM descending pathways block dynorphin upregulation, enhanced CGRP release, and abnormal pain. Antibodies to dynorphin also block CGRP release in model systems.[198]

Opioid analgesic tolerance is a pharmacological phenomenon that occurs after prolonged opioid administration, in part due to activation of the NMDA receptor (NMDAR). Excess activation of NMDARs can lead to neurotoxicity. Mao et al.[200] showed that spinal neuronal apoptosis was induced in rats made tolerant to morphine administered through intrathecal boluses or continuous infusion. The apoptotic cells were predominantly located in the superficial spinal cord dorsal horn. Most apoptotic cells expressed glutamic acid decarboxylase, a key enzyme for the synthesis of the inhibitory neurotransmitter GABA. This was associated with increased nociceptive sensitivity to heat stimulation. Morphine-induced neuronal apoptosis was modulated by spinal glutamatergic activity. Prolonged morphine administration resulted in up-regulation of the proapoptotic caspase-3 and Bax proteins, but down-regulation of the anti-apoptotic Bcl-2 protein in the spinal cord dorsal horn. Co-administration with morphine of a pan-caspase inhibitor or a relatively selective caspase-3 inhibitor blocked morphine-induced neuronal apoptosis. These results suggest that opioid-induced neurotoxicity depletes inhibitory GABA interneurons, a mechanism that may have clinical implications in opioid therapy and substance abuse and may account for refractoriness in CM.

The RVM modulates the activity of the TNC and dorsal horn neurons. Increased on-cell activity in the brainstem pain-modulation system enhances the response to both painful and non-painful stimuli. Opioid withdrawal results in increased firing of the on-cells, decreased firing of the off-cells, and enhanced nociception. [186,188] Descending facilitatory influences could contribute to chronic pain states and the development and maintenance of hyperalgesia.[201] Headache may be caused, in part,

by enhanced neuronal activity in the nucleus caudalis as a result of enhanced on-cell and decreased off-cell activity. In an animal study, dural inflammation produced extracranial allodynia that required the activation of pain facilitating on-cells in the RVM.[202] Inactivation of the RVM prevented the cutaneous allodynia that resulted from dural inflammation.[202] In humans, the PAG appears to be activated prominently in migraine and demonstrates significant structural abnormalities in migraine patients. The function of the nucleus cuneiformis also seems compromised in the interictal period,[203] which may explain the reduced threshold required for induction of central sensitization that exists between migraine episodes.[204]

A separate pain modulatory pathway involved in producing diffuse noxious inhibitory controls (DNIC) exists.[205–207] It is responsible for counter-irritation, the inhibition of pain produced by a noxious stimulus applied to a remote part of the body. Chronic opioid exposure inhibits DNIC. Dural-sensitive neurons in rats exposed to chronic morphine were not inhibited by noxious stimulation of the tail.[208] The loss of DNIC could be re-established by inactivating the RVM, providing evidence that morphine exposure produces an increase in descending facilitation from the RVM that masks inhibition from DNIC. The DNIC has also been found to be dysfunctional in chronic daily headache patients,[205–207] leading some to suggest that a reduction in descending inhibition may be responsible for migraine chronicity. Results from these studies suggest that the transformation of episodic migraine to CM, whether due to acute medication overuse or other factors, may be caused by an increase in descending facilitation from the RVM.[166,209–211] Other conditioned stimuli associated with pain and stress also can turn on the pain system and may account, in part, for the association between pain and stress.[186] CDH may result, to some extent, from enhanced neuronal activity in the TNC as a result of enhanced on-cell and decreased off-cell activity.

The exact mechanisms underlying MOH remain unknown. Preclinical studies have examined the neuroadaptive changes following sustained exposure to morphine. These include increased expression of CGRP in trigeminal primary afferent neurons and increased excitatory neurotransmission at the level of the dorsal horn and nucleus caudalis. They persist for long periods of time, and the evoked release of CGRP is enhanced following morphine pre-treatment. Nitric oxide donors, or stress, produce hyperalgesia in morphine-pre-treated but not in saline-pre-treated rats, even long after the discontinuation of the opioid.[212] Glial involvement in headache following opioid exposure has been evaluated pre-clinically using a rodent model of headache and morphine administration. Pre-exposure to an opioid results in facial allodynia, a surrogate for headache pain, during application of inflammatory "soup" to the dura in doses that fail to produce allodynia in opioid-naive rats.[213] When low-dose inflammatory soup was applied following morphine administration but prior to a dose of inflammatory soup able to reliably produce robust facial allodynia, no pain facilitation was observed, mirroring the clinical observation that MOH does not develop de novo in those without a pre-existing headache condition.[213] Minocycline, a tetracycline derivative that possesses anti-inflammatory effects that are independent of its antimicrobial actions,[214] selectively disrupts the activation of microglial cells to prevent allodynia without directly affecting either astrocytes or neurons.[215]

Sustained or repeated administration of triptans to rats elicited time-dependent and reversible cutaneous tactile allodynia that was maintained throughout and transiently after drug delivery. Triptan administration increased the numbers of trigeminal ganglion cell bodies expressing CGRP and modestly increased the expression of substance P.[216] The increase in CGRP was especially pronounced in dural afferent nerves; They also expressed increased nNOS. Several weeks after triptan exposure, when sensory thresholds returned to baseline levels, rats showed enhanced cutaneous allodynia and increased CGRP in the blood following challenge with a nitric oxide donor. It also produced significant elevations in CGRP plasma levels similar those found during spontaneous and NO-precipitated migraine headaches.[106,217,218] Triptan treatment induces a state of "latent sensitization," characterized by persistent pro-nociceptive neural adaptations in dural afferents and enhanced responses to established triggers of migraine headache. Latent sensitization provides a mechanistic

basis for the transformation of migraine to MOH.[219] Cutaneous allodynia was abolished by CGRP, but not by NK-1 receptor antagonists,[50] orby nNOS inhibitors.[219]

Prolonged exposure to certain acute medications produces long-lasting, pro-nociceptive, neuroplastic changes in the peripheral nerves of the trigeminal system in addition to changes in central neuromodulation.[166] Chronic opioid use has been clearly shown to activate RVM pain facilitation. By depleting inhibitory GABA interneurons, opioid-induced neurotoxicity may result in headache intractability.[166,200] MOH may, in part, prevent the occurrence of anti-nociceptive adaptive changes. The analgesic washout period could be a result of the time required for the system to reset. The failure of preventive drugs could result from the lack of endogenous anti-nociceptive agents. A similar phenomenon occurs in contingent tolerance in the seizure kindling model.

The long-term effectiveness of anticonvulsants can be studied in amygdala-kindled animals. Repeated pre-treatment with carbamazepine before kindling results in a loss of drug efficacy and constitutes a unique form of associative or contingent tolerance. Animals treated with carbamazepine after seizures occur do not show tolerance. Giving the drug after seizures occur can reverse tolerance once it has developed.[220] Some neurobiologic alterations following seizures may thus be adaptive, or anticonvulsant, in contrast to more enduring changes related to the primary pathophysiology of the kindled process.[166]

Clinical strategies based on these concepts might be used to reverse tolerance in the long-term treatment of CM. Switching a patient to a drug that has a different mechanism of action and does not show cross-tolerance, or discontinuing the ineffective drug and reintroducing it later may be effective for some migraine or CM patients.

NEUROIMAGING

Positron emission tomography (PET) in primary headaches, such as migraine[23] and cluster[221] headache, has shown activation (as measured by increased CBF) in brain areas associated with pain, such as the cingulate cortex, insulae, frontal cortex, thalamus, basal ganglia, and cerebellum. These areas are also activated by injecting capsaicin into the forehead of volunteers.[222] Using PET, patients with right-sided migraine headache showed increased rCBF in several brain regions, including the dorsolateral pons (DLP), but not the PAG. Sumatriptan relieved the headache and associated symptoms but did not normalize DLP rCBF. This suggests that activation is due to factors other than, or in addition to, increased activity of the endogenous antinociceptive system.[23] A second report corroborates these findings.[223] The rostral DLP and caudal midbrain include the mesencephalic and principal sensory trigeminal nuclei, the dorsolateral pontine reticular nucleus, locus ceruleus (LC), the parabrachial nuclei, the cuneiform nucleus, the vestibular nuclei, and the inferior colliculus.

As reviewed by Borsook and Burstein, DLP activation is not specific to migraine. It is commonly seen in patients with neuropathic pain and in subjects in whom mild somatic and visceral pain is induced experimentally. DLP activation is not specific to pain. It is activated in response to bladder distention, empathy-related recognition, and expression of emotions.[224] This area of the brainstem is rich in opioids and includes the pain control centers. [225] Dihydroergotamine and centrally penetrant triptans selectively bind to the brainstem. This area of the brainstem may integrate the phenomenon we call migraine, or it could be activated as a result of the migraine attack. If the first explanation is correct, ongoing activity in this area of the brainstem could produce recurrent or daily headache. If this area is responsible for controlling pain, then its failure to activate could explain ongoing headache activity. Acute migraine medications may induce daily headache by preventing the development of adaptive changes and perhaps by maintaining brainstem activation.[23]

Manjit et al.[226] reported eight patients with the IHS diagnosis of CM who showed a marked beneficial response to implanted bilateral suboccipital stimulators. Stimulation evoked local paresthesia, the presence of which was a criterion of pain relief. On stimulation, the headache began to improve instantaneously and was completely suppressed within 30 minutes. When the stimulation was switched off, the headache recurred instantly and peaked within 20 minutes. PET scans were performed using rCBF as a marker of neuronal activity. Each patient was scanned in the following three states: (1) stimulator at optimum settings: patient pain-free but with paresthesia; (2) stimulator off: patient in pain and no paresthesia; (3) stimulator partially activated: patient with intermediate levels of pain and paresthesia. There were significant changes in rCBF in the dorsal rostral pons, anterior cingulate cortex (ACC), and cuneus, correlated to pain scores, and correlated to stimulation-induced paresthesia scores in the ACC and left pulvinar. The activation pattern in the dorsal rostral pons is highly suggestive of a role for this structure in the pathophysiology of chronic migraine. The localization and persistence of activity during stimulation is exactly consistent with a region activated in episodic migraine and with persistent activation of that area after successful treatment. The dorsal rostral pons may be a locus of neuromodulation by suboccipital stimulation. In addition, suboccipital stimulation modulated activity in the left pulvinar.

Welch et al.[227] used high-resolution magnetic resonance techniques to map the transverse relaxation rates R2 (1/T2), R2' (1/T2°-1/T2), and R2° (1/T2°) in the brain, particularly the PAG, red nucleus (RN), and substantia nigra (SN). These measures are sensitive to free iron: R2' is a measure of non-heme iron in tissues. They evaluated patients with TM, patients with episodic migraine, and non-migraine controls. Mean R2' and R2° values in the PAG significantly increased in both the episodic migraine and TM patients. The value increased with disease duration. A decrease in mean R2' and R2° values in the RN and SN of only the TM group was observed; they attributed this to CBF changes due to head pain. Aurora et al.[228] reported normalization of SN and RN, but not PAG R2' values following detoxification.[229]

Kruit et al. randomly selected 295 migraineurs, and 140 controls were from a previously diagnosed population-based sample (n = 6039), who underwent an interview, physical examination, and a brain MRI-scan (CAMERA study). Migraineurs, notably those with aura, had higher prevalence of subclinical infarcts in the posterior circulation (OR 13.7, 95% CI [1.7–112]). Female migraineurs were at independent increased risk of white matter lesions (WML; OR 2.1, 95% CI [1.0–4.1]), and migraineurs had a higher prevalence of brainstem hyperintense lesions (4.4% vs. 0.7%, $p = 0.04$). In migraineurs aged < 50, compared to controls, they found evidence of increased iron concentration in putamen ($p = 0.02$), globus pallidus ($p = 0.03$), and red nucleus ($p = 0.03$). Higher risks in those with higher attack frequency or longer disease duration were found consistent with a causal relationship between migraine and lesions. The findings suggest that repeated migraine attacks are associated with increased iron concentration in multiple deep brain nuclei and not only in the PAG. It is unclear whether the increased iron concentration is just a physiological response induced by the repeated activation of nuclei involved in central pain processing, or whether the increased iron concentration could also damage these structures secondarily, for example due to formation of free radicals in oxidative stress.[229]

Post and Silberstein[166] suggested the kindling model for epilepsy as a model for nonepileptic progressive disorders, such as mania. They suggested that spontaneous recurrent migraine headaches might be analogous to the low levels of electrical stimulation in the kindling model in the process of headache transformation. Preventive migraine treatment could provide a dual benefit by preventing the occurrence of episodes and blocking the sensitization process that could lead to syndrome progression.

In CM, hypersensitivity of neurons in the TNC may be a result of supraspinal facilitation. Peripheral nociceptors may be hypersensitive as a result of sensitization. The vascular nociceptor may be hypersensitive in CM; and the myofascial nociceptor may be hypersensitive in CTTH associated with a disorder of the pericranial muscles. Less myofascial nociceptor hypersensitivity and a general increase in nociception may be present in CTTH not associated with a disorder of the pericranial muscles. CTTH and CM may result from a defective interaction between endogenous nociceptive brainstem activity and peripheral input. Physical or psychologic stress or non-physiologic working positions can increase nociception that could trigger or sustain an attack in an individual with altered pain modulation. Emotional mechanisms may also reduce endogenous anti-nociception. Long-term potentiation of nociceptive neurons and decreased activity

in the anti-nociceptive system could cause primary CDH. Sensitization of the TNC neurons can result in normally non-painful stimuli becoming painful, producing trigger spots, an overlap in the symptoms of migraine and TTH, and activation of the trigeminal vascular system.

THE AURA AND HEADACHE

The link between the migraine aura and headache is becoming clarified (Figure 5.6). Bolay showed that intrinsic brain activity (CSD) activates trigeminal meningeal afferents, causing long-lasting increase in middle meningeal artery (MMA) blood flow and PPE within the dura mater.[230] MMA flow increase was observed at around 5 minutes, or after CSD spread across the entire cortex. Trigeminal or parasympathetic transaction suppressed this response. SD also caused unilateral plasma protein leakage within the overlying dura mater and brainstem activation. Trigeminal transection suppressed this response, whereas parasympathetic transaction did not. Thus the blood-flow response and edema formation were generated by distinct neuronal mechanisms. CSD release of H^+, K^+, NO, and other agents into the extracellular space depolarizes adjacent perivascular trigeminal axons surrounding local blood vessels. CSD results in upregulation of inducible nitric oxide synthetase and inflammatory cytokines. CSD also activates matrix metalloproteinases (MMPs) and mildly disrupts the blood–brain barrier.[231] MMPs belong to a superfamily of endopeptidases that are involved in opening the blood–brain barrier, edema formation, invasion of neural tissue by blood-derived immune cells, and shedding cytokines and cytokine receptors. NFκB and pro-inflammatory cytokines, like TNF-α and IL-1β, which are elevated after CSD, bind to the promoter region of the MMP-9 gene. The data are consistent with the formulation that intense neuro-glial depolarization facilitates the access of hydrophilic molecules to approximate and discharge meningeal trigeminovascular afferents.[39] This mechanism couples meningeal blood flow and NI to CSD but does not explain headache ipsilateral to the aura.[32,230]

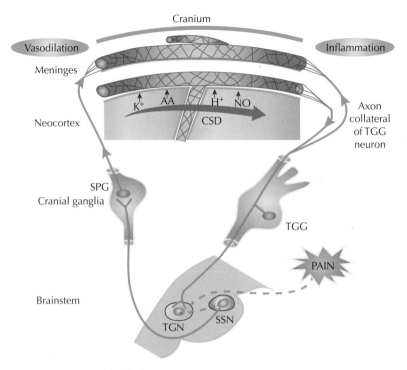

Figure 5.6. CSD and headache.

CSD can also give rise to the activation of nociceptors that innervate the meninges, an event believed to set off migraine headache. [232] CSD was induced in anesthetized male rats by stimulating the visual cortex with electrical pulses, pinprick, or KCl; single-unit activity of meningeal nociceptors was monitored *in vivo* in the rat before and after CSD. CSD was recorded in 64 trials: in 31 of those trials, CSD induced a twofold increase in the meningeal nociceptor firing rate that persisted for 37.0±4.6 minutes in trials in which activity returned to baseline, or > 68 minutes in trials in which activity remained heightened at the time recording was interrupted. In two-thirds of the trials, the onset of long-lasting neuronal activation began ~14 minutes after the wave of CSD. The authors demonstrated for the first time that the induction of CSD by focal stimulation of the rat visual cortex can lead to long-lasting activation of nociceptors that innervate the meninges. The results of this study suggest that migraine with aura is initiated by waves of CSD that lead to delayed activation of the trigeminovascular pathway.

It was previously believed that CSD activates perivascular trigeminal afferents by way of potassium, protons, nitric oxide (NO), arachidonic acid, and adenosine 5′-triphosphate release. However, sufficient concentrations of these mediators may not be sustained in the perivascular space for trigeminal sensitization and long-lasting headache to occur because of the glia limitans barrier and continuous CSF flow. Trigeminal meningeal nociceptors and central neurons start firing ~ 14 and 25 minutes after CSD in the rat.[10,13] Such time lags may be required for transduction of algesic signals over the glia limitans via inflammatory mediators. Intense depolarization and N-methyl-D-aspartate (NMDA) receptor overactivation, present during CSD, open neuronal pannexin 1 (Panx1) megachannels. CSD, by activating Panx1 and downstream inflammasome formation, may trigger inflammation. Stress-induced Panx1 activation may cause headache by releasing pro-inflammatory mediators such as high-mobility group box 1 (HMGB1) from neurons, which initiates a parenchymal inflammatory response that leads to sustained release of inflammatory mediators from the glia limitans and, hence, prolonged trigeminal stimulation.

Pannexin 1, encoded by PANX1, represents a class of vertebrate membrane channels that bear significant sequence homology to the invertebrate gap junction proteins, the innexins, and more distant similarities in the membrane topologies and pharmacologic sensitivities with gap junction proteins of the connexin family. In contrast to connexins, pannexins do not form gap junction channels, but instead function as unpaired membrane channels. Pannexin 1 and pannexin 2 are abundantly expressed in the CNS and are co-expressed in various neuronal populations. There is cooperation between pannexin channels, adenosine receptors, and K (ATP) channels that modulate neuronal excitability via ATP and adenosine. ATP release through Panx1 channels plays a critical role in maintaining synaptic strength and plasticity in CA1 neurons of the adult hippocampus. [233] Propidium iodide (PI) is a membrane-impermeable fluoroprobe used to monitor activity as it passes through megachannels. Multiple CSDs cause PI influx to cortical and dentate neurons. PI uptake is inhibited by the Panx1 channel blockers carbenoxolone (CBX), probenecid, 10Panx, or Panx1–small interfering RNA. Vehicle alone or non-silencing small interfering RNA had no effect. CBX and 10Panx did not affect CSD generation and propagation, suggesting that CSD suppression does not cause prevention of PI uptake.

Panx1 megachannels may play a role as a reporter linking neuronal stress to inflammatory response. CSD opens neuronal Panx1 channels, whose activation stimulates the inflammasome complex, subsequent caspase-1 activation, and IL-1b production. CSD causes neuronal Panx1 megachannel opening and caspase-1 activation, followed by high-mobility group box 1 (HMGB1) release from neurons and nuclear factor kB activation in astrocytes. HMGB1 is a member of the alarmin family, which mediates the communication between injured cells and surrounding cells. It is passively released from necrotic cells and actively secreted by cells under distress; it behaves like a cytokine and promotes inflammation. HMGB1 and IL-1b released during CSD may take part in initiating the inflammatory response. Subsequent NF-kB activation in astrocytes may induce the formation of cytokines, prostanoids, and inducible NO synthase-derived NO (as suggested by the inhibition of MMA response by naproxen and CSD-induced COX2 and iNOS expression in the glia limitans), which may be released to the subarachnoid space via the glia limitans

and, hence, stimulate trigeminal nerve endings around pial vessels. Suppression of this cascade abolished CSD-induced trigeminovascular activation, dural mast cell degranulation, and headache. This pathway may function to alarm an organism with headache when neurons are stressed.[234]

Alterations in cortical excitability are implicated in migraine pathophysiology. A direct relationship between cortical excitability disturbances and the activities of brainstem trigeminocervical complex neurons involved in meningeal sensory processing in the rat has been found.[235] Descending cortical projections to brainstem areas innervated by the ophthalmic branch of the trigeminal nerve originate contralaterally from insular and primary somatosensory cortices and terminate in laminae I–II and III–V of the brainstem trigeminocervical complex, respectively. CSD initiated in insular and primary somatosensory cortices induced the facilitation and inhibition of meningeal-evoked responses, respectively. CSD triggered in the primary visual cortex had different effects on insular and somatosensory cortices. Primary visual cortex CSD enhanced or inhibited meningeal-evoked responses of brainstem trigeminocervical complex neurons, without affecting cutaneous-evoked nociceptive responses. This suggests that "top-down" influences from insular and primary somatosensory cortices selectively affect interoceptive (meningeal) over exteroceptive (cutaneous) nociceptive inputs onto brainstem trigeminocervical complex neurons. Corticofugal influences could contribute to the development and location of migraine pain. Corticotrigeminal influences on brainstem trigeminocervical complex neurons could then act as modulators, once the triggering of migraine pain was produced by the direct activation of meningeal nociceptors.[235] Migraine patients may experience bilateral headaches, ipsilateral visual aura, or simultaneous aura at the onset of pain. [32] These observations appear to challenge the idea of strict unilateral CSD-like events at the origin of migraine pain.[236] Perhaps corticotrigeminal dysfunction attributable to altered cortical excitability phenotypes in genetically susceptible individuals could contribute to the development of migraine pain.

Lambert et al. tested the idea that migraine triggers cause cortical activation, which could disinhibit craniovascular sensation through the nucleus raphe magnus (NRM), producing the headache of migraine. They stimulated the dura mater or facial skin; neurons in the NRM and the trigeminal nucleus were activated. NRM stimulation suppressed the response of trigeminal neurons to electrical and mechanical stimulation of the dura mater, but not of the skin. Electrical stimulation of the NRM excites on-cells, off-cells, neutral cells, and fibers of passage. The suppression was antagonized by the iontophoretic application of the 5-HT1B/1D receptor antagonist GR127935 to trigeminal neurons. Migraine trigger factors, simulated by CSD and light flash, inhibited NRM neuronal activity. Multiple waves of CSD antagonized the inhibitory effect of NRM stimulation on responses of trigeminal neurons to dural mechanical stimulation but not to skin mechanical stimulation. Cortical activation produced by CSD may produce long-term hyperpolarization of a subset of NRM neurons, reducing their basal discharge rate and rendering them less susceptible to depolarization imposed by a nearby stimulating electrode and thus facilitating nociception.[237]

Microembolism can produce small brain foci of ischemia, which can trigger CSD in mice.[238] Microscopic infarcts were found in less than half of the other animals. CSD occurrence was associated with the depth and duration of blood flow deficit but did not correlate with the presence of microscopic lesions regardless of whether air (0.8 μL), microspheres (10 μm), or cholesterol crystals (<70 μm) were injected. Air microbubbles triggered CSD but did not cause any tissue damage. These findings may be relevant to migraine in patients who have patent foramen ovale (PFO) with right-to-left cardiac shunts, wherein the filtering capacity of the lungs is bypassed. In patients with migraine with aura and PFO, injection of air bubbles into a peripheral vein induced multiple focal or bilateral temporo-occipital electroencephalographic disturbances.[239] Bubble injection induced an attack of migraine with aura in one of the seven patients, as is occasionally reported during the microbubbles studies used to detect PFO.[240,241]

The risk of developing a migraine attack during microembolization depends not only on the location, size, and duration of transient vascular micro-occlusion, but also on the susceptibility of the brain to developing CSD. The fact that PFO closure reduces attack frequency but does not eliminate migraine attacks is not surprising, although published case series of PFO closure were not properly controlled. A shared genetic predisposition for the inter-atrial defect and the tendency for migraine with aura has also been suggested.[242]

What Could Initiate Activation of Trigeminovascular Afferents in the Absence of a Clinical Aura?

Potential mechanisms include CSD in *less eloquent* areas of the cerebral cortex, subcortical regions, or cerebellum. In addition, trigeminal afferents may be activated by events initiated in the brainstem due to descending facilitation, as suggested by Lambert. Stress can also activate meningeal plasma cells via a parasympathetic mechanism, leading to nociceptor activation.[243]

Migraine headaches are often precipitated by stress and may involve NI of the dura mater. Trigeminal nerve stimulation activates rat dura mast cells and increases vascular permeability, effects inhibited by neonatal pretreatment with capsaicin implicating sensory neuropeptides, such as SP. The role of NI (assessed by extravasation of 99-technetium-gluceptate) as well as the role of mast cells and SP and its receptor (NK-1R) in the dura mater of mice in response to acute stress has been investigated.[243] Restraint stress for 30 minutes significantly increased technetium-gluceptate extravasation in the dura mater of C57BL mice. This effect was absent in mast cell–deficient mice and NK-1 receptor knockout mice, but was unaltered in SP knockout mice. Acute restraint stress also resulted in increased dural mast cell activation in C57BL mice, but not in NK-1 receptor knockout mice. Thus, acute stress triggers NI and mast cell activation in mouse dura mater through the activation of NK-1 receptors. SP knockout mice had intact vascular permeability response to stress, which indicates that perhaps other NK-1 receptor agonist may substitute for SP. These results may help explain initial events in the pathogenesis of stress-induced migraines.[243] Alternatively, stress can cause cortical activation, which could disinhibit craniovascular sensation through the NRM producing the headache of migraine.[237]

The role of parasympathetic nerve fibers in the generation of plasma extravasation is not yet clear. Parasympathetic agonists can activate mast cells and/or sensory C-fibers, inducing pain and inflammation. Direct electrical stimulation of the sphenopalatine ganglion (SPG) of rats increased plasma extravasation of bovine serum albumin in the dura mater. Activation of the intracranial parasympathetic system by electrical stimulation of the SPG results in NI in the rat dura mater.[244] The development of NI was estimated either by microscopic examination or by quantitative measurement of PPE in the dura. SPG stimulation increased PPE by 200% in the stimulated side. Extravasation was significantly reduced by capsaicin pre-treatment and completely abolished by atropine. Carbachol infusion in the common carotid artery induced PPE in the ipsilateral dura (comparable to that induced by electrical stimulation of the SPG). The parasympathetic nervous system may trigger NI in the dura via muscarinic cholinergic receptors.[245] Trigeminal transaction blocks PPE after SD, while parasympathetic transaction does not, suggesting that they work by parallel mechanisms.[230] The release of parasympathetic vasodilator substances involved in meningeal blood flow regulation may in turn be regulated by stimuli acting at parasympathetic nerve terminals.[244]

Clinically silent CSD occurred in migraine without aura.[33] Can CSD-like events be demonstrated in functional imaging studies of subjects with migraine without aura, in addition to the subject with visually triggered migraine without aura? CSD is present in a number of disorders, including epilepsy, transient global amnesia, head trauma, and stroke,[246] in the absence of aura.

CSD occurs in damaged cortical tissue. Electrocorticographic (ECoG) activity has been recorded for up to 129 hours from 12 acutely brain-injured human patients using six platinum electrodes placed near foci of damaged cortical tissue.[247] Six of the12 patients displayed a total of 73 spontaneous episodes of spreading depression of the ECoG. Slow potential changes (0.005–0.05 Hz) were measured to test the hypothesis that the ECoG depressions were identical to Leao's CSD. (Changes in the slow potential indicate brain tissue depolarization.) Spreading ECoG depressions were always accompanied by stereotyped slow potential changes, which spread across the cortical mantle at 3.3 (0.41–10) mm/min (median, range), that is, at the same speed of spread as the depression of the ECoG activity. This is the first direct recording of peri-infarct depolarizations in an acutely injured human brain. CSD was recorded in four of five traumatic brain injury patients, and in two of seven patients with spontaneous hemorrhages.

Prospective studies suggest that headache and associated migraine symptoms are often present during aura.[248] How does one explain the onset of aura during or even after the headache, if aura generates the headache? How does one explain migraine aura without headache? CSD may be due, in part, to calcium waves, which may not always trigger CSD. Astrocytic calcium signaling is expressed as slowly propagating waves of intracellular calcium increases.[249] Astrocytic calcium waves have been implicated in a variety of physiologic and pathologic processes. A role for astrocytic calcium waves has also been proposed in migraine headache and the spread of seizures. [250] The identification of connexin hemichannels as a pathway for stimulus-evoked release of small molecules[251] raises the possibility that other intercellular messengers, in addition to ATP, may be released via this pathway. Calcium plays a role in CSD initiation and propagation. CSD is associated with elevated intracellular and reduced extracellular calcium.[252] CSD shares some similarities with astrocytic calcium waves, including the velocity of propagation, the stimulation and inhibition pattern, and the pattern of migration.[253] CSD was associated with increases in intracellular calcium that had a wave-like appearance in hippocampal slices. This calcium dynamic is attributable in part to astrocytic contributions.[254] Studying SD in hippocampal organ cultures revealed that two distinct calcium waves precede SD. The first spreads rapidly along the basilar pyramidal cell dendrites, whereas the second travels slowly and mostly perpendicular to the pyramidal cell layer.[255 Glial calcium waves are observed in conjunction with electrophysiological spreading depression in brain slices.[256] Glial calcium waves can be dissociated from spreading depression in these preparations. Thus they are related but distinct phenomena with independent mechanisms of propagation.

There is an interaction between CSD and calcium waves within the astrocyte population in slices from mouse neocortex.[256] After local KCl ejection as a trigger for CSD, the propagation of calcium increases was recorded within a large population of identified astrocytes in synchrony with CSD measured as intrinsic optical signal or negative DC-potential shift. The two events spread with 39.2±3.3 μm/sec until the intrinsic optical signal and negative DC-potential shift decayed after ~ 1 mm. However, the astrocyte calcium wave continued to propagate for up to another 500 μm, but with a reduced speed of 18.3±2.5 μm/sec, which is also typical for glial calcium waves in white matter or culture. When CSD was blocked using MK-801 (an NMDA-receptor antagonist), the astrocytic calcium wave persisted with a reduced speed. The specific gap junction blocker, carbenoxolon, did not prevent CSD but decelerated the speed of the astrocytic calcium wave. CSD determines the velocity of an accompanying astrocytic calcium response, but the astrocytic calcium wave penetrates a larger territory and represents a self-reliant phenomenon with a different mechanism of propagation.[256] Thus, calcium waves may occur and be silent and may not always accompany CSD. There may be continuous runs of CSD and/or calcium waves that may not always trigger cortical neurons, but could trigger trigeminal afferents.

CSD may occur in the cerebellum. Preliminary data have shown that blood flow decreases in the cerebellum and in the brain during a migraine attack. The decrease in the cerebellar rCBF (15%–30%) is compatible with a cerebellar CSD-like event. This can produce the common symptoms of dizziness and disequilibrium seen during a migraine attack and meningeal nociceptor activation.

In summary, calcium signaling can be part of and can lead to CSD. Both can be clinically silent. Waves of both may occur during migraine with aura; only some may trigger cortical neuronal activation and aura. In migraine without aura, SD could occur in the cerebellum. Or could CSD be silent? The presence of bilateral calcium waves activating trigeminal afferents could account for headache ipsilateral to aura. Hypotheses include the following:

- Migraine with/without aura could all be secondary to CSD.
  - Only symptomatic CSD occurring in cortex is experienced as aura.
  - CSD in subcortical structures and cerebellum may not manifest with aura symptoms.
- Migraine with/without aura could all be secondary to calcium waves.
  - Migraine with aura could be secondary to symptomatic CSD.
- All migraine in patients with migraine with aura probably has the same mechanism.

How does this relate to therapy? Ayata et al. [257] showed that migraine preventive medications given chronically, but not acutely, block CSD. Ayata et al. treated rats, either acutely or chronically, with topiramate, valproate, propranolol, amitriptyline, and methysergide, vehicle, or D-propranolol, a clinically ineffective drug. The impact of treatment was determined by the frequency of evoked CSDs after topical potassium application or by the incremental cathodal stimulation threshold to evoke CSD. They found that chronic administration of migraine prophylactic drugs dose-dependently suppressed CSD frequency by 40%–80% and increased the cathodal stimulation threshold, whereas acute treatment was ineffective. Longer treatment durations produced stronger CSD suppression. Chronic D-propranolol treatment did not differ from saline control. These data suggest that CSD provides a common therapeutic target for widely prescribed migraine prophylactic drugs.

How generalized are these results? Bogdanov et al. tested the effect on CSD of three drugs used in migraine prevention: lamotrigine, which is selectively effective on the aura but not on the headache, and valproate and riboflavin, which have a non-selective effect. Rats received intraperitoneal injections of one of the three drugs daily for 4 weeks. After treatment, CSDs were elicited for 2 hours by occipital KCl application. Lamotrigine suppressed CSDs by 37% and 60% at posterior and anterior electrodes. Valproate had no effect on posterior CSDs, but reduced anterior ones by 32% and slowed propagation velocity. Riboflavin had no significant effect at either recording site. Frontal fos expression was decreased after lamotrigine and valproate, but not after riboflavin. This study shows that preventive anti-migraine drugs have differential effects on CSD and are compatible with a causal role of CSD in migraine with aura, but not in migraine without aura.[258]

ASSOCIATED SYMPTOMS OF MIGRAINE

Photophobia

Migraine headache is exacerbated by exposure to light (photophobia). In a now-landmark study, 20 legally blind migraineurs, some with the ability to perceive light (they maintain non–image-forming photoregulation) and others without this ability, were exposed to light during a migraine headache.[259] In patients with light perception, but not in those unable to perceive light, migraine headache intensity was greater during light exposure. In migraine patients with normal eyesight, the exacerbation of headache by light involves both extrinsic photoactivation of intrinsically photosensitive retinal ganglion and intrinsic photoactivation of melanopsin. Melanopsin is a photopigment found in specialized photosensitive ganglion cells of the retina that are involved in the regulation of circadian rhythms, pupillary light reflex, and other non-visual responses to light. Entrainment to light, by which periods of behavioral activity or inactivity (sleep) are synchronized with the light-dark cycle, is not as effective in melanopsin knockout mice, but mice lacking rods and cones still exhibit circadian entrainment. The pupillary reflex is also retained in mice lacking rods and cones but has severely reduced sensitivity, identifying a crucial input from the rods and cones.

Blind people who entrain to the 24-hour light/dark cycle have eyes with functioning operative non-visual light-sensitive cells, which convey their signals to the circadian clock via the retinohypothalamic tract. The presence of migraine photophobia in blind patients was associated with the preservation of pupillary light reflex and circadian photoentrainment. Histological examination demonstrated preservation of the inner layer of the melanopsin-expressing intrinsically photosensitive retinal ganglion cells. Using single-unit recording and neural tract tracing in the rat, a retino-thalamic-cortical pathway was identified: specifically, dura-sensitive neurons in the posterior thalamus whose activity was distinctly modulated by light and whose axons projected extensively across layers I–V of somatosensory, visual, and associative cortices.[259] During exposure to ambient light, there was a doubling of activity in these thalamic neurons compared with their activity during no light exposure (dark). Cortical projections were mapped from these dura-sensitive and light-sensitive thalamic neurons to the primary somatosensory cortex, motor cortex, retrosplenial cortex, primary association cortex, primary visual cortex, and secondary visual cortex. The cell bodies and dendrites of such dura/light-sensitive neurons were opposed by axons originating from retinal ganglion cells (RGCs), predominantly from intrinsically photosensitive RGCs, the principle conduit of non–image-forming photoregulation. Photoregulation of migraine headache may be exerted by a non–image-forming retinal pathway that modulates the activity of dura-sensitive thalamocortical neurons. This is a mechanism for the exacerbation of migraine headache by light, whereby the activity of a nociceptive pathway is modulated at the level of the thalamus by retinal photoactivation. This photomodulation is exerted by axonal projections of RGCs that converge on dura-sensitive neurons in a discrete area in the posterior thalamus. The retinal projection to lateral posterior thalamic nuclei and the posterior thalamic nuclear group is distinct from the main visual pathway.

Noseda and Burstein distinguish the aforementioned classical migraine-type photophobia I from type II, wherein migraineurs describe photophobia as an increased perception of light intensity.[260] This aversion to light may be mediated the flow of nociceptive signals along the trigeminovascular pathway to light/dura-sensitive thalamic neurons that project directly to the primary and secondary visual cortices (Figure 5.7).

A third type of photophobia, termed photooculodynia, is manifest as ocular pain induced by exposure to bright light and likely mediated by indirect activation of intraocular trigeminal nociceptors. A novel reflex circuit necessary for bright light to excite nociceptive neurons in superficial laminae of trigeminal subnucleus caudalis (Vc/C1) exists.[261] Vc/C1 neurons encode light intensity and display a long delay (> 10 sec) for activation. Microinjection of lidocaine into the eye or trigeminal root ganglion (TRG) inhibited light responses completely, whereas topical application onto the ocular surface had no effect. This light-evoked Vc/C1 activity was mediated

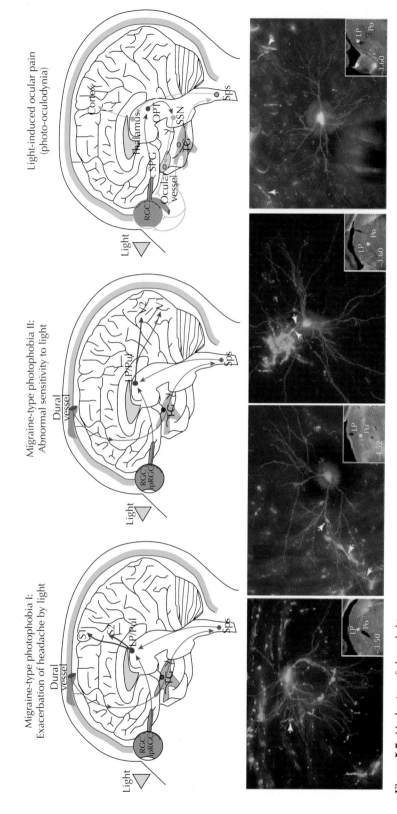

Figure 5.7. Mechanism of photophobia.

by an intraocular mechanism and transmission through the TRG. Disrupting local vasomotor activity by intraocular microinjection of vasoconstrictive agents (norepinephrine or phenylephrine) blocked light-evoked neural activity, whereas ocular surface or intra-TRG microinjection of norepinephrine had no effect. Pupillary muscle activity did not contribute, since light-evoked responses were not altered by atropine. Microinjection of lidocaine into the superior salivatory nucleus diminished light-evoked Vc/C1 activity and lacrimation, suggesting that increased parasympathetic outflow was critical for light-evoked responses. The reflex circuit required input through accessory visual pathways since both Vc/C1 activity and lacrimation were prevented by local blockade of the olivary pretectal nucleus. Thus bright light activates trigeminal nerve activity through an intraocular mechanism driven by a luminance-responsive circuit and increased parasympathetic outflow to the eye. This is one mechanism in which a reflex (light-aversive behavior) is elicited to guard against retinal damage.

PET has been used to study cortical responses to light stimulation alone and light stimulation combined with painful trigeminal stimulation. Cortical responses of seven migraineurs between attacks and the responses of seven matched control subjects to luminous stimulations were studied at three luminance intensities: 0, 600, and 1800 Cd/m2 with and without concomitant trigeminal pain stimulation.[262] To facilitate habituation, the stimulations were started 30 seconds before PET acquisitions. Light stimulation alone caused activations of bilateral visual cortices in migraineurs, but no activation in controls. Concomitant pain stimulation allowed visual cortex activation in control subjects and potentiated its activation in migraineurs. These activations were luminance-intensity-dependent in both groups. Concomitant stimulation by pain was associated with activation of the posterior parietal cortex (Brodmann's Area 7) in migraineurs and controls. Concomitant pain and light stimulation was associated with activation of the posterior parietal cortex (Brodmann's Area 7) in migraineurs but not in controls. Migraineurs had a lack of habituation and/or cortical hyperexcitability to light. The activation by light of several visual cortex

areas (including the primary visual cortex) was potentiated by trigeminal pain, demonstrating multisensory integration in these areas.[262]

Functional magnetic resonance imaging of a non-migraine patient with photophobia has detected activations within the trigeminal system. Moulton et al.[263] studied a healthy subject with transient photophobia (induced by the overuse of contact lenses). While being scanned in a darkened environment, the subject was presented with intermittent 6-s blocks of bright light. The subject was scanned twice, once during his photophobic state and once after recovery. The visual stimuli produced pain (pain intensity = 3/10 and unpleasantness = 7/10) only during the photophobic state. Specific activation patterns in the trigeminal system were seen at the level of the trigeminal ganglion, TNC, and ventroposteromedial thalamus. The anterior cingulate cortex, a brain structure associated with unpleasantness, was also active during photophobia. After recovery from photophobia, no significant activations were detected in these areas. It is uncertain whether the results are generalizable to photophobia related to migraine.

Phonophobia

There is evidence for an association between trigeminal pain and phonophobia. Sound aversiveness was investigated using a rodent model of recurrent headaches.[264] In this model, repetitive inflammatory stimulation of the rat dura was carried out over weeks. The acoustic startle reflex was used to determine sound sensitivity, and periorbital pressure thresholds were measured to detect development of sensitization. Recurrent dural stimulation resulted in a decrease in the sound intensity (12 ± 1.7 dB) needed to cause the startle reflex, suggesting that the rats had in fact become hypersensitive to sound. The timing of the decrease in startle threshold correlated with the onset of allodynia, measured as a reduction in periorbital pressure thresholds. In control rats (saline infusions), there was no change in the intensity of sound needed to cause the startle reflex, and there were no changes in periorbital pain thresholds. Investigators concluded that repetitive attacks of headache may lead to phonophobia.

Nausea/Emesis

Nausea (with or without vomiting) is highly prevalent in migraine and can cause patients to delay or avoid taking oral medication with a resultant loss or reduction of therapeutic efficacy. Nausea can occur before, during, or after the headache of migraine. It is uncertain what generates the nausea and vomiting of migraine. Both peripheral (glosophararyngeal and vagal nerves) and central (cortical and cerebellar) pathways can activate neuronal nuclei in the brainstem and trigger the vomiting reflex. Ingestion of toxin, traumatic events, adverse drug reactions, and motion can all result in nausea and emesis. Chemosensitive receptors in the chemoreceptor trigger zone (CRTZ) in the area postrema outside the blood–brain barrier detect emetic agents in the blood and relay this information to the adjacent nucleus tractus solitarius (NTS). Abdominal vagal afferents that detect intestinal luminal contents and gastric tone also terminate in the NTS. Neurons from the NTS project to a central pattern generator (CPG), which coordinates the act of emesis, and to neurons in the ventral medulla and hypothalamus. The 5-HT3 receptor antagonists work on the peripheral terminals of vagal afferents in the gastrointestinal tract and in the CRTZ. Neurokinin-1 receptor (SP) antagonists are potent antiemetics that inhibit the NTS. Neurokinin-1 receptor antagonists are antiemetics, because they act at a site in the dorsal vagal complex.[265,266]

CONCLUSION

The migraine aura may be due to CSD or calcium waves. Headache probably results from activation of meningeal and blood vessel nociceptors, combined with a change in central pain modulation. Headache and its associated neurovascular changes are subserved by the trigeminal system. Stimulation results in the release of SP and CGRP from sensory C-fiber terminals and NI.[86] NI sensitizes nerve fibers (peripheral sensitization), which now respond to previously innocuous stimuli, such as CSF, or perhaps blood vessel pulsations, causing, in part, the pain of migraine. Ahn found the throbbing pain rate was substantially slower than the arterial pulse rate and, among the few individuals in whom the rates were the same, the occurrences of throbbing and arterial pulsations fell in and out of phase with each other.[158]

Central sensitization of TNC neurons can also occur. Central sensitization may play a key role in maintaining the headache. Brainstem activation also occurs in migraine without aura, in part due to increased activity of the endogenous anti-nociceptive system. The migraine aura can trigger headache: CSD activates trigeminovascular afferents. Stress can also activate meningeal plasma cells via a parasympathetic mechanism, leading to nociceptor activation.[243] Migraine may be a result of abnormal modulation of pain and sensory input. The aura is triggered in the hyperexcitable cortex (CSD). Headache is generated by central pain facilitation and NI. Central sensitization can occur, in part mediated by supraspinal facilitation. Decreased anti-nociceptive system activity and increased peripheral input may be present.

REFERENCES

1. Giffin NJ, Ruggiero L, Lipton RB, et al. Premonitory symptoms in migraine: an electronic diary study. *Neurology*. 2003;60:935–940.
2. Hauge AW, Kirchmann M, Olesen J. Characterization of consistent triggers of migraine with aura. *Cephalalgia*. 2011;31:416–438.
3. Coppola G, Pierelli F, Schoenen J. Is the cerebral cortex hyperexcitable or hyperresponsive in migraine? *Cephalalgia*. 2007;27:1427–1439.
4. Goadsby PJ, Lipton RB, Ferrari MD. Migraine-current understanding and treatment. *N Engl J Med*. 2002;346:257–270.
5. Ray BS, Wolff HG. Experimental studies on headache. Pain sensitive structures of the head and their significance in headache. *Arch Surg*. 1940;41:813–856.
6. Penfield W. A contribution to the mechanism of intracranial pain. *Proc Assoc Res Nerv Men Dis*. 1934;15:399–415.
7. Arbab MA, Wiklund L, Svendgaard NA. Origin and distribution of cerebral vascular innervation from superior cervical, trigeminal and spinal ganglia investigated with retrograde and anterograde WGA-HRP tracing in the rat. *Neuroscience*. 1986;19:695–708.
8. Uddman R, Hara H, Edvinsson L. Neuronal pathways to the rat middle meningeal artery revealed by retrograde tracing and immunocytochemistry. *J Auton Nerv Syst*. 1989;26:69–75.
9. Messlinger K, Strassman AM, Burstein R. Anatomy and physiology of pain-sensitive cranial structures. In: Silberstein SD, Lipton RB, Dodick DW, eds. *Wolff's headache and other head pain*. 8th ed. New York: Oxford University Press, 2008:95–104.

10. Levy D. Migraine pain and nociceptor activation—where do we stand? *Headache*. 2010;50:909–916.
11. Strassman AM, Weissner W, Williams W, Ali S, Levy D. Axon diameters and intradural trajectories of the dural innervation in the rat. *J Comp Neurol*. 2004;473:364–376.
12. Strassman AM, Vos BP, Mineta Y, Naderi S, Borsook D, Burnstein R. Fos-like immunoreactivity in the superficial medullary dorsal horn induced by noxious and innocuous themal stimulation of the facial skin in the rat. *J Neuropysiol*. 1993;70:1821.
13. Yokota T, Nishikawa Y, Koyama N. Tooth pulp input to the shell region of nucleus ventralis posteromedialis of the cat thalamus. *J Neurophysiol*. 1986;56:80–98.
14. Sessle BJ, Hu JW, Dubner R, Lucier GE. Functional properties of neurons in cat trigeminal subnucleus caudalis (medullary dorsal horn). II. Modulation of responses to noxious and nonnoxious stimuli by periaqueductal gray, nucleus raphe magnus, cerebral cortex, and afferent influences, and effect of naloxone. *J Neurophysiol*. 1981;45:193–207.
15. Kruger L, Young RF. Specialized features of the trigeminal nerveand its central connections. In: Samii M, Janetta PJ, eds. *The cranial nerves*. Berlin: Springer-Verlag, 1981:273–301.
16. Wise SP, Jones EG. Cells of origin and terminal distribution of descending projections of the rat somatic sensory cortex. *J Comp Neurol*. 1977;175:129–157.
17. Jacquin MF, Chiaia NL, Haring JH, Rhoades RW. Intersubnuclear connections within the rat trigeminal brainstem complex. *Somatosens Mot Res*. 1990;7:399–420.
18. Renehan WE, Jacquin MF, Mooney RD, Rhoades RW. Structure-function relationships in rat medullary and cervical dorsal horns. II. Medullary dorsal horn cells. *J Neurophysiol*. 1986;55:1187–1201.
19. DaSilva AF, Becerra L, Makris N, et al. Somatotopic activation in the human trigeminal pain pathway. *J Neurosci*. 2002;22:8183–8192.
20. Sweatt JD, Weeber EJ, Levenons JM. Central neural mechanisms that interrelate sensory and affective dimensions of pain. *Mol Interven*. 2002;2:393–402.
21. Messlinger K, Burstein R. Anatomy of central nervous system pathways related to head pain. In: Olesen J, Tfelt-Hansen P, Welch KMA, eds. *The headaches*. 2nd ed. Philadelphia: Lippincott, Williams & Wilkins, 1999:77.
22. Schueler M, Messlinger K, Dux M, Neuhuber WL, de CR. Extracranial projections of meningeal afferents and their impact on meningeal nociception and headache. *Pain*. 2013;154:1622–1631.
23. Weiller C, May A, Limmroth V, et al. Brainstem activation in spontaneous human migraine attacks. *Nat Med*. 1995;1:658–660.
24. Cutrer FM. Pathophysiology of migraine. *Semin Neurol*. 2010;30:120–130.
25. Ambrosini A, Schoenen J. The electrophysiology of migraine. *Curr Opin Neurol*. 2003;16:327–331.
26. Maniyar FH, Sprenger T, Monteith T, Schankin C, Goadsby PJ. Brain activations in the premonitory phase of nitroglycerin-triggered migraine attacks. *Brain*. 2014;137:232–241.
27. Wolff HG. *Headache and other head pain*. New York: Oxford University, 1963.
28. Olesen J, Friberg L, Skyhoj-Olsen T. Timing and topography of cerebral blood flow, aura and headache during migraine attacks. *Ann Neurol*. 1990;28:791–798.
29. Sanchez del RM, Bakker D, Wu O, et al. Perfusion weighted imaging during migraine: spontaneous visual aura and headache. *Cephalalgia*. 1999;19:701–707.
30. Cutrer FM, O'Donnell A. Recent advances in functional neuroimaging. *Curr Opin Neurol*. 1999;12:255–259.
31. Hadjikhani N, Sanchez del RM, Wu O, et al. Mechanisms of migraine aura revealed by functional MRI in human visual cortex. *Proc Natl Acad Sci USA*. 2001;98:4687–4692.
32. Pietrobon D, Striessnic J. Neurobiology of migraine. *Nat Rev Neurosci*. 2003;4:386–398.
33. Woods RP, Iacoboni M, Mazziotta JC. Bilateral spreading cerebral hypoperfusion during spontaneous migraine headaches. *N Eng J Med*. 1994;331:1689–1692.
34. Denuelle M, Fabre N, Payoux P, Chollet F, Geraud G. Posterior cerebral hypoperfusion in migraine without aura. *Cephalalgia*. 2008;28:856–862.
35. Lashley KS. Patterns of cerebral integration indicated by the scotomas of migraine. *Arch Neurol*. 1941;46:331–339.
36. Leao AAP. Spreading depression of activity in cerebral cortex. *J Neurophysiol*. 1944;7:359–390.
37. Otori T, Greenberg JH, Welsh FA. Cortical spreading depression causes a long-lasting decrease in cerebral blood flow and induces tolerance to permanent focal ischemia in rat brain. *J Cereb Blood Flow Metab*. 2003;23:43–50.
38. Strong AJ. Detecting and characterizing spreading depression in the injured human brain. *J Cereb Blood Flow Metab*. 2003;23:748.
39. Haerter-Eikermann K, Moskowitz M. Pathophysiology of aura. In: Silberstein SD, Lipton RB, Dodick DW, eds. *Wolff's headache and other head pain*. 8th ed. New York: Oxford University Press, 2007:121–132.
40. Somjen GG. Mechanisms of spreading depression and hypoxic spreading depression-like depolarization. *Physiol Rev*. 2001;81:1065–1096.
41. Takano T, Tian GF, Peng W, et al. Cortical spreading depression causes and coincides with tissue hypoxia. *Nat Neurosci*. 2007;10:754–762.
42. Olesen J, Larsen B, Lauritzen M. Focal hyperemia followed by spreading oligemia and impaired activation of RCBF in classic migraine. *Ann Neurol*. 1981;9:344–352.
43. Olesen J. Cerebral and extracranial circulatory disturbances in migraine: pathophysiological implications. *Cerebrovasc Brain Metab Rev*. 1991;3:1–28.
44. Milner PM. Note on a possible correspondence between the scotomas of migraine and spreading depression of Leao. *Electroencephalography Clin Neurophysiol*. 1958;10:705.
45. Andersen AR, Friberg L, Skyloj-Olsen T, Olesen J. Delayed hyperemia following hypoperfusion in classic migraine: single photon emission tomographic demonstration. *Arch Neurol*. 1988;45:154–159.
46. Cao Y, Welch KM, Aurora S, Vikingstad EM. Functional MRI-BOLD of visually triggered headache in patients with migraine. *Arch Neurol*. 1999;56:548–554.
47. Cutrer FM, Sorensen AG, Weisskoff RM, et al. Perfusion-weighted imaging defects during spontaneous migrainous aura. *Ann Neurol*. 1998;43:25–31.
48. Barkley GL, Tepley N, Nagel L, Moran J, Simkins R, Welch KMA. Magnetoencephalographic studies of migraine. *Headache*. 1990;30:428–434.

49. Bowyer SM, Aurora KS, Moran JE, Tepley N, Welch KM. Magnetoencephalographic fields from patients with spontaneous and induced migraine aura. *Ann Neurol*. 2001;50:582–587.

50. Siniatchkin M, Gerber WD, Kropp P, Vein A. Contingent negative variation in patients with chronic daily headache. *Cephalalgia*. 1998;18:565–569.

51. Chen WT, Wang SJ, Fuh JL, Lin CP, Ko YC, Lin YY. Persistent ictal-like visual cortical excitability in chronic migraine. *Pain*. 2011;152:254–258.

52. Stankewitz A, May A. The phenomenon of changes in cortical excitability in migraine is not migraine-specific: a unifying thesis. *Pain*. 2009;145:14–17.

53. Chen WT, Lin YY, Fuh JL, Hamalainen MS, Ko YC, Wang SJ. Sustained visual cortex hyperexcitability in migraine with persistent visual aura. Brain. 2011; 134(8):2387–2395.

54. Aurora SK, Cao Y, Bowyer SM, Welch KM. The occipital cortex is hyperexcitable in migraine: experimental evidence. *Headache*. 1999;39:469–476.

55. Young WB, Oshinsky ML, Shechter AL, Wassermann EM. Consecutive transcranial magnetic stimulation induced phosphene thresholds in migraineurs and controls. *Neurology*. 2001;56:A142(Abstract).

56. Afra J, Mascia A, Gerard P, DeNoordhout AM, Schoenen J. Interictal cortical excitability in migraine: a study using transcranial magnetic stimulation of motor and visual cortices. *Ann Neurol*. 1998;44:209–215.

57. Aurora SK, Barrodale P, Chronicle EP, Mulleners WM. Cortical inhibition is reduced in chronic and episodic migraine and demonstrates a spectrum of illness. *Headache*. 2005;45:546–552.

58. Aurora SK, Barrodale PM, Tipton RL, Khodavirdi A. Brainstem dysfunction in chronic migraine as evidenced by neurophysiological and positron emission tomography studies. *Headache*. 2007;47:996–1003.

59. Siniatchkin M, Reich AL, Shepherd AJ, van BA, Siebner HR, Stephani U. Peri-ictal changes of cortical excitability in children suffering from migraine without aura. *Pain*. 2009;147:132–140.

60. Sand T, Zhitniy N, White LR, Stovner LJ. Visual evoked potential latency, amplitude and habituation in migraine: a longitudinal study. *Clin Neurophysiol*. 2008;119:1020–1027.

61. Afra J. Intensity dependence of auditory evoked cortical potentials in migraine. Changes in the peri-ictal period. *Funct Neurol*. 2005;20:199–200.

62. Coppola G, Vandenheede M, Di CL, et al. Somatosensory evoked high-frequency oscillations reflecting thalamo-cortical activity are decreased in migraine patients between attacks. *Brain*. 2005;128:98–103.

63. De Tommaso, M, Libro G, Guido M, Losito L, Lamberti P, Livrea P. Habituation of single CO2 laser-evoked responses during interictal phase of migraine. *J Headache Pain*. 2005;6:195–198.

64. Grosser K, Oelkers R, Hummel T, et al. Olfactory and trigeminal event-related potentials in migraine. *Cephalalgia*. 2000;20:621–631.

65. Katsarava Z, Giffin N, Diener HC, Kaube H. Abnormal habituation of "nociceptive" blink reflex in migraine: evidence for increased excitability of trigeminal nociception. *Cephalalgia*. 2003;23:814–819.

66. Ambrosini A, De Noordhout AM, Sandor PS, Schoenen J. Electrophysiological studies in migraine: a comprehensive review of their interest and limitations. *Cephalalgia*. 2003;23(Suppl 1):13–31.

67. Aurora SK, Wilkinson F. The brain is hyperexcitable in migraine. *Cephalalgia*. 2007;27:1442–1453.

68. Schoenen J, Thomsen LL. Neurophysiology and autonomic dysfunction in migraine. In: Olesen J, Tfelt-Hansen P, Welch KMA, eds. *The headaches*. 2nd ed. Philadelphia: Lippincott Williams & Wilkins, 2000:301–312.

69. Lang E, Kaltenhauser M, Neundorfer B, Seidler S. Hyperexcitability of the primary somatosensory cortex in migraine: a magnetoencephalographic study. *Brain*. 2004;127:2459–2469.

70. Siniatchkin M, Averkina N, Andrasik F, Stephani U, Gerber WD. Neurophysiological reactivity before a migraine attack. *Neurosci Lett*. 2006;400:121–124.

71. Ozkul Y, Uckardes A. Median nerve somatosensory evoked potentials in migraine. *Eur J Neurol*. 2002;9:227–232.

72. Coppola G, Curra A, Di Lorenzo C, et al. Abnormal cortical responses to somatosensory stimulation in medication-overuse headache. *BMC Neurol*. 2010;10:126(Abstract).

73. Curra A, Copolla G, Gorini M, et al. Drug-induced changes in cortical inhibition in medication overuse headache. *Cephalalgia*. 2011;31:1282–1290.

74. Peters ML, Schmidt AJ, Van den Hout MA. Chronic low back pain and the reaction to repeated acute pain stimulation. *Pain*. 1989;39:69–76.

75. Flor H. The modification of cortical reorganization and chronic pain by sensory feedback. *Appl Psychophysiol Biofeedback*. 2002;27:215–227.

76. Flor H, Diers M, Birbaumer N. Peripheral and electro-cortical responses to painful and non-painful stimulation in chronic pain patients, tension headache patients and healthy controls. *Neurosci Lett*. 2004;361:147–150.

77. Flor H, Nikolajsen L, Staehelin JT. Phantom limb pain: a case of maladaptive CNS plasticity? *Nat Rev Neurosci*. 2006;7:873–881.

78. May A. Chronic pain may change the structure of the brain. *Pain*. 2008;137:7–15.

79. Walpurger V, Hebing-Lennartz G, Denecke H, Pietrowsky R. Habituation deficit in auditory event-related potentials in tinnitus complainers. *Hear Res*. 2003;181:57–64.

80. Meincke U, Light GA, Geyer MA, Braff DL, Gouzoulis-Mayfrank E. Sensitization and habituation of the acoustic startle reflex in patients with schizophrenia. *Psychiatry Res*. 2004;126:51–61.

81. Schestatsky P, Kumru H, Valls-Sole J, et al. Neurophysiologic study of central pain in patients with Parkinson disease. *Neurology*. 2007;69:2162–2169.

82. Woolf CJ, Mitchell MB. Mechanism-based pain diagnosis issues for analgesic drug development. *Anesthesiology*. 2001;95:241–249.

83. Messlinger K. Migraine: where and how does the pain originate. *Exp Brain Res*. 2009;196:179–193.

84. Pietrobon D, Moskowitz MA. Pathophysiology of migraine. *Annu Rev Physiol*. 2013;75:365–391.

85. Uddman R, Edvinsson L, Ekman R, Kingman T, McCulloch J. Innervation of the feline cerebral vasculature by nerve fibers containing calcitonin gene-related peptide: trigeminal origin an co-existence with substance P. *Neurosci Letter*. 1985;62:131–136.

86. Dimitriadou V, Buzzi MG, Theoharides TC, Moskowitz MA. Ultrastructural evidence for neurogenically mediated changes in blood vessels of the rat aura mater and tongue following antidromic trigeminal stimulation. *Neuroscience*. 1992;48:187–203.

87. Moskowitz MA. Basic mechanisms in vascular headache. *Neurol Clin*. 1990;8:801–815.

88. Moskowitz MA. Neurogenic versus vascular mechanisms of sumatriptan and ergot alkaloids in migraine. *Trends Pharmacol Sci*. 1992;13:307–311.

89. Montalcini RL, Daltos R, Dellavalle F, Skaper SD, Leon A. Update of the NGF saga. *J Neurol Sci*. 1995;130:119–127.

90. Rang HP, Urban L. New molecules in analgesia. *Br J Anaesth*. 1995;75:145–156.

91. Edelman GM, Gally JA. Nitric oxide: linking space and time in the brain. *Proc Natl Acad Sci USA*. 1992;89:11651–11652.

92. Nozaki K, Boccalini P, Moskowitz MA. Expression of c-fos-like immunoreactivity in brainstem after meningeal irritation by blood in the subarachnoid space. *Neuroscience*. 1992;49:669–680.

93. Kaube H, Keay K, Hoskin KL, Bandler R, Goadsby PJ. Expression of c-fos like immunoreactivity in the trigeminal nucleus caudalis and high cervical cord following stimulation of the sagittal sinus in the cat. *Brain Res*. 1993;629:95–102.

94. Goadsby PJ, Hoskin KL. The distribution of trigeminovascular afferents in the non-human primate brain. *J Anatomy*. 1997;190:367–375.

95. Mungliani R, Hunt SP. Molecular biology of pain. *Br J Anaesth*. 1995;75:186–192.

96. Buzzi MG, Moskowitz MA, Shimizu t, Heath HH. Dihydroergotamine and sumatriptan attenuate levels of CGRP in plasma in rat superior sagittal sinus during electrical stimulation of the trigeminal ganglion. *Neuropharmacol*. 1991;30:1193–1200.

97. Edvinsson L, Ekman R, Jansen I, McCulloch J, Uddman R. Calcitonin gene-related peptide and cerebral blood vessels: distribution and vasomotor effects. *J Cereb Blood Flow Metab*. 1987;7:720–728.

98. Ellrich J, Messlinger K, Escott KJ, Beattie DT, Connor HE, Brain SD. Trigeminal ganglion stimulation increases facial skin blood flow in the rat: a major role for calcitonin gene-related peptide. *Brain Res*. 1995;669:93–99.

99. Ottosson A, Edvinsson L. Release of histamine from dural mast cells by substance P and calcitonin gene-related peptide. *Cephalalgia*. 1997;17:166–174.

100. Buzzi MG, Moskowitz MA. Evidence for 5-HT1B/1D receptors mediating the antimigraine effect of sumatriptan and dihydroergotamine. *Cephalalgia*. 1991;11:165–168.

101. Pappagalo M, Szabo Z, Esposito G, Lokesh A, Velez L. Imaging neurogenic inflammation inpatients with migraine headaches. *Neurology*. 2002;52:274–275.

102. May A, Gijsman HJ, Wallnoefer A, Jones R, Diener HC, Ferrari MD. Endothelin antagonist bosentan blocks neurogenic inflammation, but is not effective in aborting migraine attacks. *Pain*. 1996;67:375–378.

103. Roon KI, Olesen J, Diener HC. No acute antimigraine efficacy of CP-122,288, a highly potent inhibitor of neurogenic inflammation: results of two randomized double-blind, placebo-controlled clinical trials. *Ann Neurol*. 2000;47:238–241.

104. Williamson DJ, Hargreaves RJ. Neurogenic inflammation in the context of migraine. *Microsc Res Tech*. 2001;53:167–178.

105. Zagami AS, Goadsby PJ, Edvinsson L. Stimulation of the superior sagittal sinus in the cat causes release of vasoactive peptides. *Neuropeptides*. 1990;16:69–75.

106. Goadsby PJ, Edvinsson L, Ekman R. Vasoactive peptide release in the extracerebral circulation of humans during migraine headache. *Ann Neurol*. 1990;28:183–187.

107. Goadsby PJ, Edvinsson L. The trigeminovascular system in migraine: studies characterizing cerebrovascular and neuropeptide changes seen in humans and cats. *Ann Neurol*. 1993;33:48–56.

108. Edvinsson L, Goadsby PJ. Neuropeptides in headache. *Eur J Neurol*. 1998;5:329–341.

109. Hoffmann J, Wecker S, Neeb L, Dirnagl U, Reuter U. Primary trigeminal afferents are the main source for stimulus-induced CGRP release in jugular vein blood and CSF. *Cephalalgia*. 2012;32:659–667.

110. O'Connor TP, Van der Kooy D. Enrichment of vasoactive neuropeptide (calcitonin gene related peptide) in trigeminal sensory projection to the intracranial arteries. *J Neurosci*. 1988;8:2468–2476.

111. O'Connor TP, vanderKooy D. Pattern of intracranial and extracranial projections of trigeminal ganglion cells. *J Neurosci*. 1986;6:2200–2207.

112. Olesen J, Diener HC, Husstedt IW, et al. Calcitonin gene-related peptide receptor antagonist BIBN 4096 BS for the acute treatment of migraine. *N Engl J Med*. 2004;350:1104–1110.

113. Negro A, Lionetto L, Simmaco M, Martelletti P. CGRP receptor antagonists: an expanding drug class for acute migraine? *Expert Opin Investig Drugs*. 2012;21:807–818.

114. Ho TW, Mannix LK, Fan X, et al. Randomized controlled trial of an oral CGRP receptor antagonist, MK-0974, in acute treatment of migraine. *Neurology*. 2008;70:1304–1312.

115. Ho TW, Ferrari MD, Dodick DW, et al. Efficacy and tolerability of MK-0974 (telcagepant), a new oral antagonist of calcitonin gene-related peptide receptor, compared with zolmitriptan for acute migraine: a randomised, placebo-controlled, parallel-treatment trial. *Lancet*. 2008;372:2115–2123.

116. Tfelt-Hansen P. Excellent tolerability but relatively low initial clinical efficacy of telcagepant in migraine. *Headache*. 2011;51:118–123.

117. Connor KM, Shapiro RE, Diener HC, et al. Randomized, controlled trial of telcagepant for the acute treatment of migraine. *Neurology*. 2009;73:970–977.

118. De KJ, Mostert JP, Koch MW. Dysfunctional astrocytes as key players in the pathogenesis of central nervous system disorders. *J Neurol Sci*. 2008;267:3–16.

119. Farahani R, Pina-Benabou MH, Kyrozis A, et al. Alterations in metabolism and gap junction expression may determine the role of astrocytes as "good samaritans" or executioners. *Glia*. 2005;50:351–361.

120. Nedergaard M, Cooper AJ, Goldman SA. Gap junctions are required for the propagation of spreading depression. *J Neurobiol*. 1995;28:433–444.

121. Chao CC, Gekker G, Sheng WS, Hu S, Tsang M, Peterson PK. Priming effect of morphine on the production of tumor necrosis factor-alpha by microglia: implications in respiratory burst activity and human immunodeficiency virus-1 expression. *J Pharmacol Exp Ther*. 1994;269:198–203.

122. Hains LE, Loram LC, Weiseler JL, et al. Pain intensity and duration can be enhanced by prior challenge: initial evidence suggestive of a role of microglial priming. *J Pain*. 2010;11:1004–1014.

123. Frank MG, Watkins LR, Maier SF. Stress—and glucocorticoid-induced priming of neuroinflammatory responses: potential mechanisms of stress-induced vulnerability to drugs of abuse. *Brain Behav Immun*. 2011;25(Suppl 1):S21–S28.

124. Watkins LR, Hutchinson MR, Rice KC, Maier SF. The "toll" of opioid-induced glial activation: improving the clinical efficacy of opioids by targeting glia. *Trends Pharmacol Sci*. 2009;30:581–591.

125. White FA, Jung H, Miller RJ. Chemokines and the pathophysiology of neuropathic pain. *Proc Natl Acad Sci USA*. 2007;104:20151–20158.

126. Wei F, Guo W, Zou W, Ren K, Dubner R. Supraspinal glial-neuronal interactions contribute to descending pain facilitation. *J Neurosci*. 2008;28(42):10482–10495.

127. Tanga FY, Nutile-McMenemy N, deLeo JA. The CNS role of Toll-like receptor 4 in innate neuroimmunity and painful neuropathy. *Proc Natl Acad Sci USA*. 2005;102:5856–5861.

128. Bettoni I, Comelli F, Rossini C, et al. Glial TLR4 receptor as new target to treat neuropathic pain: efficacy of a new receptor antagonist in a model of peripheral nerve injury in mice. *Glia*. 2008;56:1312–1319.

129. Hutchinson MR, Zhang Y, Brown K, et al. Non-stereoselective reversal of neuropathic pain by naloxone and naltrexone: involvement of toll-like receptor 4 (TLR4). *Eur J Neurosci*. 2008;28:20–29.

130. Hutchinson MR, Loram LC, Zhang Y, et al. Evidence that tricyclic small molecules may possess toll-like receptor and myeloid differentiation protein 2 activity. *Neuroscience*. 2010;168:551–563.

131. Okun E, Griffioen KJ, Mattson MP. Toll-like receptor signaling in neural plasticity and disease. *Trends Neurosci*. 2011;34:269–281.

132. Lehnhardt S, Massillon L, Follett P. Activation of innate immunity in the CNS triggers neurodegeneration through a toll-like receptor. *Proc Nat Acad Sci USA*. 2003;100:8514–8519.

133. Hutchinson MR, Bland ST, Johnson KW, et al. Opioid-induced glial activation: mechanisms of activation and implications for opioid analgesia, dependence, and reward. *ScientificWorldJournal*. 2007;7:98–111.

134. Hutchinson MR, Northcutt AL, Chao LW, et al. Minocycline suppresses morphine-induced respiratory depression, suppresses morphine-induced reward, and enhances systemic morphine-induced analgesia. *Brain Behav Immun*. 2008;22:1248–1256.

135. Hutchinson MR, Zhang Y, Shridhar M, et al. Evidence that opioids may have toll-like receptor 4 and MD-2 effects. *Brain Behav Immun*. 2010;22:83–95.

136. Bartley J, Watkins LR. Comment on: excessive opioid use and the development of chronic migraine. *Pain*. 2009;145:262–263.

137. Rolan P, Gibbons JA, He L, et al. Ibudilast in healthy volunteers: safety, toberability and pharmokinetics with single and multiple doses. *Br J Clin Pharmacol*. 2008;66:792–801.

138. Hutchinson MR, Northcutt AL, Hiranita T, et al. Opioid activation of toll-like receptor 4 contributes to drug reinforcement. *J Neurosci*. 2012;32:11187–11200.

139. Sarchielli P, Alberti A, Floridi A, Gallai V. Levels of nerve growth factor in cerebrospinal fluid of chronic daily headache patients. *Neurology*. 2001;57:132–134.

140. Ashina M, Bendtsen L, Jensen R, Schifter S, Jansen-Olesen I, Olesen J. Plasma levels of calcitonin gene-related peptide in chronic tension-type headache. *Neurology*. 2000;55:1335–1340.

141. Lambert GA. The lack of peripheral pathology in migraine headache. *Headache*. 2010;50:895–908.

142. Kruuse C, Thomsen LL, Birk S, Olesen J. Migraine can be induced by sildenafil without changes in middle cerebral artery diameter. *Brain*. 2003;126:241–247.

143. Schoonman GG, van der GJ, Kortmann C, van der Geest RJ, Terwindt GM, Ferrari MD. Migraine headache is not associated with cerebral or meningeal vasodilatation: a 3T magnetic resonance angiography study. *Brain*. 2008;X.

144. Evers S, Vollmer-Haase J, Schwaag S, Rahmann A, Husstedt IW, Frese A. Botulinum toxin A in the prophylactic treatment of migraine: a randomized, double-blind, placebo-controlled study. *Cephalalgia*. 2004;24:838–843.

145. Rahmann A, Wienecke T, Hansen JM, Fahrenkrug J, Olesen J, Ashina M. Vasoactive intestinal peptide causes marked cephalic vasodilation, but does not induce migraine. *Cephalalgia*. 2008;28:226–236.

146. Asghar MS, Hansen AE, Amin FM, et al. Evidence for a vascular factor in migraine. *Ann Neurol*. 2011;69:635–645.

147. Levy D, Jakubowski M, Burstein R. Disruption of communication between peripheral and central trigeminovascular neurons mediates the antimigraine action of 5HT 1B/1D receptor agonists. *Proc Natl Acad Sci USA*. 2004;101:4274–4279.

148. Levy D, Strassman AM, Burstein R. A critical view on the role of migraine triggers in the genesis of migraine pain. *Headache*. 2009;49:953–957.

149. Selby G, Lance JW. Observation on 500 cases of migraine and allied vascular headaches. *J Neurol Neurosurg Psychiatry*. 1960;23:23–32.

150. Burstein R, Yarnitsky D, Goor-Aryeh I, Ransil BJ, Bajwa ZH. An association between migraine and cutaneous allodynia. *Ann Neurol*. 2000;47:614–624.

151. Burstein R, Cutrer MF, Yarnitsky D. The development of cutaneous allodynia during a migraine attack clinical evidence for the sequential recruitment of spinal and supraspinal nociceptive neurons in migraine. *Brain*. 2000;123(Pt 8):1703–1709.

152. Burstein R, Collins B, Bajwa Z, Jakubowski M. Triptan therapy can abort migraine attacks if given before the establishment or in the absence of cutaneous allodynia and central sensitization: clinical and preclinical evidence. *Headache*. 2002;42:390(Abstract).

153. Julius D, Basbaum AI. Molecular mechanisms of nociception. *Nature*. 2001;413:203–210.

154. Ji RR, Samad TA, Jin SX, Schmoll R, Woolf CJ. p38 MAPK activation by NGF in primary sensory neurons after inflammation increases TRPV1 levels and maintains heat hyperalgesia. *Neuron*. 2002;36:57–68.

155. Strassman AM, Raymond SA, Burstein R. Sensitization of meningeal sensory neurons and the origin of headaches. *Nature*. 1996;384:560–564.

156. Anthony M, Rasmussen BK. Migraine without aura. In: Olesen J, Tfelt-Hansen P, Welch MA, eds. *The headaches*. New York: Raven Press, 1993:255–261.

157. Moskowitz MA, Cutrer FM. SUMATRIPTAN: a receptor-targeted treatment for migraine. *Annu Rev Med*. 1993;44:145–154.

158. Ahn AH. On the temporal relationship between throbbing migraine pain and arterial pulse. *Headache*. 2010;50:1507–1510.

159. Battaglia G, Rustioni A. Coexistence of glutamate and substance P in dorsal root ganglion neurons of the rat and monkey. *J Comp Neurol*. 1988;277:302–312.

160. Murase K, Ryu PD, Randic M. Substance P augments a persistent slow inward calcium-sensitive current in voltage-clamped spinal dorsal horn neurons of the rat. *Brain Res*. 1986;365:369–376.

161. Sivilotti LG. The rate of rise of the cumulative depolarization evoked by repetitive stimulation of small-calibre afferents is a predictor of action potential windup in rat spinal neurones in vitro. *J Neurophysiol*. 1993;69:1621–1631.

162. Price DD, Mao J, Mayer DJ. Central neural mechanisms of normal and abnormal pain states. In: Fields HL, Liebeskind JC, eds. *Progress in pain research and management*. Washington, DC: IASP Press, 1994:61–84.

163. Thompson SW. Activity-dependent changes in rat ventral horn neurones in vitro: summation of prolonged afferent evoked postsynaptic depolarizations produce a D-APV sensitive windup. *Eur J Neurosci*. 1990;2:638–649.

164. Woolf CJ. Somatic pain: pathogenesis and prevention. *Br J Anaesth*. 1995;75:169–176.

165. Dray A, Urban L, Dickenson A. Pharmacology of chronic pain. *Trends Pharmacol Sci*. 1994;15:190–197.

166. Post RM, Silberstein SD. Shared mechanisms in affective illness, epilepsy, and migraine. *Neurology*. 1994;44:S37–S47.

167. Woolf CJ. Evidence for a central component of postinjury pain hypersensitivity. *Nature*. 1983;306:686–688.

168. Woolf CJ, Wall PD. The relative effectiveness of C primary afferent fibres of different origins in evoking a prolonged facilitation of the flexor reflex in the rat. *J Neurosci*. 1986;6:1433–1443.

169. Cook AJ. Dynamic receptive field plasticity in rat spinal cord dorsal horn following C primary afferent input. *Nature*. 1987;325:151–153.

170. Woolf CJ, King AE. Subthreshold components of the cutaneous mechanoreceptive fields of dorsal horn neurons in the rat lumbar spinal cord. *J Neurophysiol*. 1989;62:907–916.

171. Woolf CJ, King AE. Dynamic alterations in the cutaneous mechanoreceptive fields of dorsal horn neurons in the rat spinal cord. *J Neurosci*. 1990;10:2717–2726.

172. Sarkar S, Aziz Q, Woolf CJ, Hobson AR, Thompson DG. Contribution of central sensitisation to the development of non-cardiac chest pain. *Lancet*. 2000;356:1154–1159.

173. Burstein R, Yamamura H, Malick A, Strassman AM. Chemical stimulation of the intracranial dura induces enhanced responses to facial stimulation in brainstem trigeminal neurons. *J Neurophysiol*. 1998;79:964–982.

174. Yamamura H, Malick A, Chamberlin NL, Burstein R. Cardiovascular and neuronal responses to head stimulation reflect central sensitization and cutaneous allodynia in a rat model of migraine. *J Neurophysiol*. 1999;81:479–493.

175. Bendtsen L, Jensen R, Olesen J. Qualitatively altered nociception in chronic myofascial pain. *Pain*. 1996;65:259–264.

176. Gallai V, Alberti A, Gallai B, Coppola F, Floridi A, Sarchielli P. Glutamate and nitric oxide pathway in chronic daily headache: evidence from cerebrospinal fluid. *Cephalalgia*. 2003;23:166–174.

177. Perrotta A, Arce-Leal N, Tassorelli C, Gasperi V, Sances G, Blandini F, Serrao M, Bolla M, Pierelli F, Nappi G, Maccarrone ME. Acute Reduction of Anandamide-Hydrolase (FAAH) Activity is Coupled With a Reduction of Nociceptive Pathways Facilitation in Medication-Overuse Headache Subjects After Withdrawal Treatment. *Headache: The Journal of Head and Face Pain*. 2012;52(9):1350–1361.

178. Heinricher MM, Tavares I, Leith JL, Lumb BM. Descending control of nociception: Specificity, recruitment and plasticity. *Brain Res Rev*. 2009;60:214–225.

179. Porreca F, Ossipov MH, Gebhart GF. Chronic pain and medullary descending facilitation. *Trends Neurosci*. 2002;25:319–325.

180. Zhuo M, Gebhart GF. Characterization of descending inhibition and facilitation from the nuclei reticularis gigantocellularis and gigantocellularis pars alpha in the rat. *Pain*. 1990;42:337–350.

181. Zhuo M, Gebhart GF. Characterization of descending facilitation and inhibition of spinal nociceptive transmission from the nuclei reticularis gigantocellularis and gigantocellularis pars alpha in the rat. *J Neurophysiol*. 1992;67:1599–1614.

182. Zhuo M, Gebhart GF. Biphasic modulation of spinal nociceptive transmission from the medullary raphe nuclei in the rat. *J Neurophysiol*. 1997;78:746–758.

183. Urban MO, Gebhart GF. Characterization of biphasic modulation of spinal nociceptive transmission by neurotensin in the rat rostral ventromedial medulla. *J Neurophysiol*. 1997;78:1550–1562.

184. Urban MO, Coutinho SV, Gebhart GF. Biphasic modulation of visceral nociception by neurotensin in rat rostral ventromedial medulla. *J Pharmacol Exp Ther*. 1999;290:207–213.

185. Urban MO, Coutinho SV, Gebhart GF. Involvement of excitatory amino acid receptors and nitric oxide in the rostral ventromedial medulla in modulating secondary hyperalgesia produced by mustard oil. *Pain*. 1999;81:45–55.

186. Fields HL, Heinricher MM, Mason P. Neurotransmitters as nociceptive modulatory circuits. *Annu Rev Neurosci*. 1991;219–245.

187. Kim DH, Fields HL, Barbaro NM. Morphine analgesia and acute physical dependence: rapid onset of two opposing, dose-related processes. *Brain Res*. 1990;516:37–40.

188. Bederson JB, Fields HL, Barbaro NM. Hyperalgesia during naloxone-precipitated withdrawal from morphine is associated with increased on-cell activity in the rostral ventromedial medulla. *Somatosens Mot Res*. 1990;7:185–203.

189. Kaplan H, Fields HL. Hyperalgesia during acute opioid abstinence: evidence for a nociceptive facilitating function of the rostral ventromedial medulla. *J Neurosci*. 1991;11:1433–1439.

190. Heinricher MM, Roychowdhury SM. Reflex-related activation of putative pain facilitating

neurons in rostral ventromedial medulla requires excitatory amino acid transmission. *Neuroscience*. 1997;78:1159–1165.

191. Meng ID, Harasawa I. Chronic morphine exposure increases the proportion of on-cells in the rostal ventromedial medulla in rats. *Life Sci.* 2007;80(20):1915–1920.

192. Ma QP, Woolf CJ. Noxious stimuli induce an N-methyl-D-aspartate receptor-dependent hypersensitivity of the flexion withdrawal reflex to touch: implications for the treatment of mechanical allodynia. *Pain*. 1995;61:383–390.

193. Kovelowski CJ, Ossipov MH, Sun H, Lai J, MalanJr. TP, Porreca F. Supraspinal cholecystokinin may drive tonic descending facilitation mechanisms to maintain neuropathic pain in the rat. *Pain*. 2000;87:265–273.

194. Heinricher MM, McGaraughty S, Tortorici V. Circuitry underlying antiopioid actions of cholecystokinin within the rostral ventromedial medulla. *J Neurophysiol*. 2001;85:280–286.

195. Dourish CT, O'Neill MF, Coughlan J, Kitchener SJ, Hawley D, Iversen SD. The selective CCK-B receptor antagonist L-365,260 enhances morphine analgesia and prevents morphine tolerance in the rat. *Eur J Pharmacol*. 1990;176(1):35–44.

196. Vanderah TW, Gardell LR, Burgess SE, et al. Dynorphin promotes abnormal pain and spinal opioid antinociceptive tolerance. *J Neurosci*. 2000;20:7074–7079.

197. Arcaya JL, Cano G, Gomez G, Maixner W, Suarez-Roca H. Dynorphin A increases substance P release from trigeminal primary afferent C-fibers. *Eur J Pharmacol*. 1999;366:27–34.

198. Gardell LR, Wang R, Burgess SE, et al. Sustained morphine exposure induces a spinal dynorphin-dependent enhancement of excitatory transmitter release from primary afferent fibers 5. *J Neurosci*. 2002;22:6747–6755.

199. Draisci G, Kajander KC, Dubner R, Bennett GJ, Iadarola MJ. Up-regulation of opioid gene expression in spinal cord evoked by experimental nerve injuries and inflammation. *Brain Res*. 1991;560:186–192.

200. Mao J, Sung B, Ji RR, Lim G. Neuronal apoptosis associated with morphine tolerance: evidence for an opioid-induced neurotoxic mechanism. *J Neurosci*. 2002;22:7650–7661.

201. Urban MO, Gebhart GF. Supraspinal contributions to hyperalgesia. *PNAS*. 1999;96:7687–7692.

202. Edelmayer RM, Vanderah TW, Majuta L, et al. Medullary pain facilitating neurons mediate allodynia in headache-related pain. *Ann Neurol*. 2009;65:184–193.

203. de TM, Difruscolo O, Sardaro M, et al. Effects of remote cutaneous pain on trigeminal laser-evoked potentials in migraine patients. *J Headache Pain*. 2007;8:167–174.

204. de Tomasso M, Valeriani M, Guido M, et al. Abnormal brain processing of cutaneous pain in patients with chronic migraine. *Pain*. 2003;101:25–32.

205. Cathcart S, Winefield AH, Lushington K, Rolan P. Noxious inhibition of temporal summation is impaired in chronic tension-type headache. *Headache*. 2010;50:403–412.

206. Cathcart S, Winefield AH, Lushington K, Rolan P. Stress and tension-type headache mechanisms. *Cephalalgia*. 2010;30(10):1250–1267.

207. Pielsticker A, Haag G, Zaudig M, Lautenbacher S. Impairment of pain inhibition in chronic tension-type headache. *Pain*. 2005;118:215–223.

208. Okada-Ogawa A, Porreca F, Meng ID. Sustained morphine-induced sensitization and loss of diffuse noxious inhibitory controls in dura-sensitive medullary dorsal horn neurons. *J Neurosci*. 2009;29:15828–15835.

209. Saper JR, VanMeter MJ. Ergotamine habituation: analysis and profile. *Headache*. 1980;20:159(Abstract).

210. Saper JR. *Headache disorders: current concepts in treatment strategies*. Littleton, CO: Wright-PSG, 1983.

211. Saper JR, Jones JM. Ergotamine tartrate dependency: features and possible mechanisms. *Clin Neuropharmacol*. 1986;9:244–256.

212. De FM, Porreca F. Opiate-induced persistent pronociceptive trigeminal neural adaptations: potential relevance to opiate-induced medication overuse headache. *Cephalalgia*. 2009;29:1277–1284.

213. Wieseler, J. L., Mcfadden, A., Miles, N., and et al. Facial allodynia potentiation by supradural inflammatory mediators and morphine: a model of medication overuse headache. Program No. 178.09/NN19 2011 Neuroscience meeting planner. Washington, DC: Society for Neuroscience, 2011. Available at: http://www.abstractsonline.com/Plan/ViewAbstract.aspx?mID=2773&sKey=09c68eef-d953-455a-bc08-fb75a9980f4b&cKey=d85ed1b6-789c-488e-8458-a5ed5de401b6&mKey=%7B8334BE29-8911-4991-8C31-32B32DD5E6C8%7D (accessed 13 February 2011).

214. Watkins L, Maier S. Glia: a novel drug discovery target for clinical pain. *Nat Rev Drug Discov*. 2003;2:973–985.

215. Ledeboer A, Sloane EM, Milligan ED, et al. Minocycline attenuates mechanical allodynia and proinflammatory cytokine expression in rat models of pain facilitation. *Pain*. 2005;115:71–83.

216. De FM, Ossipov MH, Wang R, et al. Triptan-induced latent sensitization: a possible basis for medication overuse headache. *Ann Neurol*. 2010;67:325–337.

217. Juhasz G, Zsombok T, Modos EA, et al. NO-induced migraine attack: strong increase in plasma calcitonin gene-related peptide (CGRP) concentration and negative correlation with platelet serotonin release. *Pain*. 2003;106:461–470.

218. Juhasz G, Zsombok T, Jakab B, Nemeth J, Szolcsanyi J, Bagdy G. Sumatriptan causes parallel decrease in plasma calcitonin gene-related peptide (CGRP) concentration and migraine headache during nitroglycerin induced migraine attack. *Cephalalgia*. 2005;25:179–183.

219. De FM, Ossipov MH, Wang R, et al. Triptan-induced enhancement of neuronal nitric oxide synthase in trigeminal ganglion dural afferents underlies increased responsiveness to potential migraine triggers. *Brain*. 2010;133:2475–2488.

220. Pazzaglia PJ, Post RM. Contingent tolerance and reresponse to carbamazepine: a case study in a patient with trigeminal neuralgia and bipolar disorder. *J Neuropsychiat Clin Neurosci*. 1992;4:76–81.

221. May A, Bahra A, Buchel C, Frackowiak RS, Goadsby PJ. Hypothalamic activation in cluster headache attacks. *Lancet*. 1998;352:275–278.
222. May A, Kaube H, Buchel C, et al. Experimental cranial pain elicited by capsaicin: A PET study. *Pain*. 1998;74:61–66.
223. Bahra A, Matharu MS, Buchel C, Frackowiak RS, Goadsby PJ. Brainstem activation specific to migraine headache. *Lancet*. 2001;357:1016–1017.
224. Borsook D, Burstein R. The enigma of the dorsolateral pons as a migraine generator. *Cephalalgia*. 2012; 32(11):803–12.
225. Ren K, Dubner R. Descending modulation in persistent pain: an update. *Pain*. 2002;100:1–6.
226. Manjit SM, Thorsten B, Ward N, Frackowiak RS, et al. Central neuromodulation in chronic migraine patients with suboccipital stimulators: a PET study. *Brain*. 2003;1:220–230.
227. Welch KMA, Nagesh V, Rozell K, et al. Functional MRI of chronic daily headache. *Cephalalgia*. 1999;19:462(Abstract).
228. Aurora SK. Imaging chronic daily headache. *Curr Pain Headache Rep*. 2003;7:209–211.
229. Kruit MC, van Buchem MA, Launer LJ, Terwindt GM, Ferrari MD. Migraine is associated with an increased risk of deep white matter lesions, subclinical posterior circulation infarcts and brain iron accumulation: the population-based MRI CAMERA study. *Cephalalgia*. 2010;30:129–136.
230. Bolay H, Reuter U, Dunn AK, Huang Z, Boas DA, Moskowitz MA. Intrinsic brain activity triggers trigeminal meningeal afferents in a migraine model. *Nat Med*. 2002;8:136–142.
231. Gursoy-Ozdemir Y, Qiu J, Matsuoka N, et al. Cortical spreading depression activates and upregulates MMP-9. *J Clin Invest*. 2004;113:1447–1455.
232. Zhang X, Levy D, Noseda R, Kainz V, Jakubowski M, Burstein R. Activation of meningeal nociceptors by cortical spreading depression: implications for migraine with aura. *J Neurosci*. 2010;30:8807–8814.
233. Prochnow N, Abdulazim A, Kurtenbach S, et al. Pannexin1 stabilizes synaptic plasticity and is needed for learning. *PLoS One*. 2012;7:e51767.
234. Karatas H, Erdener SE, Gursoy-Ozdemir Y, et al. Spreading depression triggers headache by activating neuronal Panx1 channels. *Science*. 2013;339:1092–1095.
235. Noseda R, Constandil L, Bourgeais L, Chalus M, Villanueva L. Changes of meningeal excitability mediated by corticotrigeminal networks: a link for the endogenous modulation of migraine pain. *J Neurosci*. 2010;30:14420–14429.
236. Goadsby PJ. Migraine, aura, and cortical spreading depression: why are we still talking about it? *Ann Neurol*. 2001;49:4–6.
237. Lambert GA, Hoskin KL, Zagami AS. Cortico-NRM influences on trigeminal neuronal sensation. *Cephalalgia*. 2008;28:640–652.
238. Nozari A, Dilekoz E, Sukhotinsky I, et al. Microemboli may link spreading depression, migraine aura, and patent foramen ovale. *Ann Neurol*. 2010;67:221–229.
239. Sevgi, E. A study on the effect of air micro embolism on cerebral bioelectrical activity with spectral EEG in migraine patients with aura and patent foramen ovale. 2008. Dissertation, Hacettepe University.
240. Dinia L, Roccatagliata L, Bonzano L, Finocchi C, Del SM. Diffusion MRI during migraine with aura attack associated with diagnostic microbubbles injection in subjects with large PFO. *Headache*. 2007;47:1455–1456.
241. Zaletel M, Zvan B, Kozelj M, et al. Migraine with aura induced by artificial microbubbles. *Cephalalgia*. 2009;29:480–483.
242. Azarbal B, Tobis J, Suh,W, Chan V, Dao C, Gaster R. Association of interatrial shunts and migraine headaches: impact of transcatheter closure. *J Am Coll Cardiol*. 2005;45(4):489–492.
243. Kandere-Grzybowska K, Gheorghe D, Priller J, et al. Stress-induced dura vascular permeability does not develop in mast cell-deficient and neurokinin-1 receptor knockout mice. *Brain Res*. 2003;980:213–220.
244. Drummond PD. Sweating and vascular responses in the face: normal regulation and dysfunction in migraine, cluster headache and harlequin syndrome. *Clin Auton Res*. 1994;4:273–285.
245. Delepine L, Aubineau P. Plasma protein extravasation induced in the rat dura mater by stimulation of the parasympathetic sphenopalatine ganglion. *Exp Neurol*. 1997;147:389–400.
246. Gorji A. Spreading depression: a review of the clinical relevance. *Brain Res Brain Res Rev*. 2001;38:33–60.
247. Fabricius M, Fuhr S, Bhatia R, et al. Cortical spreading depression and peri-infarct depolarization in acutely injured human cerebral cortex. *Brain*. 2006;129:778–790.
248. Hansen JM, Lipton RB, Dodick DW, et al. Migraine headache is present in the aura phase: a prospective study. *Neurology*. 2012;79:2044–2049.
249. Cornell-Bell AH, Finkbeiner SM, Cooper MS, Smith SJ. Glutamate induces calcium waves in cultured astrocytes: long-range glial signaling. *Science*. 1990;247:470–473.
250. Charles A. Intercellular calcium waves in glia. *Glia*. 1998;24:39–49.
251. Bruzzone S, Guida L, Zocchi E, Franco L, De FA. Connexin 43 hemi channels mediate Ca2+-regulated transmembrane NAD+ fluxes in intact cells. *Faseb J*. 2001;15:10–12.
252. Nicholson C. Modulation of extracellular calcium and its functional implications. *Fed Proc*. 1980;39:1519–1523.
253. Martins-Ferreira H, Nedergaard M, Nicholson C. Perspectives on spreading depression. *Brain Res Brain Res Rev*. 2000;32:215–234.
254. Basarsky TA, Duffy SN, Andrew RD, MacVicar BA. Imaging spreading depression and associated intracellular calcium waves in brain slices. *J Neurosci*. 1998;18:7189–7199.
255. Kunkler PE, Kraig RP. Calcium waves precede electrophysiological changes of spreading depression in hippocampal organ cultures. *J Neurosci*. 1998;18:3416–3425.
256. Peters O, Schipke CG, Hashimoto Y, Kettenmann H. Different mechanisms promote astrocyte Ca2+ waves and spreading depression in the mouse neocortex. *J Neurosci*. 2003;23:9888–9896.

257. Ayata C, Jin H, Kudo C, Dalkara T, Moskowitz MA. Suppression of cortical spreading depression in migraine prophylaxis. *Ann Neurol.* 2006;59:652–661.

258. Bogdanov VB, Multon S, Chauvel V, et al. Migraine preventive drugs differentially affect cortical spreading depression in rat. *Neurobiol Dis.* 2011;41:430–435.

259. Noseda R, Kainz V, Jakubowski M, et al. A neural mechanism for exacerbation of headache by light. *Nat Neurosci.* 2010;13:239–245.

260. Noseda R, Burstein R. Migraine pathophysiology: anatomy of the trigeminovascular pathway and associated neurological symptoms, cortical spreading depression, sensitization, and modulation of pain. *Pain.* 2013;154:S44–S53.

261. Okamoto K, Tashiro A, Chang Z, Bereiter DA. Bright light activates a trigeminal nociceptive pathway. *Pain.* 2010;149:235–242.

262. Boulloche N, Denuelle M, Payoux P, Fabre N, Trotter Y, Geraud G. Photophobia in migraine: an interictal PET study of cortical hyperexcitability and its modulation by pain. *J Neurol Neurosurg Psychiatry.* 2010;81:978–984.

263. Moulton EA, Becerra L, Borsook D. An fMRI case report of photophobia: activation of the trigeminal nociceptive pathway. *Pain.* 2009;145(3):358–363.

264. Oshinsky MD, Gonzalez DM, Maxwell C. Repeated dural inflammation induces phonophobia. *Cephalalgia.* 2009;29:116(Abstract).

265. Hornby PJ. Central neurocircuitry associated with emesis. *Am J Med.* 2001;111 Suppl 8A:106S–112S.

266. Hargreaves R, Ferreira JC, Hughes D, et al. Development of arepitant, the first neurokinin-1 receptor antagonist for the prevention of chemotherapy-induced nausea and vomiting. *Ann NY Acad Sci.* 2011;(Abstract) 1222:40–8.

Chapter 6

Non-Pharmacologic Therapy

In our opinion . . . it is the joint province of both social and physical (medical) scientists to work on the central linkage, namely, how specified stresses work to evoke particular (psychophysiological) reaction patterns.

Simmons and Wolff,[1] pp. 144–145

Effective migraine treatment must address the impact of the disorder on the patient. Patients with recurrent headaches often believe that their complaints have not been taken seriously. Just as they want headache relief, patients want to know what is wrong with them, and they want to be assured that their physician is committed to relieving their distress. A treatment plan needs to consider patient expectations, needs, and goals. Patient commitment improves compliance and fosters the patient-physician relationship. Migraineurs should be educated about their condition and its treatment and encouraged to participate in its management. A variety of non-pharmacologic techniques may be used alone or to augment the effects of pharmacologic treatment (Table 6.1). Non-pharmacologic treatment includes education and reassurance; non-pharmacologic treatments, such as relaxation

Table 6.1 Behavioral and Mind-Body Treatment Options

Behavioral	Mind-Body
Cognitive behavioral therapy	Yoga
Biofeedback	Tai chi
Relaxation therapy	Medication
	Hypnosis
	Progressive muscular relaxation
	Deep breathing
	Qi gong

and biofeedback, and lifestyle regulation, such as maintaining a regular schedule, getting adequate sleep and exercise, and discontinuing the consumption of caffeine, tobacco, alcohol, and others that may be triggering or exacerbating their symptoms.

Stress is common in life, and it impacts migraine. Stress can be defined as a state of mental or emotional strain or tension resulting from the *perception* of adverse, demanding, threatening, or dangerous circumstances. The relationship between stress and headache can take multiple forms: from an etiologic factor, contributing to the first onset of a primary headache disorder, to an exacerbating factor, associated with increasing migraine attack frequency/severity; as a potential trigger, increasing the probability of a migraine attack, or as the earliest symptom of an attack occurrence during the premonitory phase. Imaging studies have shown that individual symptoms that occur during the premonitory phase are associated with localized activation in the relevant brain region.[2] Functional MRI studies suggest that migraine changes the functional connectivity of the brain. Over time, such perceived stress becomes a more permanent "state" of the migraine brain.[3,4]

There is a close relationship between stress and migraine. In a prospective observational cohort study involving 5417 migraine patients, stress was identified as the strongest predictor for anxiety (OR 1.64), while other maladaptive coping strategies, including avoidance (OR 1.15) and catastrophizing (OR 1.10), were also predictive.[5] Anxious patients, especially those who were also depressed, had higher levels of stress, functional impairment, and maladaptive coping than migraine patients without

anxiety or depression. Headache was magnified by psychological factors. Migraineurs with stress and anxiety/depression were as functionally impaired as those with chronic migraine. Anxious and depressive symptoms were also associated with increased consumption of acute treatments and low treatment effectiveness. These results illustrate the importance of routine screening for anxiety and depression when evaluating a patient with migraine.

In a longitudinal population-based German Headache Consortium (GHC) study, Schramm and colleagues investigated the association between stress intensity and headache frequency for tension-type headache (TTH), migraine, and migraine with coexisting TTH for different age groups.[6] A population of 5159 participants (aged 21–71 years) were asked questions on a quarterly basis between March 2010 and April 2012 about headache and stress. Participants who reported headache had more stress compared to those without headache. Participants with migraine experienced more stress than participants with TTH. Stressful events could increase the risk of onset of migraine attacks, or migraineurs could be more likely to perceive events as stressful. Increased stress was associated with increasing headache frequency for all headache subtypes. The American Migraine Prevalence and Prevention study found that individuals with chronic migraine (> 15 headache days per month) had a higher number of major life events in the preceding year compared to those with episodic migraine.[7] These events were rated as more stressful. These results suggest an association between stress intensity and headache frequency.

The biological underpinnings between stress and migraine are yet to be fully clarified. Stress can affect diverse physiological processes throughout the body and many of these processes are mediated by increases in endogenous sympathetic efferent activity and circulating stress hormones such as epinephrine, norepinephrine and cortisol. The meninges and cerebral vasculature are densely innervated by sympathetic fibers and the release of norepinephrine from these efferents may activate nociceptive afferent trigeminal fibers. In fact, in a recent preclinical study in a rat model of migraine, norepinephrine was shown to induce headache-like behavior when applied to the meninges and that the pro-nociceptive effects of norepinephrine are mediated by an increase in excitability of dural afferents.[7a] Norepinephrine also led to the release of pronociceptive substances such as interleukin-6 from dural fibroblasts, possibly by activating adrenergic receptors on fibroblasts. This elegant animal study provides a link that may in part explain the frequent association between stress and migraine headache.

There is abundant evidence that supports the role of self-management and bio-behavioral therapy in improving headache treatment outcomes. Self-management requires the active involvement of the patient in the management of his or her disorder. Holroyd and Creer emphasized that effective self-management requires patients to self-monitor early headache warning signs, triggers, and medication use and efficacy, to maximize behaviors that minimize exacerbations, and to implement medication and behavioral treatment strategies when attacks occur.[8]

Many behavioral treatments can be used in the self-management of headache disorders, both acutely as well as for prevention. Behavioral treatment should be strongly considered in all patients, but especially in those who have been poorly tolerant or responsive to drug therapies, possess contraindications for drug therapy, have a planned pregnancy or are pregnant or lactating, have a preference for non-pharmacologic strategies, use excessive amounts of acute medications, identify life stress, or have deficient coping skills or comorbid psychological disorders that trigger or amplify suffering during headache attacks. The long-term goals of behavior therapy include reducing the frequency, severity, and progression of headaches, headache-related disability, and affective distress; reducing reliance on poorly tolerated drugs; and enhancing self-efficacy or personal control of headaches.[9–11]

RELAXATION TRAINING

Relaxation training is a fundamental skill that should be a component in all self-management programs to facilitate the potential for patients to exert some control over migraine-associated physiological responses and lower physiological and mental arousal.[12] Patients are instructed to practice a graduated hierarchy of relaxation techniques (diaphragmatic breathing, progressive muscle relaxation, relaxation imagery, meditation) for 20–30 minutes per day. With time and mastery of the strategies, brief (e.g., 30 seconds) relaxation techniques can be used throughout the day, especially when patients recognize mental or bodily signs of tension or premonitory symptoms.

COGNITIVE BEHAVIORAL THERAPY

There is abundant evidence that cognitive behavioral therapy (CBT) reduces migraine symptoms and migraine-related disability. CBT is recommended by the US Headache Consortium guidelines based on a Grade A level of evidence (Table 6.2). CBT enhances behavioral coping (actions used to prevent attacks and manage individual attacks) and cognitive responses to attacks (automatic ways of thinking about migraine). CBT can reduce the frequency of attacks as well as reduce the pain intensity and disability associated with individual attacks. Adjusting maladaptive cognitive response styles can improve outcomes, especially those associated with catastrophizing, since it has been associated with poorer quality of life, chronicity of headache, and poorer treatment response.

Coping strategies helpful to a migraine sufferer may be either active (relaxation, stress management) or passive/palliative (trigger avoidance). The addition of behavioral migraine management to optimized acute treatment reduced catastrophizing compared to migraine drug therapy alone; both significantly increased the

Table 6.2 **US Headache Consortium Guidelines for the Prevention of Migraine**

Grade A Evidence	Grade B Evidence
Relaxation training	Behavioral treatments plus drug prevention
Thermal biofeedback with relaxation	
Electromyography biofeedback	
Cognitive behavioral therapy	

number of positive coping strategies while significantly reducing migraine-related disability. The authors suggested that reducing catastrophizing is likely an important component of cognitive behavioral treatments for migraine.[13]

BIOFEEDBACK

A variety of biofeedback techniques are used in the management of migraine. Thermal feedback of skin temperature (hand warming) and electromyography feedback (electrical activity from muscles of the scalp, neck, and/or upper body) are the most commonly employed biofeedback modalities. Electroencephalographic (EEG) biofeedback (*neurofeedback*) is another technique whose objective is to teach self-regulation of cortical excitability.[14] After training sessions, patients are instructed to use a home biofeedback training system and to practice the skills for 20–30 minutes per day. Patients are expected to integrate their biofeedback skills into their daily routine.

BEHAVIORAL TREATMENT APPROACHES

The choice of behavioral treatment depends on patient preference, patient and provider availability, and cost. High-contact treatment typically involves 6 to 12 weekly sessions, 45 to 60 minutes long, for individuals,[15] and 60 to 120 minutes for a group.[16] This approach requires more provider time and attention, while the disadvantage is patient time and cost. Limited-contact treatment involves one visit or several monthly treatment sessions, followed by the acquisition and refinement of skills using home video or audio recordings, with the option of clinician assistance via phone calls, or web-based sessions. [15,17] No-contact training is designed to enable individuals to acquire and successfully use behavioral headache management skills without either clinic visits or face-to-face instruction from a behavioral clinician. Learning in a personal environment may be supervised by a behavioral clinician through telephone or the Internet. This may be a particularly attractive option for providers without access to a behaviorally trained clinician

to make behavioral therapy options available to their patients.

EFFICACY OF BEHAVIORAL TREATMENTS

The evidence base supporting the efficacy of behavioral interventions for patients with headache disorders has grown considerably and has facilitated the development of systematic reviews of well-designed, randomized controlled trials. In one comprehensive meta-analysis, 355 articles were identified that described behavioral and physical treatments for migraine. Of these, 70 reported controlled trials of behavioral migraine treatments for adults and 39 trials satisfied the rigorous inclusion/exclusion criteria. Outcome data were available for 60 different treatment groups with summary effect size estimates and mean percentage headache improvement as the main primary outcomes. Relaxation training, thermal biofeedback combined with relaxation, electromyography biofeedback, and cognitive behavioral therapy were all statistically more effective than wait-list control, with 32%–49% reduction in migraine frequency compared to a 5% reduction for controls. On the basis of this exhaustive review, the US Headache Consortium[11] made the following recommendations pertaining to behavioral interventions for migraine: (1) relaxation training, thermal biofeedback combined with relaxation training, electromyography biofeedback, and cognitive behavioral therapy may be considered as treatment options for prevention of migraine (Grade A Evidence); and (2) behavioral therapy may be combined with preventive drug therapy to achieve added clinical improvement for migraine (Grade B Evidence) (http://www.aan.com/).[18]

Previous meta-analyses that employed less rigorous inclusion/exclusion criteria found similar outcomes (35%–55% improvement).[15,19–21] A meta-analysis of 55 controlled biofeedback trials[22] demonstrated higher efficacy compared to control conditions with a medium effect size ($d = 0.58$, 95% CI [0.52, 0.64]) and durable results with an average follow-up of 17 months. Biofeedback, in combination with home training, was more effective than therapies without home training.

Behavioral therapies appear comparable to preventive drug therapy for migraine prevention. While head-to-head comparative studies are scarce, meta-analytic comparisons have shown similar levels of improvement in migraine with propranolol (32 trials) and combined relaxation and biofeedback training (35 trials).[20,23]

Long-term outcomes appear to be favorable. At least 45% reductions in headache activity have been reported in 14 of 15 studies that used daily headache recordings to assess improvement 1 to 3 years following psychological treatment, and in three studies that assessed improvement 5 to 7 years following treatment.[24–26]

LIMITED AND NO-CONTACT BEHAVIORAL INTERVENTIONS

The intensity of treatment contact is important for clinicians and patients given the difficulty with access in certain locations and clinical settings. In a meta-analysis of 20 randomized controlled trials that evaluated limited-contact (three clinic visits) and clinic-based (nine clinic visits) treatment formats,[27] limited-contact treatment was more effective than control conditions and equivalent or superior to clinic-based treatment. The percentage of patients showing clinically meaningful improvements with limited-contact treatment (53%) was similar to clinic-based treatment (52%) for patients with migraine. This meta-analysis was consistent with previous meta-analyses. [28,29] Similarly, when comparing group versus individual format treatment approaches, a meta-analysis of 10 studies demonstrated comparable efficacy with an approximately 53% reduction in headache activity for both formats.[29]

The use of non-professional individuals to deliver headache education or behavioral treatment has also been evaluated. In a randomized trial involving 100 patients at a tertiary-care headache center, 100 consecutive patients were randomized to medical treatment by a headache specialist with or without receiving headache education classes. The headache education classes (three 90-minute didactic lectures and discussion sessions about migraine and treatments) were led by two trained volunteers with a history of migraine. Medical

management plus headache education led to significantly greater reductions in overall and functionally disabling headache frequency compared to medical management alone. The combination of medical management plus headache education also led to reductions in patient calls (54 vs. 244), unscheduled headache clinic or emergency department visits (25 vs. 50), acute therapy use (5.3 vs. 15.6 days/month), analgesic overuse (0% vs. 36% of patients), and an increase in adherence with preventive medication higher (96% vs. 59% of patients).[30]

In another study, 129 migraineurs were randomized to a wait-list control or home-based, small group behavioral treatment sessions led by non-professionals with migraine who had completed behavioral migraine management and leadership training.[31] There was a small reduction in migraine attack frequency (21%), which was not significantly different from the control group (6%; $p < 0.07$). Long-term follow-up at 6 months and 2–4 years was reported in 127 of the participants in this study.[32] Short-term improvements in attack frequency and self-efficacy post-training were maintained at long-term follow-up. Quality of life and migraine-related disability improved gradually over time. The authors concluded that lay behavioral management training for migraine may be beneficial over the long term.

The optimal approach may be a combination of behavioral treatments led by a behavioral health professional and headache education classes led by trained volunteers, but this will require further research.

TELEPHONE-ADMINISTERED TREATMENT

A controlled study randomized 87 children (aged 11–18 years) to receive an 8-week behavioral program consisting of education, relaxation training, stress management, pain-coping strategies, assertiveness, and problem-solving by either home study (workbook and audiotapes) with weekly telephone calls, versus a behavioral therapist–administered program.[33] Significant reductions in migraine attack frequency were similar in both groups (66% vs. 44%), and both formats were more effective than a one-session controlled condition that included weekly phone calls. Similar improvements were demonstrated in another comparable study with adolescents preferring the telephone-administered format over clinic treatment.[34] In a study that compared an interactive, computer-administered, home study program, plus drug therapy and weekly telephone contact (preventive and acute medications), children receiving the computer-administered program were more likely to show clinically significant reductions (≥ 50%) in migraine than children who received drug therapy alone.[35]

INTERNET- AND MASS MEDIA–ADMINISTERED TREATMENT

Studies evaluating the acquisition of behavioral headache management skills via the Internet found only modest efficacy and have been hampered by high dropout rates.[36–40] In a mass media intervention effort in the Netherlands,[41] approximately 15,000 participants purchased home-study materials that presented relaxation and cognitive behavioral skills for managing headaches. A small number (164) of participants who completed the program evaluation reported a 50% reduction in headache frequency and a reduction of about 4.5 days of lost work over 4 months.

In a recent randomized controlled trial, 195 received online behavioral management compared to 195 subjects who served as a wait-list control group.[42] An online ICHD-2 headache diary and questionnaires were completed at baseline, post-training, and at 6 months. At 6 months, attack frequency had improved significantly in both the active (–23%, ES = 0.66) and wait-list group (–19%; ES = 0.52). However, self-efficacy, internal and external control in migraine management, and triptan use improved only in the active group. These results suggest that behavioral management skills can be effectively taught via mass media and positively influence patient outcomes.

MINDFULNESS-BASED STRESS REDUCTION

Mindfulness-based stress reduction (MBSR) is a mind/body intervention technique that enables individuals to focus on a stimulus while simultaneously allowing intruding thoughts/feelings to be acknowledged but not judged. MBSR utilizes mindfulness meditation and yoga in a standardized 8-week protocol involving group instruction by certified instructors.[43] In a small, randomized controlled pilot study of 19 migraineurs randomized to either MBSR or usual care, MBSR was found to be safe, feasible, and associated with a significant reduction in headache duration and disability; it was also associated with significant improvements in self-efficacy and mindfulness.[44]

EXERCISE

Exercise is recommended for the benefit of a variety of health conditions, including migraine. Exercise may be defined as physical activity that is planned, structured, repetitive, and purposeful, where the improvement or maintenance of physical fitness is the objective. While exercise is well known to be a trigger for migraine in up to 20% of migraineurs,[45] aerobic exercise has been associated with alterations in relevant biomarkers, including elevations in endorphins, and improvements in the frequency, intensity, and duration of migraine attacks.[46–48] Evidence for both the unique effect of exercise on migraine, as well as the complementary effect when combined with bio-behavioral therapies, is emerging. In one study, 80 patients were randomized to receive either standard medical therapy from their primary care physician (with or without referral to a specialist), or an 18 group-supervised exercise therapy session, two group stress management and relaxation therapy lectures, one group dietary lecture, and two massage therapy sessions.[49] Outcome measures, including self-perceived pain intensity, frequency, and duration, functional status, quality of life, health status, depression, prescription and non-prescription medication use, and work status, were analyzed at the end of the 6-week intervention and at 3 months. The intervention group had statistically significant changes in self-perceived pain frequency ($p < 0.000$), pain intensity ($p < 0.001$), pain duration ($p < 0.000$), functional status ($p < 0.000$), quality of life ($p < 0.000$), health status ($p < 0.000$), pain-related disability ($p < 0.000$), and depression ($p < 0.000$). This study demonstrated that aerobic exercise, combined with bio-behavioral techniques and standard medical therapy, may be complementary and maximize patient outcomes. A recent systematic review evaluated the outcome in studies where aerobic exercise was part of a multicomponent treatment for headache.[50] Nine studies met the inclusion criteria. The authors concluded that incorporating exercise into behavioral headache treatments appears to be promising. Studies included in the analysis did not evaluate the individual contribution of exercise; thus further work is needed to evaluate the unique role of exercise in migraine management. To that end, in a recent randomized controlled trial, 91 subjects were randomized to exercise for 40 minutes, three times a week, and were given a structured relaxation program or topiramate prophylaxis.[51] Exercise consisted of indoor cycling. Each training session included a 15-minute warm-up period, followed by a 20-minute exercise period, and a 5-minute cool-down period. In the third month after randomization, all groups showed improvement in the primary endpoint (mean reduction in migraine attacks), without a significant difference between the groups with regard to the primary endpoint, or on many secondary endpoints. Topiramate was associated with a significant reduction in pain intensity ($p < 0.044$), whereas exercise was associated with significant improvement in maximal oxygen uptake ($p < 0.008$). This study demonstrated the ability of aerobic exercise alone to improve migraine.

COMBINING BEHAVIORAL AND DRUG THERAPY

The combination of behavioral and drug therapy is often employed in clinical practice, and a recent study demonstrated the effectiveness of this approach. A randomized trial of behavioral management and preventive (beta-blocker) drug therapy, compared to either treatment alone, was done in 232 migraine sufferers experiencing six monthly migraine attacks on average, despite optimal acute therapy.[9] Combination therapy resulted in significantly higher responder

rates ($\geq 50\%$ reduction in migraines) than either behavioral or preventive drug therapy alone. Improvements in quality of life measures were similar in the combination and behavior therapy alone groups, and larger than that observed with the preventive drug therapy alone group. Holroyd and colleagues have proposed a combination of behavioral and drug treatments if migraine attacks are frequent or severe, or psychological problems complicate treatment.[52] In those with less frequent attacks not complicated by psychological factors, behavioral and drug therapies may be equally viable treatment alternatives. Patient preference, treatment costs, and presence of medication contraindications (e.g., the possibility of pregnancy, or breastfeeding) may influence the treatment chosen.

Behavioral therapy also enhances compliance and adherence to drug therapy. Adherence is a significant health problem in the United States and it is estimated that non-adherence is associated with more than $290 billion in additional healthcare costs per year.[53] Non-adherence is a major problem with migraine preventive drug therapy; it undermines drug effectiveness and compromises patient outcomes. In a recent database study of 8,688 adult patients with chronic migraine who were started on an oral drug for migraine prevention, adherence ranged from 26% to 29% at 6 months and 17% to 20% at 12 months, depending on the calculation used to classify adherence.[54]

There is a decline in adherence with multiple medications, more frequent or complex medication dosing regimens, higher medication costs, side effects, psychiatric comorbidity, as well as psychological factors, for example, low internal locus of control and self-efficacy.[55]

Dedicated behavioral interventions may facilitate the use of medications in patients with migraine. In one study evaluating the influence of behavioral intervention to enhance adherence with ergotamine, patients were randomized to an adherence-enhancing group, participated in a one-half hour education session, received three brief phone calls to identify and remedy problems with medication use, and were provided a self-management workbook to assist the patient in monitoring and identifying adherence problems, improve decision-making, and correct adherence problems.[56] Patients receiving the adherence intervention attempted to abort 70% of migraine attacks and showed clinically significant reductions in headache activity (40% improvement at post-treatment). In contrast, the control group who received standard medication management attempted to abort only about 40% of their migraine attacks and showed smaller reductions in migraine activity (26% improvement at post-treatment). While more research is required to determine whether behavioral interventions can enhance adherence to migraine preventive therapies, these preliminary results appear promising.

COMORBID MOOD DISORDERS

Mood and anxiety disorders are comorbid with migraine and influence the selection of behavioral and drug treatments as well as patient outcomes. Screening for mood disorders should be part of every new clinical encounter and should be followed over time. The most widely used screening instruments for depression are the Primary Care Evaluation of Mental Disorders (PRIME-MD), available as both a clinician structured interview[57] and as a patient completed questionnaire (Patient Health Questionnaire or PHQ).[58] These instruments were designed (and validated) for use in medical settings and can be used to screen for multiple psychiatric disorders or for a single disorder. A positive screening result should be followed by a diagnostic workup, and clinicians should be aware of the overlap of somatic symptoms associated with headache, depression, and anxiety disorders in order to avoid inappropriate or incorrect psychiatric diagnoses.[59] More sophisticated data regarding mood can be ascertained from the Beck Depression Inventory II (BDI-II)[60] and the Hamilton Rating Scale for Depression (HRSD).[61] While they are typically used in psychiatric/psychological settings where patients are often already diagnosed with depression, these inventories are often used in tertiary headache treatment centers where the chronicity of the disease in the patient population is often associated with depression. Tertiary treatment centers generally also have affiliations with mental health professionals qualified to interpret clinical instruments. The BDI-II is self-administered, while the

Hamilton ratings are done by a trained health-care professional who is working with the patient. The two instruments correlate at the .71 level. The Generalized Anxiety Disorder Scale (GAD-7) is also commonly used in clinical headache practice to screen for anxiety disorders.[62] The GAD-7 is a 7-item anxiety scale that has been demonstrated to have good reliability, as well as criterion, construct, factorial, and procedural validity. Scores of 5, 10, and 15 are taken as the cutoff points for mild, moderate, and severe anxiety, and when used as a screening tool, further evaluation is recommended when the score is 10 or greater. A threshold score of 10 has a sensitivity of 89% and a specificity of 82% for generalized anxiety disorder, and it is also a tool that can screen effectively for other common anxiety disorders, including panic disorder (sensitivity 74%, specificity 81%), social anxiety disorder (sensitivity 72%, specificity 80%), and post-traumatic stress disorder (sensitivity 66%, specificity 81%).[63]

CBT is effective for primary mood and anxiety disorders. CBT consistently produces outcomes that equal (and often exceed) those of pharmacotherapy for depression, anxiety disorders (including panic disorder;[64] generalized anxiety disorder;[65] obsessive-compulsive disorder;[66–68] and post-traumatic stress disorder[69]). Improvements may be maintained longer with CBT than with pharmacotherapy. [65,70] CBT prevents relapses in the long-term treatment of both mood and anxiety disorders. [71,72] CBT is a first-line treatment for mild to moderately severe unipolar depression,[73] anxiety disorders, and obsessive-compulsive disorder.[74–76]

OLDER ADULTS

Behavioral management of migraine in older adults is particularly attractive given polypharmacy and the potential for drug interactions, reduced renal clearance of medications, and increasing contraindications that occur with advancing age. Prospective studies evaluating interventions adapted for elderly patients have reported positive results with CBT, relaxation training, and biofeedback training for both migraine and tension-type headache.[77–81] Mosley and colleagues found CBT, combined with relaxation training, to be more effective than relaxation training alone in elderly headache patients aged 60–78 years, with 64% of CBT participants achieving clinically significant improvement.[80]

CHILDREN AND ADOLESCENTS

The evidence base for behavioral migraine management is less robust in children and adolescents compared to adults, but published studies raise the possibility that behavioral treatments may be more effective in this age group.[25,82–85] Trautmann and colleagues examined the effectiveness of the primary behavioral interventions (relaxation, biofeedback and cognitive-behavior therapy) for pediatric headache (migraine and tension-type headache) in a meta-analysis of 22 studies.[85] Behavioral treatment was associated with a large treatment effect (ES = .87), corresponding to clinically significant improvement in 70% versus 30% of children who received behavior therapy versus control, with stable improvement at 1-year follow-up.

Behavioral therapy may be more effective than drug prevention in children and adolescents. A combination of relaxation and self-hypnosis training proved superior than both placebo and propranolol in children aged 6–12 years with migraine with aura[86,87] compared the efficacy of metoprolol and two behavioral treatments (stress-management plus either relaxation training or cephalic vasomotor biofeedback) in children aged 8–16 years with migraine. Combined relaxation/stress-management training resulted in > 50% improvement in 80% of patients, while only 42% of patients treated with metoprolol had a > 50% improvement. However, compliance was not measured.

SCHOOL-BASED BEHAVIORAL INTERVENTIONS

Relaxation training for headache management has been taught in secondary schools in Uppsala, Sweden, for 20 years. In a summary of seven relaxation training trials conducted in the school setting (n = 228, aged 10–18 years),

Larsson and colleagues reported clinically significant improvements ($\geq 50\%$) in about half of students with migraine who participated in a 6- to 10-session, therapist-administered, group relaxation training program.[88] Expertise is required for positive outcomes since only 15% of students improved when the training program was conducted by a school nurse or with a self-help relaxation training program that included a relaxation manual and audiotapes of relaxation.[88] Ineffective results were also found when relaxation training was conducted by school gym instructors.[89] Methods of teaching school personnel the clinical skills necessary to effectively administer relaxation training is crucial if behavioral headache management programs are to be offered to the large number of adolescents with migraine in the school setting.

PREGNANCY

Behavioral approaches are a treatment option for managing migraine during pregnancy and lactation. They prevent exposing the developing fetus to medications, some of which have teratogenic effects.[90,91] The majority of pregnancies are unplanned and the majority of women do not know that they are pregnant until several weeks after conception. Thus, behavioral self-management skills should be introduced early when patients are considering pregnancy to allow them time to practice and acquire the skill. Data on the efficacy of behavioral approaches for headache management for pregnant and postpartum/lactating migraineurs is limited. Attack frequency often decreases during the second and third trimesters, making causal interpretation difficult in uncontrolled studies. Only one controlled study[92] randomized pregnant migraineurs to a behavioral intervention (education, relaxation training, thermal biofeedback training, and physical therapy exercises) or a pseudotherapy control condition (educational plus biofeedback training to decrease finger temperature). The interventions were initiated during the second trimester and completed before delivery. Significant symptom improvement was found in 79% of subjects with migraine and the behavioral intervention resulting in larger reductions in headache activity (81% vs. 33%) and a greater number of patients with clinically significant improvements (73% vs. 29%) relative to the control group. Treatment improvements were maintained throughout the perinatal period and at 3- and 6-month follow-up evaluations and up to 1 year postpartum in 68% of the treated patients. This study supports the use of behavioral interventions as an important non-pharmacological treatment option for the pregnant or lactating migraineur.

REFERENCES

1. Simmons LW, Wolff HG. *Social science in medicine*. New York: Russell Sage Foundation, 1954.
2. Maniyar FH, Sprenger T, Montieth T, Schankin C, Goadsby PJ. Brain activations in the premonitory phase of nitroglycerin-triggered migraine attacks. *Brain*. 2014; 137(Pt 1):232–241.
3. Schwedt TJ, Chong CD, Chia-Chun Chiang CC, Baxter L, Schlaggar BL, DodickDW. Enhanced pain-induced activity of pain-processing regions in a case-control study of episodic migraine. *Cephalalgia*. 2014;34(12):947–958.
4. Hadjikhani N, Ward N, Boshyan J, Napadow V, Maeda Y, Truini A, et al. The missing link: enhanced functional connectivity between amygdala and visceroceptive cortex in migraine. *Cephalalgia*. 2013;33:1264–1268.
5. Radat F, Mekies C, Geraud G, et al. Anxiety, stress and coping behaviors in primary care migraine patients: results of the SMILE study. *Cephalalgia* 2008;28:1115–25
6. Schramm SH, Moebus S, Lehmann N, Galli U,Obermann M, Bock E, Yoon M-S, Diener HC, Katsarava A.The association between stress and headache: a longitudinal population-based study. *Cephalalgia*. 2015;35:853–863.
7. Manack AN, Buse DC, Serrano D, Turkel CC, Lipton RB. Major life events, stress appraisal and migraine: results of the American Migraine Prevalence and Prevention (AMPP) Study. *Headache*. 2012;52:871.
7a. Wei X, Yan J, Tillu D, Asiedu M, Weinstein N, Melemedjian O, et al. Meningeal norepinephrine produces headache behaviors in rats via actions both on dural afferents and fibroblasts. *Cephalalgia*. 2015; DOI: 10.1177/0333102414566861.
8. Holroyd KA, Creer TL, eds. *Self-management of chronic disease: handbook of clinical interventions and research*. Orlando, FL: Academic Press, 1986:29–58.
9. Holroyd, Wolff, Bigal, Lipton (2006).
10. Lipton RB, Pan J. Is migraine a progressive disease? *JAMA*. 2004;291(4):493–494.
11. Silberstein SD. Practice parameter: evidence-based guidelines for migraine headache (an evidence-based review): report of the Quality Standards Subcommittee of the American Academy of Neurology. *Neurology* 2000;55(6):754–762.
12. Bernstein DA, Borkovec TD, Hazlett-Stevens H. *New directions in progressive relaxation training: a guidebook for helping professions*. Westport, CT: Praeger, 2000.
13. Seng EK, Holroyd KA. Behavioral migraine management modifies behavioral and cognitive coping in people with migraine. *Headache*. 2014;54:1470–1483.
14. Schwartz MS, Andrasik F. *Biofeedback: a practitioner's guide*. 3rd ed. New York: Guilford Press, 2003.
15. Blanchard EB, Andrasik F. (1985). *Management of chronic headaches: a psychological approach*. Elmsford, NY: Pergamon Press, 1985.
16. Scharff L, Marcus DA. Interdisciplinary outpatient group treatment of intractable headache. *Headache*. 1994;34:73–78.
17. Lipchik GL, Holroyd KA, Nash JM. Cognitive-behavioral management of recurrent headache disorders: a minimal-therapist contact approach. In: Turk DC, Gatchel RS, eds. *Psychological approaches to pain management* (2nd ed.) New York: Guilford Press, 2002:356–389.
18. Campbell JK, Penzien DB, Wall EM. Evidence-based guidelines for migraine headache: Behavioral and physical treatments. Prepared for the US Headache Consortium. 1999. http://www.aan.com/professionals/practice/pdfs/gl0089.pdf. Accessed March 2007.
19. Blanchard EB, Andrasik F, Ahles TA, et al. Migraine and tension-type headache: A meta-analytic review. *Behav Ther.* 1980;11:613–31.
20. Holroyd KA, Penzien DB. Pharmacological vs. non-pharmacological prophylaxis of recurrent migraine headache: A meta-analytic review of clinical trials. *Pain*. 1990;42:1–13.
21. Penzien DB, Holroyd KA, Hursey KG, et al. *Behavioral treatment of recurrent migraine: a meta-analysis of over five-dozen group outcome studies*. Paper presented at the Association for Advancement of Behavior Therapy, Houston, TX, 1985.
22. Nestoriuc Y, Martin A. Efficacy of biofeedback for migraine:a meta-analysis.*Pain.* 2007;128(1–2):111–127.
23. Holroyd KA, Penzien DB, Cordingley GA. Propranolol in the prevention of recurrent migraine: a meta-analytic review. *Headache*. 1991;31:333–340.
24. Blanchard EB. Long-term effects of behavioral treatment of chronic headache. *Behav Ther.* 1987;23:375–385.
25. Blanchard EB. Psychological treatment of benign headache disorders. *J Consul Clin Psychol.* 1992;60:537–551.
26. Gauthier JG, Fournier A, Roberge C. The differential effects of biofeedback in the treatment of menstrual and non-menstrual migraine. *Headache*. 1991;31:82–90.
27. Haddock CK, Rowan AB, Andrasik F, et al. Home-based behavioral treatments for chronic benign headache: a meta-analysis of controlled trials. *Cephalalgia* 1997;17(2):113–118.
28. Rowan AB, Andrasik F. Efficacy and cost-effectiveness of minimal therapist contact treatments for chronic headache: A review. *Behav Ther.* 1996;27:207–234.
29. Rains JC, Penzien DB, Holroyd KA. Meta-analysis of alternative behavioral treatments for recurrent headache. *Headache*. 1993;33:279–280.
30. Rothrock J, Parada V, Sims C, Key K, et al. The impact of intensive patient education on clinical outcome in a clinic-based migraine population. *Headache*. 2006;46:726–731.
31. Merelle SY, Sorbi MJ, et al. Migraine patients as trainers of their fellow-patients in non-pharmacological

preventive attack management: short-term effects of a randomized controlled trial. *Cephalagia* 2008; 28(2):127–138.

32. Voerman JS, de Klerk C, Merelle SYM, Aartsen E, Timman R, Sorbi MJ, et al. Long-term follow-up of home-based behavioral management training provided by migraine patients. *Cephalalgia.* 2014;34(5):357–364.

33. McGrath PJ, Humphreys P, Keene D, et al. The efficacy and efficiency of a self-administered treatment for adolescent migraine. *Pain.* 1992;49(3):321–324.

34. Cottrell C, Drew J, Holroyd K, et al. Feasibility of telephone administered behavioral treatment for adolescent migraine. *Headache.* 2007;47:1293–1302.

35. Connelly M, Rapoff M, Thompson N, et al. Headstrong: a pilot study of a CD-ROM Intervention for recurrent pediatric headache. *J Pediatr Psychol.* 2005;31(7):737–747.

36. Andersson G, Lundstom P, Strom L. A controlled trial of self-help treatment of recurrent headache conducted via the Internet. *Headache.* 2003;43:353–361.

37. Devineni T, Blanchard EB. A randomized controlled trial of an Internet-based treatment for chronic headache. *Behav Res Ther.* 2005;43:277–292.

38. Hicks C, von Baeyer C, McGrath P. Online psychological treatment for pediatric recurrent pain: a randomized evaluation. *J Pediatr Psychol.* 2006;31(7):1–13.

39. Schneider WJ, Furth PA, Blalock TH, et al. A pilot study of a headache program in the workplace. *J Occup Environ Med.* 1999;41:868–871.

40. Strom L, Peterson R, Andersson G. A controlled trial of self-help treatment of recurrent headache conducted via the Internet. *J Consult Clin Psychol.* 2000;68:722–727.

41. de Bruin-Kofman AT, van de Wiel H, Groenman NH, et al. Effects of a mass media behavioral treatment for chronic headache: a pilot study. *Headache.* 1997;37:415–20.

42. Sorbi MJ, Kleiboer AM, van Silfhout HG, Vink G, Passchier J. Medium-term effectiveness of online behavioral training in migraine self-management: a randomized trial controlled over 10 months. *Cephalalgia;* 2015;35:608–618.

43. Rosenzweig S, Greeson JM, Reibel DK, Green JS, Jasser SA, Beasley D. Mindfulness-based stress reduction for chronic pain conditions: variation in treatment outcomes and role of home meditation practice. *J Psychosomatic Res.* 2010;68:29–36.

44. Wells RE, Burch R, Paulsen RH, Wayne PM, Houle TT, Loder E. Meditation for migraines: a pilot randomized controlled trial. *Headache.* 2014;54:1484–1495.

45. Kelman L. The triggers or precipitants of the acute migraine attack. *Cephalalgia.* 2007;27(5):394–402.

46. Koseoglu E, Akboyraz A, Soyuer A, Ersoy AO. Aerobic exercise and plasma beta endorphin levels in patients with migrainous headache without aura. *Cephalalgia.* 2003;23(10):972–976.

47. Lockett DM, Campbell JF. The effects of aerobic exercise on migraine. *Headache.* 1992;32(1):50–54.

48. Narin SO, Pinar L, Erbas D, Ozturk V, Idiman F. The effects of exercise and exercise-related changes in blood nitric oxide level on migraine headache. *Clin Rehabil.* 2003;17(6):624–630.

49. Lemstra M, Stewart B, Olszynski WP. Effectiveness of multidisciplinary intervention in the treatment of migraine: a randomized clinical trial *Headache.* 2002;42:845–854.

50. Baillie LE, Gabriele JM, Penzien DB. A systematic review of behavioral headache interventions with an aerobic exercise component. *Headache.* 2014;54:40–53.

51. Varkey E, sa Cider A, Carlsson J, Linde M. Exercise and migraine prophylaxis: a randomized study using relaxation and topiramate as controls. *Cephalalgia.* 2011;31(14):1428–1438.

52. Holroyd KA, Lipchik GL, Penzien DB. Psychological management of recurrent headache disorders: empirical basis for clinical practice. In Dobson KS, Craig, KD, eds. *Empirically supported therapies: best practice in professional psychology.* Thousand Oaks, CA: SAGE, 1998:187–236.

53. Yeaw J, Benner JS, Walt JG, et al. Comparing adherence and persistence across 6 chronic medication classes. *J Manag Care Pharm.* 2009;15:728–740

54. Hepp Z, Dodick DW, Varon SF, Gillard P, Hansen RN, Devine EB. Adherence to oral migraine preventive medications among patients with chronic migraine. *Cephalalgia* 2014; 0333102414547138.

55. Rains JC, Lipchik GA, Penzien DB. Behavioral facilitation of medical treatment for headache. Part I: Review of headache treatment compliance. *Headache* 2006;46(9):1387–1394.

56. Holroyd KA, Cordingley GE, Pingel JD, et al. Enhancing the effectiveness of abortive therapy: A controlled evaluation of self-management training. *Headache.* 1989;29(3):148–153.

57. Spitzer RL, Williams JBW, Kroenke K, et al. Utility of a new procedure for diagnosing mental disorders in primary care: the PRIME MD 1000 study. *JAMA.* 1994;272:1749–1756.

58. Spitzer AL, Kroenke K, Williams JBW. Validation and utility of a self-report version of the PRIME-MD: The PHQ primary care study. *JAMA.* 1999;282:1737–44.

59. Maizels M, Smitherman TA, Penzien DB. A review of screening tools for psychiatric comorbidity in headache patients. *Headache.* 2006;46(suppl 3):S98–S109.

60. Beck AT, Steer RA, Brown GK. Manual for the Beck Depression Inventory-II. San Antonio, TX: Psychological Corporation, 1996.

61. Hamilton M. Rating depressive patients. *J Clin Psychiatry.* 1980;41:21–24.

62. Spitzer RL, Kroenke K, Williams JB, et al. A brief measure for assessing generalized anxiety disorder: the GAD-7. *Arch Intern Med.* 2006 May 22;166(10):1092–1097.

63. Kroenke K, Spitzer RL, Williams JB, et al. Anxiety disorders in primary care: prevalence, impairment, comorbidity, and detection. *Ann Intern Med.* 2007;146(5):317–325.

64. Gould RA, Otto MW, Pollack MH. A meta-analysis of treatment outcome for panic disorder. *Clin Psychol Rev.* 1995;15:819–844.

65. Gould RA, Otto MW, Pollack MH, et al. Cognitive behavioral and pharmacological treatment of generalized anxiety disorder: a preliminary meta-analysis. *Behav Ther.* 1997;28:285–305.

66. Franklin ME, Foa EB. (2002). Cognitive behavioral treatments for obsessive compulsive disorder. In: Nathan PE, Gorman JM, eds., *A guide to treatments that work.* 2nd ed. New York: Oxford University Press; 367–386.

67. Kobak KA, Greist JH, Jefferson JW, Katzelnick DJ, Henk HJ. Behavioral versus pharmacological treatments of obsessive compulsive disorder: a meta-analysis. *Psychopharmacol.* 1998;136:205–216.

68. Sousa MB, Isolan LR, Oliveira RR, et al. A randomized clinical trial of cognitive-behavioral group therapy and sertraline in the treatment of obsessive-compulsive disorder. *J Clin Psychiatry.* 2006;67:1133–1139.

69. Foa EB. Psychosocial treatment of posttraumatic stress disorder. *J Clin Psychiatry.* 2000;61(suppl 5):43–48.

70. Brown TA, Barlow DH. Long-term outcome in cognitive-behavioral treatment of panic disorder: clinical predictors and alternative strategies for assessment. *J Consult Clin Psychol.* 1995;63:754–765.

71. Ball JR, Mitchell PB, Corry JC, et al. A randomized controlled trial of cognitive therapy for bipolar disorder: focus on long-term change. *J Clin Psychiatry.* 2006;67:277–286.

72. Mitte K. Meta-analysis of cognitive-behavioral treatments for generalized anxiety disorder: a comparison with pharmacotherapy. *Psychol Bull.* 2005; Sep;131(5):785–795.

73. Lau MA. New developments in psychosocial interventions for adults with unipolar depression. *Curr Opin in Psych.* 2008;21:30–36.

74. Sheehan DV, Mao CG. Paroxetine treatment of generalized anxiety disorder. *Psychopharmacol Bull.* 2003;37(suppl 1):64–75.

75. Royal Australian and New Zealand College of Psychiatrists. Australian and New Zealand clinical practice guidelines for the treatment of panic disorder and agoraphobia. *Aust N Z J Psychiatry.* 2003;37:641–656.

76. Cloos JM. The treatment of panic disorder. *Curr Opin Psychiatry.* 2005;18:45–50.

77. Arena JG, Hightower NE, Chong GC. Relaxation therapy for tension headache in the elderly: a prospective study. *Psychol Aging* 1988;3(1):96.

78. Arena JG, Hannah SL, Bruno GM, et al. Electromyographic biofeedback training for tension headache in the elderly: a prospective study. *Biofeedback Self Reg.* 1991;35:187–195.

79. Kabela E, Blanchard EB, Appelbaum KA, et al. Self-regulatory treatment of headache in the elderly. *Biofeedback Self Reg.* 1989;14(3):219–228.

80. Mosley TH, Grotheus CA, Meeks WM. Treatment of tension headache in the elderly: a controlled evaluation of relaxation training and relaxation combined with cognitive-behavior therapy. *J Clin Geropsychol.* 1995;1:175–188.

81. Nicholson NL, Blanchard EB. A controlled evaluation of behavioral treatment of chronic headache in the elderly. *Behav Ther.* 1993;24(3):67–76.

82. Blanchard EB, Andrasik F. Psychological assessment and treatment of headache: Recent developments and emerging issues. *J Consult Clin Psychol.* 1982;50(6):859–879.

83. Hermann C, Kim M, Blanchard EB. Behavioral and prophylactic pharmacological intervention studies of pediatric migraine: an exploratory meta-analysis. *Pain.* 1995;60:239–255.

84. Holroyd KA. Assessment and psychological treatment of recurrent headache disorders. *J Consult Clin Psychol.* 2002;70:656–677.

85. Trautmann E, Lackschewitz H, Kroner-Herwig B. Psychological treatment of recurrent headache in children and adolescents: a meta-analysis. *Cephalalgia.* 2006;26(12):1411–1426.

86. Olness K, MacDonald JT, Uden DL. Comparison of self-hypnosis and propranolol in the treatment of juvenile migraine. *Pediatrics.* 1987;79:593–597.

87. Sartory G, Muller B, Metsch J, et al. A comparison of psychological and pharmacological treatment of pediatric migraine. *Behav Res Ther.* 1998;36(12):1155–1170.

88. Larsson B, Carlsson J, Fichtel A, et al. (2005). Relaxation treatment of adolescent headache sufferers: results from a school-based replication series. *Headache.* 2005;45(6):692–704.

89. Passchier J, van den Bree MBM, Emmen HH, et al. Relaxation training in school classes does not reduce headache complaints. *Headache.* 1990;30:660–664.

90. Marcus DA. Headache in pregnancy. *Curr Treat Options Neurol.* 2007;9(1):23–30.

91. Pfaffenrath V, Rehm M. Migraine in pregnancy: what are the safest treatment options? *Drug Saf.* 1998;19(5):383–388.

92. Marcus DA, L. Scharff L, Turk DC. Nonpharmacological management of headache during pregnancy. *Psychosomatic Medicine.* 1995;57:527–35.

Chapter 7

Acute Migraine Therapy

INTRODUCTION

The majority of patients use pharmacologic agents for the acute treatment of migraine headache. In a recent longitudinal population-based study, 91.7% of 11,388 people with episodic migraine reported using pharmacologic treatment for their acute migraine attacks. [1] The objectives of acute treatment are to treat attacks early while pain is still mild, to achieve rapid and complete relief of pain and associated symptoms, to minimize or eliminate adverse events, to restore the patient's ability to function, to minimize recurrence and the need for rescue medications, to optimize self-care, and to reduce the use of and dependence on medical resources.[2]

Acute pharmacologic migraine therapy includes both "migraine-specific" medications, such as triptans and dihydroergotamine, and "non-specific" medications such as ASA, acetaminophen, and non-steroidal anti-inflammatory drugs (NSAIDs). It also includes adjunctive medications for relief of both pain and associated symptoms, particularly nausea. Adjunctive medications include anti-emetics, such as dopamine antagonists (e.g., metoclopramide or prochlorperazine), and corticosteroids.

The introduction of subcutaneous sumatriptan in 1991 represented a significant advance in the acute treatment of migraine. Over the past two decades, many triptans in a variety of formulations have become available.[3] They have improved the quality of life for countless migraineurs and have led to important insights into the anatomy, physiology, and molecular pharmacology of migraine.[3–7] They are considered the treatment of choice for moderate and severe migraine and have been identified as.[2] the most important therapeutic advance in neurology over the past 25 years.[8]

Despite these advances, the proportion of patients using triptans for the acute treatment of migraine has remained relatively modest. [9–11] In a recent epidemiologic study among persons with episodic migraine, only 18% of migraineurs in the United States and 8% in Canada use triptans for acute migraine treatment.[1] Their use is significantly associated with certain demographic and clinical factors, including female gender, Caucasian race, age (40–49 years), higher levels of education (college or higher), annual household income less than $40,000, having health insurance, the presence of cutaneous allodynia, high headache-related disability, and the use of migraine-preventive medication. The higher prevalence of cardiovascular risk factors and the increased risk of ischemic stroke and other adverse cardiovascular outcomes in migraineurs limits those who are eligible for treatment with triptans and other migraine-specific drugs.[12–21]

GENERAL PRINCIPLES

A number of principles apply to the use of acute medications for migraine treatment.

Acute Treatment Strategy

It is important to select the most appropriate treatment strategy to maximize success. Three general strategies are used to choose the most appropriate treatment, and choice is based largely on the average severity and disability associated with attacks.[22,23] The first strategy is step-care across attacks, wherein the provider prescribes an acute treatment to be tried for several attacks. If this is not effective, care is "stepped up," or escalated, to another type of treatment; however, most patients have already tried several over-the-counter (OTC) medications, including simple analgesics and NSAIDS, before they seek medical attention. In essence, the patient has already initiated his or her own care, and the provider will likely need to escalate his or her acute treatment. Continuing a step-care strategy across attacks is not recommended when patients present with migraine that is poorly responsive to the usual acute therapy. The chance of failure is high and the patient will continue to suffer, become discouraged, and lapse from care.

The second strategy is step-care within attacks, wherein patients are instructed to escalate therapy within a single attack if the first medication is ineffective. This strategy is commonly employed when attacks are severe and disabling. This is an appropriate strategy for patients whose attacks begin with mild pain that lasts at least 30 minutes, when the treatment can be administered before pain escalates, and for patients who are able to recognize attacks that have a high likelihood of responding to non-specific therapy. This would not be an appropriate strategy for patients who have failed to respond to simple analgesics, even if used early, because it may render the attack less responsive to higher-end therapy when the attack progresses and pain becomes moderate or severe. This is important, since successful early treatment, while the pain is mild, predicts response; attacks that progress often respond less favorably to all acute medications. Since inadequate acute treatment has been shown to be an independent risk factor for progression from episodic to chronic migraine, optimal acute treatment should be a treatment priority and patients should be educated in this regard, although many have discovered this for themselves over time.[24]

The third option, stratified care, is the most appropriate strategy for many migraine patients who present with a chief complaint of headache. These patients experience pain and associated symptoms that are moderate or severe, have failed to respond to simple and mixed analgesics, and have a moderate or severe degree of migraine-related disability.[22,23,25] Stratified care has been shown to be cost-effective and has been recommended by the US Headache Consortium and the European Federation of Neurological Societies.[2,26–28] In the recent acute treatment guidelines from the Canadian

Headache Society, stratified care is the model of care recommended for patients with the most severe migraine attacks, while a modified, or "hybrid," model of care, which incorporates features of both stratified care and the "step-care-across-attacks" model, is recommended for less disabled patients with migraine.[29] We believe that the most effective strategy for patients with attacks of different severity is a step-care-within-attack strategy, provided that patients can readily distinguish their attacks and have responded to lower-end therapies. Because the ultimate goals are to rapidly achieve freedom from pain and associated symptoms with minimal or no adverse events, the consistent and early administration of this treatment is most appropriate for patients with consistently moderate or severe attacks that respond well to triptans or other higher-end therapies.

Timing of Administration

The second general principle is to encourage patients to administer treatment soon after the attack has started, while pain is still mild. The biological rationale for early administration is the inability of most acute treatments to reverse established central sensitization of second-order trigeminovascular neurons in the trigeminal nucleus caudalis.[30–38] Central sensitization, which is the physiological basis for cutaneous allodynia, usually develops over 20–60 minutes,[35,36] and once established, the attack is less responsive to triptans and other acute medications. There is ample evidence that administering triptans while pain is mild results in substantially higher 2-hour pain-free results.[39–46] The recommendation to treat early, while pain is mild, should be guided by the frequency of the headache and should be offered to patients with episodic migraine. For those with high-frequency episodic migraine (10–14 headache days per month) or chronic migraine (>15 headache days per month), caution is needed to avoid acute medication overuse.

Formulation

Most patients prefer oral medications, but for some patients a non-oral route of administration

may be necessary. The route of administration depends on the prior response to oral therapy, the temporal characteristics of the attack, especially the time from onset to peak pain intensity, and the presence and timing of nausea and vomiting. Early nausea and vomiting during an attack may impair absorption and bioavailability and diminish the efficacy and/or consistency of acute medications.[47] Non-oral routes of administration include nasal spray, suppository, transcutaneous patch, subcutaneous or transcutaneous injection, and inhalation. Several triptans, dihydroergotamine, ergotamine tartrate, and non-specific medications are available in non-oral formulation. These should be considered when individuals do not respond to oral triptans or achieve a partial or suboptimal response. They are also effective for patients who have an attack profile that is characterized by pain intensity that has a very short "time to peak" (attacks rapidly escalate, the mild pain phase is missed, or individuals awaken from sleep with a headache that is already moderate or severe).[48] In these cases, drugs associated with rapid absorption (subcutaneous sumatriptan, zolmitriptan nasal spray, or DHE inhalation or injection) may be more effective than an oral formulation.[49–62] Non-oral routes are preferable when attacks are associated with prominent nausea, especially if it occurs early in the course of an attack. Oral medications may be poorly absorbed or expelled, and a non-oral route may provide more rapid and consistent relief. Prokinetic medications may be used if the patient prefers oral medication, but there is no evidence that these agents enhance absorption or result in more consistent or rapid relief of pain and associated symptoms.

Use of Adjunctive Medications

The use of adjunctive medications is useful for patients who respond partially to a single medication. Patients who do not consistently achieve a rapid pain-free or sustained pain-free response to a triptan, for example, may require concomitant therapy to treat nausea (antiemetic) or to achieve a more sustained response by reducing the risk of recurrence within a 24–48 hour period (NSAID).[39,63–65] This is particularly true for patients who develop allodynia or have pain that escalates rapidly. While triptans have not been shown to reverse central sensitization, NSAIDs, particularly when given by the parenteral route, may reverse central sensitization and amplify a partial response to a triptan.[63]

Rescue Therapy

All patients need rescue therapy when acute therapy is not effective, even if they typically respond to a particular medication or strategy.[3,29,66,67] A rescue strategy will reduce suffering and disability and the need to seek care from urgent care clinics or emergency departments. Rescue strategies may include escalation of therapy (step-care within attack); a second dose of the same medication, sometimes in a different formulation (e.g., sumatriptan injection in the event that oral sumatriptan is not effective); or another medication class by oral (e.g., oral dexamethasone), nasal (e.g., intranasal zolmitriptan), inhalation (e.g., orally inhaled dihydroergotamine), suppository (e.g., prochlorperazine, indomethacin), or parenteral administration (e.g., intramuscular or nasal ketorolac). When patients have cardiovascular contraindications to migraine-specific medications or contraindications to the use of corticosteroids, NSAIDs, or dopamine antagonists, opioid medication can be provided for rescue therapy.

Avoid Acute Medication Overuse

The overuse of acute medications may result in medication overuse headache (MOH), as well as cause hepatic, renal, or gastrointestinal toxicity. Simple analgesics, including acetaminophen, aspirin, and NSAIDs, should not be used more than 14 days a month, while triptans, ergotamine, opioids, and combination analgesics should not be used more than nine days a month.[68–73] In the event that patients use a combination of two or more acute medications for some or all attacks, they should not be used for more than 14 days.[73] These limits are somewhat arbitrary, and not all patients who exceed them experience frequent headache that is induced by acute medication overuse, but exceeding these limits is an indication that new or modified preventive strategies are required, and the patient may be at risk for acute medication systemic toxicity.

ACUTE MEDICATIONS

Migraine Specific Medications

MIGRAINE-SPECIFIC DRUGS: TRIPTANS

Triptans are selective serotonin (5HT) agonists that are highly specific for the $5HT_{1B}$ and $5HT_{1D}$ receptors; many act at the $5HT_{1F}$ receptor.[74–76] There are seven serotonin receptors (5-HT_1, 5-HT_2, 5-HT_3, 5-HT_4, 5-HT_5, 5-HT_6, and 5-HT_7), and five 5-HT_1 receptor subtypes occur in humans: 5-HT_{1A}, 5-HT_{1B}, 5-HT_{1D}, 5-HT_{1E}, and 5-HT_{1F}.[74,77,78] 5-HT_{1B} receptors are located on intracranial, extracranial, and systemic blood vessels, as well as on central nervous system neurons; 5-HT_{1F} receptors are located on trigeminal nerve endings; and 5-HT_{1D} receptors are located on central nervous system neurons and trigeminal nerve endings.[6,79,80] Triptans and ergotamine inhibit the release of calcitonin gene-related peptide (CGRP), substance P, neurokinin A, glutamate, and other vesicle-bound neuropeptides and neurotransmitters by binding at presynaptic 5-HT_{1B}, 5-HT_{1D}, and 5-HT_{1F} inhibitory autoreceptors. At the peripheral neurovascular junction, the inhibition of neuropeptide release from activated sensory trigeminal afferents prevents neurogenic vasodilation and neurogenic inflammation at the neurovascular junction, while in the central nervous system, the presynaptic inhibition of neuropeptide release from first-order trigeminal neurons prevents the activation and/or sensitization of central second-order neurons in the trigeminal nucleus caudalis.[74,81–83] Considerable controversy exists as to whether triptans cross the blood–brain barrier and act centrally; 5-HT_{1B}, 5-HT_{1D}, and 5-HT_{1F} receptors are present on neurons located throughout the central nervous system in areas important for pain modulation [84–88] and could be a site of triptan action. Animal model iontophoresis experiments have demonstrated that triptans can modulate activity and ascending transmission of nociceptive traffic from the trigeminal nucleus caudalis when applied to the thalamus and periacqueductal gray matter.[89,90] The presence of central side effects (e.g., sedation, dizziness) commonly seen with some triptans clinically also reinforces the notion that they access central nervous system sites. PET studies demonstrating binding within the brain after the administration of intranasal zolmitriptan confirm access to CNS sites. In a recent fMRI study in human subjects, sumatriptan increased BOLD signal intensity within the trigemino-thalamo-cortical pathway and the authors suggested that specific functional inhibition of trigemino-thalamic-cortical projections is one of the reasons that triptans, unlike pain killers, act highly specifically on headache and migraine but not pain as such.[90a]

There are currently seven triptans available in different formulations (Table 7.1). The selection of a triptan requires a knowledge of the evidence base, characteristics of an individual patient's attacks (time to peak severity, presence and timing of nausea, the usual time of onset [e.g., nocturnal versus daytime]), pharmacokinetics of each triptan (Table 7.2), and patient preference of the attributes of the triptan. The response to and tolerability of a triptan is highly variable from one individual to another; before a patient is deemed a nonresponder, based on either lack of efficacy or intolerable side effects, different triptans, in different formulations, administered early while pain is still mild, should be tried.[91–94]

Because of their avid binding to $5HT_{1B}$ receptors, triptans are contraindicated in patients with coronary, cerebrovascular, and peripheral vascular disease or poorly controlled hypertension. However, numerous controlled trials and hundreds of millions of patient exposures indicate that the triptans are generally very safe in patients without vascular disease.[11] Concern has been expressed about the risk of serotonin syndrome when triptans are used by patients who are on medications, such as selective serotonin reuptake inhibitors (SSRIs) and selective serotonin and norepinephrine reuptake inhibitors (SNRIs), that increase the release, prevent the reuptake, or reduce the synaptic clearance of serotonin. However, the inhibitory effect of triptans on the presynaptic release of neurotransmitters, combined with the results of analyses of large patient databases that include patients who are exposed both to triptans and other serotonergic drugs, indicate that serotonin syndrome due to triptans is very rare, and possibly biologically implausible, based on their mechanism of action.[95–98] Since depression and anxiety and migraine are frequently comorbid, patients using antidepressants that increase serotonergic tone are seen often in clinical practice. These patients should not be prohibited from using triptans, as the benefit far exceeds the risk.

Over the past two decades, a large body of evidence that supports the use of triptans for the acute treatment of moderate or severe migraine headaches has accumulated. In a landmark meta-analysis of 53 randomized, double-blind, placebo- or active comparator-controlled trials, all oral triptans (with the exception of frovatriptan, which was not available at the time) were found to be effective for the acute treatment of migraine.[7] From a comparative standpoint, even though head-to-head trials were not available, rizatriptan 10 mg, eletriptan 80 mg, and almotriptan 12.5 mg appeared to provide superior efficacy (2-hour headache response and pain-free endpoints) compared with sumatriptan 100 mg, which was used as the reference drug comperator in this meta-analysis. Recurrence rates were lowest for frovatriptan (17%), eletriptan (24%), and naratriptan (25%).[7]

Almotriptan 12.5 mg and naratriptan 2.5mg showed superior tolerability compared with sumatriptan 100 mg. A later systematic review of 38 double-blind, randomized clinical trials

Table 7.1 Triptans: Dosage and Formulations

Medication	Formulation and Dose (mg)			
	Tablet	**Oral Disintegrating Tablet**	**Nasal Spray**	**Injection**
Sumatriptan	50, 100		20	4, 6
Zolmitriptan	2.5	2.5	5	
Rizatriptan	5, 10	5, 10		
Naratriptan	1.0, 2.5			
Eletriptan	20, 40			
Almotriptan	12.5			
Frovatriptan	2.5			

Table 7.2 Triptans Pharmacokinetics[29]

Variable	Almotriptan	Eletriptan	Frovatriptan	Naratriptan	Rizatriptan	Sumatriptan	Zolmitriptan
Bioavailability	70%	50%	Males: 20% Females: 30%	Males: 63% Females: 74%	45%	SC: 96% Oral: 14% Nasal: 16%	Oral: 40% Nasal: 41%
T_{max}	1–3 h	1–2 h	2–4 h	2–3 h	Oral: 1–1.5 h ODT: 1.6–2.5 h	SC: 15 min Oral: 2.5 h Nasal: 1–1.5 h	Oral/ODT: 2 h Nasal: 2 h
Onset	0.5–2 h	0.5–1 h	precise data not available; slow onset for most patients	1–3 h	0.5–1 h	SC: 10–15 min Oral (fast dissolving): 30 min Nasal: 15 min	Oral/ ODT: 45 min Nasal: 10–15 min
Elimination half-life	3–4 h	3.8 h	~26 h	5–8 h	2–3 h	2 h	2.5–3 h
Metabolism and elimination	MAO-A, CYP3A4, CYP2D6; inactive metabolites; 40% unchanged in urine	CYP3A4; active N-demethylated metabolite; 90% non-renal clearance	CYP1A2; several metabolites; active desmethyl frovatriptan	CYP 450 (various isoenzymes); inactive metabolites; 50% unchanged in urine	MAO-A: inactive & one active metabolites; 8–16% unchanged in urine	MAO-A: inactive metabolites	CYP1A2, MAO-A; inactive & one active metabolites; 8% unchanged in urine
Significant drug interactions*	None	CYP 3A4 inhibitors: contraindicated within 72 h of potent CYP3A4 inhibitors (e.g., ketoconazole, itraconazole)	None (CYP1A2 inhibitors have minimal potential to affect kinetics of frovatriptan)	None	MAOIs (avoid use within 14 days) Propranolol (↑ AUC of R; max. 5 mg single doses & 10 mg/24 h of R)	MAOIs (avoid use within 14 days)	MAOIs (avoid use within 14 days) CYP 1A2 inhibitors (e.g., cimetidine, fluvoxamine, ciprofloxacin); ↑ AUC & $t_{1/2}$ of Z; max. 5 mg/24 h of Z)

*All triptans: do not use within 24 hours of an ergot derivative (e.g., ergotamine, DHE) or another triptan (due to possibility of additive vasoconstriction); there is a theoretical possibility of serotonin syndrome (rare) when combined with other serotonergic drugs (e.g., SSRIs, lithium)—however, this is controversial.

AUC = area under the curve; MAOI = monoamine oxidase inhibitor; E = eletriptan; R = rizatriptan; Z = zolmitriptan; ODT = orally disintegrating tablet that included data on all seven oral triptans revealed similar results, with all oral triptans demonstrating headache relief and/or freedom from pain at 2 hours and pain relief at 1 hour, when compared with placebo.[99] Fast-dissolving sumatriptan 50 and 100 mg, sumatriptan 50 mg, and rizatriptan 10 mg showed significant relief at 1 hour when compared with placebo. The fast-dissolving formulation of sumatriptan 100 mg was the only oral triptan that provided freedom from pain at 1 hour compared with placebo. Fast-dissolving sumatriptan 50 and 100 mg and eletriptan 40 mg had significantly lower rates of recurrence compared with placebo, while rizatriptan 10 mg was the only triptan with a significantly higher rate of recurrence between 2 and 24 hours after an initial headache response. Sumatriptan and zolmitriptan were associated with a significantly higher number of adverse events compared with placebo.

A quantitative systematic review/meta-analysis of 54 trials (21,022 patients) involving 73 placebo comparisons included the following medications: rizatriptan (5 and 10 mg), naratriptan (2.5 mg), sumatriptan (6, 20, 50, and 100 mg), aspirin (900 mg) plus metoclopramide (10 mg), zolmitriptan (2.5 and 5 mg), dihydroergotamine mesylate (2 mg), Excedrin (paracetamol 500 mg plus aspirin 500 mg plus caffeine 130 mg), tolfenamic acid rapid release (200 to 400 mg), eletriptan (40 and 80 mg), Cafergot (ergotamine tartrate 2 mg plus caffeine 200 mg), and placebo.[100] All were oral formulation, except for subcutaneous sumatriptan (6 mg), intranasal sumatriptan (20 mg), and dihydroergotamine mesylate (2 mg). Ergotamine tartrate was not found to be statistically significantly superior to placebo for headache response at 1 and 2 hours or for pain-free at 2 hours. The number of patients needed to treat (NNT) to achieve a 2-hour headache response in one individual ranged from 2.0 (95% CI [1.8, 2.2]) for sumatriptan 6 mg to 5.4 (95% CI [3.8, 9.2]) for naratriptan 2.5 mg. The NNT at 1 hour (which didn't include aspirin [900 mg] plus metoclopramide [10 mg] and tolfenamic acid [200 to 400 mg]), ranged from 2.1 (95% CI [1.9, 2.2]) for sumatriptan (6 mg) to 10.0 (95% CI [7.3, 17.0]) for Excedrin. The NNT for a 2-hour pain-free response (with the exception of dihydroergotamine, which was not included in the analysis) ranged from 2.1 (95% CI [1.9, 2.4]) for subcutaneous sumatriptan

(6 mg) to 8.6 (95% CI [6.2, 14.0]) for aspirin (900 mg) plus metoclopramide (10 mg). There was a statistically significant dose-response for eletriptan (40 mg versus 80 mg, $p = 0.024$), rizatriptan (5 mg versus 10 mg, $p < 0.0001$), zolmitriptan (2.5 mg versus 5 mg, $p < 0.0059$), and sumatriptan (50 mg versus 100 mg, $p < 0.0002$). For sustained headache relief over 24 hours (headache response at 2 hours and no recurrence within 24 hours), NNT ranged from 2.8 for eletriptan 80 mg (most effective) to 8.3 for rizatriptan 5 mg (least effective) (Table 7.3).

Based on the efficacy of both triptans and NSAIDs for the acute treatment of migraine, the presumed different mechanisms of action, the evidence and clinical experience for adjunctive relief when both are used in combination, and the potential role of NSAIDs to inhibit the development of central sensitization or reverse the presence of established central sensitization and provide sustained pain relief, combinations of triptans and NSAIDs have been evaluated for the acute treatment of migraine. The combination of separate tablets of oral sumatriptan 50 mg and naproxen sodium 500 mg was evaluated in a multicenter, randomized, double-blind, double-dummy, placebo-controlled, four-arm study in 972 patients who treated a moderate or severe migraine

Table 7.3 Number Needed to Treat (NNT) for Triptans in the Acute Treatment of Migraine[29]

Drug and Dosage	Route	NNT (for 2-h pain-free vs. placebo)**
Sumatriptan 6 mg	subcutaneous	2.3
Sumatriptan 20 mg	intranasal	4.7
Zolmitriptan 5 mg	intranasal	4.6
Almotriptan 12.5	oral	4.3
Eletriptan 20 mg	oral	10
Eletriptan 40 mg	oral	4.5
Frovatriptan 2.5 mg	oral	8.5
Naratriptan 2.5 mg	oral	8.2
Rizatriptan 10 mg	oral	3.1
Sumatriptan 50 mg	oral	6.1
Sumatriptan 100 mg	oral	4.7
Zolmitriptan 2.5 mg	oral	5.9

** Note: Migraine attacks were treated at moderate or severe intensity. NNTs may be lower for individual drugs when treatment is taken early in the migraine attack

attack with placebo, naproxen sodium 500 mg, sumatriptan 50 mg, or a combination of sumatriptan 50 mg and naproxen sodium 500 mg. Sumatriptan plus naproxen sodium was superior (46%) to sumatriptan alone (29%), naproxen sodium alone (25%), or placebo (17%; $p < 0.001$) for the primary endpoint, sustained 24-hour headache relief.[101] This proof of concept was extended in two randomized, placebo-controlled trials where a fixed combination of sumatriptan (85 mg)/naproxen sodium (500 mg) was more effective than placebo for headache relief at 2 hours and superior for sustained pain-free response compared with sumatriptan monotherapy, naproxen sodium monotherapy, and placebo.[64] In addition, in two other replicate, multicenter, randomized, double-blind, placebo-controlled, two-attack, crossover trials, the fixed-dose formulation of sumatriptan 85 mg and naproxen sodium 500 mg was demonstrated to be superior to placebo when administered while pain was mild, in patients who were historically considered non-responders to oral triptans.[102]

While most triptan clinical trials have evaluated efficacy and tolerability when administered for moderate to severe headache, it has been clear from clinical practice that drug efficacy and patient outcomes are improved when the medication is administered early. This widely practiced approach is now supported by abundant evidence from randomized controlled trials that sustained pain-free outcomes, and a rapid return to normal function is enhanced when triptans are administered early, while pain is mild. The distinction between early and mild is important, since early treatment when pain is moderate or severe is not associated with improved outcomes.[103] The *key predictor* of outcome is the pain intensity at the time the drug is administered. Placebo-controlled early intervention trials have been done with almotriptan (12.5 mg) zolmitriptan (2.5 mg), frovatriptan (2.5 mg), sumatriptan (50 and 100 mg), eletriptan (20 and 40 mg), sumatriptan fast-disintegrating tablets (50 and 100 mg), and rizatriptan (10 mg).[41,103–105]

An iontophoretic transdermal sumatriptan patch is effective for the acute treatment of migraine.[106] This may prove useful for patients who have prominent nausea at the onset of attack, have shown inconsistent or poor response to oral triptans, or do not wish to use the intranasal, inhalation, or parenteral routes of administration.[107,108] In a randomized, placebo-controlled, parallel-group study, 469 patients received either transdermal sumatriptan or placebo after pain became moderate or severe. Active drug was superior to placebo for 2-hour pain-free and 24-hour sustained pain-free. The treatment was reasonably well tolerated. Mild to moderate application-site reactions were reported by 50% and 44% of patients treated with transdermal sumatriptan and placebo, respectively.

Other Migraine-Specific Medications

ERGOTAMINE

Ergotamine tartrate (ET) was one of the first ergot alkaloids to be isolated and used for migraine treatment and had been a cornerstone in the acute management of migraine for much of the twentieth century since its isolation and before the introduction of triptans in the early 1990s. Dihydroergotamine (DHE) is a semi-synthetic, hydrogenated ergot alkaloid, synthesized by reducing an unsaturated bond in ergotamine (E).[109] Both ET and DHE have significant activity at monoaminergic receptors, but their antimigraine efficacy, like the triptans, is considered to be mainly due to their agonist activity at 5-HT_{1B}, 5-HT_{1D}, and 5-HT_{1F} receptors. Their activity at 5-HT_{1B} receptors contraindicates their use for patients with established vascular disease and uncontrolled hypertension. Their side effect profiles differ from the triptans, likely due to their agonist activity at 5-HT_{1A}, 5-HT_{2A}, and dopamine D_2 receptors.[109] Because of very high first-pass metabolism, both ET and DHE have very low oral bioavailability (oral 1%, rectal 1%–2%), but several of their metabolites are present in concentrations several times higher than that of the parent compound and have biologic activity similar to that of the parent drug. The major metabolite of DHE is 8'-OH DHE, which is present at a concentration five to seven times greater than that of DHE.[109] The pharmacologic effects of the active metabolites are qualitatively similar to those of the parent compound. They are also avidly sequestered by tissues, which may contribute to delayed and sustained activity after the parent drug or metabolites can no longer be detected in plasma. DHE has much higher bioavailability via the intramuscular (100%), intranasal (40%), and inhalation (100%) routes. Peak plasma levels occur approximately 1–2 minutes after intravenous administration, 24 minutes after intramuscular administration, 30–60 minutes after intranasal administration, and 10 minutes following inhalation administration. Intranasal and inhalation DHE administration, which avoids first-pass hepatic metabolism, delivers adequate plasma concentrations of the drug and eliminates the need for parenteral administration. The major route of elimination is the feces following biliary excretion of unchanged drug and metabolites. Dihydroergotamine is eliminated in a biphasic manner, with mean half-lives of approximately 0.7–1 and 10–13 hours.[109] The long half-life, potent and active metabolites, high tissue sequestration, and kinetics of receptor binding may account for the lower headache recurrence rate observed in DHE-treated patients compared to triptan-treated patients.[110]

Ergot alkaloid trials are dated and highly variable in their design, outcomes, and formulation of ergotamine tartrate used. A review of 23 trials included numerous treatment comparisons involving ergotamine, ergotamine-containing compounds, and ergostine-containing compounds.[109] Comparisons with placebo included five trials of ergotamine tartrate, three trials of ergotamine plus caffeine, and single trials of ergotamine plus caffeine plus cyclizine, ergotamine plus caffeine plus pentobarbital plus Bellafoline (Cafergot PB), ergotamine plus caffeine plus butalbital plus belladonna alkaloids (Cafergot Compound), and ergostine plus caffeine.[109] Only one study (1961) of ergotamine tartrate demonstrated significant efficacy, but this study used a high dose that is not used in clinical practice because of prohibitive side effects. Two ergotamine tartrate-containing proprietary combinations (Cafergot Compound and Cafergot PB) were found to be superior to placebo. In general, oral ergotamine has been shown to be inferior to oral triptans. In a multicenter, randomized, double-blind, double-dummy, parallel-group trial ($n = 580$), oral ergotamine (2 mg plus caffeine 200 mg) was inferior to oral sumatriptan (100 mg dispersible tablet) for 2-hour headache relief (48% vs. 66%, respectively; $p < 0.001$) and 2-hour pain-free (13% vs. 35%, respectively; $p < 0.001$).[111] Recurrence rates were significantly higher ($p = 0.009$) in the sumatriptan-treated patients (41%) within 48 hours compared with the ergotamine/caffeine group (30%). Oral eletriptan 40 mg and 80 mg was superior to ergotamine tartrate for 2-hour headache response (33% vs. 54% for eletriptan 40 mg; $p < 0.001$),[112] and almotriptan 12.5 mg was more effective than caffeine/ergotamine for both 2-hour headache (58% vs. 45%; $p < 0.01$) and 2-hour pain-free response (21% vs. 14%, respectively; $p < 0.05$).[113] Finally, a meta-analysis of oral sumtriptan indicated that ergotamine (plus caffeine) was significantly less effective than oral sumatriptan.[114]

Intranasal DHE was superior to placebo in a pooled analysis of four randomized, placebo-controlled studies evaluating higher dosages of DHE (1–4mg).[115–118] The summary effect size from these studies was comparable in magnitude with the results reported in the DHE nasal spray multicenter investigators' trial, which found a difference of 0.4 points (on a 5-point scale) in mean 2-hour headache relief scores between DHE and placebo. Comparator trials with intranasal DHE and intranasal sumatriptan indicate that intranasal sumatriptan is superior. In a multicenter, randomized, two-attack, double-blind, double-dummy, crossover study ($n = 368$), significantly ($p < 0.001$) more patients (53%) treated with a single spray of intranasal sumatriptan 20 mg achieved headache relief at 1 hour compared to 41% of patients treated with intranasal DHE 1 mg (0.5 mg spray in each nostril plus optional 0.5 mg in each nostril after 30 minutes).[119] In a similar multicenter, randomized, double-blind, double-dummy, crossover study ($n = 266$), subcutaneous sumatriptan (6 mg) was significantly better than intranasal DHE (1 mg plus optional 1 mg) at providing headache relief and freedom from pain at each time point measured between 15 minutes and 2 hours after drug administration ($p < 0.001$). While 24-hour sustained headache relief rates were significantly ($p < 0.001$) higher in the subcutaneous sumatriptan-treated patients (54%) compared with those patients treated with intranasal DHE (39%), recurrence rates were higher with subcutaneous sumatriptan (31%) compared to intranasal DHE (17%).[118]

Adverse events reported in association with intranasal DHE are generally mild to moderate and were related to the intranasal route of administration. The most common events reported were nasal congestion or irritation, throat irritation, unpleasant taste, and other local reactions related to the route of administration.

The use of parenteral DHE is common in tertiary care centers in the United States, but the evidence base is not robust. Two of three small trials comparing intravenous DHE with intramuscular meperidine suggest that DHE was significantly better at relieving head pain at 30 and 60 minutes.[120,121] The most rigorous clinical trial was a multicenter, randomized, double-blind clinical trial (n = 295) that demonstrated superior efficacy for subcutaneous sumatriptan 6 mg compared with SC DHE 1 mg for both 1-hour (78% vs. 57%) and 2-hour response rates (85% vs. 73%). However, 4-hour headache relief rate with DHE was similar to that of sumatriptan 6 mg (85.5% vs. 83.3%), and the recurrence rate was significantly lower (p < 0.001) in the DHE-treated patients (18%) compared to the sumatriptan-treated patients (45%). Therefore, subcutaneous sumatriptan provides faster relief, but subcutaneous DHE provides lower recurrence and higher sustained relief rates over a 24-hour period.

MAP0004 (Levadex™) is an orally inhaled formulation of DHE that delivers 0.6 mg emitted dose (1.0-mg nominal dose) to the lungs using a TEMPO inhaler. MAP0004 is quickly absorbed into the systemic circulation with a maximum concentration (Cmax) in approximately 10 minutes.[122,123] This is significantly lower than the Cmax associated with intravenous DHE and results in fewer adverse events.[123] In a randomized, 86-subject, double-blind, placebo-controlled, two-period, dose-ranging, multicenter study, MAP0004 0.5 or 1.0 mg systemic equivalent dose (1.0 or 2.0 mg nominal dose), MAP0004 (0.5 mg) was found to be superior for headache response at 2-hour (72%, p = .019) and 1.0 mg (65%, p = .071) compared to placebo (33%).[61,62] Pain relief at 10 (32%), 15 (46%), and 30 (55%) minutes was significantly (p < .05) greater with MAP0004 0.5 mg than with placebo (respectively, 0%, 7%, and 14%). Pain-free at 2 hours was significantly greater with MAP0004 0.5 mg (44%, p = .015) and 1.0 mg (35%, p = .050) than with placebo (7%). In a larger double-blind, placebo-controlled, parallel group, single attack of moderate or severe intensity study, 903 patients were randomized to receive either MAP0004 (0.63 mg emitted dose; 1.0 mg nominal dose) or placebo. MAP0004 was superior to placebo for all four co-primary endpoints, including pain relief (58.7% vs. 34.5%, p < .0001) and the absence of phonophobia (52.9% vs. 33.8%, p < .0001), photophobia (46.6% vs. 27.2%, p < .0001), and nausea (67.1% vs. 58.7%, p = .0210). (62;62) Significantly more patients were pain-free at 2 hours following treatment with MAP0004 than with placebo (28.4% vs. 10.1%, p < .0001).[62] MAP0004 (now known as Semprana; formerly Levadex) has not yet received regulatory approval.

NON-SPECIFIC MEDICATIONS

Simple Analgesics and NSAIDs

About 60% of migraine patients use only OTC analgesics for their attacks. In a qualitative systematic review of the literature from January 1966 through April 2002, acetaminophen, aspirin, ibuprofen, and an aspirin-acetaminophen-caffeine combination product were shown to be more effective than placebo in 2-hour headache response rates.[124] Similar to trials that evaluated migraine-specific treatments, these trials evaluated efficacy for treatment of moderate or severe pain. However, published trials of OTC agents have evaluated less severely affected patient populations by excluding patients who experience attack-related disability with at least 50% of attacks and/or vomiting with at least 20% of attacks. The conclusion was that treatment with only OTC products is a reasonable option for patients with migraine who encounter disability with less than 50% of attacks and/or vomiting with less than 20% of attacks.[124] NSAIDs, including ibuprofen, naproxen sodium, and diclofenac potassium, have been evaluated for migraine acute treatment and are effective for migraine at all levels of severity. The pharmacokinetic profile of the NSAIDs typically used for the acute treatment of migraine headache are reviewed in Table 7.4. A meta-analysis of five trials of low-dose ibuprofen concluded that ibuprofen (200 and 400 mg) is effective for the 2-hour pain-free endpoint compared to placebo (NNT = 13 for 200 mg; NNT = 9 for 400 mg); photophobia and phonophobia improved only with the 400 mg dose.[125] Adverse events were similar for ibuprofen and placebo.[125] In a Cochrane review based on nine studies (4273 participants,

Table 7.4 Non-Steroidal Anti-Inflammatory Drugs: Pharmacokinetics and Dosage[29]

Drug	T_{max} (hours)	Elimination Half-Life (hours)	Dose (mg)*	Dosage Interval (if repeated) and Maximum Daily Dose*
Acetylsalicylic acid (ASA) (tablet)	1–2	ASA: 0.25 Salicylate (active): 5–6 (after 1 g dose)	975–1,000	Every 4–6 h; max: 5.4 g/day (varies depending on indication)
Acetylsalicylic acid (ASA)(effervescent)	~20 min	as above	975–1,000	Every 4 h; max: 8 (325 mg) tablets
Ibuprofen (tablet)	1–2	2	400	Every 4 h; max: 2,400 mg
Ibuprofen (solubilized)	< 1	2	400	Every 4 h; max: 2,400 mg
Naproxen sodium°°	2	14	500–550 (up to 825 mg)	Twice a day; max: 1,375 mg
Diclofenac potassium (tablet)	< 1	2	50	3–4 times a day; max: 150 mg
Diclofenac potassium (powder for oral solution)	15 min	2	50	Single dose recommended for migraine attack
Ketorolac°°°	< 1	5	10	3–4 times a day; max: 40 mg

T_{max} = time to maximum plasma concentration
°Note: for acute migraine treatment, only one or two doses are usually recommended; doses are for adults.
°°Absorbed more quickly than naproxen
°°°No controlled trial evidence for efficacy in migraine

5223 attacks), the NNT for ibuprofen 400 mg versus placebo for 2-hour pain-free, 2-hour headache relief, and 24-hour sustained headache relief were 7.2, 3.2, and 4.0, respectively[126] (Table 7.5). The NNT for ibuprofen 200 mg versus placebo for 2-hour pain-free and 2-hour headache relief were 9.7 and 6.3, respectively.

Table 7.5 Number Needed to Treat (NNT) for Simple Analgesics/NSAIDs in the Acute Treatment of Migraine[29]

Analgesic or NSAID (tablets)	NNT (2-hour relief)	NNT (2-hour pain-free)
Acetaminophen 1000 mg	5.0	12.0
ASA 900–1000 mg	4.9	8.1
ASA 900 mg + metoclopramide 10 mg	3.3	8.8
Ibuprofen 400 mg	3.2	7.2
Naproxen sodium 500–825 mg	7.0	15.0
Diclofenac potassium (tablet)	6.2	8.9
Diclofenac potassium powder for oral solution	4.5	7.1

Ibuprofen 400 mg is consistently superior to 200 mg, and solubilized formulations of ibuprofen 400 mg are superior to standard tablets (Table 7.4). The Cochrane review concluded that ibuprofen is an effective treatment for acute migraine headache, providing pain relief in about half of sufferers; however, it only provided a pain-free response in approximately 25% of those taking 400 mg, and it only provided relief of associated symptoms in a minority of subjects.[126]

A meta-analysis of four trials of naproxen sodium also showed that dosages between 500 mg and 825 mg showed superior 2-hour pain-free results (pooled risk ratio for headache relief at 2 hours = 1.58 [$p < 0.00001$], and pain-free at 2 hours = 2.22 [$p = 0.0002$]) compared with placebo for the treatment of moderate or severe pain.[127] Pain-free at 2 hours and sustained pain-free at 24 hours were higher with naproxen sodium 825 mg compared to 500 mg. Naproxen sodium is preferred over naproxen (base) due to its faster onset of action. NSAIDs should be avoided in patients with a history of peptic ulceration, gastrointestinal hemorrhage, renal failure, and aspirin- or NSAID-related allergic disorders.

Oral diclofenac potassium was evaluated in five placebo-controlled studies (n = 1356) for acute treatment for moderate or severe migraine headache pain; the evaluation was summarized in a Cochrane review.[128] Headache response (55%; NNT 6.2), pain-free (22%; NNT 8.9), and sustained pain-free (19%; NNT 9.5) rates were superior to placebo. Adverse effects were mostly mild to moderate in intensity, self-limiting, and not significantly different from placebo. In a single comparator study, no significant difference was found between diclofenac potassium (50 and 100 g) and sumatriptan 100 mg for headache relief at 2 hours, though both doses of diclofenac potassium were significantly better than placebo and sumatriptan in reducing nausea at 2 hours.[129]

A European multicenter, randomized, placebo-controlled, crossover trial compared single doses of 50 mg diclofenac potassium sachets (a novel water-soluble buffered powder formulation for oral solution) and tablets with placebo in 328 migraine patients (888 attacks). [130] Significant treatment differences were shown for diclofenac potassium sachets versus placebo (p < 0.0001), tablets versus placebo (p = 0.0040), and sachets versus tablets (p = 0.0035). The NNT for 2-hour pain-free were 7.75 (95% CI [5.46, 13.35]) for sachets and 15.83 (95% CI [8.63, 96.20]) for tablets. Sachets were also superior to tablets for sustained headache response, sustained pain-free, and reduction in headache intensity within the first 2 hours post-dose (p < 0.05). Sachets provided faster onset of pain relief (15 minutes) compared to tablets (60 minutes). No safety issues were identified with either tablets or sachets. The study concluded that sachets are more effective than tablets, with a faster onset of analgesia.

In another randomized, double-blind, parallel-group, placebo-controlled study conducted in 23 US centers, 690 subjects were randomized to either 50 mg diclofenac potassium (dissolved in approximately 2 ounces of water) solution or matching placebo for the treatment of a migraine headache of moderate or severe intensity. Significantly more subjects treated with diclofenac potassium solution (n = 343) compared to placebo achieved a

2-hour pain-free (25% vs. 10%, p < .001) and 24-hour sustained pain-free response (19% vs. 7%, p < .0001). The absence of nausea (65% vs. 53%, p = .002), photophobia (41% vs. 27%, p < .001) and phonophobia (44% vs. 27%, p < .001) was also superior for diclofenac potassium oral solution compared to placebo. Significant differences in pain relief were seen in the patients treated with active drug starting at 30 minutes post-treatment (p = .013) and at all subsequent time-points (p < .001). The most common adverse event considered to be treatment related was nausea, but the rates for both active drug and placebo were identical (diclofenac potassium for oral solution [4.6%]; placebo [4.3%]).[131]

Based upon an exhaustive review of the evidence (Table 7.6), the Canadian Headache Society has made a strong recommendation for the following based upon evidence that was judged to be of high quality: aspirin (975–1000 mg tablets or effervescent formulation), given with oral metoclopramide (10 mg) if nausea is present; ibuprofen (400 mg tablet or solubilized liquid containing capsules); naproxen sodium in immediate release formulation (500 or 550 mg; up to 825 mg); diclofenac potassium (50 mg tablet or powder for oral solution); and acetaminophen (1,000 mg), alone or in combination with oral metoclopramide (10 mg), are recommended for the acute treatment of mild or moderate migraine attacks.[29]

Opioids

There is limited evidence for oral opioids, including codeine, morphine, hydromorphone, meperidine, and opioid-containing combination products such as ASA/acetaminophen plus codeine, for the acute treatment of migraine. Acetaminophen-codeine combination was compared to aspirin in a placebo-controlled study; there was no difference between the two active drugs, but both were superior to placebo.[132]

Butorphanol tartrate is a potent, synthetic, mixed agonist-antagonist opioid analgesic with activity at the kappa opioid receptor that can give rise to significant dysphoria.[133] The drug has a stronger evidence base for its use for the acute treatment of migraine headache

Table 7.6 **Summary of Canadian Headache Society Guidelines and Recommendations for Acute Treatments* of Migraine Headache[29]**

Drug and Route(s)	Recommendation	Quality of Evidence
Recommended for use in episodic migraine** (Use)		
Triptans and other migraine-specific medications		
Almotriptan (oral)	Strong	High
Eletriptan (oral)	Strong	High
Frovatriptan (oral)	Strong	High
Naratriptan (oral)	Strong	High
Rizatriptan (oral)	Strong	High
Sumatriptan (SC, oral, intranasal)	Strong	High
Zolmitriptan (oral, intranasal)	Strong	High
Dihydroergotamine (intranasal, SC self-injection)	Weak	Moderate
Ergotamine (oral)	Weak (not recommended for routine use)	Moderate
ASA / NSAIDs		
ASA (oral)	Strong	High
Diclofenac potassium (oral)	Strong	High
Ibuprofen (oral)	Strong	High
Naproxen sodium (oral)	Strong	High
Other		
Acetaminophen (oral)	Strong	High
Opioids and Tramadol (not recommended for routine use)		
Opioid (i.e., codeine)–containing medications (oral)	Weak	Low
Tramadol-containing medications (oral)	Weak	Moderate
Anti-emetics		
Domperidone (oral)	Strong	Low
Metoclopramide (oral)	Strong	Moderate
Not recommended for use in episodic migraine** (Do not use)***		
Butalbital-containing medications (oral)	Strong	Low
Butorphanol (intranasal)	Strong	Low

*Utilizing GRADE criteria
**Migraine with headache on less than 15 days a month
***Except under exceptional circumstances

based upon two two randomized, double-blind, placebo-controlled trials that have shown it to be effective in rapidly relieving pain associated with acute moderate or severe migraine. [2,134,135] In a randomized, controlled, double-blind, parallel-group trial, butorphanol (1 mg) nasal spray was compared to a combination of butalbital 50 mg, caffeine 40 mg, aspirin 325 mg, and codeine phosphate 30 mg in patients with moderate or severe migraine. [134] Butorphanol was more effective in treating migraine pain with a rapid time to onset of relief at 15 minutes.

Tramadol inhibits the reuptake of serotonin and norepinephrine and is a weak u-opioid receptor agonist. Although the abuse potential of tramadol is considered to be less than that of other more potent opioids, the side effect profile is similar and abuse has been demonstrated in migraine patients.[137–139]

A single placebo-controlled trial in 305 patients compared the combination of tramadol (75 mg) and acetaminophen (650 mg) (n = 305) in acute migraine, and it was found to be significantly better than placebo for headache relief (55.8% vs. 33.8%, $p < 0.001$) and freedom from pain (22.1% vs. 9.3%, $p \leq 0.007$) at 2 hours.[136] Tramadol-related adverse events included nausea, dizziness, vomiting, and somnolence.

The Canadian Headache Society recommends against the routine use of oral opioids because of the risk of habituation, addiction, and tolerance; withdrawal syndromes; the high rate of side effects, including sedation, dizziness, and constipation; and the high risk of medication overuse headache with as few as five doses per month.[29] However, when patients do not respond to or cannot tolerate NSAIDS, triptans, or ergots, their use as acute or rescue therapy, with close monitoring, may be considered.

Butalbital-Containing Products

Butalbital-containing analgesics, like opioids, are associated with significant adverse effects, including sedation, intoxication, risk of dependence, abuse, risk of MOH with frequent use, and severe withdrawal syndromes (including seizures) on discontinuation of high doses.[140–142] A qualitative systematic search (1966–2001) concluded that although butalbital-containing products are commonly prescribed for migraine, no evidence in the literature has demonstrated their benefit over other agents or placebo.[143] In a randomized, controlled acute treatment trial (n = 275), butorphanol nasal spray was superior to a combination of butalbital 50 mg, caffeine 40 mg, aspirin 325 mg, and codeine phosphate 30 in relieving migraine pain.[135] In an enriched (butalbital responders), randomized, double-blind, placebo-controlled trial involving 442 subjects, sumatriptan-naproxen sodium compound was found to be superior to placebo and the butalbital compound on most secondary endpoints, although not for the primary endpoint of sustained pain-free.[144] This study demonstrated that while butalbital-containing analgesics may have efficacy in the treatment of acute migraine attacks, the evidence is limited

and the risks substantial, and their use should be limited both in frequency and in those for whom triptans, NSAIDS, simple analgesics, and ergots are contraindicated, poorly tolerated, or not effective.

Neuroleptics (Dopamine Antagonists)

Dopamine antagonists are widely used for acute migraine therapy, often as adjuncts to triptans, NSAIDS, or ergots to augment their efficacy or to relieve nausea or vomiting. They are also commonly used as parenteral or suppository treatments for patients with prolonged attacks of migraine that do not respond to usual therapies and episodes of status migrainosus. Neuroleptics encompass different classes of medications, including the phenothiazines (e.g., prochlorperazine, chlorpromazine, promethazine), butyrophenones (e.g., droperidol and haloperidol), and metoclopramide. Clinicians must be alert to their idiosyncratic and potentially severe side effects, including extrapyramidal side effects (especially dystonia and akathisia). Extrapyramidal side effects may be prevented or treated by administering anticholinergic agents such as benztropine, diphenhydramine, or trihexyphenidyl. Hypotension infrequently occurs with the phenothiazines. Rare but serious side effects include neuroleptic malignant syndrome and QT interval prolongation with ventricular arrhythmia. Nine cases of torsade de pointes have been reported in 30 years, and all have been with droperidol at doses of 5 mg IV or greater.[145,146] Electrocardiogram and electrolytes should therefore be checked before a patient receives a neuroleptic for the first time to ensure that the QTc interval is not prolonged.

Droperidol, in four intramuscular dosages (0.1, 2.75, 5.5, and 8.25 mg), was evaluated in a randomized placebo-controlled trial in which patients treated moderate or severe pain. The percentages of subjects pain-free at 2 hours for placebo and droperidol doses 0.1, 2.75, 5.5, and 8.25 mg were 16%, 27%, 49%, 37%, and 34%, respectively ($p < .01$).[147] Serious side effects occurred in 30% of those receiving droperidol and included anxiety, akathisia, and somnolence. No patient had electrocardiogram changes showing QT prolongation.

Prochlorperazine has been evaluated in placebo-controlled trials using three different routes of administration. Rectal prochlorperazine 25 mg was superior to placebo in reducing pain according to an 11-point pain scale (11-PPS) (–7.6 vs. -4.3, $p = .018$); no adverse events were reported.[148] Intravenous prochlorperazine 10 mg was superior to intravenous normal saline (placebo) for a 1-hour pain-free endpoint (74% vs. 13%, $p < .001$).[149] No extrapyramidal reactions were reported. Drowsiness was the most frequent side effect in both groups (prochlorperazine 17% vs. placebo 7%). In a placebo-controlled active comparator study, intravenous prochlorperazine 10 mg was compared to intravenous metoclopramide and was shown to be superior for a 30-minute pain-free endpoint (82% vs. 48%, $p = .03$). Metoclopramide was not shown to be superior to placebo (48% vs. 29%, $p = .14$).[150] Intramuscular prochlorperazine (10 mg) was compared to intramuscular metoclopramide and 10 mg intramuscular saline in 86 subjects with moderate or severe migraine headache and was shown to be superior for the mean reduction in headache severity (respectively 67% vs. 34% vs. 16%). Symptoms of nausea and vomiting were significantly relieved in the prochlorperazine group ($p < 0.001$). However, rescue analgesic therapy was necessary in the majority of patients treated with prochlorperazine (16/28) and metoclopramide (23/29) after the 60-minute study period. The authors concluded that although intramuscular prochlorperazine appears to provide more effective relief than metoclopramide, the results do not support either drug as a single-agent therapy for acute migraine headache.[151]

In one study, the combination of prochlorperazine and dihydroergotamine, a combination frequently used in infusion centers and emergency departments as rescue therapy for an intractable migraine attack (e.g., status migrainosus), was evaluated using different dosages of each drug.[152] The percentage of patients pain-free at 4 hours was 80% for IV prochlorperazine 5 mg plus IV DHE 0.5 mg, 89% for IV prochlorperazine 3.5 mg plus IV DHE 1 mg, 95% for IV prochlorperazine 10 mg plus IV DHE 1 mg, and 83% for IV DHE 1 mg alone. Side effects occurred in all patients receiving IV DHE alone, the most common being chest discomfort (75%), nausea (67%), and sedation (30%). Higher doses of prochlorperazine were associated with a higher frequency of side effects, although all doses yielded fewer side effects than were recorded with DHE alone.

Two small, prospective, randomized, double-blind, placebo-controlled studies have evaluated the efficacy of intravenous chlorpromazine for the acute treatment of migraine. In a 36-subject trial involving patients presenting to the emergency department, there was no significant difference ($p = 0.18$) in the ability to return to usual activities within 1 hour between those who received intravenous chlorpromazine 1 mg/kg (9/19) or placebo 4/17 (23.5%). However, chlorpromazine was more often effective in achieving relief of headache ($p < 0.005$) and nausea ($p < 0.001$). The only significant side effects were drowsiness (79% vs. 35%, $p < 0.01$) and an asymptomatic drop in blood pressure (10 mm Hg systolic) (53% vs. 20%, $p < .05$).[153] In a second trial, the effect of intravenous chlorpromazine 1 mg/kg or placebo on pain and associated symptoms was evaluated in 68 patients with migraine with aura and 68 patients with migraine without aura.[154] Significant ($p < 0.01$) improvement in pain relief (66.7% vs. 6.7%, $p < .01$ for migraine with aura; and 63.2% vs 10%, $p < .01$ for migraine without aura) and for all associated symptoms (nausea, photophobia, and phonophobia) was demonstrated at the 60-minute time point with NNT of 2. The need for rescue medication and rate of recurrence at 24 hours was also significantly reduced in both groups. Treatment with chlorpromazine was associated with drowsiness and postural hypotension. The authors concluded that chlorpromazine is an excellent option for the treatment of migraine with and without aura in the emergency department.

Three placebo-controlled studies of parenteral metoclopramide were negative, and one study revealed metoclopramide 10 mg IV to be inferior to prochlorperazine 10 mg IV.[150,151,155] However, metoclopramide 10 mg IV was superior to placebo for pain relief at 1 hour (67% vs. 19%, $p = .02$).[156] As a single or adjunctive medication, metoclopramide 10 mg IV and metoclopramide plus ibuprofen 600 mg orally was superior to placebo for pain relief as measured on a visual analogue scale; the combination was superior to treatment with ibuprofen alone or placebo (both -25, $p < .01$).[157] A number of positive uncontrolled and/or open-label studies comparing metoclopramide in IV dosages between 10 and 20 mg in combination with diphenhydramine 25 mg IV and DHE IV 1 mg with other parenteral therapies have been reported,[121,158–163] but controlled evidence to support these combinations is still not available.

Oral metoclopramide has demonstrated efficacy as an adjunctive medication.[164–166] A Cochrane systematic review concluded that the addition of metoclopramide (10 mg po) to oral aspirin 1000 mg improves relief of nausea and vomiting.[167] In a small, double-blind, randomized, crossover study in 16 patients who had failed to receive adequate relief from triptans, meaningful relief was attained in 10 of 16 (63%) migraine attacks treated with the combination of sumatriptan 50 mg plus metoclopramide 10 mg, compared with 5 of 16 (31%) migraines treated with sumatriptan plus placebo.[168] Overall, the data suggest that metoclopramide, either as a 10 mg oral dose or 10–20 mg IV dose, may be useful as an adjunctive medication to provide relief of nausea and possibly to enhance the pain relief associated with other medications.

ACUTE TREATMENT GUIDELINES

The evidence base supporting the use and adverse event profile of a medication or class of medication is the principle of evidence-based medicine and the basis for clinical decision-making. This evidence, combined with the clinical experience of experts, also forms the basis of authoritative evidence-based guidelines and recommendations. According to a recent authoritative evidence-based guideline from the American Headache Society (Table 7.9), the published literature suggests that all currently available triptans, in various formulations, are effective (Level A) for the acute treatment of migraine for pain that is moderate or severe at the time of treatment. Dihydroergotamine nasal spray and inhalation (MAP004) are effective (Level A), and ergotamine and intravenous ergotamine are probably effective (Level B) for the acute treatment of migraine.

Multiple comparator trials have evaluated the relative efficacy of one migraine-specific acute treatment to another. Rizatriptan 10 mg is probably more effective than ergotamine 2 mg + 200 mg caffeine (Class B),[169] sumatriptan 25 mg or 50 mg,[170] and naratriptan

Table 7.7 Levels of Evidence: GRADE System[176]

Level of Evidence	Definition
High quality	We are confident that the true effect lies close to the estimate given by the evidence available.
Moderate quality	We are moderately confident in the effect estimate, but there is a possibility it is substantially different.
Low quality	Our confidence in the effect estimate is limited. The true effect may be substantially different.
Very low quality	We have little confidence in the effect estimate.

2.5 mg.[171] Eletriptan 40 mg or 80 mg is more effective than sumatriptan 50 mg or 100 mg (Class A).[172–174] Eletriptan 40 mg and 80 mg are probably superior to naratriptan 2.5 mg[175], and eletriptan 80 mg is probably superior to zolmitriptan 2.5 mg.[112]

Multiple non-specific medications are effective in acute migraine, including aspirin 500 mg, acetaminophen 1000 mg, diclofenac 50 or 100 mg, ibuprofen, metamizole (dipyrone) 1 mg, naproxyn 500 or 550 mg, rofecoxib 25 mg, butorphenol nasal spray, codeine, and the combination of acetaminophen/aspirin/caffeine (Level A). Ketoprofen, intravenous ketorolac, intravenous magnesium, and the combination of both isometheptene compounds and tramadol/acetominphen are probably effective (Level B) for migraine. There is not enough information available to determine if celecoxib 400 mg is effective in migraine (Level U). The anti-emetics prochlorpromazine, droperidol, chlorpromazine, and metoclopramide are probably effective (Level B).

Dexamethasone is probably effective when given with rizatriptan 10 mg (Level B). There is inadequate evidence for the use of other corticosteroids, including monotherapy with intravenous dexamethasone, and there is inadequate evidence for intravenous valproic acid (Level U). Butalbital is possibly effective (Level C) for the acute treatment of migraine. Octreotide is probably not effective for the acute treatment of migraine (Level B).

Table 7.8 **Recommendation Grades: Meaning and Clinical Implications[29]**

Recommendation Grade	Benefit versus Risks	Clinical Implications
Strong—high-quality evidence	Benefits clearly outweigh risks and burden for most patients	Can apply to most patients in most circumstances
Strong—moderate-quality evidence	Benefits clearly outweigh risks and burden for most patients	Can apply to most patients, but there is a chance the recommendations may change with more research
Strong—low-quality evidence	Benefits clearly outweigh risks and burden for most patients	Can apply to most patients, but there is a good chance the recommendations could change with more research
Weak—high-quality evidence	Benefits are more closely balanced with risks and burdens for many patients	Whether a medication is used will depend upon patient circumstances
Weak—moderate-quality evidence	Benefits are more closely balanced with risks and burdens for many patients	Whether a medication is used will depend upon patient circumstances, but there is less certainty about when it should be used
Weak—low-quality evidence	Benefits are more closely balanced with risks and burdens	There is considerable uncertainty about when to use this medication

The Canadian Headache Society guidelines used the GRADE system to assess the level of evidence (Table 7.7).[176] The recommendations given are based not only on the level of evidence but also based on the adverse event profile, risk-benefit analysis, and the clinical experience and consensus of the expert panel (Table 7.8).[29]

The Canadian Headache Society also recently reported a systematic review and recommendations on the treatment of migraine pain in emergency settings. From a review of 831 titles and abstracts and 120 full text articles, 44 papers were considered eligible and were included in this systematic review. [177] Individual studies were assigned US Preventive Services Task Force quality rating. The GRADE scheme was used to assign a level of evidence and recommendation strength for each intervention (Table 7.10). Strong recommendations were given for the use of prochlorperazine, based on a high level of evidence; lysine acetylsalicylic acid, metoclopramide and sumatriptan, based on a moderate level of evidence; and ketorolac, based on a low level of evidence. They presented weak recommendations for the use of chlorpromazine, based on a moderate level of evidence, and ergotamine, dihydroergotamine, lidocaine intranasal, and meperidine, based on a low level of evidence. This group also strongly recommended against the use of dexamethasone for the acute treatment of migraine pain, based on a moderate level of evidence, and granisetron, haloperidol, and trimethobenzamide, based on a low level of evidence. Weak recommendations against the use of acetaminophen and magnesium sulfate, based on moderate-quality evidence, and based on a low level of evidence, weak recommendations were issued against the use of diclofenac, droperidol, lidocaine intravenous, lysine clonixinate, morphine, propofol, and tramadol for this indication.

EMERGING ACUTE THERAPIES

While the triptans have significantly advanced the acute treatment of migraine, approximately one-fifth of migraineurs have cardiovascular contraindications that limit their use. Their efficacy is limited when considering the most robust patient-centered outcomes. About 30% achieve a pain-free response at 2 hours, and only about 20% achieve a sustained pain-free response at 24 hours. In addition, triptans induce latent central sensitization and may promote the development of medication overuse headache.[178] Therefore, there is a large unmet treatment

Table 7.9 Summary of US Headache Consortium Guidelines (Adapted)[2]

Group 1*	Group 2¥	Group 3€	Group 4£	Group 5δ
Migraine-specific				
Almotriptan°° (oral)	Acetaminophen plus codeine (oral)	Butalbital, aspirin, plus caffeine (oral)	Acetaminphen PO	Dexamethasone IV
Eletriptan°° (oral)	Butalbital, aspirin, caffeine, plus codeine (oral)	Ergotamine (oral)	Chlorpromazine IM	Hydrocortisone IV
Frovatriptan°° (oral)	Butorphanol IM	Ergotamine plus caffeine (oral)	Granisotron IV	
Naratriptan (oral)	Chlorpromazine IM/IV	Metoclopramide IM/PR	Lidocaine IV	
Rizatriptan (oral)	Diclofenac-K PO (tablet)			
Sumatriptan (SC, oral, intranasal)	Ergotamine plus caffeine plus pentobarbital, plus Bellafline (oral)			
Zolmitriptan (oral, intranasal°°)	Flurbiprofen			
Dihydroergotamine (intranasal, SC self-injection, intravenous intramuscular)	Isomethaptine			
Dihydroergotamine inhalation°°	Ketorolac IM			
	Lidocaine intranasal			
Acetaminophen, aspirin, plus caffeine (oral)	Meperidine IM/IV			
Diclofenac potassium (oral/sachets°°)	Methadone IM			
Ibuprofen (oral)	Metaclopramide IV			
Naproxen sodium (oral)	Naproxen (oral)			
Neuroleptics				
Prochlorperazine (intravenous)	Prochlorperazine IM/PR			

° Proven, pronounced statistical and clinical benefit (at least two double-blind, placebo-controlled studies and clinical impression of effect).

°° Modified based on data since 2000

¥ Moderate statistical and clinical benefit (one double-blind, placebo-controlled study and clinical impression of effect).

€ Statistically but not proven clinically *or* clinically but not proven statistically effective (conflicting or inconsistent evidence).

£ Proven to be statistically or clinically ineffective (failed efficacy versus placebo).

δ Clinical and statistical benefits unknown (insufficient evidence available).

US Headache Consortium Rating

The assignment of medications to treatment groups is based on the quality of evidence, based on the ratings of each study for each medication. The rating of each study followed recommendations from the Clinical Practice Guidelines Manual, ranging from Class I to IV. Class I studies, usually double-blind, randomized placebo-controlled trials, were considered the best, while class IV studies are often retrospective studies or case reports with unclear outcomes data. Based on the quality of studies, a level of evidence was assigned for each drug as follows:

Level A: Established as effective (or ineffective) for acute migraine (supported by at least 2 class I studies)

Level B: Probably effective (or ineffective) for acute migraine (supported by 1 class I study or 2 class II studies)

Level C: Possibly effective (or ineffective) for acute migraine (supported by 1 class II study or 2 class III studies)

Level U: Evidence is conflicting or inadequate to support or refute the use of the following medications for acute migraine

Table 7.10 **Canadian Headache Society Evidence-Based Recommendations for Acute Migraine Treatment in Emergency Settings[177]**

Recommended for Use in Acute Migraine in ED or Similar Settings (Use)

Treatment	Recommendation Strength	Level of Evidence
Prochlorperazine	Strong	High
Lysine acetylsalicylic acid	Strong	Moderate
Metoclopramide	Strong	Moderate
Sumatriptan subcutaneous	Strong	Moderate
Ketorolac	Strong	Low
Chlorpromazine	Weak	Moderate
Ergotamine	Weak	Low
Dihydroergotamine	Weak	Low
Lidocaine intranasal	Weak	Low
Meperidine	Weak	Low

Not Recommended for Use in Acute Migraine in ED or Similar Settings (Do Not Use)

Treatment	Recommendation Strength	Level of Evidence
Dexamethasone	Strong	Moderate
Trimethobenzamide	Strong	Moderate
Granisetron	Strong	Low
Haloperidol	Strong	Low
Acetaminophen	Weak	Moderate
Magnesium sulfate	Weak	Moderate
Octreotide	Weak	Moderate
Diclofenac intramuscular	Weak	Low
Droperidol	Weak	Low
Lidocaine intravenous	Weak	Low
Lysine clonixinate intravenous	Weak	Low
Morphine	Weak	Low
Propofol	Weak	Low
Tramadol	Weak	Low

need for safe and effective acute migraine drugs that do not constrict vascular beds or have the potential to induce medication overuse headache.

5-HT 1F RECEPTOR ANTAGONISTS

The presence of 5-HT_{1F} receptor mRNA in trigeminal ganglia neurons led to the speculation that this receptor could be a therapeutic target for migraine. Lasmiditan (COL-144) is a new, highly selective, 5-HT_{1F} receptor agonist that has been shown in pre-clinical animal models to inhibit dural plasma protein extravasation and reduce trigeminal nucleus caudalis c-Fos expression following trigeminal ganglion stimulation.[179] It is highly potent 5-HT_{1F} receptor

agonist, with a Ki at human 5-HT1F receptors of 2.21 nM and an affinity more than 470-fold higher for 5-HT_{1F} receptors compared to other 5-HT1 receptor subtypes.[180] Lasmiditan was shown to have no vasoconstrictor effect on the rabbit saphenous vein, a surrogate assay for human coronary vasoconstrictor liability.[179] An intravenous formulation was effective in a proof-of-concept migraine study. This study was a randomized, multicenter, placebo-controlled, double-blind, group-sequential, adaptive treatment-assignment, proof-of-concept, and dose-finding study. Intravenous lasmiditan at a starting dose of 2.5 mg was evaluated for the acute treatment of migraine in 130 subjects in a hospital setting.[180] The study was designed to explore the overall dose response relationship but was not powered to differentiate individual doses from placebo on the primary endpoint of headache response at 2 hours or on any other migraine associated symptom. Forty-two subjects received placebo and 88 received lasmiditan in doses ranging from 2.5 mg to 45 mg. Of subjects treated in the 10, 20, 30 and 45 mg lasmiditan dose groups, 54%–75% showed a 2-hour headache response, compared to 45% in the placebo group ($p < 0.0126$) for the linear association between response rates and dose levels. Patient global impression at 2 hours and lack of need for rescue medication also showed statistically significant linear correlations with dose. Adverse events were reported by 65% of subjects on lasmiditan and by 43% on placebo. Dizziness, paresthesia, and sensations of limb heaviness were more common on lasmiditan. The authors concluded that at intravenous doses of 20 mg and higher, lasmiditan proved effective in the acute treatment of migraine, but further studies to assess the optimal oral dose and full efficacy and tolerability profile are required.

The efficacy and safety of oral lasmiditan (50, 100, 200, and 400 mg) in acute migraine treatment was studied in a multicenter, double-blind, parallel-group, dose-ranging study.[181] All doses were superior to placebo, and there was a linear association between headache response rate at 2 hours and the dose of lasmiditan. Treatment-emergent adverse events were dose-dependent and mild or moderate in intensity. The most common adverse events were vertigo, dizziness, fatigue, paresthesia, and somnolence. Vestibular adverse events could be due to activation of 5-HT_{1F} receptors in the lateral vestibular nucleus, temporoparietal cortex, and cerebellum. Controlled phase III trials are necessary to confirm the efficacy and safety of lasmiditan, but the preliminary efficacy from these studies establish the potential for drugs that have no vasoconstrictor activity to be effective acute anti-migraine drugs.

CGRP RECEPTOR ANTAGONISTS

In humans, CGRP exists in two forms: α-CGRP and β-CGRP. The 37-amino-acid neuropeptide α-CGRP, which is produced by alternative RNA splicing of the calcitonin gene, is the main form expressed in trigeminal ganglia neurons.[182] Functional CGRP receptors are composed of a G protein–coupled receptor

known as the calcitonin-like receptor, a single transmembrane domain protein called receptor activity–modifying protein type 1, and a receptor component protein that defines the G-protein to which the receptor couples.[183] CGRP receptors are found on meningeal blood vessels, trigeminal ganglia, primary dural sensory afferents, and in the periaqueductal gray and other areas of the brain associated with migraine.[182]

Ample evidence now supports a critical role of CGRP in the pathophysiology of migraine; CGRP infusion triggers attacks of migraine that are indistinguishable from spontaneous attacks in migraineurs;[184] triptans potently inhibit the release of CGRP[185] and the relief of pain associated with migraine parallels the decline in circulating CGRP levels;[186] and plasma CGRP levels are elevated in external jugular venous blood during an acute migraine attack.[186] The most compelling evidence that supports a crucial role of CGRP in the pathophysiology of migraine is the result of several trials that have evaluated the efficacy of selective CGRP receptor antagonists (*gepants*) for the acute treatment of migraine. Gepants have no vasoconstrictor properties and few adverse events, and five chemically unrelated small molecule CGRP receptor antagonists have demonstrated efficacy for the acute treatment of migraine.[187–191] The first gepant, olcegepant (BIBN4096BS), was effective in migraine, but because it could only be administered intravenously it was abandoned after phase II.[189] Intravenous administration of 2.5 mg of olcegepant produced a response rate of 66% compared with 27% for placebo. A second gepant, telcagepant, was orally available, and six positive phase III trials have been reported.[182,192,193] The adverse event profile of telcagepant was similar to that of placebo. However, the pooled results of four randomized controlled trials with telcagepant (300 mg orally) showed that it acted less rapidly than triptans: 26% of patients were pain-free at 2 hours (11% with placebo, NNT 6.7) as compared with 41% in rizatriptan (10 mg) and 35% in almotriptan (12.5 mg) trials.[193] Telcagepant development has been stopped. In a phase IIa exploratory study, a small number of patients taking telcagepant twice daily for 3 months for migraine prevention showed significant elevations in liver transaminase levels. Similar elevations in liver transaminase were found in a short-term study of menstrual migraine. The development of another gepant, MK-3207, was also terminated following review of phase I and II clinical trial results that showed asymptomatic liver enzyme abnormalities.[190] Boehringer Ingelheim completed a phase II trial wherein 341 migraine subjects were treated with the oral CGRP receptor antagonist BI 44370 TA.[188] It compared 50, 200, and 400 mg of BI 44370 TA with eletriptan (40 mg) as an active comparator and placebo. The number of patients reaching the primary endpoint—pain freedom after 2 hours—was significant exclusively in the 400-mg group (27.4%) and the eletriptan group (34.8%) as compared with placebo. A potent, orally active CGRP receptor antagonist (BMS-846372) was synthesized with limited aqueous solubility. A derivative was then created (BMS-927711) by adding a primary amine to the cycloheptane ring of BMS-846372 to increase solubility. This drug was tested in a double-blind, placebo controlled, dose-ranging study,[191] in which 885 patients were randomized using an adaptive design to BMS-927711 (10, 25, 75, 150, 300, or 600 mg), sumatriptan 100 mg (active comparator), or placebo. Significantly more patients in the BMS-927711 75 mg (31.4%, $p < 0.002$), 150 mg (32.9%, $p < 0.001$), and 300 mg (29.7%, $p < 0.002$) groups and the sumatriptan group (35%, $p < 0.001$) were free of pain at two hours post-dose versus placebo (15.3%). For the secondary endpoint of sustained pain freedom at 24 hours, BMS-927711 doses (25–600 mg) were also statistically significant compared with placebo. The tolerability profile was very favorable, no treatment-related serious adverse events were reported, and no patients discontinued because of adverse events.

In aggregate, these studies confirm that CGRP receptor antagonists are effective acute migraine therapies and, like lasmiditan, lack vasoconstrictor activity and represent a promising therapeutic target.

REFERENCES

1. Chu MK, Buse DC, Bigal ME, Serrano D, Lipton RB. Factors associated with triptan use in episodic migraine: results from the American Migraine Prevalence and Prevention Study. *Headache*. 2011;52:213–223.

2. Silberstein SD. Practice parameter—evidence-based guidelines for migraine headache (an evidence-based review): report of the Quality Standards Subcommittee of the American Academy of Neurology for the United States Headache Consortium. *Neurology*. 2000;55:754–762.

3. Silberstein S.D. Emerging target-based paradigms to prevent and treat migraine. *Clin Pharmacol Ther*. 2013;93(1):78–85.

4. Bigal ME, Ferrari M, Silberstein SD, Lipton RB, Goadsby PJ. Migraine in the triptan era: lessons from epidemiology, pathophysiology, and clinical science. *Headache*. 2009 Feb;49(Suppl 1):S21–S33.

5. May A, Goadsby PJ. The trigeminovascular system in humans: pathophysiological implications for primary headache syndromes of the neural influences on the cerebral circulation. *J Cereb Blood Flow Metabol*. 1999;19:115–127.

6. Goadsby PJ, Lipton RB, Ferrari MD. Migraine-current understanding and treatment. *N Engl J Med*. 2002 Jan 24;346(4):257–270.

7. Ferrari MD, Goadsby PJ, Roon KI, Lipton RB. Triptans (serotonin, 5-HT1B/1D agonists) in migraine: detailed results and methods of a meta-analysis of 53 trials. *Cephalalgia*. 2002 Oct;22(8):633–658.

8. Kesselheim AS, Avorn J. The most transformative drugs of the past 25 years: a survey of physicians. *Nat Rev Drug Discov*. 2013;12:425–431.

9. Bigal ME, Borucho S, Serrano D, Lipton RB. The acute treatment of episodic and chronic migraine in the USA. *Cephalalgia*. 2009 Aug;29(8):891–897.

10. Bigal M, Krymchantowski AV, Lipton RB. Barriers to satisfactory migraine outcomes: what have we learned, where do we stand? *Headache*. 2009 Jul;49(7):1028–1041.

11. Dodick DW, Martin VT, Smith T, Silberstein S. Cardiovascular tolerability and safety of triptans: a review of clinical data. *Headache*. 2004 May;44(Suppl 1):S20-S30.

12. Kurth T, Gaziano JM, Cook NR, Bubes V, Logroscino G, Diener HC, et al. Migraine and risk of cardiovascular disease in men. *Arch Intern Med*. 2007 Apr 23;167(8):795–801.

13. Kurth T. Migraine and ischaemic vascular events. *Cephalalgia*. 2007 Aug;27(8):965–975.

14. Kurth T, Ridker PM, Buring JE. Migraine and biomarkers of cardiovascular disease in women. *Cephalalgia*. 2008 Jan;28(1):49–56.

15. Schurks M, Rist PM, Bigal ME, Buring JE, Lipton RB, Kurth T. Migraine and cardiovascular disease: systematic review and meta-analysis. *BMJ*. 2009;339:b3914.

16. Kurth T, Schurks M, Logroscino G, Buring JE. Migraine frequency and risk of cardiovascular disease in women. *Neurology*. 2009;73:581–588.

17. Peterlin BL, Rapoport AM, Kurth T. Migraine and obesity: epidemiology, mechanisms, and implications. *Headache*. 2010 Apr;50(4):631–648.

18. Schurks M, Buring JE, Kurth T. Migraine, migraine features, and cardiovascular disease. *Headache*. 2010 Jun;50(6):1031–1040.

19. Kurth T, Diener HC, Buring JE. Migraine and cardiovascular disease in women and the role of aspirin: subgroup analyses in the Women's Health Study. *Cephalalgia*. 2011 Jul;31(10):1106–1115.

20. Scher AI, Gudmundsson LS, Sigurdsson S, et al. Migraine headache in middle age and late-life brain infarcts. *JAMA*. 2013;301(24):2563–2570.

21. Scher AI, Terwindt GM, Picavet HS, Verschuren WM, Ferrari MD, Launer LJ. Cardiovascular risk factors and migraine: the GEM population-based study. *Neurology*. 2005 Feb 22;64(4):614–620.

22. Lipton RB, Stewart WF, Sawyer J. Stratified care is a more effective migraine treatment strategy than stepped care: results of a randomized clinical trial. *Neurology*. 2000;54:A14.

23. Lipton RB, Stewart WF, Stone AM, Lainez MJ, Sawyer JP. Stratified care vs step care strategies for migraine: the disability in strategies of care (DISC) study: A randomized trial. *JAMA*. 2000;284(20):2599–2505.

24. Lipton RB, Buse DC, Fanning KM, Serrano D, Reed ML. Suboptimal acute treatment of episodic migraine (EM) is associated with an increased risk of progression to chronic migraine (CM): results of the American Migraine Prevalence and Prevention (AMPP) Study. *Cephalalgia*. 2013;33(11):954–955.

25. Lipton RB. Disability assessment as a basis for stratified care. *Cephalalgia*. 1998;18(Suppl 22):40–46.

26. Williams P, Dowson AJ, Rapoport AM, Sawyer J. The cost effectiveness of stratified care in the management of migraine. *Pharmacoeconomics*. 2001;19(8):819–829.

27. Sculpher M, Millson D, Meddis D, Poole L. Cost-effectiveness analysis of stratified versus stepped care strategies for acute treatment of migraine: The Disability in Strategies for Care (DISC) Study. *Pharmacoeconomics*. 2002;20(2):91–100.

28. Evers S, Afra J, Frese A, Goadsby PJ, Linde M, May A, et al. EFNS guideline on the drug treatment of migraine: report of an EFNS task force. *Eur J Neurol*. 2006 Jun;13(6):560–572.

29. Worthington I, Pringsheim T, Gawel MJ, Gladstone JP, Cooper P, Dilli E, et al. Canadian Headache Society Guideline: acute drug therapy for migraine headache. *Can J Neuro Sci*. 2013;40(5 Suppl 3):S1–S80.

30. Burstein R, Collins B, Jakubowski M. Defeating migraine pain with triptans: a race against the developing allodynia. *Ann Neurol*. 2004;55 (1):19–26.

31. Burstein R, Jakubowski M. Analgesic triptan action in an animal model of intracranial pain: a race against the development of central sensitization. *Ann Neurol*. 2004 Jan;55(1):27–36.

32. Levy D, Jakubowski M, Burstein R. Disruption of communication between peripheral and central trigeminovascular neurons mediates the antimigraine action of 5HT 1B/1D receptor agonists. *Proc Natl Acad Sci USA*. 2004 Mar 23;101(12):4274–4279.

33. Burstein R, Collins B, Bajwa Z, Jakubowski M. Triptan therapy can abort migraine attacks if given before the establishment or in the absence of cutaneous allodynia and central sensitization: clinical and preclinical evidence. *Headache*. 2002;42[5]:390–391(Abstract).

34. Burstein R, Woolf CJ. Central sensitization and headache. In: Olesen J, Tfelt-Hansen P, Welch KMA, eds. *The headaches*. 2nd ed. Philadelphia: Lippincott Williams & Wilkins, 2000:125–132.

35. Burstein R, Yarnitsky D, Goor-Aryeh I, Ransil BJ, Bajwa ZH. An association between migraine and cutaneous allodynia. *Ann Neurol*. 2000;47(5):614–624.

36. Burstein R, Cutrer MF, Yarnitsky D. The development of cutaneous allodynia during a migraine attack clinical

37. Malick A, Burstein R. Peripheral and central sensitization during migraine. *Funct Neurol*. 2000;15(Suppl 3):28–35.

38. Burstein R. Deconstructing migraine headache into peripheral and central sensitization. *Pain*. 2001 Jan;89(2–3):107–110.

39. Silberstein SD, Mannix LK, Goldstein J, Couch JR, Byrd SC, Ames MH, et al. Multimechanistic (sumatriptan-naproxen) early intervention for the acute treatment of migraine. *Neurology*. 2008 Jul 8;71(2):114–121.

40. Freitag F, Smith T, Mathew N, Rupnow M, Greenberg S, Mao L, et al. Effect of early intervention with almotriptan vs placebo on migraine-associated functional disability: results from the AEGIS Trial. *Headache*. 2008 Mar;48(3):341–354.

41. Goadsby PJ, Zanchin G, Geraud G, De KN, Diaz-Insa S, Gobel H, et al. Early vs. non-early intervention in acute migraine—'Act when Mild (AwM)': a double-blind, placebo-controlled trial of almotriptan. *Cephalalgia*. 2008 Apr;28(4):383–391.

42. Cady RK, Sheftell F, Lipton RB. Effect of early intervention with sumatriptan on migraine pain: retrospective analyses of data from three clinical trials. *Clin Therap*. 2000;22:1035–1048.

43. Mathew NT. Early intervention with almotriptan improves sustained pain-free response in acute migraine. *Headache*. 2003 Nov;43(10):1075–1079.

44. Moschiano F, D'Amico D, Allais G, Rigamonti A, Melzi P, Schieroni F, et al. Early triptan intervention in migraine: an overview. *Neurol Sci*. 2005 May;26(Suppl 2):s108–s110.

45. Dowson AJ, Mathew NT, Pascual J. Review of clinical trials using early acute intervention with oral triptans for migraine management. *Int J Clin Pract*. 2006 Jun;60(6):698–706.

46. Mathew NT, Finlayson G, Smith TR, Cady RK, Adelman J, Mao L, et al. Early intervention with almotriptan: results of the AEGIS trial (AXERT Early Migraine Intervention Study). *Headache*. 2007 Feb;47(2):189–198.

47. Aurora S, Kori S, Barrodale P, Nelsen A, McDonald S. Gastric stasis occurs in spontaneous, visually induced, and interictal migraine. *Headache*. 2007 Nov;47(10):1443–1446.

48. Pryse-Phillips W, Aube M, Bailey P, Becker WJ, Bellavance A, Gawel M, et al. A clinical study of migraine evolution. *Headache*. 2006 Nov;46(10):1480–1486.

49. Cady RK, Wendt JK, Kirchner JR, Sargent J, Rothrock JF, Skaggs H. Treatment of acute migraine with subcutaneous sumatriptan. *JAMA*. 1991;265:2831–2835.

50. Hardebo JE. Subcutaneous sumatriptan in cluster headache: a time study in the effect of pain and autonomic symptoms. *Headache*. 1993;33:18–21.

51. Linde M, Mellberg A, Dahlof C. Subcutaneous sumatriptan provides symptomatic relief at any pain intensity or time during the migraine attack. *Cephalalgia*. 2006 Feb;26(2):113–121.

52. Dowson AJ, Hansen SB, Farkkila AM. Zolmitriptan nasal spray is fast acting and highly effective in the acute treatment of migraine. *Neurology*. 2000;7(Suppl 3):82.

53. Sorensen J, Bergstrom M, Antoni A. Distribution of 11C-zolmitriptan nasal spray assessed by positron emission tomography (PET). *Eur J Neurology.* 2000;7(Suppl 3):82.

54. Nairn K, Yates R, Kemp J, Dane A. Rapid, dose-proportional absorption of zolmitriptan nasal spray: comparison with the oral tablet. *Neurology.* 2001;56: A356(Abstract).

55. Becker WJ, Lee D. Zolmitriptan nasal spray is effective, fast-acting and well tolerated during both short- and long-term treatment. *Cephalalgia.* 2001;21(4):271(Abstract).

56. Abu-Shakra S, Becker W, Lee D. Zolmitriptan nasal spray is effective, fast-acting and well tolerated in the acute treatment of migraine. Headache. 2002;42(5):389(Abstract).

57. Dodick DW, Brandes J, Elkind A, Mathew N, Rodichok L. Speed of onset, efficacy and tolerability of zolmitriptan nasal spray in the acute treatment of migraine: a randomised, double-blind, placebo-controlled study. *CNS Drugs.* 2005;19:125–136.

58. Gawel M, Aschoff J, May A, Charlesworth BR. Zolmitriptan 5 mg nasal spray: efficacy and onset of action in the acute treatment of migraine—results from phase 1 of the REALIZE study. *Headache.* 2005;45:7–16.

59. Dowson AJ, Charlesworth BR, Green J, Farkkila M, Diener HC, Hansen SB, et al. Zolmitriptan nasal spray exhibits good long-term safety and tolerability in migraine: results of the INDEX trial. *Headache.* 2005 Jan;45(1):17–24.

60. Silberstein SD, Kori SH, Aurora S, Tepper SJ, Borland SW, Wang M, et al. LEVADEXT, a novel orally inhaled treatment for acute migraine: efficacy and tolerability results of a phase 3 study. 14th Congress of the International Headache Society, Philadelphia, PA, September 10–13, 2009.

61. Aurora SK, Rozen TD, Kori SH, Shrewsbury SB. A randomized, double blind, placebo-controlled study of MAP0004 in adult patients with migraine. *Headache.* 2009 Jun;49(6):826–837.

62. Aurora SK, Silberstein SD, Kori SH, Tepper SJ, Borland SW, Wang M, et al. MAP0004, orally inhaled DHE: a randomized, controlled study in the acute treatment of migraine. *Headache.* 2011 Apr;51(4):507–517.

63. Jakubowski M, Levy D, Goor-Aryeh I, Collins B, Bajwa Z, Burstein R. Terminating migraine with allodynia and ongoing central sensitization using parenteral administration of COX1/COX2 inhibitors. *Headache.* 2005 Jul;45(7):850–861.

64. Brandes JL, Kudrow D, Stark SR, O'Carroll CP, Adelman JU, O'Donnell FJ, et al. Sumatriptan-naproxen for acute treatment of migraine: a randomized trial. *JAMA.* 2007 Apr 4;297(13):1443–1454.

65. Rapoport AM. Acute treatment of headache. *J Headache Pain.* 2006 Oct;7(5):355–359.

66. Malik SN, Hopkins M, Young WB, Silberstein SD. Acute migraine treatment: patterns of use and satisfaction in a clinical population. *Headache.* 2006 May;46(5):773–780.

67. Bigal ME, Ho TW. Is there an inherent limit to acute migraine treatment efficacy? *J Headache Pain.* 2009 Dec;10(6):393–394.

68. Dodick D, Silberstein S. Central sensitization theory of migraine: clinical implications. *Headache.* 2006 Nov;46 Suppl 4:S182–S191.

69. Olesen J, Bousser MG, Diener HC, Dodick D, First M, Goadsby PJ, et al. New appendix criteria open for a broader concept of chronic migraine. *Cephalalgia.* 2006 Jun;26(6):742–746.

70. Diener HC, Limmroth V, Katsarava Z. Medication overuse headache. In: Goadsby PJ, Dodick D, Silberstein SD, editors. *Chronic daily headache for clinicians.* Philadelphia: B. C. Decker, 2004:117–128.

71. Headache Classification Committee. The International Classification of Headache Disorders, 2nd edition. *Cephalalgia.* 2004;24(Suppl 1):1–160.

72. Diener HC, Limmroth V. Medication-overuse headache: a worldwide problem. *Lancet Neurol.* 2004 Aug;3(8):475–483.

73. The International Classification of Headache Disorders, 3rd edition (beta version). *Cephalalgia.* 2013;33(9):629–808.

74. Goadsby PJ. Serotonin receptors and the acute attack of migraine. *Clin Neurosci.* 1998;5(1):18–23.

75. Buzzi MG, Moskowitz MA. Evidence for 5-HT1B/1D receptors mediating the antimigraine effect of sumatriptan and dihydroergotamine. *Cephalalgia.* 1991 Sep;11(4):165–168.

76. Goadsby PJ, Knight YE. Naratriptan inhibits trigeminal neurons after intravenous administration through an action at the serotonin (5HT1B/1D) receptors. *Br J Pharmacol.* 1997;122:918–922.

77. Silberstein SD. Emerging target-based paradigms to prevent and treat migraine. *Clin Pharm Ther.* 2012;(93):78–85.

78. Martin GR, Humphrey PP. Receptors for 5-hydroxytryptamine: current perspectives on classification and nomenclature. *Neuropharmacology.* 1994 Mar;33(3–4):261–273.

79. Goadsby PJ, Akerman S, Storer RJ. Evidence for postjunctional serotonin (5-HT1) receptors in the trigeminocervical complex. *Ann Neurol.* 2001 Dec;50(6): 804–807.

80. Storer RJ, Goadsby PJ. Direct evidence using microiontophoresis that neurons of the caudal trigeminal nucleus contain 5HT1B/1D receptors. *Cephalalgia.* 1997;17:241.

81. Kaube H, Hoskin KL, Goadsby PJ. Sumatriptan inhibits central trigeminal neurons only after blood-brain barrier disruption. *Br J Pharmacol.* 1993;109:788–792.

82. Goadsby PJ, Edvinsson L. Peripheral and central trigeminovascular activation in cat is blocked by serotonin (5HT)-1D receptor agonist 31 1C90. *Headache.* 1994;34(7):394–399.

83. Goadsby PJ, Hoskin KL. Serotonin inhibits trigeminal nucleus activity evoked by craniovascular stimulation through a 5-HT1B/1D receptor: a central action in migraine? *Ann Neurol.* 1998;43:711–718.

84. Thomsen LL, Dixon R, Lassen LH. 311C90 (zolmitriptan), a novel centrally and peripheral acting oral 5-nydroxytryptamine-1D agonist: a comparison of its absorption during a migraine attack and in a migraine-free period. *Cephalalgia.* 1996;16(4):270–275.

85. Edmeads JG, Millson DS. Tolerability profile of zolmitriptan (Zomig; 311C90), a novel dual central and peripherally acting 5HT1B/1D agonist. International clinical experience based on >3000 subjects treated with zolmitriptan. *Cephalalgia.* 1997;16(Suppl 18):41–52.

86. Cumberbatch MJ, Hill RG, Hargreaves RJ. rizatriptan has central antinociceptive effects against durally evoked responses. *Eur J Pharmacol*. 1997;328:37–40.

87. Goadsby PJ, Knight YE. Direct evidence for central sites of action of zolmitriptan (311C90): an autoradiographic study in cat. *Cephalalgia*. 1997;17(3):153–158.

88. Schoenen J, Sawyer J. Zolmitriptan (Zomigr, 311C90), a novel dual central and peripheral 5-HT1B/1D agonist: an overview of efficacy. *Cephalalgia*. 1997;17:28–40.

89. Shields KG, Goadsby PJ. Serotonin receptors modulate trigeminovascular responses in ventroposteromedial nucleus of thalamus: a migraine target? *Neurobiol Dis*. 2006;23(3):491–501.

90. Bartsch T, Knight YE, Goadsby PJ. Activation of 5-HT(1B/1D) receptor in the periaqueductal gray inhibits nociception. *Ann Neurol*. 2004;56(3):371–381.

90a. Kröger IL, May A. Triptan-induced disruption of trigemino-cortical connectivity. *Neurology*. 2015;84:2124–2131.

91. Dodick DW. Triptan nonresponder studies: implications for clinical practice. *Headache*. 2005 Feb;45(2):156–162.

92. Seeburger JL, Taylor FR, Friedman D, Newman L, Ge Y, Zhang Y, et al. Efficacy and tolerability of rizatriptan for the treatment of acute migraine in sumatriptan non-responders. *Cephalalgia*. 2011 May;31(7):786–796.

93. Diener HC, Gendolla A, Gebert I, Beneke M. Almotriptan in migraine patients who respond poorly to oral sumatriptan: a double-blind, randomized trial. *Headache*. 2005 Jul;45(7):874–882.

94. Farkkila M, Olesen J, Dahlof C, Stovner LJ, ter Bruggen JP, Rasmussen S, et al. Eletriptan for the treatment of migraine in patients with previous poor response or tolerance to oral sumatriptan. *Cephalalgia*. 2003 Jul;23(6):463–471.

95. Rothrock JF. Triptans, SSRIs/SNRIs and serotonin syndrome. *Headache*. 2010 Jun;50(6):1101–1102.

96. Evans RW, Tepper SJ, Shapiro RE, Sun-Edelstein C, Tietjen GE. The FDA alert on serotonin syndrome with use of triptans combined with selective serotonin reuptake inhibitors or selective serotonin-norepinephrine reuptake inhibitors: American Headache Society position paper. *Headache*. 2010 Jun;50(6):1089–1099.

97. Evans RW. Concomitant triptan and SSRI or SNRI use: what is the risk for serotonin syndrome? *Headache*. 2008 Apr;48(4):639–640.

98. Gillman PK. Triptans, serotonin agonists, and serotonin syndrome (serotonin toxicity): a review. *Headache*. 2010 Feb;50(2):264–272.

99. Pascual J, Mateos V, Roig C, Sanchez-Del-Rio M, Jimenez D. Marketed oral triptans in the acute treatment of migraine: a systematic review on efficacy and tolerability. *Headache*. 2007 Sep;47(8):1152–1168.

100. Oldman AD, Smith L.A, McQuay HJ, Moore RA. Pharmacological treatments for acute migraine: quantitative systematic review. *Pain*. 2002;97(3):247–257.

101. Smith TR, Sunshine A, Stark SR, Littlefield DE, Spruill SE, Alexander WJ. Sumatriptan and naproxen sodium for the acute treatment of migraine. *Headache*. 2005 Sep;45(8):983–991.

102. Mathew NT, Landy S, Stark S, Tietjen GE, Derosier FJ, White J, et al. Fixed-dose sumatriptan and naproxen in poor responders to triptans with a short half-life. *Headache*. 2009 Jul;49(7):971–982.

103. Brandes JL, Kudrow D, Cady R, Tiseo PJ, Sun W, Sikes CR. Eletriptan in the early treatment of acute migraine: influence of pain intensity and time of dosing. *Cephalalgia*. 2005 Sep;25(9):735–742.

104. Klapper JA, Rosjo O, Charlesworth B, Jergensen AP, Soisson T. Treatment of mild migraine with oral zolmitriptan 2.5mg provides high pain free response rates in patients with significant migraine related disability. *Neurology*. 2002;58(7)[Suppl 3]:A416(Abstract).

105. Tfelt-Hansen P. Early responses in randomized clinical trials of triptans in acute migraine treatment: are they clinically relevant? A comment. *Headache*. 2010 Jul;50(7):1198–200.

106. Goldstein J, Smith TR, Pugach N, Griesser J, Sebree T, Pierce M. A sumatriptan iontophoretic transdermal system for the acute treatment of migraine. *Headache*. 2012;52(9):1402–1410.

107. Pierce M, Marbury T, O'Neill C, Siegel S, Du W, Sebree T. Zelrix: a novel transdermal formulation of sumatriptan. *Headache*. 2009 Jun;49(6):817–825.

108. Goldstein J, Pugach N, Smith T, Nett R, Angelov AS, Pierce MW. Acute anti-migraine efficacy and tolerability of Zelrix™, a novel iontophoretic transdermal patch of sumatriptan. *Cephalagia*. 2009;29:20 (Abstract).

109. Silberstein SD, McCrory DC. Ergotamine and dihydroergotamine: history, pharmacology, and efficacy. *Headache*. 2003 Feb 1;43(2):144–166.

110. Winner P, Ricalde O, Leforce B, Saper J, Margul B. A double-blind study of subcutaneous dihydroergotamine vs subcutaneous sumatriptan in the treatment of acute migraine. *Arch Neurol*. 1996;53(2):180–184.

111. Multinational Oral Sumatriptan and Cafergot Comparative Study Group. A randomized, double-blind comparison of sumatriptan and cafergot in the acute treatment of migraine. *Eur Neurol*. 1991;31(5):314–322.

112. Diener HC, Jansen JP, Reches A, Pascual J, Pitei D, Steiner TJ. Efficacy, tolerability and safety of oral eletriptan and ergotamine plus caffeine (Cafergot) in the acute treatment of migraine: a multicentre, randomised, double-blind, placebo-controlled comparison. *Eur Neurol*. 2002;47(2):99–107.

113. Dowson AJ, Massiou H, Lainez JM, Cabarrocas X. Almotriptan is an effective and well-tolerated treatment for migraine pain: results of a randomized, double-blind, placebo-controlled clinical trial. *Cephalalgia*. 2002;22:453–461.

114. Derry CJ, Derry S, Moore RA. Sumatriptan (oral route of administration) for acute migraine attacks in adults. *Cochrane DB Syst Rev*. 2012;2:008615.

115. Paiva T, Esperanca P, Marcelino L, Assis G. A double-blind trial with dihydroergotamine nasal spray in migraine crisis. *Cephalalgia*. 1985;5(Suppl 3):140–141.

116. Tulunay FC, Karan O, Aydin N, Culcuoglu A, Guvener A. Dihydroergotamine nasal spray during migraine attacks: a double-blind crossover study with placebo. *Cephalalgia*. 1987;7(2):131–133.

117. Ziegler D, Ford R, Kriegler J, Gallagher RM, Peroutka S, Hammerstad J, et al. Dihydroergotamine

nasal spray for the acute treatment of migraine. *Neurology*. 1994;44(3):447–453.

118. Touchon J, Bertin L, Pilgrim AJ, Ashford E, Bes A. A comparison of subcutaneous sumatriptan and dihydroergotamine nasal spray in the acute treatment of migraine. *Neurology*. 1996;47(2):361–365.

119. Boureau F, Kappos L, Schoenen J, Esperanca P, Ashford E. A clinical comparison of sumatriptan nasal spray and dihydroergotamine nasal spray in the acute treatment of migraine. *Int J Clin Pract*. 2000;54:281–286.

120. Klapper JA, Stanton J. Current emergency treatment of severe migraine headaches. *Headache*. 1993;33(10):560–562.

121. Belgrade MJ, Ling LJ, Schleevogt MB, Ettinger MG, Ruiz E. Comparison of single-dose meperidine, butorphanol, and dihydroergotamine in the treatment of vascular headache. *Neurology*. 1989;39:590–592.

122. Shrewsbury SB, Cook RO, Taylor G, Edwards C, Ramadan NM. Safety and pharmacokinetics of dihydroergotamine mesylate administered via a novel (Tempo) inhaler. *Headache*. 2008 Mar;48(3):355–367.

123. Cook RA, Shrewsbury SB, Ramadan NM. Reduced AE profile of orally inhaled DHE (MAP004) versus IV DHE: potential mechanism. *Headache*. 2009.

124. Wenzel RG, Sarvis CA, Krause ML. Over-the-counter drugs for acute migraine attacks: literature review and recommendations. *Pharmacotherapy*. 2003 Apr;23(4):494–505.

125. Suthisisang C, Poolsup N, Kittikulsuth W, Pudchakan P. Efficacy of low-dose ibuprofen in acute migraine treatment: systematic review and meta-analysis. *Ann Pharmacother*. 2007;1782–1791.

126. Rabbie R., Derry S, Moore RA, McQuay HJ. Ibuprofen with or without an antiemetic for acute migraine headaches in adults. *Cochrane DB Syst Rev*. 2010;0080039.

127. Suthisisang CC, Poolsup N, Suksomboon N, Lertpipopmetha V, Tepwitukgid B. Meta-analysis of the efficacy and safety of naproxen sodium in the acute treatment of migraine. *Headache*. 2010 May;50(5):808–818.

128. Derry S, Rabbie R, Moore RA. Diclofenac with or without an antiemetic for acute migraine headaches in adults. *Cochrane DB Syst Rev*. 2012;2:008783.

129. The Diclofenac-K/Sumatriptan Study Group. Acute treatment of migraine attacks: efficacy and safety of a nonsteroidal anti-inflammatory drug, diclofenac-potassium, in comparison to oral sumatriptan and placebo: The Diclofenac-K/Sumatriptan Migraine Study Group. *Cephalalgia*. 1999;19:232–240.

130. Diener HC, Montagna P, Gacs G, Lyczak P, Schumann G, Zoller B, et al. Efficacy and tolerability of diclofenac potassium sachets in migraine: a randomized, double-blind, cross-over study in comparison with diclofenac potassium tablets and placebo. *Cephalalgia*. 2006 May;26(5):537–547.

131. Lipton RB, Grosberg B, Singer RP, Pearlman SH, Sorrentino JV, Quiring JN, et al. Efficacy and tolerability of a new powdered formulation of diclofenac potassium for oral solution for the acute treatment of migraine: results from the International Migraine Pain Assessment Clinical Trial (IMPACT). *Cephalalgia*. 2010 Nov;30(11):1336–1345.

132. Boureau F, Joubert JM, Lasserre V, Prum B, Delecoeuillerie G. Double-blind comparison of an acetaminophen 400mg-codeine 25mg combination versus aspirin 1000mg and placebo in acute migraine attack. *Cephalalgia*. 1994;14(2):156–161.

133. Loder E. Post-marketing experience with an opioid nasal spray for migraine: lessons for the future. *Cephalalgia*. 2006 Feb;26(2):89–97.

134. Hoffert MJ, Couch JR, Diamond S, Elkind AH, Goldstein J, Kohlerman NJ. Transnasal butorphanol in the treatment of acute migraine. *Headache*. 1995;35(2):65–69.

135. Goldstein J, Gawel MJ, Winner P, Diamond S, Reich L, Davidson WJ, et al. Comparison of butorphanol nasal spray and fiorinal with codeine in the treatment of migraine. *Headache*. 1988;38:516–522.

136. Silberstein SD, Freitag FG, Rozen TD, Kudrow DB, Hewitt DJ, Jordan DM, et al. Tramadol HCl/acetaminophen versus placebo in the treatment of acute migraine pain. *Headache*. 2005;45(10):1317–1327.

137. Cicero TJ, Adams EH, Geller A, Inciardi JA, Munoz A, Schnoll SH, et al. A postmarketing surveillance program to monitor Ultram (tramadol hydrochloride) abuse in the United States. *Drug Alcohol Depend*. 1999 Nov 1;57(1):7–22.

138. Raffa RB. Basic pharmacology relevant to drug abuse assessment: tramadol as example. *J Clin Pharm Ther*. 2008;33:101–108.

139. Tjaderborn M, Jonsson AK, Ahlner J, Hagg S. Tramadol dependence: a survey of spontaneously reported cases in Sweden. *Pharmacoepidem Dr S*. 2009;18:1192–1198.

140. Silberstein SD, McCrory DC. Butalbital in the treatment of headache: history, pharmacology, and efficacy. *Headache*. 2001;41(10):953–967.

141. Pryse-Phillips WEM, Dodick DW, Edmeads JG, Gawel MJ, Nelson RF, Purdy RH, et al. Guidelines for the diagnosis and management of migraine in clinical practice. *Can Med Assoc J*. 1997;156(9):1273–1287.

142 Silberstein SD; McCrory DC.Butalbital in the treatment of headache: history, pharmacology, and efficacy. *Headache*. 2001;41(10):953–967.

143. Wenzel RG, Sarvis CA. Do butalbital-containing products have a role in the management of migraine? *Pharmacotherapy*. 2002;22:1029–1035.

144. Derosier F, Sheftell F, Silberstein S., et al. Sumatriptan-naproxen and butalbital: a double-blind, placebo-controlled crossover study. *Headache*. 2012;52:530–543.

145. Kao LW, Kirk MA, Evers SJ, Rosenfeld SH. Droperidol, QT prolongation, and sudden death: what is the evidence? *Ann Emerg Med*. 2003;41:546–558.

146. Lischke V, Behne M, Doelken P, Schledt U, Probst S, Vetterman J. Droperidil causes a dose-dependent prolongation of the QT interval. *Anesth Analg*. 1994;79:983–986.

147. Silberstein SD, Young WB, Mendizabal JE, Rothrock JF, Alam AS. Acute migraine treatment with the dopamine receptor antagonist, droperidol: results of a randomized, double-blind, placebo-controlled, multicenter trial. *Neurology*. 2003;60:315–321.

148. Jones EB, Gonzales ER, Boggs JG, Grillo JA, Elswick RK, Jr. Safety and efficacy of rectal prochlorperazine for the treatment of migraine in the emergency department. *Ann Emerg Med*. 1994;24:237–241.

149. Jones J, Sklar D, Dougherty J, White W. Randomized double-blind trial of intravenous prochlorperazine for the treatment of acute headache. *JAMA*. 1989;261(8):1174–1176.

150. Coppola M, yealy DM, Leibold RA. Randomized, placebo-controlled evaluation of prochlorperazine versus metoclopramide for emergency department treatment of migraine headache. *Ann Emerg Med*. 1995 Nov;26(5):541–546.

151. Jones J, Pack S, Chun E. Intramuscular prochlorperazine versus metoclopramide as single-agent therapy for the treatment of acute migraine headache. *Am J Emerg Med*. 1996 May;14(3):262–264.

152. Saadah HA. Abortive headache therapy in the office with interavenous dihydroergotamine plus prochlorperazine. *Headache*. 1992;32:143–146.

153. McEwen JI, O'Connor HM, Dinsdale HB. Treatment of migraine with intramuscular chlorpromazine. *Ann Emerg Med*. 1987 Jul;16(7):758–763.

154. Bigal ME, Bordini CA, Speciali JG. Intravenous chlorpromazine in the emergency department treatment of migraines: a randomized controlled trial. *J Emerg Med*. 2002 Aug;23(2):141–148.

155. Cete Y, Dora B, Ertan C, Ozdemir C, Oktay C. A randomized prospective placebo-controlled study of intravenous magnesium sulphate vs. metoclopramide in the management of acute migraine attacks in the Emergency Department. *Cephalalgia*. 2005 Mar;25(3):199–204.

156. Tek DS, McClellan DS, Olshaker JS, Allen CL, Arthur DC. A prospective, double-blind study of metoclopramide hydrochloride for the control of migraine in the emergency department. *Ann Emerg Med*. 1990;19(10):1083–1087.

157. Ellis GL, Delaney J, Dehart DA, Owens A. The efficacy of metoclopramide in the treatment of migraine headache. *Ann Emerg Med*. 1993 Feb;22(2):191–195.

158. Friedman BW, Corbo J, Lipton RB, Bijur PE, Esses D, Solorzano C, et al. A trial of metoclopramide vs sumatriptan for the emergency department treatment of migraines. *Neurology*. 2005 Feb 8;64(3):463–468.

159. Edwards KR, Norton J, Behnke M. Comparison of intravenous valproate versus intramuscular dihydroergotamine and metoclopramide for acute treatment of migraine headache. *Headache*. 2001;41(10):976–980.

160. Klapper JA, Stanton JS. Ketorolac versus DHE and metoclopramide in the treatment of migraine headaches. *Headache*. 1991;31:523–524.

161. Klapper JA, Stanton JS. The emergency treatment of acute migraine headache: a comparison of intravenous dihydroergotamine, dexamethasone, and placebo. *Cephalalgia*. 1991;11(Suppl 11):159–160.

162. Scherl ER, Wilson JF. Comparison of dihydroergotamine with metoclopramide versus meperidine with promethazine in the treatment of acute migraine. *Headache*. 1995;35(5):256–259.

163. Friedman BW, Esses D, Solorzano C, et.al. A randomized controlled trial of prochlorperazine versus metoclopramide for treatment of acute migraine. *Ann Emerg Med*. 2008;52:399–406.

164. Geraud G, Compagnon A, Rossi A. Zolmitriptan versus a combination of acetylsalicylic acid and metoclopramide in the acute oral treatment of migraine: a double-blind, randomised, three-attack study. *Eur Neurol*. 2002;47(2):88–98.

165. Tfelt-Hansen P, Henry P, Mulder LJ, Scheldewaert RG, Schoenen J, Chazot G. The effectiveness of combined oral lysine acetylsalicylate and metoclopramide compared with oral sumatriptan for migraine. *Lancet*. 1995;346(8980):923–926.

166. Chabriat H, Joire JE, Danchot J, Grippon P, Bousser MG. Combined oral lysine acetylsalicylate and metoclopramide in the acute treatment of migraine: a multicenter double-blind placebo-controlled study. *Cephalalgia*. 1994;14:297–300.

167. Kirthi V, Derry S, Moore RA, McQuay HJ. Aspirin with or without an antiemetic for acute migraine headaches in adults. *Cochrane DB Syst Rev*. 2010;4:008041.

168. Schulman EA, Dermott KF. Sumatriptan plus metoclopramide in triptan-nonresponsive migraineurs. *Headache*. 2003 Jul;43(7):729–733.

169. Christie S, Gobel H, Mateos V, Allen C, Vrijens F, Shivaprakash M. Crossover comparison of efficacy and preference for rizatriptan 10 mg versus ergotamine/caffeine in migraine. *Eur Neurol*. 2003;49(1):20–29.

170. Kolodny A, Polis A, Battisti WP, Johnson-Pratt L, Skobieranda F. Rizatriptan Protocol:.052 Study Group.Comparison of rizatriptan 5 mg and 10 mg tablets and sumatriptan 25 mg and 50 mg tablets. *Cephalalgia*. 2004;24:540–546.

171. Bomhof M, Paz J, Legg N, Allen C, Vandormael K, Patel K. Comparison of rizatriptan 10 mg vs. naratriptan 2.5 mg in migraine. *Eur Neurol*. 1999;42(3):173–179.

172. Goadsby PJ, Ferrari MD, Olesen J, Stovner LJ, Senard JM, Jackson NC, et al. Eletriptan in acute migraine: a double-blind, placebo-controlled comparison to sumatriptan. Eletriptan Steering Committee. *Neurology*. 2000;54(1):156–163.

173. Sandrini G, Farkkila M, Burgess G, Forster E, Haughie S. Eletriptan vs sumatriptan: a double-blind, placebo-controlled, multiple migraine attack study. *Neurology*. 2002 Oct 22;59(8):1210–1217.

174. Mathew NT, Schoenen J, Winner P, Muirhead N, Sikes CR. Comparative efficacy of eletriptan 40 mg versus sumatriptan 100 mg. *Headache*. 2003 Mar;43(3):214–222.

175. Garcia-Ramos G, MacGregor EA, Hilliard B, Bordini CA, Leston J, Hettiarachchi J. Comparative efficacy of eletriptan vs. naratriptan in the acute treatment of migraine. *Cephalalgia*. 2003;23(9):869–876.

176. Guyatt GH, Oxman AD, Vist GE, et.al. GRADE: an emerging consensus on rating quality of evidence and strength of recommendations. *BMJ*. 2008;336:924–926.

177. Orr SL, Aube M, Becker WJ, Davenport J, Dilli E, Dodick DW, et al. Canadian Headache Society systematic review & recommendations on the treatment of migraine pain in emergency settings. *Cephalalgia*. 2015;35(3):271–284.

178. De FM, Ossipov MH, Wang R, Dussor G, Lai J, Meng ID, et al. Triptan-induced enhancement of neuronal nitric oxide synthase in trigeminal ganglion dural afferents underlies increased responsiveness to potential migraine triggers. *Brain*. 2010 Aug;133(Pt 8):2475–2488.

179. Nelson DL, Phebus LA, Johnson KW, Wainscott DB, Cohen ML, Calligaro DO, et al. Preclinical pharmacological profile of the selective 5-HT1F receptor agonist lasmiditan. *Cephalalgia*. 2010 Oct;30(10):1159–1169.

180. Ferrari MD, Farkkila M, Reuter U, Pilgrim A, Davis C, Krauss M, et al. Acute treatment of migraine with the selective 5-HT1F receptor agonist lasmiditan: a randomised proof-of-concept trial. *Cephalalgia*. 2010 Oct;30(10):1170–1178.

181. Farkkila M., Diener HC, Geraud G, et.al. Efficacy and tolerability of lasmiditan, and oral 5-HT(1F) receptor agonist, for the acute treatment of migraine: a phase 2 randomized, placebo-controlled, parallel-group, dose-ranging study. *Lancet Neurol*. 2012;11:405–413.

182. Ho TW, Edvinsson L, Goadsby PJ. CGRP and its receptors provide new insights into migraine pathophysiology. *Nat Rev Neurol*. 2010;(6):573–582.

183. Eftekhari S, Edvinsson L. Calcitonin gene-related peptide (CGRP) and its receptor components in human and rat spinal trigeminal nucleus and spinal cord at C1-level. *BMC Neurosci*. 2011;12:112.

184. Hansen JM, Hauge AW, Olesen J, Ashina M. Calcitonin gene-related peptide triggers migraine-like attacks in patients with migraine with aura. *Cephalalgia*. 2010 Oct;30(10):1179–1186.

185. Amrutkar DV, Ploug KB, Hay-Schmidt A, Porreca F, Olesen J, Jansen-Olesen I. mRNA expression of 5-hydroxytryptamine 1B, 1D, and 1F receptors and their role in controlling the release of calcitonin gene-related peptide in the rat trigeminovascular system. *Pain*. 2012;153:830–838.

186. Goadsby PJ, Edvinsson L. Sumatriptan reverses the changes in calcitonin gene-related peptide seen in the headache phase of migraine. *Ann Neurol*. 1993;33:48–56.

187. Ho TW, Ferrari MD, Dodick DW, Galet V, Kost J, Fan X, et al. Efficacy and tolerability of MK-0974 (telcagepant), a new oral antagonist of calcitonin gene-related peptide receptor, compared with zolmitriptan for acute migraine: a randomised, placebo-controlled, parallel-treatment trial. *Lancet*. 2008 Dec 20;372(9656):2115–2123.

188. Diener HC, Barbanti P, Dahlof C, Reuter U, Habeck J, Podhorna J. BI 44370 TA, an oral CGRP antagonist for the treatment of acute migraine attacks: results from a phase II study. *Cephalalgia*. 2011 Apr;31(5):573–584.

189. Olesen J, Diener HC, Husstedt IW, Goadsby PJ, Hall D, Meier U, et al. Calcitonin gene-related peptide receptor antagonist BIBN 4096 BS for the acute treatment of migraine. *N Engl J Med*. 2004 Mar 11;350(11):1104–1110.

190. Hewitt DJ, Aurora SK, Dodick DW, Goadsby PJ, Ge YJ, Bachman R, et al. Randomized controlled trial of the CGRP receptor antagonist MK-3207 in the acute treatment of migraine. *Cephalalgia*. 2011 Apr;31(6):712–722.

191. Marcus R, Goadsby P, Dodick D, Stock D, Manos G, Fischer T. BMS-927711 for the acute treatment of migraine: a double-blind, randomized, placebo controlled, dose-ranging trial. *Cephalalgia*. 2013;34:114–125.

192. Ho AP, Dahlof CG, Silberstein SD, Saper JR, Ashina M, Kost JT, et al. Randomized, controlled trial of telcagepant over four migraine attacks. *Cephalalgia*. 2010 Dec;30(12):1443–1457.

193. Tfelt-Hansen P. Excellent tolerability but relatively low initial clinical efficacy of telcagepant in migraine. *Headache*. 2011 Jan;51(1):118–123.

Chapter 8

Preventive Treatment

INTRODUCTION

Migraine is a chronic neurologic disease that varies in its frequency, severity, and impact on patients' quality of life. A treatment plan should consider not only the patient's diagnosis, symptoms, and coexistent or comorbid conditions, but also his or her expectations, needs,

163

and goals.[1] Effective migraine treatment begins with making an accurate diagnosis, ruling out alternate causes, ordering appropriate studies, and addressing the headache's impact on the patient, educating the patient with regard to treatment options, side-effect profile, duration of therapy, expectations for improvement, and developing a treatment plan that considers coincidental and comorbid conditions.[2] Comorbidity is the presence of two or more disorders, the association of which is more likely than chance. Conditions that occur in migraineurs with a higher prevalence than coincidence include stroke, comorbid pain disorders, angina, patent foramen ovale (aura), epilepsy, and certain psychiatric disorders, which include depression, mania, anxiety, and panic disorder (see Chapter 4).

The pharmacologic treatment of migraine may be acute (abortive) or preventive (prophylactic), and patients with frequent severe headaches require both approaches. Preventive therapy is used to reduce the frequency, duration, or severity of attacks. Additional benefits may include the following: enhancement of response to acute treatments; improvement of a patient's ability to function; reduction of disability.[2] Preventive treatment may also result in the reduction of healthcare costs.[3]

IMPACT OF PREVENTIVE TREATMENT

Silberstein et al.[3] found that the addition of migraine preventive drug therapy to therapy that consisted of only an acute medication was effective in reducing resource consumption. During the second 6 months after the initial preventive medication, as compared with the 6 months preceding preventive therapy, migraine diagnosis-related office and other outpatient visits decreased by 51.1%, emergency department visits with a migraine diagnosis decreased 81.8%, CT scans decreased 75.0%, MRIs decreased 88.2%, and other migraine medication dispensements decreased 14.1%.[3]

The cost and consumption of triptan medications is also an important factor and has been evaluated after the addition of preventive medication.[4] Silberstein et al. evaluated the medical resource utilization and overall cost of care among patients treated with topiramate for migraine prevention in a commercially insured population that included 2645 plan members. Topiramate utilization was associated with significantly less triptan utilization. In addition, in post-index period 1, there was a 46% decrease in emergency department visits, a 39% decrease in diagnostic procedures (e.g., CT scans and MRIs), and a 33% decrease in hospital admissions; physician office visits were unchanged. In post-index period 2, there was a 46% decrease in emergency department visits, a 72% decrease in diagnostic procedures, a 61% decrease in hospital admissions, and a 35% decrease in physician office visits.[5]

While controlling healthcare costs is of significant importance to insurers and patients, so too are the employment-related costs to businesses. A British study examined the impact of topiramate treatment for migraine and found that not only was treatment associated with a decrease in the number of migraine attacks per month, but also with improved quality of life and a significant reduction in lost work time that would more than compensate for the cost of treatment.[6] Educational programs added to acute and preventive drug therapy resulted in greater productivity, less time lost from work, and a significant reduction in total medical migraine-related costs.[7]

Several studies have examined the impact of migraine prevention therapy on patients' quality of life. These have included specific therapies, such as topiramate, as well a more far-reaching assessment. Using the SF36 to examine quality of life, studies[8.9] showed highly statistically significant changes across the range of scores with as little as 6 months of treatment. With a migraine-specific quality-of-life assessment,[10] broad improvements were found across domains of at least moderate size and an effect that persisted over a prolonged period of observation.

PRINCIPLES OF PREVENTIVE TREATMENT

Preventive treatment can be pre-emptive, short-term, or maintenance.

- Pre-emptive treatment is used when there is a known headache trigger, such as exercise or sexual activity. Patients can be instructed to pre-treat prior to the exposure or activity. For example, a single dose of indomethacin can be used to prevent exercise-induced migraine.

- Short-term prevention is used when patients are undergoing a time-limited exposure to a provoking factor, such as ascent to a high altitude or menstruation. These patients can be treated with daily medication just before and during the exposure.[11] For example, the perimenstrual use of an NSAID or triptan for 3–5 days may prevent the emergence of menstrually associated migraine.
- Maintenance prevention is used when patients need ongoing treatment.Recent US, Canadian, and European Guidelines[12–17] have established the circumstances under which migraine preventive treatment should be considered. These include the following:

1. Recurring migraine attacks that significantly interfere with a patient's quality of life and daily routine despite appropriate use of acute medications, trigger management, and/or lifestyle modification strategies;
2. Frequent headaches (≥ 4 attacks/month or ≥ 8 headache days a month) because of the risk of CM;
3. Failure of, contraindication to, overuse, or troublesome side effects from acute medications;
4. Patient preference, that is, the desire to have as few acute attacks as possible;
5. Presence of certain migraine conditions: hemiplegic migraine; basilar migraine; frequent, prolonged, or uncomfortable aura symptoms; or migrainous infarction. [12.13,18]

A preventive migraine drug is considered successful if it reduces migraine attack frequency or days by at least 50% within 3 months. Additional benefits include reduced attack duration or severity, enhanced response to acute treatments, improved ability to function, and reduced disability. A migraine diary is useful to evaluate treatment response. [12,13,18] According to the American Migraine Prevalence and Prevention (AMPP) Study, 38.8% of patients with migraine should be considered for (13.1%) or offered (25.7%) preventive migraine therapy.[19] Unfortunately, the underutilization of migraine preventive medications is underscored by the fact that only 13% of all migraineurs currently use preventive therapy to control their attacks.[13]

The following classes of medications are used for migraine prevention: anti-epileptic drugs (AEDs), antidepressants, ß-adrenergic blockers, calcium channel antagonists, serotonin antagonists, botulinum neurotoxins, non-steroidal anti-inflammatory drugs, and others (including riboflavin, magnesium, and petasides). A drug is chosen based on its efficacy, its adverse event (AE) profile, the patient's preference, and the presence of any coexistent or comorbid conditions. Preventive drugs with the best proven efficacy are selected ß-blockers, divalproex, and topiramate. The chosen drug should have the best risk-to-benefit ratio for the individual patient and, where possible, take advantage of the drug's side effect profile[11,20,21] An underweight patient would be a candidate for one of the medications that commonly produce weight gain, such as a tricyclic antidepressant (TCA); in contrast, one would try to avoid these drugs and consider topiramate when the patient is overweight. Tertiary TCAs that have a sedating effect would be useful at bedtime for patients with insomnia. Older patients with cardiac disease or patients with significant hypotension may not be able to use TCAs or calcium channel or ß-blockers, but could use divalproex or topiramate. The following principles will help increase the chance of success.

GENERAL PRINCIPLES FOR INSTITUTING PREVENTIVE THERAPY

- Start the chosen drug at a low dose and increase it slowly until therapeutic effects develop, the ceiling dose is reached, or AEs become intolerable.
- Consider comorbidity and coexistent illnesses in drug choice. Conditions comorbid with migraine are shown in Table 8.1. [14,22–29]
- Avoid exacerbating, overused, and contraindicated drugs (because of coexistent or comorbid illnesses).
- Give each treatment an adequate trial. A full therapeutic trial may take 2–6 months

Table 8.1 **Migraine Comorbid Disease**

Cardiovascular

Raynaud's
Patent Foramen Ovale (Migraine with aura)
Atrial Septal Defects (ASD), Pulmonary AVMs
Mitral Valve Prolapse
Angina/Myocardial Infarction
Stroke

Psychiatric

Depression
Mania
Panic Disorder
Anxiety Disorder

Neurologic

Epilepsy
Fibromyalgia
Bells Palsy
Positional Vertigo
Restless Legs Syndrome

GI

Irritable Bowel Syndrome

Other

Asthma
Allergies

before the maximal response to a treatment is evident.
- Set realistic goals. Success is defined as a 50% reduction in attack frequency or headache days, a significant decrease in attack duration, or an improved response to acute medication.
- Re-evaluate therapy: migraine may improve or remit independent of treatment.
- Be sure that a woman of childbearing potential is aware of any potential risks, and choose the medication that will have the least potential for adverse effect on a fetus.[30]
- To maximize compliance, involve patients in their care. Discuss the rationale for a particular treatment, when and how to use it, and what AEs are likely. Address patient expectations. Set realistic goals.
- Set realistic expectations regarding AEs. Most are self-limited and dose-dependent, and patients should be encouraged to tolerate the early AEs that may develop when a new medication is started.

While monotherapy is a treatment goal, and taking advantage of comorbid and/or coexistent illness may facilitate treatment of both disorders with a single drug, there are limitations to using a single medication to treat two illnesses. Giving a single medication may not treat two different conditions optimally: although one of the conditions may be adequately treated, the second illness may require a higher or lower dose, and, therefore, there is a risk that the second illness is not being adequately treated. Therapeutic independence may be needed should monotherapy fail. Avoiding drug interactions or increased AEs is a primary concern when using polypharmacy. Polytherapy may enable therapeutic adjustments based on the status of each illness. For example, TCAs are often recommended for patients with migraine and depression.[31] However, appropriate management of depression often requires higher doses of TCAs, which may be associated with more AEs. A better approach might be to treat the depression with an SSRI or SNRI and treat the migraine with an anti-epileptic. Migraine and epilepsy[32] may both be controlled with an anti-epileptic drug, such as topiramate or divalproex sodium, which are also the drugs of choice for the patient with migraine and bipolar illness[33,34] When individuals have more than one disease, certain categories of treatment may be relatively contraindicated. For example, ß-blockers should be used with caution for the depressed migraineur, while TCAs or neuroleptics may lower the seizure threshold and should be used with caution for the epileptic migraineur.
- Although monotherapy is preferred, it often does not yield the desired therapeutic effect, and it may be necessary to combine preventive medications. Antidepressants are often used with ß-blockers or calcium-channel blockers, and topiramate or divalproex sodium may be used in combination with any of these medications.

GUIDELINES FOR STOPPING PREVENTIVE THERAPY

- The patient develops intolerable AEs or a severe drug reaction.

- The drug does not demonstrate even partial efficacy after 2 months of therapy and disorders such as acute medication overuse have not been eliminated.
- The patient has shown significant benefit. If the headaches are well controlled for at least 6 months, slowly taper and, if possible, discontinue the drug.

Preventive treatment is often recommended for 6–9 months, but until now no randomized, placebo-controlled trials have been performed to investigate migraine frequency after the preventive treatment has been discontinued. Diener et al.[35] assessed 818 migraine patients who were treated with topiramate for 6 months to see the effects of topiramate discontinuation. Patients received topiramate in a 26-week, open-label phase. They were then randomly assigned to continue topiramate or switch to placebo for a 26-week, double-blind phase. Of the 559 patients who completed the open-label phase, 514 entered the double-blind phase and were assigned to topiramate (*n* = 255) or placebo (*n* = 259). The mean increase in number of migraine days was greater in the placebo group (1.19 days in 4 weeks, 95% CI [0.71–1.66]; *p* < 0.0001) than in the topiramate group (0.10, –0.36–0.56, *p* = 0.5756). Patients in the placebo group had a greater number of days on acute medication than did those in the topiramate group (mean difference between groups –0.95 [–1.49 to –0.41], *p* = 0.0007). Sustained benefit was reported after topiramate was discontinued, although the number of migraine days did increase. In a subsequent analysis of this study, no factors were identified that predicted consistent relapse after withdrawal of topiramate therapy.[36] While the authors did find evidence that the likelihood of sustained relapse was higher when the initial response to migraine preventive treatment had been more pronounced, the same effect was found in the placebo group, leading the authors to speculate that this observation likely reflected "regression to the mean." Woeber et al. found that 75% of patients developed increased migraine frequency after flunarizine or ß-blockers were stopped.[37] Relapse occurred on average 6 months after cessation of the medication. These findings suggest that patients may relapse after the discontinuation of preventive treatment; patients should be cautioned in this regard, and should be followed carefully for an escalating frequency of attacks. It is unclear which factors increase the risk of relapse or sustained remission.

SPECIFIC MIGRAINE PREVENTIVE AGENTS

ß-Adrenergic Blockers for the Prevention of Migraine

ß-blockers are the most widely used class of drugs in prophylactic migraine treatment, and are about 50% effective in producing a greater than 50% reduction in attack frequency (Tables 8.2 and 8.3). Evidence has consistently demonstrated the efficacy[38,39] of the non-selective ß-blocker propranolol[23–25,38–44] and of the selective ß1-blocker metoprolol.[23,24,40,45–49] Atenolol,[50] bisoprolol,[47,51] nadolol,[52,53] and timolol[38,54] are also likely to be effective. β-blockers with intrinsic sympathomimetic activity (acebutolol, alprenolol, oxprenolol, pindolol) are not effective for migraine prevention.

The combination of propranolol and topiramate versus topiramate alone was recently examined as a preventive treatment for chronic migraineurs, in the National Institute of Neurological Diseases and Stroke (NINDS) Clinical Research Collaboration Chronic Migraine Treatment Trial (CMTT). This was a randomized, double-blind, placebo-controlled, parallel study to examine the safety and efficacy of topiramate (up to 100 mg/day) and propranolol (up to 240 mg/day LA formulation) taken in combination, compared with treatment with topiramate (up to 100 mg/day) and placebo. The trial was terminated in September 2010, when an interim analysis determined that the combination of topiramate and propranolol offered no additional advantage over topiramate alone.[55]

The action of ß-blockers is probably central and could be mediated by (1) inhibiting central ß-receptors that interfere with the vigilance-enhancing adrenergic pathways; (2) interacting with 5-HT receptors (but not all effective ß-blockers bind to the 5-HT receptors); and (3) cross-modulation of the serotonin system. [41] Propranolol inhibits nitrous oxide production by blocking inducible nitric oxide synthase. Propranolol also inhibits kainate-induced

Table 8.2 Classification of Migraine Preventive Therapies

Level A:Effective (≥2 Class I Trials)	Level B: Probably Effective (1 Class I or 2 Class II Studies)	Level C: Possibly Effective (1 Class II Study)	Level U: Inadequate or Conflicting Data	Ineffective, Probably or Possibly Ineffective
AEDs	Antidepressants	ACE inhibitors	α-Agonists	Ineffective
Divalproex sodium	Amitriptyline	Lisinopril	Clonidine	Lamotrigine
Sodium valproate	Venlafaxine	**Angiotensin blockers**	**Antidepressants**	**Probably ineffective**
Topiramate	**ß-Blockers**	Candesartan	Fluoxetine	Clomipramine[a]
ß-Blockers	Atenolol	**AEDs**	Fluvoxamine	**Possibly ineffective**
Metoprolol	Nadolol[a]	Carbamazepine	Protriptyline[a]	Acebutolol
Propranolol		**Antihistamines**	**AEDs**	Clonazepam
Timolol[a]		Cyproheptadine	Gabapentin	Nabumetone[a]
		ß-Blockers	**ß-Blockers**	Oxcarbazepine
		Nebivolol	Bisoprolol[a]	Telmisartan
			Pindolol[a]	
			Ca++ blockers	
			Cyclandelate	
			Nicardipine	
			Nifedipine	
			Nimodipine	
			Verapamil	

Abbreviations: ACE = angiotensin-converting-enzyme; Ca++ blockers = calcium channel blockers; MRM = menstrually related migraine; SSNRI = selective serotonin–norepinephrine reuptake inhibitor; SSRI = selective serotonin reuptake inhibitor; TCA = tricyclic antidepressant.
[a] Classification based on original guideline and new evidence not found for this report.

Table 8.3 ß-Blockers and Antidepressants in the Preventive Treatment of Migraine

Agent	Daily Dose	Comment
ß-blockers		
Atenolol	50 mg to 200 mg	• Use qid • Fewer side effects than propranolol
Metoprolol	100 mg to 200 mg	• Use the short-acting form bid • Use the long-acting form qid
Nadolol	20 mg to 160 mg	• Use qid • Fewer side effects than propranolol
Propranolol	40 mg to 240 mg	• Use the short-acting form bid or tid • Use the long-acting form qid or bid • 1 to 2 mg/kg in children
Timolol	20 mg to 60 mg	• Divide the dose • Short half-life
Antidepressants		
Tertiary Amines		
Amitriptyline	10 mg to 200 mg	• Start at 10 mg at bedtime
Doxepin	10 mg to 200 mg	• Start at 10 mg at bedtime
Secondary Amines		
Nortriptyline	10 mg to 150 mg	• Start at 10–25 mg at bedtime • If insomnia, give early in the morning
Protriptyline	5 mg to 60 mg	• Start at 10–25 mg at bedtime
Selective Serotonin and Norepephrine Reuptake Inhibitors		
Venlafaxine	75 mg to 225 mg	• Start 37.5 mg in a.m.

currents and is synergistic with N-methyl D-aspartate blockers, which reduce neuronal activity and have membrane-stabilizing properties.[42]

Contraindications to the use of ß-blockers include asthma and chronic obstructive lung disease, congestive heart failure, atrioventricular conduction defects, Raynaud's disease, peripheral vascular disease, and severe diabetes mellitus. All ß-blockers can produce behavioral AEs, such as drowsiness, fatigue, lethargy, sleep disorders, nightmares, depression, memory disturbance, and hallucinations.[38] Other potential AEs include gastrointestinal complaints, decreased exercise tolerance, orthostatic hypotension, bradycardia, and impotence. Although stroke has been reported to occur after patients with migraine with aura were started on ß-blockers, there is neither an absolute nor a relative contraindication to their use by patients with migraine, either with or without aura.

SUMMARY: EVIDENCE FOR SS-BLOCKERS IN THE PREVENTION OF MIGRAINE[14]

- Strong evidence establishes the effectiveness of metopralol, propranolol, and timolol (Level A—See Appendix 2 for definitions of levels of evidence).
- Evidence exists (Level B) to suggest that atenolol and nadolol are probably effective and should be considered.
- Nebivolol and pindolol are possibly effective (Level C) and may be considered.
- There is inadequate evidence to support or refute the use of bisoprolol.

Antidepressant Medication for Migraine Prevention

Antidepressants consist of a number of different drug classes with different mechanisms of action (Table 8.3). Although the mechanism by which antidepressants work to prevent migraine headache is uncertain, it does not result from treating latent or undiagnosed depression. Antidepressants are useful in treating many chronic pain states, including headache, independent of the presence of depression, and the response occurs sooner and at lower dosages than that expected for an antidepressant effect.

[47,50] In animal pain models, antidepressants potentiate the effects of co-administered opioids.[51] The antidepressants that are clinically effective in headache prevention either inhibit noradrenaline and 5-HT reuptake or are antagonists at the 5-HT_2 receptors.[52]

TRICYCLIC ANTIDEPRESSANTS

Tricyclic antidepressants (TCAs) are used for migraine prevention. Only one TCA (amitryptyline) has proven efficacy in migraine.[39] Amitriptyline has been used for migraine prevention for over 35 years.[56] Jackson et al. performed a meta-analysis in which adults with migraine or tension-type headache were treated with a TCA as a single intervention for at least 4 weeks. Contol groups included placebo or another preventive, such as ß-blockers, serotonin reuptake inhibitors (SSRIs), or alternative/complimentary strategies, such as spinal manipulation or behavioral therapy. Although the analyses were performed on studies that were heterogeneous with respect to study population, study design, and study quality, the study did demonstrate the effectiveness of amitriptyline over placebo for both migraine and tension-type headache. When pooling data from studies that compared TCAs and SSRIs, the authors found that TCAs were superior to SSRIs in subjects with both migraine and tension-type headache. The subjects in the tricyclic arms had higher rates of adverse effects than those in SSRI arms, although the rates of study withdrawal did not differ in the two treatment arms. An analysis of studies that compared TCAs with ß-blockers found no difference in the reduction of the number of headache days or attacks.[57]

Couch[56] published the results of a randomized, double-blind, placebo-controlled study ($n = 391$) on the efficacy of amitriptyline in preventing intermittent migraine and chronic daily headache. Although the study took place between 1976 and 1979, the results had not been reported previously. Results for the entire study group (i.e., both intermittent migraine and chronic daily headache) revealed that there was a statistically significant improvement in the frequency of headache from the end of the titration period (week 4) to the end of the first 4 weeks on maintenance dose (week 8) between the amitriptyline arm and the placebo arm ($p = 0.018$ in favor of amitriptyline).

However, when week 4 was compared with subsequent weeks of treatment (i.e., weeks 12, 16, and 20), the differences in the decrease in headache frequency between the amitriptyline and placebo groups did not persist, probably because of the large placebo effect that continued to increase with the duration of study participation. Additionally, there was a large attrition rate, whereby Couch suggests that subjects in the placebo group who did not improve may have preferentially withdrawn, thus diminishing the difference between the treatment and placebo groups. When subgroups were examined, there was no difference between the amitriptyline and placebo groups in reducing episodic migraine headache frequency. Amitriptyline was effective in reducing headache frequency in subjects with chronic daily headache. When headaches did occur in either subjects with episodic migraine or chronic daily headache, there was no significant difference in pain intensity or duration between placebo and amitriptyline groups. This may have been because headache duration was assessed independent of severity (e.g., duration of a mild headache contributed the same as a disabling headache). The importance of this recently published older study is that it is the largest placebo-controlled study of amitriptyline for migraine prevention.

The most rigorous evidence for amitriptyline may be found in a 26-week, multicenter, randomized, double-blind, double-dummy, parallel-group noninferiority study that randomized 331 subjects to either treatment with amitriptyline 100 mg or topiramate 100 mg.[93] The change from baseline in the mean monthly number of migraine episodes was not significantly different between the topiramate and amitriptyline groups (–2.6 and –2.7, respectively; 95% CI [–0.6–0.7]). Moreover, there were no significant differences between treatment groups in any of the pre-specified secondary outcome measures. Treatment emergent AEs were reported in 118 subjects (66.7%) in the topiramate group and 112 subjects (66.3%) in the amitriptyline group. Among the most common treatment-emergent adverse events (TEAEs) (reported in ±5% of subjects during the double-blind phase) in the topiramate group were paresthesia (29.9%), fatigue (16.9%), somnolence (11.9%), hypoesthesia (10.7%), and nausea (10.2%). The most commonly reported TEAEs in the amitriptyline group were dry mouth (35.5%), fatigue (24.3%), somnolence (17.8%), weight increase (13.6%), dizziness (10.7%), and sinusitis (10.7%). Subjects receiving topiramate had a mean weight loss of 2.4 kg, compared with a mean weight gain of 2.4 kg in subjects receiving amitriptyline.

The dose range for TCAs is wide and must be individualized. Amitriptyline and doxepin are sedating TCAs. Patients with coexistent depression may require higher doses of these drugs to treat underlying depression. Start at a dose of 10–25 mg at bedtime. The usual effective dosage for migraine ranges from 25 to 200 mg. Nortriptyline, a major metabolite of amitriptyline, is a secondary amine that is less sedating than amitriptyline. Start at a dose of 10–25 mg at bedtime. The dose ranges from 10 to 150 mg a day. Protriptyline is a secondary amine that is similar to nortriptyline. Start at a dose of 5 mg in the morning. The dose ranges from 5 to 60 mg a day, as a single or split dose. Start with a low dose of the chosen TCA at bedtime, except when using protriptyline, which should be administered in the morning. If the TCA is too sedating, switch from a tertiary TCA (amitriptyline, doxepin) to a secondary TCA (nortriptyline, protriptyline). AEs are common with TCA use. Antimuscarinic AEs include dry mouth, a metallic taste, epigastric distress, constipation, dizziness, mental confusion, tachycardia, palpitations, blurred vision, and urinary retention. Other AEs include weight gain (rarely seen with protriptyline), orthostatic hypotension, reflex tachycardia, and palpitations. Antidepressant treatment may change depression to hypomania or frank mania (particularly in bipolar patients). Older patients may develop confusion or delirium. [53] The muscarinic and adrenergic effects of these agents may pose increased risks for cardiac conduction abnormalities, especially in the elderly, and these patients should be carefully monitored or other agents considered.

SELECTIVE SEROTONIN AND NOREPINEPHRINE REUPTAKE INHIBITORS

Evidence for the use of SSRIs or other antidepressants for migraine prevention are mixed and overall are poor.

The efficacy analysis summarized in the AHCPR Evidence Report did not indicate a clear benefit of the racemic mixture of fluoxetine over placebo. One Class II study showed fluoxetine (racemic) was significantly better than placebo for migraine prevention,[58] but the results were not duplicated in a second study.[59] An additional Class II study showed fluoxetine 20 mg/day was more effective than placebo in reducing total pain index; however, differences were noted between treatment groups for baseline measures.[60] Anecdotal reports and our experience seem to indicate its benefit in migraine prophylaxis where coexistent depression is a prominent issue.

Other antidepressants not effective in placebo-controlled trials were clomipramine and sertraline; for other antidepressants, only open or non-placebo-controlled trials are available. Because their tolerability profile is superior to that of tricyclics, SSRIs may be helpful for patients with comorbid depression.[61] The most common AEs include sexual dysfunction, anxiety, nervousness, insomnia, drowsiness, fatigue, tremor, sweating, anorexia, nausea, vomiting, and dizziness or lightheadedness. The combination of an SSRI and a TCA can be beneficial in treating refractory depression[34] and, in our experience, resistant cases of migraine. The combination may require the TCA dose to be adjusted, because TCA plasma levels may significantly increase.

Venlafaxine, a selective serotonin and norepinephrine reuptake inhibitor, has been shown to be effective in a double-blind, placebo-controlled trial[62] and a separate placebo- and amitriptyline-controlled trial.[63] The usual effective dose is 150 mg a day. Start with the extended release tablet of 37.5 mg for 1 week, then 75 mg for 1 week, and then 150 mg extended release in the morning. AEs include insomnia, nervousness, mydriasis, and seizures.

SUMMARY: EVIDENCE FOR ANTIDEPRESSANTS IN THE PREVENTION OF MIGRAINE[14]

- There is no strong evidence (Level A) for any.
- Evidence exists (Level B) to suggest that amitriptyline and venlafaxine are probably effective and should be considered.
- There is conflicting Class II evidence for fluoxetine.

- There is inadequate evidence to support or refute (Level U) the use of fluvoxamine and protriptyline.

Calcium Channel Antagonists for the Prevention of Migraine

Two types of calcium channels exist: calcium entry channels, which allow extracellular calcium to enter the cell, and calcium release channels, which allow intracellular calcium (in storage sites in organelles) to enter the cytoplasm.[64] Calcium entry channel subtypes include voltage-gated, opened by depolarization; ligand-gated, opened by chemical messengers, such as glutamate; and capacitative, activated by depletion of intracellular calcium stores. The mechanism of action of the calcium channel antagonists in migraine prevention (Table 8.4) is uncertain, but possibilities include the inhibition of 5-HT release, neurovascular inflammation, or the initiation and propagation of cortical spreading depression.[65]

Flunarizine, a non-selective calcium channel antagonist with antidopaminergic properties, was superior to placebo in six of seven randomized clinical trials.[43,46,62–70] The dose is 5–10 mg at night (women seem to need lower doses than men). The most prominent AEs include weight gain, somnolence, dry mouth, dizziness, hypotension, occasional extrapyramidal reactions, and exacerbation of depression. Because of its side-effect profile, flunarizine should be considered as a second-line drug for migraine prevention, after ß-blockers. Flunarizine is widely used in Europe, but is not available in the United States, where verapamil is the recommended calcium-channel antagonist.

Verapamil was more effective than placebo in two of three trials, but both positive trials were very small and dropout rates were high, rendering the findings uncertain.[71–73] The original studies on verapamil and nimodipine were found to have conflicting Class III evidence on the basis of current classification criteria yielding Level U recommendations.

CONCLUSIONS

Data from older studies regarding verapamil, nimodipine, nicardipine, diltiazem,

Table 8.4 **Selected Calcium-Channel Blockers and Selected Anti-epileptics in the Preventive Treatment of Migraine**

Agent	Daily Dose	Comment
Selected Calcium Channel Blockers		
Verapamil	120 mg to 480 mg	• Start 80 mg bid or tid • Sustained release can be given qid or bid
Flunarizine	5 mg to 10 mg	• qid at bedtime • Weight gain is the most common side effect.
Selected Anti-epileptics		
Carbamazepine	600 mg to 1200 mg	• tid
Gabapentin	600 mg to 3600 mg	• Dose can be increased to 3000 mg
Topiramate	50 mg to 200mg	• Start 15–25 mg at bedtime • Increase 15–25 mg per week • Attempt to reach 50–100 mg • Increase further if necessary • Associated with weight loss, not weight gain
Valproate/Divalproex	500 mg to 2000 mg/day	• Start 250–500 mg day • Monitor levels if compliance is an issue • Max dose is 60 mg/kg day

cyclandelate, and other non-selective calcium-channel antagonists have not shown superiority over placebo in well-designed clinical trials and cannot be recommended for migraine prophylaxis.

SUMMARY: EVIDENCE FOR CALCIUM-CHANNEL BLOCKERS IN THE PREVENTION OF MIGRAINE[14]

• Flunarizine has strong evidence (Level A) (European guidelines).
• There is inadequate evidence (Level U) to support or refute the use of cyclandelate, nimodipine, verapamil, nicardipine, or nifedipine.

Anti-epileptic Drugs for the Prevention of Migraine

Anti-epileptic drugs (AEDs) are increasingly recommended for migraine prevention (Table 8.4) because of well-conducted placebo-controlled trials. With the exception of valproic acid, topiramate (doses < 200 mg./day), and zonisamide, AEDs may substantially interfere with the efficacy of oral contraceptives.[71,74]

CARBAMAZEPINE

The only placebo-controlled trial of carbamazepine that suggested a significant benefit suffered from methodologic issues in several respects, including the absence of a washout phase between the two treatment arms in the crossover design.[72] Carbamazepine, 600–1200 mg a day, may be effective preventive migraine treatment, but it is rarely used in clinical practice for this purpose, because of the absence of rigorous data concerning efficacy and because of adverse hematologic, hepatic, and cardiovascular effects (Table 8.4).

GABAPENTIN

Gabapentin (1800–2400 mg) showed efficacy in a placebo-controlled, double-blind trial only when a modified intent-to-treat analysis was used (Table 8.4). Migraine attack frequency was reduced by 50% in about one-third of patients.[73] The most common AEs were dizziness or giddiness and drowsiness. Results of another double-blind, placebo-controlled trial[75] was positive; however, the ability to draw conclusions from the placebo-controlled studies is limited because of their methodologic and analytical limitations. Recent reviews, including a Cochrane review, conclude that further evaluation of gabapentin in migraine prophylaxis is warranted in order to inform clinical practice.[76]

Silberstein et al.[77] conducted a randomized, double-blind, placebo-controlled trial of gabapentin enacarbil (GEn), a transported prodrug of gabapentin that provides sustained, dose-proportional exposure to gabapentin. GEn is rapidly converted to gabapentin upon absorption from the intestinal lumen. Patients were randomized 2:1:2:2:1 to one of the following five groups during the 20-week treatment period: placebo, GEn 1200 mg, GEn 1800 mg, GEn 2400 mg, or GEn 3000 mg. No statistically significant difference between active treatment and placebo was found. Pharmacokinetic data demonstrate that patients had adequate estimated exposure to GEn. GEn did not significantly differ from placebo for migraine headache prevention.

VALPROIC ACID

Valproic acid is a simple 8-carbon, 2-chain fatty acid. Divalproex sodium (approved by the FDA) is a combination of valproic acid and sodium valproate. Both are effective,[78,79] as is an extended release form of divalproex sodium.[80] In 1992, Hering and Kuritzky[81] evaluated sodium valproate's efficacy in migraine treatment in a double-blind, randomized, crossover study. Sodium valproate was effective in preventing migraine or reducing the frequency, severity, and duration of attacks in 86.2% of 29 patients, whose attacks were reduced from 15.6 to 8.8 a month. In 1994, Jensen et al.[82] studied 43 patients with migraine without aura in a triple-blind, placebo- and dose-controlled, crossover study of slow-release sodium valproate. In the valproate group, 50% of the patients had a reduction in migraine frequency to 50% or less, compared with 18% for placebo.

Several subsequent randomized, placebo-controlled studies have confirmed these results, with significant responder rates ranging between 43% and 48%[69,82] with dosages ranging from 500 to 1500 mg per day. Extended-release (ER) divalproex sodium has also been shown to be effective for migraine prevention, and compliance and side-effect profile may be more favorable with this formulation.[83] Since the 2000 publication, one double-blind, randomized, Class I placebo-controlled 12-week trial showed migraine headache rate from 4.4/week (baseline) to 3.2/week (± 1.2 attacks/week) in the ER divalproex sodium group and from 4.2/week to 3.6/week (± 0.6 attacks/week) in the placebo group (CI 0.2–1.2, $p < 0.006$).[80] No significant differences were detected between groups in the number of treatment-emergent AEs.

Clinical Context

In most headache trials, patients taking divalproex sodium or sodium valproate reported no more AEs than those on placebo. However, weight gain has been clinically observed with divalproex sodium long-term use. Treatment with these agents requires careful follow-up and testing because of pancreatitis, liver failure, and teratogenicity risks.[84,85]

Nausea, vomiting, and gastrointestinal distress are the most common AEs; their incidence decreases, however, particularly after 6 months. Tremor and alopecia can, however, occur later. Valproate has little effect on cognitive functions and rarely causes sedation. Rare, severe AEs include hepatitis and pancreatitis. The frequency varies with the number of concomitant medications used, the patient's age, the presence of genetic and metabolic disorders, and the patient's general state of health. These idiosyncratic reactions are unpredictable.[86] Valproate is teratogenic.[33] In addition to well-known teratogenic effects, including neural tube defects, the US Food and Drug Administration recently issued an alert to healthcare providers and patients that medications including and related to valproate sodium can cause decreased IQ scores in children whose mothers took the medication during pregnancy. These drugs continue to be contraindicated for (should never be used by) pregnant women for the prevention of migraine headaches. Valproate products include valproate sodium (Depacon), divalproex sodium (Depakote, Depakote CP, and Depakote ER), valproic acid (Depakene and Stavzor), and their generics. In fact, in women of childbearing potential, valproate sodium and all related drugs should be used with extreme caution. Hyperandrogenism, ovarian cysts, and obesity are of concern in young women with epilepsy who use valproate.[87] Absolute contraindications are pregnancy and a history of pancreatitis or a hepatic disorder. Other contraindications are thrombocytopenia, pancytopenia, and bleeding disorders.

Valproic acid is available as 250 mg capsules and as syrup (250 mg/5 ml) (Table 8.4). Divalproex sodium is available as 125, 250, and 500 mg capsules and a sprinkle formulation.

Start with 250 to 500 mg a day in divided doses and slowly increase the dose. Monitor serum levels if there is a question of toxicity or compliance. The maximum recommended dose is 60 mg/kg/day.

TOPIRAMATE

Topiramate was originally synthesized as part of a research project to discover structural analogs of fructose-1, 6-diphosphate capable of inhibiting the enzyme fructose 1, 6-bisphosphatase, thereby blocking gluconeogenesis, but it has no hypoglycemic activity. Topiramate and divalproex sodium are the only two anti-epileptics that have FDA approval for migraine prevention. Topiramate is not associated with significant reductions in estrogen exposure at doses below 200 mg per day. At doses above 200 mg per day, there may be a dose-related reduction in exposure to the estrogen component of oral contraceptives.

Four Class I studies[88–91] and 7 Class II studies[92–98] report topiramate (50–200 mg/day) is effective in migraine prevention.

Two large, pivotal, multicenter, randomized, double-blind, placebo-controlled clinical trials assessed the efficacy and safety of topiramate (50, 100, and 200 mg/day) in migraine prevention. In the first trial, the responder rate (patients with ≥ 50% reduction in monthly migraine frequency) was 52% with topiramate 200 mg/day ($p < 0.001$); 54% with topiramate 100 mg ($p < 0.001$); and 36% with topiramate 50 mg/day ($p = 0.039$); compared with 23% with placebo.[99] The 200 mg dose was not significantly more effective than the 100 mg dose. The second pivotal trial[92] had significantly more patients who exhibited at least a 50% reduction in mean monthly migraines in the groups treated with 50 mg/day of topiramate (39%, $p = .009$), 100 mg/day of topiramate (49%, $p = .001$), and 200 mg/day of topiramate (47%, $p = .001$).

A third randomized, double-blind, parallel-group, multicenter trial[93] compared two doses of topiramate (100 mg/day or 200 mg/day) to placebo or propranolol (160 mg/day). Topiramate 100 mg/day was superior to placebo, as measured by average monthly migraine period rate, average monthly migraine days, rate of rescue medication use, and percentage of patients with a 50% or greater decrease

in average monthly migraine period rate (responder rate 37%). The topiramate 100 mg/day and propranolol groups were similar in change from baseline to the core double-blind phase in average monthly migraine period rate and other secondary efficacy variables.

Topiramate's most common AE is paresthesia; other common AEs are fatigue, decreased appetite, nausea, diarrhea, weight decrease, taste perversion, hypoesthesia, and abdominal pain. In the migraine trials, body weight was reduced an average of 2.3% in the 50 mg group, 3.2% in the 100 mg group, and 3.8% in the 200 mg group. Patients on propranolol gained 2.3% of their baseline body weight. The most common CNS AEs were somnolence, insomnia, mood problems, anxiety, difficulty with memory, language problems, and difficulty with concentration. Renal calculi can occur with topiramate use. The reported incidence is about 1.5%, representing a two-to fourfold increase over the estimated occurrence in the general population.[100] In 2011, the FDA notified healthcare professionals and patients of an increased risk of development of cleft lip and/or cleft palate (oral clefts) in infants born to women treated with topiramate during pregnancy. Because of new human data that show an increased risk for oral clefts, topiramate is being placed in Pregnancy Category D. Pregnancy Category D means there is positive evidence of human fetal risk based on human data but the potential benefits from the use of the drug in pregnant women may be acceptable in certain situations despite its risks.

A very rare AE is acute myopia associated with secondary angle closure glaucoma. No cases of this condition were reported in the clinical studies.[101] Oligohidrosis has been reported in association with an elevation in body temperature. Most reports have involved children.

Start topiramate at a dose of 15–25 mg at bedtime (Table 8.4). Increase by a dose of 15–25 mg/week. Do not increase the dose if bothersome AEs develop; wait until they resolve (they usually do). If they do not resolve, decrease the drug to the last tolerable dose, then increase by a lower dose more slowly. Attempt to reach a dose of 50–100 mg/day given twice a day. It is our experience that patients who tolerate the lower doses with only partial improvement often have increased benefit with higher doses. The dose can be increased to 600 mg/day or higher.

Dodick et al.[94] in a multicenter, randomized, double-blind double-dummy, parallel group, non-inferiority trial comparing topiramate and amitriptyline for the prevention of episodic migraine, demonstrated that topiramate was as effective as amitriptyline in reducing the frequency of migraine headache. The primary efficacy variable, change from baseline in the mean monthly number rate of migraine episodes, was –2.6 in the topiramate arm and –2.7 in the amitriptyline arm (NS). There also was no significant difference between the two preventives with respect to the pre-specified secondary outcome measures. However, the topiramate group showed statistically greater improvement in mean functional disability during migraine attacks (LSM change: –0.33 vs. –0.19; 95% CI [–0.3–0.0], $p = 0.040$) and experienced an improvement in weight satisfaction, while subjects on amitriptyline experienced weight satisfaction deterioration ($p < 0.001$).

Very recently, the National Institute of Neurological Diseases and Stroke (NINDS) Clinical Research Collaboration conducted the Chronic Migraine Treatment Trial (CMTT) to examine the safety and efficacy of topiramate (up to 100 mg/day) and propranolol (up to 240 mg/day LA formulation) taken in combination, compared with treatment with topiramate (up to 100 mg/day) and placebo. This double-blind, placebo-controlled, randomized clinical trial was terminated in September 2010, when an interim analysis determined that the combination of topiramate and propranolol offered no additional advantage over topiramate alone.[102]

LAMOTRIGINE

Lamotrigine blocks voltage-sensitive sodium channels, leading to inhibition of neuronal glutamate release of glutamate. Chen et al. [103] reported two patients with migraine with persistent aura-like visual phenomena for months to years. After 2 weeks of lamotrigine treatment, both had resolution of the visual symptoms.

Although open-label studies have suggested that lamotrigine may have a select role in the treatment of patients with frequent or prolonged aura, results from a placebo-controlled study in migraine without aura was negative.

Steiner et al.[104] compared the safety and efficacy of lamotrigine (200 mg/day) and placebo in migraine prophylaxis in a double-blind, randomized, parallel-groups trial. Although improvements were greater with placebo, these changes were not statistically significant, and indicate that lamotrigine was ineffective for migraine prophylaxis. There were more AEs with lamotrigine than placebo, most commonly rash. With slow dose escalation, their frequency was reduced, and the rate of withdrawal due to AEs was similar in both treatment groups.

Open-label studies have suggested that lamotrigine may have a select role in the treatment of migraine with aura, but no placebo-controlled studies have yet been conducted in this patient population. Both lamotrigine and topiramate[105] may have a special role in the treatment of migraine with aura. A more recent Class II study comparing lamotrigine 50 mg/d to placebo or topiramate 50 mg/d reported that lamotrigine was not more effective than placebo (for both primary endpoints) and was less effective than topiramate in reducing the frequency and intensity of migraine.[88] The primary outcome measure (responder rate of ≥ 50% reduction in monthly migraine frequency) was 46% for lamotrigine versus 34% for placebo ($p = .093$, CI 0.02–0.26), and 63% for topiramate versus 46% for lamotrigine ($p = .019$, CI 0.03–0.31).

OXCARBAZEPINE

In a multicenter, double-blind, randomized, placebo-controlled, parallel-group trial, 170 patients were randomized to receive oxcarbazepine 1200 mg/day or placebo.[106] Oxcarbazepine was initiated at 150 mg/day and increased by 150 mg/day every 5 days, and the primary outcome measure was change from baseline in the number of migraine attacks during the last 28-day period of the 16-week double-blind phase. There was no difference between the oxcarbazepine and placebo groups in mean change in number of migraine attacks from baseline during the last 28 days of double-blind phase. Adverse events were reported for 68 oxcarbazepine-treated patients (80%) and 55 placebo-treated patients (65%). The majority of adverse events were mild or moderate in severity. The most common adverse events (≥ 15% of patients) in the oxcarbazepine-treated group were fatigue (20.0%), dizziness (17.6%), and nausea (16.5%); no adverse event occurred in more than 15% of the placebo-treated patients.

SUMMARY: EVIDENCE FOR ANTI-EPILEPTIC DRUGS IN THE PREVENTION OF MIGRAINE[14]

- There is strong evidence (Level A) establishing the effectiveness of divalproex sodium, sodium valproate, topiramate.
- Carbamazepine is possibly effective (Level C).
- There is inadequate evidence (Level U) to support or refute the use of gabapentin.
- Lamotrigine is ineffective (Level A Negative) and should not be offered for migraine prevention, although there is anectodal evidence that it may have some efficacy for patients with migraine with aura.
- Oxcarbazepine is possibly ineffective for migraine prevention.

SEROTONIN ANTAGONISTS

The antiserotonin migraine-preventive drugs are potent 5-HT_{2B} and 5-HT_{2C} receptor antagonists.

Methysergide

Methysergide is a semisynthetic ergot alkaloid that is structurally related to methylergonovine. It is a 5-HT_2 receptor antagonist and a $5\text{-HT}_{1B/D}$ agonist. It was probably the first drug developed for migraine prevention,[107] but its usefulness is limited by reports of retroperitoneal and retropleural fibrosis associated with long-term, mostly uninterrupted, administration.[108] It is no longer available in the United States. Methysergide is effective.[38,109] AEs include transient muscle aching, claudication, abdominal distress, nausea, weight gain, and hallucinations. The major complication is rare (1/2500) retroperitoneal, pulmonary, or endocardial fibrosis.[109] To prevent this, a 4-week medication-free interval is recommended after 6 months of continuous treatment.

Methysergide is indicated for the treatment of migraine and cluster headache. The dose ranges from 2 to 8 mg a day, with the higher doses being given two or three times a day. Some clinicians find they can use higher doses, up to 14 mg a day, without AEs and with higher efficacy.[110] To minimize early AEs, patients can start with a dose of 1 mg a day and increase the dose gradually by 1 mg every 2 to 3 days. Methysergide, in general, should not be taken continuously for long periods, since doing so may produce retroperitoneal fibrosis.[108,111,112] Instead, the drug should be given for 6 months, stopped for 1 month, and then restarted. To avoid an increase in headache when methysergide is stopped, the patient should be weaned off the drug over a 1-week period. Some authorities use methysergide on a continuous basis with careful monitoring,[110] which includes auscultation of the heart and yearly echocardiography, chest X-ray, and abdominal MRI. The drug should be discontinued immediately on suspicion of pulmonary or cardiac retroperitoneal fibrosis.[110]

Cyproheptadine

Cyproheptadine, an antagonist at the 5-HT2, histamine H1, and muscarinic cholinergic receptors, is widely used in the prophylactic treatment of migraine in children.[110,113,114] Cyproheptadine is available as 4 mg tablets. The total dose ranges from 12 to 36 mg a day (given two to three times a day or at bedtime). Common AEs are sedation and weight gain; dry mouth, nausea, lightheadedness, ankle edema, aching legs, and diarrhea are less common. Cyproheptadine may inhibit growth in children[115] and reverse the effects of SSRIs. A single Class II study showed cyproheptadine (4 mg/day) was as effective as propranolol (80 mg/day) in reducing migraine frequency and severity.[44]

OTHER DRUGS FOR THE PREVENTION OF MIGRAINE

Angiotensin-Converting Enzyme Inhibitors and Angiotensin II Receptor Antagonists

Schrader et al.[116] conducted a double-blind, placebo-controlled, crossover study of lisinopril, an angiotensin-converting enzyme inhibitor in migraine prophylaxis (Table 8.5). Days with migraine were reduced by at least 50% in 14 participants for active treatment versus placebo and 17 patients for active treatment versus runin period. Days with migraine were fewer by at least 50% in 14 participants for active treatment versus placebo.

Tronvik et al.[117] performed a randomized, double-blind, placebo-controlled, crossover study of candesartan (16 mg), an angiotensin II receptor blocker, in migraine prevention (Table 8.5). In a 12-week period, the mean number of days with headache was 18.5 with placebo versus 13.6 with candesartan ($p = .001$) in the intention-to-treat analysis ($n = 57$). The number of candesartan responders (reduction of $\geq 50\%$ compared with placebo) was 18 of 57 (31.6%) for days with headache and 23 of 57 (40.4%) for days with migraine. AEs were similar in the two periods. In this study, the

angiotensin II receptor blocker candesartan was effective, with a tolerability profile comparable with that of placebo.

A second randomized, triple-blind, double cross-over, placebo-controlled with propranolol as an active comparator confirmed the preventive efficacy of candesartan.[118] The study involved 72 adult subjects with episodic or chronic migraine who were treated over three 12-week treatment periods with either candesartan 16 mg, propranolol slow-release 160 mg, or placebo. In the modified intention-to treat analysis, candesartan and propranolol were both superior to placebo: 2.95 (95% CI, 2.35–3.55) and 2.91 (2.36–3.45), versus 3.53 (2.98–4.08) for migraine days per month ($p < 0.02$ for both active drugs). Candesartan was non-inferior to propranolol. The proportion of responders was significantly higher on candesartan (43%) and propranolol (40%) than on placebo (23%) ($p < 0.025$ and < 0.050, respectively). The authors concluded that 16 mg is effective for migraine prevention, with an effect size similar to propranolol 160 mg.

In a single Class II placebo-controlled trial, telmisartan 80 mg did not show a significant difference from placebo for reduction in migraine days (–1.65 vs. –1.14).[119]

SUMMARY: EVIDENCE FOR ACE-INHIBITORS/ANTAGONISTS IN THE PREVENTION OF MIGRAINE[14]

Candesartan and lisinopril are possibly effective (Level C) and may be considered. Telmisartan is possibly ineffective for reducing the number of migraine days (1 negative Class II study).

NSAIDs and Other Complementary Treatments for Episodic Migraine Prevention in Adults

HISTAMINES/ANTIHISTAMINES/ LEUKOTRIENE RECEPTOR ANTAGONISTS

The new 2012 American Academy of Neurology (AAN) guideline includes studies of histamines, antihistamines, and leukotriene receptor antagonists for migraine prevention.

Table 8.5 Miscellaneous Medication in the Preventive Treatment of Migraine

ACE and Angiotensin Receptor Antagonists		
Agent	Daily Dose	Comment
Lisinopril	10 mg to 40 mg	• Positive small controlled trial
Candesartan	16 mg to 32mg	• Positive small controlled trial
Others		
Agent	Daily Dose	Comment
Feverfew	50 mg to 82 mg	• Controversial evidence
Petasites	225 mg	• 75 mg and 100 mg better than placebo in independent trials
Riboflavin	400 mg	• Positive small controlled trial
Coenzyme Q	300 mg	• Two positive controlled trials
Magnesium	400 mg to 600 mg	• Controversial evidence

Histamine

Three Class II single-center studies (all from the same center) show the efficacy of histamine for migraine prevention.[98,120,121] N-alpha-methyl histamine (1–10 ng two times/week) SC injections reduced attack frequency from baseline as compared with placebo.[122] Histamine was statistically superior to placebo at all treatment visits through 12 weeks for reduction in migraine frequency, severity, and duration ($p < 0.0001$). Transient itching at the injection sites was the only reported adverse effect, but it did not reach significance. In a second Class II study, histamine was shown to be as effective as sodium valproate in reducing attack frequency and better than sodium valproate in reducing headache duration and intensity.[121] A third study reported the efficacy of histamine in migraine prevention as compared with topiramate. Topiramate 100 mg/day was compared with histamine (1–10 ng two times/week SC), and both active treatments showed improvement over baseline measures for attack frequency, intensity, and use of rescue medication.[98] Eleven percent (5/45) of subjects treated with histamine withdrew from the histamine group because they were not satisfied with the speed of results, although no AEs were reported. Few subjects reported transitory burning and itching at the injection site. Similar AEs and withdrawal rates (for slow reaction speed) were reported for the sodium valproate study.[121] Histamine SC was associated with transitory burning and itching at the injection site.

Cyproheptadine

A single Class II study showed cyproheptadine (4 mg/day) was as effective as propranolol (80 mg/day) in reducing migraine frequency and severity.[44]

Montelukast

One Class I study of montelukast (20 mg) for migraine prevention reported no significant difference between treatments in the percentage of patients with a > 50% decrease in migraine attack frequency per month (15.4% for montelukast vs. 10.3% for placebo.[123]

CONCLUSIONS

Histamine SC is established as probably effective (three Class II studies) for migraine

prevention. Cyproheptadine is possibly effective for migraine prevention and possibly as effective as propranolol for migraine prevention (single Class II study). Montelukast is probably ineffective for migraine prevention (1 Class I study; table 1).

MEDICINAL HERBS, VITAMINS, AND OTHER INTERVENTIONS

Herbal Preparations, Vitamins, and Minerals

Since the original guidelines, additional studies have been identified that assess the efficacy of Co-Q10, estrogen, hyperbaric oxygen (HBO), magnesium, MIG-99, omega-3, petasites, and riboflavin for migraine prevention (Table 8.5).

PETASIDES HYBRIDUS (BUTTERBUR)

Petasites is a purified extract from the root of the butterbur plant, a perennial shrub.[124] In a double-blind, placebo-controlled trial conducted by Grossmann and Schmidramsl, 50 mg of a standardized extract of petasites was given twice a day, resulting in a statistically significant decrease in both frequency of migraine (primary endpoint) and pain intensity.[125] A three-arm, parallel-group, double-blind, placebo-controlled trial by Lipton et al. compared petasides extract at doses of 75 mg bid, 50 mg bid, and placebo, concluding that the 75 mg bid dose was superior to placebo in reducing migraine frequency; however, the 50 mg bid dose was not statistically different from placebo.[126] The most common AE was belching. While Level A evidence exists for the use of Petasites, recent studies suggest that caution should be exercised given the potential for hepatic toxicity.

TANACETUM PARTHENIUM (FEVERFEW)

Feverfew (*Tanacetum parthenium*) is a medicinal herb whose effectiveness had not been totally established.[127] MIG-99 is a stable extract of feverfew, which is reproducibly manufactured with supercritical

CO_2 from feverfew. In the original guideline, three positive studies and one negative study (feverfew given as alcohol extract) are reviewed that suggest possible efficacy for migraine prevention.[39]

Since the original AAN guideline, three new studies on MIG-99 for migraine prophylaxis have been published. In one Class I study, the migraine frequency decreased from 4.76 by 1.9 attacks/month in the MIG-99 group and by 1.3 attacks in the placebo group. In a Class II dose-finding study, MIG-99 6.25 mg tid was effective in reducing migraine frequency by 1.8 attacks/month. The placebo group reduced migraine frequency by 0.3 attacks/month. In a second Class II study, the efficacy of the combination of magnesium (300 mg), riboflavin (400 mg), and MIG-99 (100 mg) was not shown in comparison with a placebo.[128–130]

OTHER VITAMINS AND HERBAL PREPARATIONS

Riboflavin (400 mg) was effective in one placebo-controlled, double-blind trial. Over half the patients responded.[131] Coenzyme Q10 may be effective for the prevention of migraine. One small Class II study (see Appendix 1) showed that Co-Q10 100 mg tid was significantly more effective than placebo in reducing attack frequency from baseline to 4 months following treatment.[132] A phytoestrogen preparation of 60 mg soy isoflavones, 100 mg dong quai, and 50 mg black cohosh (each component standardized to its primary alkaloid) reduced migraine attack frequency versus placebo in a small Class II study.[133]

SUMMARY: EVIDENCE FOR MEDICINAL HERBS AND VITAMINS IN THE PREVENTION OF MIGRAINE[14]

- Petasites (butterbur) is effective (Level A) but caution should be exercised given the potential for hepatic toxicity before it is offered.
- Magnesium, MIG-99 (feverfew), and riboflavin are probably effective (Level B) and should be considered.
- Co-Q10 and phytoestrogens are possibly effective (Level C) and may be considered.
- Omega-3 is possibly ineffective (Level C Negative) and may not be considered.

Aspirin and Other NSAIDS

The efficacy of NSAIDs for migraine prevention was reported in the original guideline, including 23 controlled trials of 10 different NSAIDs that showed a modest but significant benefit for naproxen sodium, with similar trends for flurbiprofen, ketoprofen, and mefenamic acid.[48,134,135] In the original AAN guideline, studies of aspirin had conflicting results. Since the original report, two additional Class II studies have been reported. Aspirin was found to be as effective as metoprolol for migraine prevention.[48] In a second study, aspirin 100 mg in combination with vitamin E 600 IU every other day was compared with placebo in combination with vitamin E.[135] No differences were noted between aspirin and placebo treatments for migraine frequency or severity at 12 months or 36 months.

SUMMARY: EVIDENCE FOR ASPIRIN AND OTHER NSAIDS IN THE PREVENTION OF MIGRAINE[14]

The following NSAIDS are probably effective (Level B) for the prevention of migraine: fenoprofen, ibuprofen, ketoprofen, naproxen, or naproxen sodium[48,134,135] The efficacy of aspirin for migraine prevention is unknown. Regular or daily use of selected NSAIDs for the treatment of frequent migraine attacks may exacerbate headache because of development of a condition called medication overuse headache. Therefore, use of aspirin, selected analgesics, and NSAIDs may exacerbate headache; use of these agents in migraine prevention studies may confound the clinical interpretation of the study results.

A comprehensive series of guidelines for the prevention of migraine were also developed by the Canadian Headache Society. Randomized, double-blind, controlled trials and relevant Cochrane reviews were graded according to criteria developed by the US Preventive Services Task Force.[136] The principles of the Grading of Recommendations Assessment, Development and Evaluation (GRADE) Working Group Recommendations were used to develop recommendations, and expert consensus that incorporated the best available evidence, side-effect profile, and migraine characteristics, and comorbid and coexisting disorders was used to develop final recommendations for drug selection. In this guideline, topiramate, propranolol, nadolol, metoprolol, amitriptyline, gabapentin, candesartan, butterbur, riboflavin, coenzyme Q10, and magnesium citrate received a strong recommendation for use, while divalproex sodium, flunarizine, pizotifen, venlafaxine, verapamil, and lisinopril received a weak recommendation.

NEW PREVENTIVE MEDICATIONS

CGRP Antibody Antagonists[137]

A recent development is the creation of antibodies to CGRP and its receptor. Multiple human monoclonal antibodies that specifically target the human CGRP receptor have been generated. They have minimum activity at the rat receptor and have > 50-fold selectivity over other closely related receptors. The inhibition of capsaicin-induced increases in dermal blood flow has been used as an *in vivo* pharmacodynamic model in humans and in non-human primates during the development of CGRP receptor antagonists. Topically applied capsaicin stimulates dermal neurons to release CGRP, which in turn results in a localized increase in dermal blood flow, measured by laser Doppler imaging. The CGRP receptor antagonist monoclonal antibody (mAb) AA95 prevented capsaicin-induced increase in dermal blood flow in cynomolgus monkeys for up to 7 days.[138]

The immunochemical distribution of another antibody in the series, AA32, has been tested; this recognizes the functional CLR/RAMP1 receptor complex, but not its individual components. AA32-positive CGRP receptor complexes are expressed on multiple levels in the trigeminal vascular system of the cynomolgus monkey: (1) in the meningeal vasculature innervated by CGRP-positive nerve fibers, (2) in neurons and satellite cells in the trigeminal ganglion, and (3) in neurons in the spinal trigeminal nucleus. The CGRP receptor localization is consistent with CGRP's role in trigeminal sensitization and suggests that interfering with CGRP receptor transmission may be beneficial for the treatment of migraines.[139]

Zeller et al.[140] took another approach, using monoclonal antibodies to previously identified rat alpha-CGRP received through a licensing agreement from UCLA.[141] They investigated whether or not function-blocking CGRP antibodies would inhibit neurogenic vasodilation with a long duration of action. They used two rat blood-flow models that measure electrically stimulated vasodilation in the skin or the middle meningeal artery (MMA). These responses are largely dependent on the neurogenic release of CGRP from sensory afferents. Treatment with anti-CGRP antibodies inhibited skin vasodilation or the increase in MMA diameter to a similar magnitude as treatment with CGRP receptor antagonists, but with a slower onset of action. The inhibition was still evident 1 week after dosing. Chronic treatment with anti-CGRP antibodies had no detectable effects on heart rate or blood pressure. Anti-CGRP antibodies may be a suitable drug candidate for the preventive treatment of migraine. They are currently being developed by Pfizer.

Another humanized monoclonal antibody, LY2951742, was developed by Eli Lilly and is being further developed by Arteaus, a joint venture of Eli Lilly's Chorus unit and Atlas Venture's AVDC initiative (http://clinicaltrials.gov/ct2/show/NCT01625988). LY2951742 prevents capsaicin-induced increases in dermal blood flow in rats, non-human primates, and healthy human volunteers. It is administered by subcutaneous injection. The time to maximum serum concentration ranges from 7 to 13 days, with an elimination half-life of approximately 28 days. A Phase 2 randomized, double-blind, placebo-controlled study of LY2951742 in patients with migraine is now underway. The study comprises four trial periods: screening and washout; baseline for assessment of type, frequency, and severity of headaches (4 weeks); treatment (12 weeks); and follow-up (12 weeks). LY2951742 (150 mg) will be administered subcutaneously once every other week for 12 weeks. The primary outcome measure is the mean change from baseline in the number of migraine headache days in a 28-day period.

LBR-101(formerly known as RN-307 or PF-04427429) is a fully humanized monoclonal antibody that potently and selectively binds to both isoforms (α and β) of CGRP and blocks its binding to the CGRP receptors.[142] This antibody is being developed by Labrys in a phase IIb trial for prevention of both high-frequency episodic and chronic migraine. In phase 1 studies, LBR-101 was administered to 94 subjects in dosages ranging from 0.2 mg to 2000 mg administered once (day 1) as a single IV infusion, or up to 300 mg given twice (Day 1 and Day 14). The drug was very well tolerated with an average of 1.4 treatment-emergent adverse events on active drug compared to an average of 1.3 treatment-emergent adverse events among those receiving placebo. Overall, treatment-related adverse events occurred in 21.2% of subjects receiving LBR-101, compared to 17.7% in those receiving placebo. LBR-101 was not associated with any clinically relevant patterns of change in vital signs, ECG parameters, or laboratory findings.

ALD403 is a genetically engineered, desialylated, humanized IgG1 antibody that potently (Kd < 20pM) and selectively binds to both α and β forms of human CGRP. The plasma half-life after a single intravenous infusion of 1000 mg is 31 days. This drug, developed by Alder Biopharmaceuticals, has completed a randomized, placebo-controlled, Phase II study in subjects with moderate- to high-frequency episodic migraine, delivered as a once monthly infusion of 1000 mg. The primary endpoint was the mean change in migraine headache days between weeks 5 to 8 and the results are expected to be published in 2014.

Unlike the three monoclonal antibodies in development that target CGRP, AMG 334 (Amgen) is a fully human monoclonal immunoglobulin (IgG2) against the CGRP receptor. AMG 334 binds to the CGRP receptor complex with high affinity (Kd 20 pM), which competitively and reversibly blocks the binding of the native ligand, CGRP. AMG 334 effectively functions as a CGRP receptor antagonist and is in Phase II development in a randomized, double-blind, placebo-controlled, parallel-group study of patients with episodic migraine. The drug is delivered once monthly as a subcutaneous injection.

BOTULINUM TOXIN FOR MIGRAINE

While daily oral prophylactic treatments have proven effective for many patients, issues such as lack of compliance with daily dosing regimens and adverse effects have limited their usefulness[1,143] and have resulted in a search for other modalities and agents, including Botulinum toxins (Botulinum neurotoxins; BoNTs), as potential preventive treatments.

Formulations of Botulinum Toxin

The 7 BoNT serotypes (A, B, C1, D, E, F, and G) produced by *Clostridium botulinum* are synthesized as single-chain polypeptides. All serotypes inhibit acetylcholine release, although their intracellular target proteins, physiochemical characteristics, and potencies are different.[144,145] Botulinum toxin type A (BoNTA) is the most widely studied serotype for therapeutic purposes.[144]

Currently, BoNT is available for clinical use in the United States as onabotulinumtoxinA (Botulinum toxin type A), branded as BOTOX® (Allergan, Inc., Irvine, CA, USA) and abobotulinumtoxinA (another Botulinum toxin type A), branded as Dysport® (Ipsen Ltd., Slough, UK), and the BoNTB product rimabotulinumtoxinB, branded as Myobloc®/Neurobloc® (Solstice Neurosciences, Inc., South San Francisco, CA, USA/Solstice Neurosciences Ltd., Dublin, Ireland). Lyophilized BOTOX® is available in vials containing 100 units (U) of BoNTA and is diluted with 2 or 4 mL of preservative-free 0.9% saline to yield a concentration of 5.0 or 2.5 U per 0.1 mL, respectively.[146] Reconstituted solutions of BOTOX® can be refrigerated but must be used within 4 hours.[146] Myobloc® is available in 0.5, 1, and 2 mL vials containing 5000 U per mL.[145]

Mechanism of Action of Botulinum Toxin in Headache

BoNT acts by inhibiting the release of acetylcholine at the neuromuscular junction by binding to motor or sympathetic nerve terminals, then entering the nerve terminals and inhibiting the release of acetylcholine, thereby blocking neuromuscular transmission. This inhibition occurs as the BoNT cleaves one of several proteins integral to the successful docking and release of acetylcholine from vesicles situated within nerve endings. Following intramuscular injection, BoNT produces partial chemical denervation of the muscle, resulting in a localized reduction in muscle activity. [144,145]

The potential association between BoNTA use and the alleviation of migraine headache symptoms was observed during initial clinical trials of BoNTA treatment for hyperfunctional lines of the face.[147] BoNTA therapy has been used for a variety of disorders associated with painful muscle spasms. Because migraine attacks are frequently associated with muscle tenderness,[148] it was generally believed that intramuscular BoNTA might prevent abnormal sensory signals in the affected muscle from arriving at the central nervous system. If abnormal muscle physiology can trigger migraine, one would predict that BoNTA treatment would work prophylactically only in patients whose migraine attacks develop on the heels of episodic or chronic muscle tenderness.

Jakubowski et al. explored neurologic markers that might distinguish migraine patients who benefited from BoNTA treatment from those who did not. The prevalence of neck tenderness, aura, photophobia, phonophobia, osmophobia, nausea, and throbbing was similar between responders and non-responders. However, the two groups offered different accounts of their pain. Among non-responders, 92% described a buildup of pressure inside their head (exploding headache). Among responders, 74% perceived their head to be crushed, or clamped, or stubbed by external forces (imploding headache), and 13% attested to an eye-popping pain (ocular headache). The finding that exploding headache is not as responsive to extracranial BoNTA injections is consistent with the view that migraine pain is mediated by intracranial innervation. The amenability of imploding and ocular headaches to BoNTA treatment suggests that these types of migraine pain involve extracranial innervation as well.[149] The precise mechanisms by which BoNTA alleviates headache pain are unclear. It inhibits the release of glutamate and the neuropeptides, substance P and CGRP, from nociceptive neurons, suggesting that its anti-nociceptive properties are distinct from its neuromuscular activity.[150]

Evidence from preclinical studies suggests that BoNTA may inhibit central sensitization of trigeminovascular neurons, which is believed to be key to migraine's development and maintenance [150–153] Afferent-afferent communication happens in the nerve through axon-axon glutamate secretion, and at the level of the ganglion through non-synaptic release of glutamate and peptides (CGRP and SP). Oshinsky et al. used a preclinical model of sensitizing dorsal horn neurons in the trigeminal nucleus caudalis (TNC) following a 5-minute chemical stimulation of the dura as a model for testing the effects of BoNTA on central sensitization.[154] It was hypothesized that Botulinum toxin blocks the axon-to-axon and interganglionic communication of the afferents and thus prevents central and peripheral sensitization outside rat dura. Single neuron electrophysiological recordings of second-order sensory neurons in the TNC with cutaneous receptive fields and microdialysis of the TNC were used to evaluate the effects of pre-treatment of the periorbital region of the rat with BoNTA. In saline-treated animals, extracellular glutamate increased steadily after 100 minutes following the application of inflammatory soup to the dura. Glutamate reached ~ 3 times the basal level 3 hours after the inflammatory soup. Electrophysiologic recordings of neurons in the TNC, before and after sensitization by the inflammatory soup, showed an increase in the magnitude of the response to sensory stimuli and an increase in the cutaneous receptive field of the second sensory neurons in the TNC.

Increases in glutamate were blocked by pre-treating the face of the rat with BoNTA. Electrophysiologic studies then confirmed that, unlike saline treated animals, there was no change in the magnitude of the sensory response in the TNC neurons or their receptive field in the BoNTA-treated rats following the inflammatory soup. These data show that peripheral application of BoNTA prevents central sensitization elicited by stimulating the dura with inflammatory mediators.[154]

One mechanism by which BoNTA may prevent central sensitization is through direct inhibition of central trigeminovascular neurons. Matak et al. assessed the effects of low doses of BoNTA injected into the rat whisker pad or into the sensory trigeminal ganglion on formalin-induced facial pain and employed immunohistochemical labeling of BoNTA-truncated synaptosomal-associated protein 25 (SNAP-25) in the medullary dorsal horn of trigeminal nucleus caudalis after toxin injection into the whisker pad.[155] BoNTA-truncated

Table 8.6 BOTOX Dosing for Chronic Migraine, by Muscle

Head/Neck Area	Total Number of Units (U) (Number of IM Injection Sites)	
	Minimum Dose	Maximum Dose
Frontalis	20 U (4 sites)	20 U (4 sites)
Corrugator	10 U (2 sites)	10 U (2 sites)
Procerus	5 U (1 site)	5 U (1 site)
Occipitalis	30 U (6 sites)	≤ 40 U (5 U per site; ≤ 8 sites)
Temporalis	40 U (8 sites)	≤ 50 U (5 U per site; ≤ 10 sites)
Trapezius	30 U (6 sites)	≤ 50 U (5 U per site; ≤ 10 sites)
Cervical paraspinal muscle group	20 U (4 sites)	20 U (4 sites)
Total Dose Range	**155 U**	**195 U**
	31 sites	**≤ 39 sites**

Each IM injection site = 0.1 mL = 5 U onabotulinumtoxinA.

SNAP-25 in the medullary dorsal horn (spinal trigeminal nucleus) was evident 3 days following the peripheral treatment, and axonal transport was prevented by colchicine injection into the trigeminal ganglion. The authors concluded that axonal transport from peripheral trigeminal afferents to sensory neurons within the caudal trigeminal nucleus is obligatory for the anti-nociceptive effects of BoNTA in the pain disorders mediated by the trigeminal sensory system, such as migraine. Recently, onabotulinumtoxinA was shown to inhibit mechanical nociception in peripheral trigeminovascular neurons by interfering with neuronal surface expression of high-threshold mechanosensitive ion channels.[156] The authors concluded that the inhibition of flow of mechanical pain signals from meningeal and other trigeminovascular nociceptors to the trigeminal nucleus caudalis may be the pivotal mechanism that underlies the preventive effect of onabotulinumtoxinA in patients with chronic migraine.

BoNT Treatment Techniques

Sterile technique should be observed for the entire BoNT injection procedure. Injections do not have to be intramuscular, but the muscles can be used as reference sites for injections, which are usually administered in the glabellar and frontal regions, the cervical paraspinal region, and the temporalis and occipitalis muscles.

The following injection protocols are commonly used: (1) the fixed-site approach, which uses fixed, symmetrical injection sites and a range of predetermined doses; (2) the follow-the-pain approach, which adjusts the sites and doses depending on where the patient feels pain and where the examiner can elicit pain and tenderness when palpating the muscle, and often employs asymmetrical injections; and (3) a combination approach, using injections at fixed frontal sites, supplemented with follow-the-pain injections (this approach typically uses higher doses of BoNTA).[143] Table 8.6 lists recommended anatomical sites of injection for headache and the BoNTA (BOTOX®) dose per site used in the PREEMPT trials.

Clinical Studies of BoNT's Efficacy in Headache Disorders

Most studies of BoNT's efficacy and safety in headache treatment have used BOTOX®.[157] No large, well-controlled studies using other preparations of Botulinum toxin have been published. Clinical trial results are summarized in Table 8.7[157] and are discussed further in the following.

The results of studies evaluating the efficacy of BoNTA for the preventive treatment of episodic migraine are mixed, but are largely negative. A double-blind, vehicle-controlled trial of 123 patients with moderate-to-severe migraine found that subjects treated with a single injection of 25 U BoNTA (but not those treated with 75 U) had significantly fewer migraine attacks per month, as well as reductions in migraine severity, number of days requiring acute medication, and incidence of migraine-induced

Table 8.7 Summary of Randomized, Double-blind, Controlled Studies of the Efficacy of Botulinum Toxin Type A (BoNTA) in the Treatment of Headache

Headache Type	Study Outcome
Migraine	
Silberstein 2000 [158]	• Decreased migraine frequency and severity and acute medication use with BoNTA 25 U but not with BoNTA 75 U
Brin 2000 [169]	• Decreased migraine pain compared with PBO with simultaneous frontal and temporal BoNTA injections
Evers 2004 [159]	• No difference from PBO in decreased frequency of migraine • Greater decrease in migraine-associated symptoms with BoNTA 16 U
Saper 2007 [160]	• Decreased frequency and severity of migraine in BoNTA and PBO groups with no between-group differences
Elkind 2006 [161]	• Comparable decreases in migraine frequency in both BoNTA and PBO groups with no between-group differences
Chronic Migraine	
Mathew 2005 [170]	• No difference from PBO on primary efficacy endpoint: change in headache-free days from baseline at day 180 • A significantly higher % of BoNTA patients had a ≥ 50% decrease in headache days/month at day 180 compared with PBO.
Dodick 2005 [150]	• Greater decrease in headache frequency after 2 and 3 injections compared with PBO
Silberstein 2005 [162]	• No difference from PBO on primary efficacy endpoint—change in headache frequency from baseline at day 180 • Greater decrease in headache frequency for BoNT-A 225U and 150U than PBO
Dodick 2010 [150,163,164]	• Two large P-C, D-B trials • Follow the pain • BoNT-A both safe and effective
Chronic Tension-Type Headache	
Silberstein 2006 [166]	• No difference from PBO on primary efficacy endpoint: mean change from baseline in CTTH headache days • Greater percentage of BoNTA patients than PBO with ≥ 50% reduction in headache frequency at 90 and 120 days for several doses of BoNTA

PBO = placebo.

vomiting.[158] The lack of significant effect in the higher-dose group may be related to group differences at baseline, e.g., fewer migraines or a longer time since migraine onset in the higher-dose group.[158] Another double-blind, placebo-controlled, region-specific study found a significant reduction in migraine pain among patients who received simultaneous injections of BoNTA in the frontal and temporal regions, as well as an overall trend toward BoNTA superiority to placebo in reducing migraine frequency and duration.[158] A randomized, double-blind, placebo-controlled study compared the efficacy of placebo, 16 U BoNTA, and 100 U BoNTA as migraine prophylaxis when injected into the frontal and neck muscles.[159] There were no statistically significant differences in reduction of migraine frequency among the groups, but the accompanying migraine symptoms were reduced in the 16 U BoNTA group.[159]

Later studies, however, have not demonstrated significant improvements over placebo. A study[160] of patients (n = 232) with moderate-to-severe episodic migraine (4 to 8 episodes/month) compared placebo with regional (frontal, temporal, or glabellar) or combined (frontal/temporal/glabellar) treatment with BoNTA. Reductions from baseline in migraine frequency, maximum severity, and duration occurred with BoNTA and placebo, but there were no significant between-group differences.[160] Elkind et al.[161] conducted a series of three sequential studies of 418 patients with a history of four to eight moderate-to-severe migraines per month with re-randomization at each stage and BoNTA doses ranging from 7.5 to 50 U BoNTA and placebo. There was no comparable decrease from baseline in migraine frequency at each time-point examined, and no consistent, statistically significant, between-group differences were observed.[161]

The results in studies of chronic daily headache have also been less than robust. In a large, placebo-controlled study (n = 355), Mathew et al. found that while BoNTA did not differ from placebo in the primary efficacy measure (change from baseline in headache-free days at day 180), there were significant differences in several secondary endpoints, including a greater percentage of patients with a 50% or greater decrease in headache frequency and a greater mean change from baseline in headache frequency at day 180. A subgroup analysis of patients not taking concomitant preventive agents (n = 228) found that BoNTA patients had a greater decrease in headache frequency compared with placebo after two and three injections, and at most time-points from day 180 to 270.[150] In a similar study (n = 702) by Silberstein et al.[162] which utilized several doses of BoNTA (75, 150, 225 U), the primary efficacy endpoint (mean improvement from baseline in headache frequency at day 180) was also not met. However, all groups responded to treatment, and patients taking 150 and 225 U of BoNTA had a greater decrease in headache frequency at day 240 than those taking placebo.[162]

THE PREEMPT TRIALS

The PREEMPT clinical program confirmed onabotulinumtoxinA as an effective, safe, and well-tolerated headache prophylactic treatment for adults with chronic migraine. Two phase-3 multicenter studies (PREEMPT 1 & 2), which each had a 24-week, double-blind, parallel-group, placebo-controlled phase, followed by a 32-week open-label phase, enrolled 1384 patients with CM. All patients received the minimum intramuscular (IM) dose of 155 U of onabotulinumtoxinA administered to 31 injection sites across seven head and neck muscles using a fixed-site, fixed-dose injection paradigm. In addition, up to 40 U onabotulinumtoxinA, administered IM to eight injection sites across three head and neck

muscles, was allowed, using a modified follow-the-pain approach. Thus, the minimum dose was 155 U and the maximum dose was 195 U (Table 8.6). Statistically significant reductions from baseline for frequency of headache days after BoNTA treatment compared with placebo treatment in both PREEMPT 1 & 2 studies (p = .006; p < .001) were observed. Statistically significant improvement from baseline after onabotulinumtoxinA treatment compared with placebo was seen for headache episodes in PREEMPT 2 (p = .003). Pooled analysis demonstrated that onabotulinumtoxinA treatment significantly reduced mean frequency of headache days (–8.4 onabotulinumtoxinA, –6.6 placebo; p < .001) and headache episodes (5.2 onabotulinumtoxinA, –4.9 placebo; p = .009). Additionally, for several other efficacy variables (migraine episodes, migraine days, moderate or severe headache days, cumulative hours of headache on headache days, and proportion of patients with severe disability), there were significant between-group differences favoring onabotulinumtoxinA. The PREEMPT results showed highly significant improvements in multiple headache symptom measures and demonstrated improvement in patients' functioning, vitality, psychological distress, and overall quality of life. Multiple treatments of 155 U up to 195 U per treatment cycle administered every 12 weeks were shown to be safe and well tolerated.[163–165]

Studies evaluating the efficacy of BoNTA in CTTH have been inconsistent. A double-blind, randomized, placebo-controlled study[166] of 300 patients found that while all treatment groups, including placebo, improved in mean change from baseline in CTTH-free days per month (primary endpoint: within-group comparison) at day 60, BoNTA did not demonstrate improvement compared with placebo at any dose or regimen (50–150 U between-groups comparison). However, a significantly greater percentage of patients in three BoNTA groups at day 90 and two BoNTA groups at day 120 had a 50% or greater decrease in CTTH days than the placebo group.[166] Furthermore, a review evaluating clinical studies of TTH supports the benefit of BoNTA in reducing frequency and severity of headaches, improving quality of life and disability scales, and reducing the need for acute medication.[167] In contrast, a later review, which also included studies with both BOTOX® and Dysport®, concluded that randomized, double-blind, placebo-controlled trials present contradictory results attributable to variable doses, injection sites, and treatment frequency.[168]

Adverse Events Associated with the Use of BoNT

More than two decades of clinical use have established BoNTA as a safe drug with no systemic reactions. Side effects have been extensively summarized by Mauskop and are highlighted in this section.[145] Rash and flu-like symptoms can rarely occur as a result of an allergic reaction. However, serious allergic reactions have never been reported. Injection of anterior neck muscles can cause dysphagia in some patients. Dysphagia and dry mouth appear to be more common with injections of BoNTB (Myobloc®) because of its wider migration pattern. The most common side effects when treating facial muscles are cosmetic, and include ptosis or asymmetry of the position of the eyebrows. Another possible, but rare, side effect is difficulty holding the head erect because of neck muscle weakness. Headache patients occasionally develop a headache following the injection procedure; however, some patients have immediate relief of an acute attack. The latter is most likely due to trigger point injection effect. Worsening of headaches and neck pain can occur and last for several days or, rarely, weeks after the injections, because of the irritating effect of the needling and delay in the muscle relaxing effect of BoNT.[145]

In summary, clinical studies suggest that BoNT is a safe treatment and is effective for the prevention of some forms of migraine: that is, chronic migraine and perhaps high-frequency episodic migraine. Further research is needed to understand the mechanism of action of BoNT in headache, to establish its safety and efficacy for these indications, and to fully develop its therapeutic potential.

CONCLUSION

Preventive therapy plays an important role in migraine management. When a preventive medication is added, attack frequency may be reduced and response to acute treatment improved, which can result in reduced health-care resource utilization and improved quality of life. Despite research suggesting that a large percentage of migraine patients are candidates for prevention, only a fraction of these patients are receiving or have ever received preventive migraine medication.

Many preventive medications are available, and guidelines for their selection and use have been established. Since comorbid medical and psychological illnesses are prevalent in patients with migraine, one must consider comorbidity when choosing preventive drugs. Drug therapy may be beneficial for both disorders; however, it is also a potential confounder of optimal treatment of either.

There are no biological markers or clinical characteristics that are predictive of response to a particular migraine preventive medication. The impact of prevention on the natural history of migraine remains to be fully investigated.

APPENDIX 1: AAN CLASSIFICATION OF EVIDENCE FOR THE RATING OF A THERAPEUTIC STUDY

Class I: A randomized, controlled clinical trial of the intervention of interest with masked or objective outcome assessment, in a representative population. Relevant baseline characteristics are present and substantially equivalent among treatment groups, or there is appropriate statistical adjustment for differences.

The following are also required:

a. Concealed allocation
b. Primary outcome(s) clearly defined
c. Exclusion/inclusion criteria clearly defined
d. Adequate accounting for dropouts (with at least 80% of enrolled subjects completing the study) and crossovers, with numbers sufficiently low to have minimal potential for bias.
e. For non-inferiority or equivalence trials claiming to prove efficacy for one or both drugs, the following are also required:*
   1. The authors explicitly state the clinically meaningful difference to be excluded by defining the threshold for equivalence or non-inferiority.

2. The standard treatment used in the study is substantially similar to that used in previous studies establishing efficacy of the standard treatment. (e.g., for a drug, the mode of administration, dose, and dosage adjustments are similar to those previously shown to be effective).

3. The inclusion and exclusion criteria for patient selection and the outcomes of patients on the standard treatment are comparable to those of previous studies establishing efficacy of the standard treatment.

4. The interpretation of the results of the study is based upon a per protocol analysis that takes into account dropouts or crossovers.

Class II: A randomized controlled clinical trial of the intervention of interest in a representative population with masked or objective outcome assessment that lacks one criteria a–e above, or a prospective matched cohort study with masked or objective outcome assessment in a representative population that meets b–e above. Relevant baseline characteristics are presented and substantially equivalent among treatment groups, or there is appropriate statistical adjustment for differences.

Class III: All other controlled trials (including well-defined natural history controls or patients serving as own controls) in a representative population, where outcome is independently assessed, or independently derived by objective outcome measurement.°°

Class IV: Studies not meeting Class I, II, or III criteria, including consensus or expert opinion.

°Note that numbers 1–3 in Class Ie are required for Class II in equivalence trials. If any one of the three is missing, the class is automatically downgraded to Class III.

°°Objective outcome measurement: an outcome measure that is unlikely to be affected by an observer's (patient, treating physician, investigator) expectation or bias (e.g., blood tests, administrative outcome data).

APPENDIX 2: CLASSIFICATION OF RECOMMENDATIONS

Level A = Established as effective, ineffective, or harmful (or established as useful/predictive or not useful/predictive) for the given condition in the specified population. (Level A rating requires at least two consistent Class I studies.)°

Level B = Probably effective, ineffective, or harmful (or probably useful/predictive or not useful/predictive) for the given condition in the specified population. (Level B rating requires at least one Class I study or two consistent Class II studies.)

Level C = Possibly effective, ineffective, or harmful (or possibly useful/predictive or not useful/predictive) for the given condition in the specified population. (Level C rating requires at least one Class II study or two consistent Class III studies.)

Level U = Data inadequate or conflicting; given current knowledge, treatment (test, predictor) is unproven.

°In exceptional cases, one convincing Class I study may suffice for an "A" recommendation if (1) all criteria are met, (2) the magnitude of effect is large (relative rate improved outcome > 5 and the lower limit of the confidence interval is > 2).

REFERENCES

1. Silberstein SD. Migraine. Lancet 2004;363:381–391.
2. Lipton RB, Silberstein SD. Why study the comorbidity of migraine? *Neurology.* 1994;44(17):4–5.
3. Silberstein SD, Winner PK, Chmiel JJ. Migraine preventive medication reduces resource utilization. *Headache.* 2003 Mar 1;43(3):171–178.
4. Etemad LR, Wang W, Globe D, Barlev A, Johnson KA. Costs and utilization of triptan users who receive drug prophylaxis for migraine versus triptan users who do not receive drug prophylaxis. *J Manag Care Pharm.* 2005;11:137–144.
5. Silberstein SD, Feliu AL, Rupnow MF, Blount AC, Boccuzzi SJ. Topiramate in migraine prophylaxis: long-term impact on resource utilization and cost. *Headache.* 2007 Apr;47(4):500–510.
6. Brown JS, Papadopoulos G, Neumann PJ, Price M, Friedman M, Menzin J. Cost-effectiveness of migraine prevention: the case of topiramate in the UK. *Cephalalgia.* 2006;26:1473–1482.
7. Vicente-Herrero T, Burke TA, Lainez MJ. The impact of a worksite migraine intervention program on work productivity, productivity costs, and non-workplace impairment among Spanish postal service employees from an ermployer perspective. *Curr Med Red Opin.* 2004;20:1805–1814.
8. Bordini CA, Mariano da Silva H, Garbelini RP, Teixeira SO, Speciali JG. Effect of preventive treatment on health-related quality of life in episodic migraine. *J Headache Pain.* 2005;6:387–391.
9. D'Amico D, Solari A, Usai S, Santoro P, Bernardoni P, Frediani F, et al. Improvement in quality of life and

activity limitations in migraine patients after prophylaxis. A prospective longitudinal multicentre study. *Cephalalgia.* 2006 Jun;26(6):691–696.

10. Diamond M, Dahlof C, Papadopoulos G, Neto W, Wu SC. Topiramate improves health-related quality of life when used to prevent migraine. *Headache.* 2005;45:1023–1030.

11. Silberstein SD, Lipton RB, Goadsby PJ. Migraine: diagnosis and treatment. In: Silberstein SD, Lipton RB, Goadsby PJ, eds. *Headache in clinical practice.* 1st ed. Oxford: Isis Medical Media Ltd., 1998:61–90.

12. Silberstein SD. Headaches in pregnancy. *Neurol Clin.* 2004 Dec;22(4):727–756.

13. Lipton RB, Diamond M, Freitag F, Bigal M, Stewart WF, Reed ML. Migraine prevention patterns in a community sample: results from the American migraine prevalence and prevention (AMPP) study. *Headache.* 2005;45(6):792–793(Abstract).

14. Silberstein SD, Holland S, Freitag F, Dodick DW, Argoff C, Ashman E. Evidence-based guideline update: pharmacologic treatment for episodic migraine prevention in adults: report of the Quality Standards Subcommittee of the American Academy of Neurology and the American Headache Society. *Neurology.* 2012 Apr 24;78(17):1337–1345.

15. Holland S, Silberstein SD, Freitag F, Dodick DW, Argoff C, Ashman E. Evidence-based guideline update: NSAIDs and other complementary treatments for episodic migraine prevention in adults: report of the Quality Standards Subcommittee of the American Academy of Neurology and the American Headache Society. *Neurology.* 2012 Apr 24;78(17):1346–1353.

16. Pringsheim T, Davenport W, Mackie G, Worthington I, Aube M, Christie SN, et al. Canadian Headache Society guideline for migraine prophylaxis. *Can J Neurol Sci.* 2012 Mar;39(2 Suppl 2):S1–59.

17. Carville S, Padhi S, Reason T, Underwood M. Diagnosis and management of headaches in young people and adults: summary of NICE guidance. *BMJ.* 2012;345:e5765.

18. Lipton RB, Bigal M, Diamond M. Migraine prevalence, disease burden and the need for preventive therapy. *Neurology.* 2007;68:343–349.

19. Silberstein SD, Diamond S, Loder E, Reed ML, Lipton RB. Prevalence of migraine sufferers who are candidates for preventive therapy: results from the American migraine study (AMPP) study. *Headache.* 2005;45(6):770–771(Abstract).

20. Silberstein SD. Preventive treatment of migraine: an overview. *Cephalalgia.* 1997;17:67–72.

21. Minnesota Evidence-based Practice Center. *Comparative effectiveness review,* Number 103: Migraine in adults: preventive pharmacologic treatments. Agency for Healthcare Research and Quality, US Department of Health and Human Services, 2013 [cited 2013 Jun 3]. Available from www.ahrq.gov.

22. Olerud B, Gustavsson CL, Furberg B. Nadolol and propranolol in migraine management. *Headache.* 1986;26(10):490–493.

23. Ryan RE, Sudilovsky A. Nadolol: its use in the prophylactic treatment of migraine. *Headache.* 1983;23(1):26–31.

24. Ryan RE. Comparative study of nadolol and propranolol in prophylactic treatment of migraine. *Am Heart J.* 1984;108(4):1156–1159.

25. Sudilovsky A, Stern MA, Meyer JH. Nadolol: the benefits of an adequate trial duration in the prophylaxis of migraine. *Headache.* 1986;26:325.

26. Ifergane G, Buskila D, Simiseshvely N, Zeev K, Cohen H. Prevalence of fibromyalgia syndrome in migraine patients. *Cephalalgia.* 2006 Apr;26(4):451–456.

27. Saunders K, Merikangas K, Low NC, Von KM, Kessler RC. Impact of comorbidity on headache-related disability. *Neurology.* 2008 Feb 12;70(7):538–547.

28. Schwedt TJ. The migraine association with cardiac anomalies, cardiovascular disease, and stroke. *Neurol Clin.* 2009 May;27(2):513–523.

29. Schoenen J, Dodick DW, Sandor PS. *Comorbidity in migraine.* Sussex, UK: Wiley Blackwell, 2011.

30. Silberstein SD. Migraine and pregnancy. *Neurologic Clinics.* 1997;15(1):209–231.

31. Silberstein SD, Lipton RB, Breslau N. Migraine: association with personality characteristics and psychopathology. *Cephalalgia.* 1995;15:337–369.

32. Mathew NT, Saper JR, Silberstein SD, Tolander LR, Markley H, Solomon S, et al. Prophylaxis of migraine headaches with divalproex sodium. *Arch Neurol.* 1995;52:281–286.

33. Silberstein SD. Divalproex sodium in headache: literature review and clinical guidelines. *Headache.* 1996;36(9):547–555.

34. Bowden CL, Brugger AM, Swann AC. Efficacy of divalproex vs lithium and placebo in the treatment of mania. *JAMA.* 1994;271:918–924.

35. Diener HC, Agosti R, Allais G, Bergmans P, Bussone G, Davies B, et al. Cessation versus continuation of 6-month migraine preventive therapy with topiramate (PROMPT): a randomised, double-blind, placebo-controlled trial. *Lancet Neurol.* 2007 Dec;6(12):1054–1062.

36. Schoenen J, Reuter U, Diener HC, Pfeil J, Schwalen S, Schauble B, et al. Factors predicting the probability of relapse after discontinuation of migraine preventive treatment with topiramate. *Cephalalgia.* 2010 Nov;30(11):1290–1295.

37. Wober C, Wober-Bingol C, Koch G, Wessely P. Long-term results of migraine prophylaxis with flunarizine and beta-blockers. *Cephalalgia.* 1991 Dec;11(6):251–256.

38. Gray RN, Goslin RE, McCrory DC, Eberlein K, Tulsky J, Hasselblad V. Drug treatments for the prevention of migraine headache. Prepared for the Agency for Health Care Policy and Research, Contract No. 290-94-2025. Available from the National Technical Information Service 1999; Accession.

39. Silberstein SD. Practice Parameter—evidence-based guidelines for migraine headache (an evidence-based review): report of the Quality Standards Subcommittee of the American Academy of Neurology for the United States Headache Consortium. *Neurology.* 2000;55:754–762.

40. Andersson K, Vinge E. Beta-adrenoceptor blockers and calcium antagonists in the prophylaxis and treatment of migraine. *Drugs.* 1990;39(3):355–373.

41. Koella WP. CNS-related (side-)effects of ß-blockers with special reference to mechanisms of action. *Eur J Clin Pharmacol.* 1985;28(Suppl):55–63.

42. Ramadan NM. Prophylactic migraine therapy: mechanisms and evidence. *Curr Pain Headache Rep.* 2004;8:91–95.

43. Cortelli P, Sacquegna T, Albani F, Baldrati A, D'Alessandro R, Baruzi A, et al. Propranolol plasma levels and relief of migraine. *Arch Neurol.* 1985;42:46–48.

44. Rao BS, Das DG, Taraknath VR, Sarma Y. A double blind controlled study of propranolol and cyproheptadine in migraine prophylaxis. *Neurol India.* 2000 Sep;48(3):223–226.

45. Sudilovsky A, Elkind AH, Ryan RE, Saper JR, Stern MA, Meyer JH. Comparative efficacy of nadolol and propranolol in the management of migraine. Headache 1987;27:421–6.

46. Tfelt Hansen P, Standnes B, Kangasniemi P, Hakkarainen H, Olesen J. Timolol vs propranolol vs placebo in common migraine prophylaxis: a double-blind multicenter trial. *Acta Neurol Scand.* 1984;69(1):1–8.

47. Panerai AE, Monza G, Movilia P, Bianchi M, Francussi BM, Tiengo M. A randomized, within-patient, crossover, placebo-controlled trial on the efficacy and tolerability of the tricyclic antidepressants chlorimipramine and nortriptyline in central pain. *Acta Neurol Scand.* 1990;82:34–38.

48. Diener HC, Hartung E, Chrubasik J, Evers S, Schoenen J, Eikermann A, et al. A comparative study of oral acetylsalicyclic acid and metoprolol for the prophylactic treatment of migraine: a randomized, controlled, double-blind, parallel group phase III study. *Cephalalgia.* 2001 Mar;21(2):120–128.

49. Schellenberg R, Lichtenthal A, Wohling H, Graf C, Brixius K. Nebivolol and metoprolol for treating migraine: an advance on beta-blocker treatment? *Headache.* 2008 Jan;48(1):118–125.

50. Kishore-Kumar R, Max MB, Schafer SC, Gaughan AM, Smoller B, Gracely RH, et al. Desipramine relieves post-herpetic neuralgia. *Clin Pharmacol Ther.* 1990;47:305–312.

51. Feinmann C. Pain relief by antidepressants: possible modes of action. *Pain.* 1985;23:1–8.

52. Richelson E. Antidepressants and brain neurochemistry. *Mayo Clin Proc.* 1990;65:1227–1236.

53. Baldessarini RJ. Drugs and the treatment of psychiatric disorders. In: Gilman AG, Rall TW, Nies AS, Taylor P, eds. *The pharmacological basis of therapeutics.* 8th ed. New York: Pergamon, 1990:383–435.

54. Abramowicz M. Fluoxetine (Prozac) revisited. *Drugs Ther.* 1990;Medical Letter(32):83–85.

55. Dodick D, Silberstein SD, Lindblad A, Holroyd K, Mathew N, Cordell J, et al. Clinical trial design in chronic migraine: lessons learned from the NINDS CRC chronic migraine treatment trial (CMTT). *Neurology.* 2011(Abstract).

56. Couch JR. Amitriptyline in the prophylactic treatment of migraine and chronic daily headache. *Headache.* 2011 Jan;51(1):33–51.

57. Jackson JL, Shimeall W, Sessums L, Dezee KJ, Becher D, Diemer M, et al. Tricyclic antidepressants and headaches: systematic review and meta-analysis. *BMJ.* 2010;341:c5222.

58. Adly C, Straumanis J, Chesson A. Fluoxetine prophylaxis of migraine. *Headache.* 1992;32:101–104.

59. Saper JR, Silberstein SD, Lake AE, Winters ME. Double-blind trial of fluoxetine: chronic daily headache and migraine. *Headache.* 1994;34:497–502.

60. d'Amato CC, Pizza V, Marmolo T, Giordano E, Alfano V, Nasta A. Fluoxetine for migraine prophylaxis: a double-blind trial. *Headache.* 1999;39(10):716–719.

61. Lipton RB, Gobel H, Wilks K, Mauskop A. Efficacy of petasites (an extract from petasites rhizone) 50 and 75mg for prophylaxis of migraine: results of a randomized, double-blind, placebo-controlled study. *Neurology.* 2002;58:A472(Abstract).

62. Ozyalcin SN, Talu GK, Kiziltan E, Yucel B, Ertas M, Disci R. The efficacy and safety of venlafaxine in the prophylaxis of migraine. *Headache.* 2005;45(2):144–152.

63. Bulut S, Berilgen MS, Baran A, Tekatas A, Atmaca M, Mungen B. Venlafaxine versus amitriptyline in the prophylactic treatment of migraine: randomized, double-blind, crossover study. *Clin Neurol Neurosurg.* 2004;107(1):44–48.

64. Greenberg DA. Calcium channels in neurological disease. *Ann Neurol.* 1997;42(3):275–282.

65. Wauquier A, Ashton D, Marranes R. The effects of flunarizine in experimental models related to the pathogenesis of migraine. *Cephalalgia.* 1985;5(Suppl 2):119–120.

66. Solomon GD. Verapamil and propranolol in migraine prophylaxis: a double-blind crossover study. *Headache.* 1986;26:325.

67. Markley HG, Cleronis JCD, Piepko RW. Verapamil prophylactic therapy of migraine. *Neurology.* 1984;34:973–976.

68. Riopelle R, McCans JL. A pilot study of the calcium channel antagonist diltiazem in migraine syndrome prophylaxis. *Can J Neurol Sci.* 1982;9:269.

69. Smith R, Schwartz A. Diltiazem prophylaxis in refractory migraine. *N Engl J Med.* 1984;310:1327–1328.

70. Reveiz-Herault L, Cardona AF, Ospina EG, Carrillo P. Effectiveness of flunarizine in the prophylaxis of migraine: a meta-analytical review of the literature. *Rev Neurol.* 2003 May 16;36(10):907–912.

71. Hanston PP, Horn JR. Drug interaction. *Newsletter.* 1985;5:7–10.

72. Rompel H, Bauermeister PW. Aetiology of migraine and prevention with carbamazepine (Tegretol). *S Afr Med J.* 1970;44:75–80.

73. Mathew NT, Rapoport A, Saper J, Magnus L, Klapper J, Ramadan N, et al. Efficacy of gabapentin in migraine prophylaxis. *Headache.* 2001;41(2):119–128.

74. Coulam CB, Annagers JR. New anticonvulsants reduce the efficacy of oral contraception. *Epilepsia.* 1979;20:519–525.

75. Di TG, Mei D, Marra C, Mazza S, Capuano A. Gabapentin in the prophylaxis of migraine: a double-blind randomized placebo-controlled study. *Clin Ter.* 2000 May;151(3):145–148.

76. Mulleners WM, Chronicle EP. Anticonvulsants in migraine prophylaxis: a Cochrane review. *Cephalalgia.* 2008 Jun;28(6):585–597.

77. Silberstein S, Goode-Sellers S, Twomey C, Saiers J, Ascher J. Randomized, double-blind, placebo-controlled, phase II trial of gabapentin enacarbil for migraine prophylaxis. *Cephalalgia.* 2013 Jan;33(2):101–111.

78. Klapper JA. Divalproex sodium in migraine prophylaxis: a dose-controlled study. *Cephalalgia.* 1997; 17:103–108.

79. Klapper JA. An open label crossover comparison of divalproex sodium and propranolol HCl in

the prevention of migraine headaches. *Headache Quarterly*. 1995;5(1):50–53.

80. Freitag FG, Collins SD, Carlson HA, Goldstein J, Saper J, Silberstein S, et al. A randomized trial of divalproex sodium extended-release tablets in migraine prophylaxis. *Neurology*. 2002 Jun 11;58(11):1652–1659.

81. Hering R, Kuritzky A. Sodium valproate in the prophylactic treatment of migraine: a double-blind study versus placebo. *Cephalalgia*. 1992;12:81–84.

82. Jensen R, Brinck T, Olesen J. Sodium valproate has prophylactic effect in migraine without aura: a triple-blind, placebo-controlled crossover study. *Neurology*. 1994;44:241–244.

83. Mathew NT, Saper JR, Silberstein SD, Rankin L, Markley HG, Solomon S, et al. Migraine prophylaxis with divalproex. *Arch Neurol*. 1995;52:281–286.

84. Silberstein SD, Collins SD. Safety of divalproex sodium in migraine prophylaxis: an open-label, long-term study (for the long-term safety of depakote in headache prophylaxis study group). *Headache*. 1999;39(9):633–643.

85. Harden CL, Meador KJ, Pennell PB, Hauser WA, Gronseth GS, French JA, et al. Practice parameter update: management issues for women with epilepsy—focus on pregnancy (an evidence-based review): teratogenesis and perinatal outcomes: report of the Quality Standards Subcommittee and Therapeutics and Technology Assessment Subcommittee of the American Academy of Neurology and American Epilepsy Society. *Neurology*. 2009 Jul 14;73(2):133–141.

86. Pellock JM, Willmore LJ. A rational guide to routine blood monitoring in patients receiving antiepileptic drugs. *Neurology*. 1991;41:961–964.

87. Vainionpaa LK, Rattya J, Knip M, Tapanainen JS, Pakarinen AJ, Lanning P, et al. Valproate-induced hyperandrogenism during pubertal maturation in girls with epilepsy. *Ann Neurol*. 1999;45(4):444–450.

88. Gupta P, Singh S, Goyal V, Shukla G, Behari M. Low-dose topiramate versus lamotrigine in migraine prophylaxis (the Lotolamp study). *Headache*. 2007 Mar;47(3):402–412.

89. Ashtari F, Shaygannejad V, Akbari M. A double-blind, randomized trial of low-dose topiramate vs propranolol in migraine prophylaxis. *Acta Neurol Scand*. 2008 Nov;118(5):301–305.

90. Shaygannejad V, Janghorbani M, Ghorbani A, Ashtary F, Zakizade N, Nasr V. Comparison of the effect of topiramate and sodium valporate in migraine prevention: a randomized blinded crossover study. *Headache*. 2006 Apr;46(4):642–648.

91. Storey JR, Calder CS, Hart DE, Potter DL. Topiramate in migraine prevention: a double-blind, placebo-controlled study. *Headache*. 2001 Nov;41(10):968–975.

92. Brandes JL, Saper JR, Diamond M, Couch JR, Lewis DW, Schmitt J, et al. Topiramate for migraine prevention: a randomized controlled trial. *JAMA*. 2004;291(8):965–973.

93. Diener HC, Tfelt-Hansen P, Dahlof C, Lainez MJ, Sandrini G, Wang SJ, et al. Topiramate in migraine prophylaxis: results from a placebo-controlled trial with propranolol as an active control. *J Neurol*. 2004 Aug;251(8):943–950.

94. Dodick DW, Freitag F, Banks J, Saper J, Xiang J, Rupnow M, et al. Topiramate versus amitriptyline in migraine prevention: a 26-week, multicenter, randomized, double-blind, double-dummy, parallel-group noninferiority trial in adult migraineurs. *Clin Ther*. 2009 Mar;31(3):542–559.

95. Keskinbora K, Aydinli I. A double-blind randomized controlled trial of topiramate and amitriptyline either alone or in combination for the prevention of migraine. *Clin Neurol Neurosurg*. 2008 Dec;110(10):979–984.

96. Mei D, Capuano A, Vollono C, Evangelista M, Ferraro D, Tonali P, et al. Topiramate in migraine prophylaxis: a randomised double-blind versus placebo study. *Neurol Sci*. 2004 Dec;25(5):245–250.

97. Silberstein SD, Neto W, Schmitt J, Jacobs D. Topiramate in migraine prevention: results of a large controlled trial. *Arch Neurol*. 2004 Apr;61(4):490–495.

98. Millan-Guerrero RO, Isais-Millan R, Barreto-Vizcaino S, et al. Subcutaneous histamine versus topiramate in migraine prophylaxis: a double-blind study. *Eur J Neurol*. 2008;59:237–242.

99. Silberstein SD, Neto W, Schmitt J, Jacobs D. Topiramate in the prevention of migraine headache: a randomized, double-blind, placebo-controlled, multiple-dose study. For the MIGR-001 Study Group. *Arch Neurol*. 2004;61:490–495.

100. Sachedo RC, Reife RA, Lim P, Pledger G. Topiramate monotherapy for partial onset seizures. *Epilepsia*. 1997;38:294–300.

101. Thomson H. *Physicians' desk reference*. 57th ed. Montvale: Thomson PDR, 2003.

102. Silberstein SD, Dodick DW, Lindblad AS, Holroyd K, Harrington M, Mathew NT, et al. Randomized, placebo-controlled trial of propranolol added to topiramate in chronic migraine. *Neurology*. 2012 Mar 27;78(13):976–984.

103. Chen WT, Fuh JL, Lu SR, Wang SJ. Persistent migrainous visual phenomena might be responsive to lamotrigine. *Headache*. 2001;41 (8):823–825.

104. Steiner TJ, Findley LJ, Yuen AW. Lamotrigine versus placebo in the prophylaxis of migraine with and without aura. *Cephalalgia*. 1997;17(2):109–112.

105. Freitag FG. Topiramate prophylaxis in patients suffering from migraine with aura: results from a randomized, double-blind, placebo-controlled trial. *Adv Stu Med*. 2003;3:S562–S564.

106. Silberstein SD, Saper J, Berenson F, Somogyi M, McCague K, D'Souza J. Oxcarbazepine in migraine headache: a double-blind, randomized, placebo-controlled study. *Neurology*. 2008 Feb 12;70(7):548–555.

107. Sicuteri R. Prophylactic and therapeutic properties of 1-methylsergic acid butanolamide in migraine. *Int Arch Allerg*. 1959;15:300–307.

108. Graham JR, Suby HI, LeCompte PR, Sadowsky NL. Fibrotic disorders associated with methysergide therapy for headache. *N Engl J Med*. 1966;274:360–368.

109. Silberstein SD. Methysergide. *Cephalalgia*. 1998;18(7):421–435.

110. Raskin NH. *Headache*. 2nd ed. New York: Churchill-Livingstone, 1988.

111. Graham J. Cardiac and pulmonary fibrosis during methysergide therapy for headache. *Am J Med Sci*. 1967;254:1–12.

112. Bana DS, MacNeal PS, LeCompte PM, Shah Y, Graham JR. Cardiac murmurs and endocardial fibrosis associated with methysergide therapy. *Amer Heart J*. 1974;88:640–655.

113. Barlow CF. *Headaches and migraine in children.* Philadelphia: 1984.

114. Forsythe I, Hockaday JM. Management of childhood migraine. In: Hockaday JM, ed. *Migraine in childhood.* London: Butterworths, 1988:63–74.

115. Smyth GA, Lazarus L. Suppression of growth hormone secretion by melatonin and cyproheptadine. *J Clin Invest.* 1974;54:116–121.

116. Schrader H, Stovner LJ, Helde G, Sand T, Bovim G. Prophylactic treatment of migraine with angiotensin converting enzyme inhibitor (lisinopril): randomized, placebo-controlled, crossover study. *Br Med J.* 2001;322:19–22.

117. Tronvik E, Stovner LJ, Helde G, Sand T, Bovim G. Prophylactic treatment of migraine with an angiotensin II receptor blocker: a randomized controlled trial. *JAMA.* 2003;289 (1):65–69.

118. Stovner LJ, Linde M, Gravdahl GB, Trovnik E, Aamodt AH, Sand T, et al. A comparative study of candesartan versus propranolol for migraine prophylaxis: a randomised, triple-blind, placebo-controlled, double cross-over study. *Cephalalgia.* 2013;34(7):523–532.

119. Diener HC, Gendolla A, Feuersenger A, Evers S, Straube A, Schumacher H, et al. Telmisartan in migraine prophylaxis: a randomized, placebo-controlled trial. *Cephalalgia.* 2009 Sep;29(9):921–927.

120. Millan-Guerrero RO, Pineda-Lucatero AG, Hernandez-Benjamin T, Tene CE, Pacheco MF. Nalpha-methylhistamine safety and efficacy in migraine prophylaxis: phase I and phase II studies. *Headache.* 2003 Apr;43(4):389–394.

121. Millan-Guerrero RO, Isais-Millan R, Barreto-Vizcaino S., et al. Subcutaneous histamine versus sodium valproate in migraine prophylaxis: a randomized, controlled, double-blind study. *Eur J Neurol.* 2007;14:1079–1084.

122. Millan-Guerrero RO, Isais-Millan R, Benjamin TH, Tene CE. Nalpha-methyl histamine safety and efficacy in migraine prophylaxis: phase III study. *Can J Neurol Sci.* 2006 May;33(2):195–199.

123. Brandes JL, Visser H, Farmer MV, Schuhl AL, Malbecq W, Vrijens F, et al. Montelukast for migraine prophylaxis: a randomized, double-blind, placebo-controlled study. On behalf of the Protocol 125 study group. *Headache.* 2004;44(6):581–586.

124. Lipton RB, Hamelsky SW, Stewart WF. Epidemiology and impact of headache. In: Silberstein SD, Lipton RB, Dalessio DJ, eds. *Wolff's headache and other head pain.* 7th ed. New York: Oxford University Press, 2001:85–107.

125. Grossmann M, Schmidramsl H. An extract of Petasites hybridus is effective in the prophylaxis of migraine. *Int J Clin Pharmacol Therapeut.* 2000;38(9):430–435.

126. Lipton RB, Göbel H, Einh..upl KM, Wilks K, Mauskop A. *Petasites hybridus* root (butterbur) is an effective preventive treatment for migraine. *Neurology.* 2004;63(12):2240–2244.

127. Vogler BK, Pittler MH, Ernst E. Feverfew as a preventive treatment for migraine: a systematic review. *Cephalalgia.* 1998;18:704–708.

128. Maizels M, Blumenfeld A, Burchette R. A combination of riboflavin, magnesium, and feverfew for migraine prophylaxis: a randomized trial. *Headache.* 2004 Oct;44(9):885–890.

129. Pfaffenrath V, Diener HC, Fischer M, Friede M, Henneicke HH. The efficacy and safety of *Tanacetum parthenium* (feverfew) in migraine prophylaxis: a double-blind, multicenter, randomized, placebo-controlled, dose-response study. *Cephalalgia.* 2002;22(7):523–532.

130. Diener HC, Pfaffenrath V, Schnitker J, Friede M, Henneicke-von Zepelin HH. Efficacy and safety of 6.25 mg t.i.d. feverfew CO2-extract (MIG-99) in migraine prevention: a randomized, double-blind, multicentre, placebo-controlled study. *Cephalalgia.* 2005 Nov;25(11):1031–1041.

131. Schoenen J, Jacquy J, Lenaerts M. Effectiveness of high-dose riboflavin in migraine prophylaxis: a randomized controlled trial. *Neurology.* 1998;50:466–470.

132. Sandor PS, Di CL, Coppola G, Saenger U, Fumal A, Magis D, et al. Efficacy of coenzyme Q10 in migraine prophylaxis: a randomized controlled trial. *Neurology.* 2005 Feb 22;64(4):713–715.

133. Burke BE, Olson RD, Cusack BJ. Randomized, controlled trial of phytoestrogen in the prophylactic treatment of menstrual migraine. *Biomed Pharmacother.* 2002 Aug;56(6):283–288.

134. Pradalier A, Clapin A, Dry J. Treatment review: nonsteroid antiinflammatory drugs in the treatment and long-term prevention of migraine attacks. *Headache.* 1988;28:550–557.

135. Bensenor IM, Cook NR, Lee IM, Chown MJ, Hennekens CH, Buring JE. Low-dose aspirin for migraine prophylaxis in women. *Cephalalgia.* 2001 Apr;21(3):175–183.

136. Pringsheim T, Davenport W, Mackie G, Worthington I, Aube M, Christie SN, et al. Canadian Headache Society Prophylactic Guidelines Development Group. *Can J Neurol Sci.* 2012;39(2 [suppl 2]):S1–S59.

137. Lafreniere RG, Cader MZ, Poulin JF, ndres-Enguix I, Simoneau M, Gupta N, et al. A dominant-negative mutation in the TRESK potassium channel is linked to familial migraine with aura. *Nat Med.* 2010 Oct;16(10):1157–1160.

138. Zhu DXD, Zhang J, Zhou L, Smith B, Salyers K, et al. A human CGRP receptor antagonist antibody, AA95, is effective in inhibiting capsaicin-induced increase in dermal blood flow in cynomolgus monkeys. 2012 Jun 21.

139. Liu H, Xu C, Shi L, Kaufman S, Smith D, Immke D, et al. Immunohistochemical localization of the CLR/RAMP1 receptor complex in the trigeminovascular system of the cynomolgus monkey. *Headache.* 2011;51(Suppl 1):6.

140. Zeller J, Poulsen KT, Sutton JE, Abdiche YN, Collier S, Chopra R, et al. CGRP function-blocking antibodies inhibit neurogenic vasodilatation without affecting heart rate or arterial blood pressure in the rat. *Br J Pharmacol.* 2008 Dec;155(7):1093–1103.

141. Wong HC, Tache Y, Lloyd KC, Yang H, Sternini C, Holzer P, et al. Monoclonal antibody to rat alpha-CGRP: production, characterization, and in vivo immunoneutralization activity. *Hybridoma.* 1993 Feb;12(1):93–106.

142. Bigal ME, Escandon R, Bronson M, Walter S, Sudworth M, Huggins JP, et al. Safety and tolerability

of LBR-101, a humanized monoclonal antibody that blocks the binding of CGRP to its receptor: results of the Phase 1 program. *Cephalalgia*. 2014.

143. Blumenfeld AM, Binder W, Silbrestein SD, Blizter A. Procedures for administering botulinum toxin type A for migraine and tension-type headache. *Headache*. 2003;43(8):884–891.

144. Aoki KR, Guyer B. Botulinum toxin type A and other botulinum toxin serotypes; a comparative review of biochemical and pharmacological actions. *Eur J Neurol*. 2001;8(S5):21–29.

145. Mauskop A. The use of botulinum toxin in the treatment of headaches. *Pain Physician*. 2004;7:377–387.

146. BOTOX® package insert. Irvine, CA: Allergan, Inc., 2004.

147. Binder WJ, Brin MF, Blitzer A, Shoenrock LD, Pogoda JM. Botulinum toxin type A (Botox) for treatment of migraine headaches: an open-label study. *Otolaryngol Head Neck Surg*. 2000;123(6):669–676.

148. Jensen R, Bendtsen L, Olesen J. Muscular factors are of importance in tension-type headache. *Headache*. 1998;38:10–17.

149. Jakubowski M, McAllister PJ, Bajwa ZH, Ward TN, Smith P, Burstein R. Exploding vs. imploding headache in migraine prophylaxis with Botulinum Toxin A. *Pain*. 2006 Dec 5;125(3):286–295.

150. Dodick DW, Mauskop A, Elkind AH, deGryse R, Brin MF, Silberstein SD. Botulinum toxin type A for the prophylaxis of chronic daily headache: subgroup analysis of patients not receiving other prophylactic medications (a randomized, double-blind, placebo-controlled study). *Headache*. 2005;45(4):315–324.

151. Aoki KR. Evidence for antinociceptive activity of botulinum toxin Type A in pain management. *Headache*. 2003;43(Suppl 3):S109–S115.

152. Cui M, Khanijou S, Rubino J, Aoki KR. Subcutaneous administration of botulinum toxin A reduces formalin-induced pain. *Pain*. 2004 Jan;107(1–2):125–133.

153. Oshinsky ML. Botulinum toxins and migraine: how does it work. *Practical Neurol*. 2004;Suppl:10–13.

154. Oshinsky M, Poso-Rosich P, Luo J, Hyman S, Silberstein SD. Botulinum toxin A blocks sensitization of neurons in the trigeminal nucleus caudalis. *Cephalalgia*. 2004;24:781(Abstract).

155. Matak IBLFBLZ. Behaviorial and immunohistochemical evidence for central antinociceptive activity of Botulinum toxin A. *Neuroscience*. 2011;186:201–207.

156. Burstein RB, Zhang X, Levy D, Aoki R, Brin MF. Selective inhibition of meningeal nociceptors by Botulinum neurotoxin type A: therapeutic implications to migraine and other pains. *Cephalalgia*. 2014;34(11):853–869.

157. Schulte-Mattler WJ, Leinisch E. Evidence based medicine on the use of botulinum toxin for headache disorders. *J Neural Transm*. 2007;115(4):647–651.

158. Silberstein SD, Mathew N, Saper J, Jenkin S. Botulinum toxin type A as a migraine preventive treatment: for the Botox® Migraine Clinical Research Group. *Headache*. 2000;40:445–450.

159. Evers S, Vollmer-Haase J, Schwaag S, Rahmann A, Husstedt IW, Frese A. Botulinum toxin A in the prophylactic treatment of migraine: a randomized, double-blind, placebo-controlled study. *Cephalalgia*. 2004;24(10):838–843.

160. Saper JR, Mathew NT, Loder EW, deGryse R, VanDenburgh AM. A double-blind, randomized, placebo-controlled comparison of Botulinum toxin type A injection sites and doses in the prevention of episodic migraine. *Pain Med*. 2007;8(6):478–85.

161. Elkind AH, O'Carroll P, Blumenfeld A, deGryse R, Dimitrova R. A series of three sequential, randomized, controlled studies of repeated treatments with Botulinum toxin type A for migraine prophylaxis. *J Pain*. 2006 Oct;7(10):688–696.

162. Silberstein SD, Stark SR, Lucas SM, Christie SN, DeGryse RE, Turkel CC. Botulinum toxin type A for the prophylactic treatment of chronic daily headache: a randomized, double-blind, placebo-controlled trial. *Mayo Clin Proc*. 2005 Sep;80(9):1126–1137.

163. Aurora SK, Dodick DW, Turkel CC, DeGryse RE, Silberstein SD, Lipton RB, et al. OnabotulinumtoxinA for treatment of chronic migraine: results from the double-blind, randomized, placebo-controlled phase of the PREEMPT 1 trial. *Cephalalgia*. 2010 Jul;30(7):793–803.

164. Diener HC, Dodick DW, Aurora SK, Turkel CC, DeGryse RE, Lipton RB, et al. OnabotulinumtoxinA for treatment of chronic migraine: results from the double-blind, randomized, placebo-controlled phase of the PREEMPT 2 trial. *Cephalalgia*. 2010 Jul;30(7):804–814.

165. Dodick DW, Turkel CC, DeGryse RE, Aurora SK, Silberstein SD, Lipton RB, et al. OnabotulinumtoxinA for treatment of chronic migraine: pooled results from the double-blind, randomized, placebo-controlled phases of the PREEMPT clinical program. *Headache*. 2010 Jun;50(6):921–936.

166. Silberstein SD, Gobel H, Jensen R, Elkind AH, deGryse R, Walcott JM, et al. Botulinum toxin type A in the prophylactic treatment of chronic tension-type headache: a multicentre, double-blind, randomized, placebo-controlled, parallel-group study. *Cephalalgia*. 2006 Jul;26(7):790–800.

167. Mathew NT, Kaup AO. The use of botulinum toxin type A in headache treatment. *Cur Treatment Options Neurol*. 2002;4:365–373.

168. Rozen D, Sharma J. Treatment of tension-type headache with botox: a review of the literature. *Mt Sinai J Med*. 2006 Jan;73(1):493–498.

169. Brin MF, Swope DM, O'Brien C, Abbasi S, Pogoda JM. Botox for migraine: double-blind, placebo-controlled, region-specific evaluation. *Cephalalgia*. 2000;20:421–422(Abstract).

170. Mathew NT, Frishberg BM, Gawel M, Dimitrova R, Gibson J, Turkel C. Botulinum toxin type A (BOTOX) for the prophylactic treatment of chronic daily headache: a randomized, double-blind, placebo-controlled trial. *Headache*. 2005 Apr;45(4):293–307.

Chapter 9

Chronic Migraine

INTRODUCTION

Migraine can be episodic (headache < 15 days/month) or chronic (headache ≥ 15 days/month).

Chronic migraine (CM) is a subtype of chronic daily headache (CDH), a group of disorders characterized by very frequent headaches (15 or more days a month) for at least 3 months.

Table 9.1 **Classification of the More Common Primary Headache Disorders**

Duration	Frequency	
	Chronic (15+ days/month)	**Episodic (< 15 days/month)**
Long (≥ 4 hours)	Chronic daily headache of long duration • Chronic migraine • Chronic tension-type • New daily persistent headache • Hemicrania continua	Episodic headache of long duration • Episodic migraine • Episodic tension-type headache
Short (< 4 hours)	Chronic daily headache of short duration • Chronic cluster headache • Chronic paroxysmal hemicranias • SUNCT	Episodic headache of short duration • Episodic cluster headache • Episodic paroxysmal hemicrania

Modified from Silberstein et al.[15]

CDH is a significant public health concern. In population-based studies around the world, 4%–5% of the general population has primary CDH, and 0.5% has severe headaches on a daily basis.[1–6] Table 9.1 outlines the most common primary headache disorders, organized by frequency (chronic versus episodic) and duration (long attacks versus short attacks).[7] CDH can be a primary or secondary headache disorder. Primary CDH is not related to a structural or systemic illness and probably reflects an intrinsic brain disturbance.[8] Patients with CDH experience diminished quality of life and mental health (especially anxiety and depression), as well as impaired physical, social, and occupational functioning.[9–13] They frequently overuse medication.[14,15] In addition, they account for substantial direct medical costs, and are the major reason for headache subspecialty practice consultations in the United States.[16,17] In population samples, chronic tension-type headache (CTTH) is the leading cause of primary CDH.[18]

In subspecialty practices, the most common form of CDH is a form of very frequent migraine that was previously termed "transformed migraine" (TM) and is now called "chronic migraine" (CM). The estimated prevalence of CM/TM worldwide is 1%–3%; prevalence varies by case definition, case ascertainment, population, ethnicity, and other variables.[7,19–23] Patients with CM experience pain and other symptoms, including nausea, vomiting, photophobia, and phonophobia; at least half of their days and are disabled by the disorder.[17,24]

Secondary CDH (Table 9.2) has an identifiable underlying cause, although the secondary process may provoke a pre-existing primary headache entity, such as migraine. Causes of secondary CDH include head trauma, cervical spine disorders, vascular disorders, nonvascular intracranial disorders, temporomandibular joint disorders, sinus infections,[25–29] chronic meningitis, and idiopathic intracranial hypertension (IIH).[16,30–33] IIH is easily diagnosed when papilledema is present, but some patients with IIH do not have papilledema, in which case the disorder can mimic primary CDH. Cervicogenic headache is a unilateral pain disorder that does not switch sides, occurs mainly in women, and may be associated with ipsilateral blurred vision, tinnitus, lacrimation, tingling, difficulty swallowing, photophobia, arm pain, and, when more severe, nausea and anorexia.[34,35] Certain focal dystonias of the

Table 9.2 **Secondary Chronic Daily Headache**

Medication overuse headache (MOH)
Post-traumatic headache
Cervical spine disorders
    Headache associated with vascular disorders (arteriovenous malformation, arteritis [including giant cell arteritis], dissection, and subdural hematoma)
    Headache associated with nonvascular intracranial disorders (intracranial hypertension, infection [EBV, HIV], neoplasm)
    Other (temporomandibular joint disorder, sinus infection)

Modified from Silberstein et al.[15]

head and neck (pharyngeal dystonia, spasmodic torticollis, mandibular dystonia, lingual dystonia, and segmental craniocervical dystonia) are often accompanied by daily headache. Medication overuse headache (MOH) was previously termed a secondary disorder; it is now classified as aggravating pre-existing migraine.

Once secondary headache has been excluded, primary daily or almost-daily headache sufferers are subdivided into two groups, based on headache duration. When the headache duration is less than 4 hours, the differential diagnosis includes cluster headache, paroxysmal hemicrania, idiopathic stabbing headache, hypnic headache, and Short-lasting unilateral neuralgiform headache attacks with conjunctival injection and tearing (SUNCT). When the headache duration is greater than 4 hours, the major primary disorders to consider are chronic migraine (CM), hemicrania continua (HC), chronic tension-type headache (CTTH), and new daily persistent headache (NDPH) (Table 9.1).[15]. CM, CTTH, NDPH, and HC are now included in the third IHS classification (ICHD-3 β).[36] In this chapter, we discuss the classification and treatment of CM, mechanisms and treatment, and the role of medication overuse.

THE HISTORY OF CM/TM CLASSIFICATION

Clinicians observed that migraine can increase in frequency over time in some patients.[16,33,37,38] Mathew introduced the term "transformed migraine" (TM) in 1987 to characterize this group of patients.[16] These patients had episodic migraine headaches that progress in severity and frequency (i.e., migraines that transform to the point of near-daily occurrence).[16,31] Others used the term "progressive migraine" [31,33,39] and "mixed or combined headache."[40,41]

Mathew[30] reported a series of patients with distinct attacks of migraine, whose headaches evolved over the years into a daily or near-daily headache. The majority were women who had menstrual aggravation of headache.[31,33,39,42] They had features of both migraine and TTH; most (90%) had migraine without aura. They had more triggers, gastrointestinal symptoms, and family history

of headaches than patients with CTTH.[30] Most overused acute medications. Stopping the overused medication frequently, but not always, resulted in distinct headache improvement.[42]

Saper[33] found that 80% of his CDH patients had prior episodic migraine (EM), with onset between the ages of 26 and 41 years. These patients were typically women. They were frequently clinically depressed and had superimposed acute bouts of migraine. Many of them overused acute headache medications and had significant long-term improvement following detoxification.

Migraine often transforms CDH as a result of medication overuse (MOH), but transformation can occur without overuse.[31,43] About 80% of CDH patients seen in subspecialty clinics overuse symptomatic medication. [16,31,33,44,45] Headache frequency often increases when medication use increases. In many, but not all, cases, stopping the overused medication results in distinct headache improvement, although it may take days to weeks. Many patients have significant long-term improvement after detoxification.

Many studies identified weaknesses in the original criteria mandated by the IHS to classify CDH[46], one of the most common disorders seen in headache centers. [19,30,38,40,41,47,48] CDH was not easily classified within the old IHS system, which did not include TM or CM.[19,30,38,41,48] When originally classified, the headaches were placed in the CTTH group. But because the daily headaches often evolved from EM and the patients had many migrainous features, it was inappropriate to classify them as CTTH. The headaches were too frequent to permit their being classified as migraine.[41]

ICHD-1 (1988)

After the publication of the TM concept, the International Headache Society (IHS) published its *International Classification of Headache Disorders* (ICHD-1), to establish consistent operational diagnostic criteria for the headache disorders.[46] The ICHD-1 did not include a classification for patients with migraine who also suffer from daily or near-daily headaches. Patients with TM required several diagnoses using ICHD-1.[49] Because these patients often had frequent headaches of variable intensity and used acute medications for treatment, they were often diagnosed with CTTH, migraine, and medication overuse headache (MOH) using ICHD-1 criteria.[19,38,41,48,49] The term "mixed tension-vascular headaches" was applied, because these headaches resembled tension-type headache (TTH). However, they are likely biologically similar, if not identical, to migraine. This is supported by studies that demonstrate that triptans effectively treat phenotypic TTH in migraineurs but not in patients with pure TTH.[50] Furthermore, in the absence of daily diary studies, it is unclear whether the milder headaches these patients experience are truly tension-type, migraine, or probable migraine. Indeed, in two large, recently conducted, randomized controlled trials of CM, participants used an interactive voice-response system daily telephone diary to record their headache symptoms.[51] They had an average of 20 headache days per month, 95% of which met criteria for migraine or probable migraine.

The difficulty in classifying patients with CDH using the original ICHD-1 approach has been demonstrated repeatedly.[19,38,41,48,49] Messinger et al.,[38] using the IHS criteria and questionnaire data from two surveys, attempted to classify a clinic-based sample of 410 subjects. They were unable to classify 35.9% of the patients. Only 9.1% had CTTH, but about 86% of these CTTH patients had two or more migrainous features. Solomon et al.[41] evaluated 100 consecutive CDH patients in a tertiary headache center with CDH. Most (61%) had continuous headache; 39% had intermittent headache, defined by pain-free intervals of at least 1 hour at least 4 days a week. More than 50% overused acute medication. While two-thirds met the criteria for CTTH, many had migrainous features. One-third could not be classified as CTTH because they had too many migrainous features. Many of these headaches would be classifiable as migraine were it not for their daily occurrence. Many patients could not be classified in the old IHS system (except as "headache of the tension-type not fulfilling above [other] criteria"). The IHS criteria did not take into account the historical features of CDH before it becomes daily. Is CDH preceded by EM or TTH, or do the headaches begin de novo? Solomon and Lipton concluded

that the IHS criteria should be modified to include TM (CDH evolving from migraine), and that subtypes with and without medication overuse should be distinguished. They did not propose specific diagnostic criteria for these disorders.

Sanin et al.[19] attempted to validate the IHS criteria in a headache clinic population. They randomly selected 400 patients and classified them using the IHS criteria. More than 55% of the patients had more than one diagnosis, and 37.7% had CDH; 110 had CTTH; 90% of them also had migraine. Sanin et al. concluded that most patients in their clinic had more than one IHS diagnosis, that CTTH occurring alone is rare, and that chronic headache classification needed revision. Pfaffenrath and Isler[48] investigated the IHS criteria for CTTH in a sample of 211 subjects participating in a clinical trial of antidepressant treatment. Fifty-six percent had daily headache. The remaining 44% experienced headaches an average of 18 days per month. More than two-thirds met the two major IHS criteria for CTTH (bilateral pain, 79%; pressure or tightening, 72%); 59% met all the IHS criteria for CTTH. Many migraine symptoms were reported: unilateral headache, 20%; throbbing, 28%; anorexia, 39%; osmophobia, 25%; phonophobia, 60%; nausea, 53%; and increased pain with physical activity, 48%. Many had migraine symptoms with headaches of mild intensity. These studies suggested that the IHS criteria needed to be revised with respect to the classification of daily headache.

Sandrini et al.[52] classified 90 consecutive CDH outpatients who attended a clinic in Italy. Most (75%) had CDH evolving from migraine, while 16.7% began de novo and 7.7% had evolved from episodic TTH. They differentiated two subsets of patients with CDH evolving from migraine. TM referred to those patients who had distinct bouts of migraine that evolved into CDH with disappearance of typical migraine attacks. "Migraine with interparoxysmal headache" was defined as recurrent bouts of migraine with a constant, low-severity headache between attacks.

Silberstein et al.[53] studied 300 patients who had CDH and were admitted to an inpatient unit. Most (216) had acute medication overuse. A subset of these patients (50) who overused medication were followed for 2 years. Most had TM (74%), some had NDPH (24%), and only 2% had CTTH with a diagnosis of prior episodic tension-type headache (ETTH). Most (80%) reverted to episodic headache following detoxification, suggesting that both TM and NDPH associated with medication overuse are perpetuated by drug overuse.

These studies showed that the ICHD-1 classification was not comprehensive, as patients with daily headache were not well classified. [49] The ICHD-1 approach did not take natural history into account, and did not include the concept of a history of transformation or a period when migraine headaches increased in frequency.

SILBERSTEIN-LIPTON CRITERIA (1994, 1996)

Based upon these and other observations, Silberstein and Lipton came to the following conclusions: (1) the IHS classification was not comprehensive, for there was a large subset of patients with daily headache who were not well classified; (2) daily headache is often TM; and (3) CDH is often associated with medication overuse but may occur without it. They recommended revising the IHS criteria for chronic, frequent primary headache disorders and proposed adding several headache types to the 1988 IHS classification.[15] They defined CDH as a group of several distinct types of primary headaches. CDH includes all of the primary headache disorders with daily or near-daily headaches that last more than 4 hours a day untreated. CDH was subdivided into TM, CTTH evolved from ETTH, NDPH, and HC.

Silberstein and Lipton proposed draft operational criteria for TM in 1994 (Table 9.3).[15] They considered TM to be a subset of migraine with a diagnosis dependent on a history of ICHD-1-defined migraine and the presence of head pain lasting more than 4 hours a day on at least 15 days a month. The 1994 draft criteria required a history of transformation. Silberstein and Lipton elected not to require particular characteristics for the daily or near-daily headaches, in part because these headaches are pleiomorphic: daily headaches may be unilateral or bilateral, mild to severe in intensity, with or without associated migrainous features. Furthermore, while patients with TM often continue to have episodes of headaches that fulfill ICHD-1 criteria for migraine (1.1 or 1.2), ICHD-1-defined migraine attacks may cease in a minority of patients. TM was subdivided into two categories, one with and one without medication overuse, using a consensus of published reports to define medication overuse.

In field tests, approximately 40% of CDH sufferers could not be classified using the 1994 Silberstein-Lipton draft criteria.[49,54] One of the major limitations was patients' difficulty in remembering the characteristics of their prior headaches and the evolution of headaches over time (i.e., whether their headaches had escalated, when they had escalated, and how long the process of escalation took). Silberstein, Lipton, and Sliwinski then modified their draft definition of TM in 1996 so that a clear history of increasing headache frequency was not required.[54] Their 1996 modified draft criteria included patients with a history of ICHD-1 migraine, a history of escalation over 3 months,

Table 9.3 Original Proposed Criteria for Transformed Migraine

1.8 Transformed Migraine (TM)
    A. History of episodic migraine meeting any IHS criteria 1.1 to 1.6
    B. Daily or almost daily (> 15 days/month) head pain for > 1 month
    C. Average headache duration of 4 hours/day (if untreated)
    D. History of increasing headache frequency with decreasing severity of migrainous features over at least 3 months
    E. At least one of the following:
        1. There is no suggestion of one of the disorders listed in groups 5–11.
        2. Such a disorder is suggested, but it is ruled out by appropriate investigations.
        3. Such disorder is present, but first migraine attacks do not occur in close temporal relation to the disorder.
1.8.1 Transformed Migraine with medication overuse
1.8.2 Transformed Migraine without medication overuse

Table 9.4 Silberstein-Lipton (Revised) Criteria for Chronic Migraine

1.8 Chronic Migraine

   A. Daily or almost daily (> 15 days/month) head pain for > 1 month

   B. Average headache duration of > 4 hours/day (if untreated)

   C. At least one of the following:

      1. History of episodic migraine meeting any IHS criteria 1.1 to 1.6

      2. History of increasing headache frequency with decreasing severity of migrainous features over at least 3 months

      3. Headache at some time meets IHS criteria for migraine 1.1 to 1.6 other than duration

   D. Does not meet criteria for new daily persistent headache (4.7) or hemicrania continua (4.8)

   E. At least one of the following:

      1. There is no suggestion of one of the disorders listed in groups 5–11.

      2. Such a disorder is suggested, but it is ruled out by appropriate investigations.

      3. Such a disorder is present, but first migraine attacks do not occur in close temporal relation to the disorder.

Modified from Silberstein et al.[15]

or a current headache that, except for duration, met the ICHD-1 criteria for migraine. This modification allowed the use of both historical and current headache features, which are crucial to diagnosis (Table 9.4). They distinguished two forms of TM, one with medication overuse and the other without medication overuse, and defined requisite levels of use. They did not attempt to define the causal role of medication-taking in the progression of headache, but instead identified it as a modifier of TM. Further, to avoid more than one diagnosis for a single headache type, they imposed a hierarchical diagnostic rule whereby patients could not be diagnosed with chronic tension-type headache if they met the criteria for TM. The 1996 Silberstein-Lipton criteria have been used around the world in clinic-based and population-based studies as well as in clinical trials.[1,3–5,25,55,56]

ICHD-2 (2004)

The IHS issued a revised *ICHD-2* in 2004. [36] The ICHD-2 added CM as a complication of migraine, nomenclature that was intended to capture patients with TM as defined by the Silberstein-Lipton criteria, and proposed operational diagnostic criteria for CM (Table 9.5). The ICHD-2 codified the term "CM," although the term "TM" has not been eliminated from usage.[7] The ICHD-2 CM criteria require migraine headache that occurs on 15 or more days per month for more than

3 months without medication overuse. It must not be attributable to another disorder, including hemicrania continua or new daily persistent headache.

Like ICHD-1, ICHD-2 classifies headaches rather than syndromes. Because this approach eliminates the possibility of incorporating patterns of evolution over time as part of classification, it is problematic for CM/TM. The ICHD-2 CM classification does not allow for the presence of medication overuse. When medication overuse is present, the diagnosis is unclear until the medication has been withdrawn and there is no subsequent improvement. These patients were coded according to the antecedent migraine subtype (usually migraine without aura), probable CM, and probable MOH. If criteria for CM are still fulfilled 2 months after acute headache medication overuse has ceased, CM and the antecedent migraine subtype become the diagnoses, and the diagnosis of probable MOH is discarded. If CM criteria are no longer fulfilled, the diagnoses are MOH and the antecedent migraine subtype, and the diagnosis of probable CM is discarded. These coding recommendations, besides being complicated

Table 9.5 Original IHS Criteria for Chronic Migraine[46]

A. Headache fulfilling criteria C and D for 1.1 *migraine without aura* on ≥ 15 days/month for > 3 months

B. Not attributed to another disorder

to implement in clinical practice, do not allow for the existence of MOH in the absence of chronic headache. A patient having high-frequency EM (occurring 14 days per month) and using triptans 10 days per month has medication overuse (which would not be coded), but by virtue of too few headache days is not eligible for a diagnosis of MOH. The same patient having 15 headache days per month would have MOH. Because medication overuse can exist in the absence of chronic headache, it is important to code for medication overuse rather than MOH in all contexts.

Results of field studies of ICHD-2 CM criteria demonstrated that most patients who meet TM criteria do not meet CM criteria, and patients meeting the ICHD-2 diagnostic criteria for CM are rare in clinical practice.[7,21] The ICHD-2 criteria for CM are so restrictive that they exclude most patients with TM. A clinic-based CDH study was conducted at the New England Headache Center. They applied alternative diagnostic approaches to 638 CDH patients.[49] Patients were classified according to the Silberstein-Lipton, ICHD-1, and ICHD-2 classification systems. Of the 158 patients with Silberstein-Lipton TM without medication overuse, only nine (5.6%) met ICHD-2 criteria for CM. Most were classified using combinations of migraine and CTTH diagnoses. Just 41 of 399 patients (10.2%) with Silberstein-Lipton TM with medication overuse were classified as ICHD-2 probable CM with probable medication overuse.

The authors concluded that, for patients who have TM according to the Silberstein-Lipton diagnostic approach, both the ICHD-1 and ICHD-2 criteria are complex to use and require multiple diagnoses. Very few patients with Silberstein-Lipton TM could be classified with a single ICHD-2 diagnosis. ICHD-2 CM was so rare that it would be virtually impossible to conduct CM clinical trials using ICHD-2 criteria.

The same group conducted a similar study in adolescents.[57] Of the 69 patients with Silberstein-Lipton TM without medication overuse, most (71%) could be classified as having ICHD-2 CM. However, of the patients with TM with medication overuse ($n = 48$), just 39.6% met criteria for probable CM. Most patients (94.2% not overusing medication and 91.6% of those overusing medication) had migraine or probable migraine on at least 50% of the headache days.

ICHD-2R (2006)

Recognizing that the ICHD-2 classification of CM inadequately described the population of patients it was meant to diagnose, the Classification Committee of the IHS proposed a revised version of the criteria for CM in 2006.[58] The ICHD-2R criteria required that patients have 15 or more headaches per month with ≥ 8 migraine days—or ≥ 8 days on which headaches were treated and relieved by a triptan or an ergot before the patient expected development of a headache with migrainous features—for at least 3 months and five or more previous attacks of migraine (Table 9.6). [58] The ICHD-2R criteria were validated in Europe and the United States,[59–61] and have been incorporated into the third edition of the ICHD: ICHD-3 β.[62] The ICHD-3 β retains the diagnostic criteria of both CM and MOH but *now allows* both diagnoses to be made concurrently, rather than medication overuse (MO) being incompatible with a diagnosis of CM.

The ICHD-2R criteria were field tested in a sample of patients from the New England Headache Center diary study.[61] The study included individuals with both TM with medication use (TM+) and TM without medication overuse (TM−) according to the criteria proposed by Silberstein and Lipton.[7] The authors concluded that the ICHD-2R criteria address many of the criticisms of the ICHD-2 with respect to the CM diagnostic criteria.

The ICHD-2R criteria were also field tested on data from the pivotal phase 3 studies of onabotulinumtoxinA for the treatment of CM (the PREEMPT program), the largest clinical trials database of CM sufferers.[51,63,64] Baseline diary data from the PREEMPT program were used to compare the epidemiologic and headache symptom profiles for three proposed diagnostic approaches for chronic migraine: the PREEMPT criteria proposed by the IHCC experts; the Silberstein-Lipton 2006 criteria stratified by medication overuse criteria (denoted as either S-L TM-MO for those without medication overuse and S-L TM+/-MO for those with and without medication overuse).

Table 9.6 Diagnostic Criteria for TM According to Silberstein-Lipton Criteria and for CM According to ICHD-2R and ICHD-3 β

Silberstein-Lipton TM	ICHD-2R CM	ICHD-3 β CM

A. Daily or almost daily (> 15 days a month) head pain for > 1 month
B. Average headache duration of > 4 hours (if untreated)
B. At least 1 of the following:
  1. History of episodic migraine meeting any IHS criterion 1.1–1.6
  2. History of increasing headache frequency with decreasing severity of migrainous features over at least 3 months
  3. Headache at some time meets IHS criteria for migraine 1.1–1.6 other than duration
D. Does not meet criteria for *new daily persistent headache (4.7) or hemicrania continua (4.8)*
	A. Headache on ≥ 15 days/month for 3 months
	B. Occurring in a patient who has had at least five attacks fulfilling criteria for 1.1 *migraine without aura*
	C. On ≥ 8 days per month, for at least 3 months, headache fulfills criteria for migraine C1 and/or C2 below, that is, has fulfilled criteria for pain and associated symptoms of *migraine without aura*
	  1. Criteria C and D for 1.1 migraine without aura
	  2. Treated or relieved with triptans or ergotamine before the expected development of C1 above
	D. No medication overuse and not attributable to other causative disorder
		A. Headache on ≥15 days per month for at least 3 months
		B. Occurring in a patient who has had at least five attacks fulfilling criteria for 1.1 *migraine without aura* and/or 1.2 *migraine with aura*
		C. On ≥ 8 days per month for at least 3 months one or more of the following criteria were fulfilled:
		  1. Criteria C and D for 1.1 *migraine without aura*
		  2. Criteria B and C for 1.2 migraine with aura
		  3. Headache considered by patient to be onset migraine and relieved by a triptan or an ergotamine derivative
		D. Not better accounted for by another ICHD-3 β diagnosis

For the purpose of analysis, ICHD-3 β is used, as it retains the diagnostic criteria of ICHD-2R CM and MOH but allows both diagnoses to be made concurrently. The ICHD-3 β CM subjects were stratified by medication overuse criteria (ICHD-3 β-MO) for those without and ICHD-3 β +/-MO for those with and without medication overuse). Medication overuse was defined as intake during baseline of simple analgesics on ≥ 15 days, or of other medication types or combination of types for ≥ 10 days, with intake ≥ 2 days/week from the category of overuse. Comparisons between the ICHD-3 β criteria and the Silberstein-Lipton 2006 criteria are summarized herein.

The analysis involved baseline diary data from two phase 3 studies (PREEMPT 1 and PREEMPT 2) that recruited chronic migraine patients between January 2006 and July 2007 from 122 study centers in six countries (Canada, United States, Croatia, Switzerland, Germany, and United Kingdom). The number of patients enrolled in the 28-day screening baseline period and having sufficient diary data (≥ 20 days) for assessment was 2736. During the 28-day screening phase, patients used an interactive voice-response system daily telephone diary to record their headache symptoms and acute headache medication use.

Demographic profiles and headache characteristics were similar across CM diagnostic criteria. Mean age ranged from 38.1 to 41.9 years, populations that did not include medication overuse (ICHD-3 β-MO = ICHD-2R and S-L TM-MO) had slightly lower estimates at 38.1 years. Body mass index (BMI) was nearly identical among case definition populations. Most were female and white.

Headache characteristics of subjects meeting the alternative diagnostic criteria features were strikingly similar (Table 9.7). No differences across CM were observed in mean frequency of headache days (per 28 days), headache episodes, or migraine days. About 64% of subjects met criteria for acute medication overuse. The mean age of onset was within the second decade (mean age range of 20.8–21.9). Those with medication overuse were more likely to have tried a preventive medication. Most (92.7%–97.5%) were currently using acute medications. Triptans use varied based on whether medication overuse was an exclusion for the case definition.

Results of analyses to validate case definitions against the gold standards are summarized in Table 9.7. ICHD-2R (which do not allow for medication overuse in CM) are denoted as ICHD-3 β; ICHD-2R criteria including those with and without medication overuse are

Table 9.7 Headache (HA) Profile by CM Criteria

	ICHD-3 β -MO n = 673	ICHD-3 β +/-MO n = 1912	S-L TM +/-MO n = 2021	S-L TM -MO n = 723
Frequency HA days, mean (SD)	18.4 (5.1)	18.2 (5.3)	18.0 (5.4)	18.3 (5.1)
Frequency HA episodes, mean (SD)	10.0 (5.0)	11.3 (5.4)	11.3 (5.4)	10.1 (4.94)
Frequency migraine days, mean (SD)	15.6 (6.1)	15.3 (6.3)	14.6 (6.8)	14.7 (6.7)
% with medication overuse	0.0	64.8	64.2	0.0
Age of onset of CM, mean (SD)	20.8 (11.1)	21.9 (11.6)	21.7 (11.5)	21.6 (11.5)
Ever tried preventive medications, %	50.8	60.6	61.5	63.5
Currently used acute medications, %	92.7	97.4	97.0	97.5
No medications, %	7.3	2.6	3.0	2.5
Single analgesics, %	66.0	66.6	67.6	67.1
Combination analgesics, %	34.5	54.1	54.7	55.5
Multiple analgesics, %	36.8	59.2	57.0	58.1
Ergots, %	1.5	2.6	2.8	2.9
Triptans, %	45.0	65.4	61.2	63.3
Opioids, %	4.0	7.9	8.4	8.3

SD = standard deviation
ICHD-3 β-MO = ICHD-2R criteria (which do not allow for medication overuse in CM)
ICHD-3 β+/-MO = ICHD-2R criteria including those with and without medication overuse
S-L TM+/-MO = Silberstein-Lipton criteria for TM (which allow for medication overuse in TM)
S-L TM-MO = Silberstein-Lipton criteria for TM excluding those with medication overuse

denoted as ICHD-3 β +/-MO; Silberstein and Lipton criteria for TM (which allow for medication overuse in TM) as S-L TM+/-MO; and Silberstein-Lipton criteria for TM excluding those with medication overuse as S-L TM-MO.

When ICHD-3 β-MO was considered the gold standard for evaluating S-L, sensitivity was high: 99.6% of those identified as having CM by ICHD-2R-MO criteria also met S-L TM+/-MO and S-L TM-MO criteria for TM. Specificity was more variable. Of those identified as not having CM by ICHD-3 β-MO, 97.4% did not meet criteria for TM by S-L TM-MO, and 34.5% did not meet S-L TM+/-MO criteria. These differences in specificity arise from differences in the way the S-L case definitions treat medication overuse. Level of agreement with ICHD-3 β-MO was highest for S-L TM-MO (Cohen's kappa 0.95), because both sets of criteria exclude medication overuse. When ICHD-3 β-MO was considered the gold standard, PPV was variable and ranged between 33.2% and 92.7%. The probability was high (92.7%) that those with S-L TM-MO would be diagnosed as having CM when using the ICHD-3 β-MO criteria, and relatively low (33.2%) that those meeting criteria for S-L TM+/-MO would be diagnosed as CM using the ICHD3 β-MO. NPV was far less variable. The probability was high (99.6% to 99.9%) that those not meeting criteria for S-L TM-MO or S-L TM+/-MO would not be diagnosed with CM when using the ICHD-3 β-MO criteria.

When S-L TM was considered the gold standard, 33.2% of those identified as TM by S-L TM+/-MO also met criteria for CM by ICHD-3 β-MO and 94.5% by ICHD-3 β +/-MO. Specificity ranged from 99.6% to 100.0%. Of those not identified as having TM by S-L TM criteria, the majority did not meet criteria for ICHD-3 β-MO or ICHD-3 β +/-MO. Level of agreement with S-L TM was highest for ICHD-3 β +/-MO (Cohen's kappa 0.90) and lowest for ICHD-3 β-MO (Cohen's kappa 0.20). When S-L TM was considered the gold standard, PPV ranged from 99.6% to 100.0%. Probability was extremely high that those with ICHD-3 β-MO, ICHD-3 β+/-MO, and S-L TM-MO would be diagnosed as having TM when using the S-L TM criteria. NPV ranged between 34.5% and 86.4%.

The ICHD criteria for CM continue to undergo field testing. Results of field tests available suggest that the ICHD-2-R criteria for CM were an improvement upon the ICHD-2 criteria. Further, the ICHD-2R criteria, now the ICHD-3 β criteria, which includes both those with and without medication overuse, agree with the Silberstein-Lipton criteria for TM.

ICHD-3 (BETA [β] VERSION)

The IHS issued a revised *ICHD* in 2013.[62] The ICHD-3 β no longer considers CM a complication of migraine and allows both migraine with and without aura (Table 9.6) and now excludes the diagnosis of TTH. It separates chronic from EM, because it is impossible to distinguish the individual episodes of headache in patients with such frequent or continuous headaches. The features of the headache and the associated symptoms often change within the same day. CM patients often use acute medication, making it difficult to observe the untreated characteristics of the headache. Attacks with and without aura and tension-type–like headaches are all counted toward the headache burden. The most common associated complication of CM is medication overuse.

The ICHD-3 β now allows patients with chronic migraine and medication overuse to have two diagnoses: 1.3 chronic migraine and 8.2 medication overuse headache. The rationale for providing a beta-version of the diagnostic criteria is to synchronize ICHD-3 β with the World Health Organization's next revision (11th edition) of the International Classification of Diseases (ICD-11) and to provide an opportunity to field test and refine the proposed diagnostic criteria in preparation for a final published version of ICHD-3 β.

RECOMMENDATIONS FOR DIAGNOSTIC CRITERIA FOR CM/TM

The ICHD-3 β criteria for CM (Table 9.6) constitute an advance over older diagnostic approaches because they allow acute medication overuse as defined by MOH criteria, and they allow both migraine with and without aura.[21,62] But areas for improvement remain. The ICHD-3 β criteria are difficult to operationalize in clinical practice. [7] The specification that patients have 15 or more headache days per month with ≥ 8 migraine days—*or ≥ 8 days on which headaches were treated and relieved by a triptan or an ergot before the patient expected development of a headache with migrainous features*—can be problematic. Recalling days with migraine and days of successfully treated attacks may be difficult. The term "relieved" is not operationally defined. Patients must not only identify and recall relief but also identify headaches that would have become full-blown migraine in the absence of treatment. [21] Even if these problems were addressed, at minimum, reliable diagnosis may require very detailed headache diaries with all pain and associated symptoms recorded, rarely available at initial consultation. In addition, conceptual problems exist. This approach assumes that response to "migraine-specific" medication implies that the attack is a migraine. The evidence suggests that a variety of primary and secondary headache disorders may respond to triptans.[65–67] This approach makes diagnosis more difficult since some patients are unable to take triptans or ergots due to contraindications, cost, or availability. How would one account for treated headache? The simplest way is to count probable migraine attacks with or without aura (as suggested in the appendix criteria).

We recommend, based on evidence available and extensive field testing already performed, that the ICHD-3 β criteria for CM be modified with the following revisions: (1) remove criterion B, which specifies that CM must occur in a patient with at least five prior migraine attacks; (2) add probable migraine to C1 and C2, and remove criterion C3 regarding treatment and relief of headache by a triptan or ergot (this is one alternative in the appendix (A1.3)); (3) add the Silberstein-Lipton criterion that the headache does not meet criteria for new daily persistent headache or hemicrania continua. Removal of criterion B is suggested because the requirement of diagnosable migraine without aura in the past appears to be an unreasonable burden given the limitations of patient recall and the fact that CM can be present for years. In addition, the requirement for five migraine attacks can be logically inconsistent.

If a patient has high-frequency EM, a diagnosis of migraine (with or without aura) can be made after five attacks. If the patient has 16 headache days/month for at least 3 months and eight separate attacks, then a diagnosis can be made. A diagnosis cannot be made in a patient with continuous headache and no discrete attacks.

We agree that further study be conducted on two additional potential subtypes of CM that have been included in the ICHD-3 β appendix. These subtypes are defined by headache pattern: continuous headaches (constant headache with no pain-free breaks) versus non-continuous headaches (headaches with pain-free breaks). The epidemiology and clinical course of continuous and non-continuous headaches need to be further defined in the context of CM, as both headache patterns are encountered in clinical practice. In addition, there could also be constant versus fluctuating subtypes.

The proposed revisions to the CM diagnostic criteria are shown in Table 9.8. With these revisions, the IHCD-3 β criteria constitute operational diagnostic criteria that represent the clinical phenotype of most primary CDH patients. With the proposed revisions, the ICHD-3 β criteria should facilitate large-scale international epidemiologic, genetic, and treatment studies on each subtype, while maintaining the clinical and biological homogeneity of this patient population.

Differentiating CM from Other Chronic Daily Headaches

To diagnose CM requires that the headaches are not attributable to another disorder, including prior trauma (chronic post-traumatic headache), cervical spine disorders, vascular disorders, chronic meningitis, IIH, temporomandibular joint disorder, and sinus infection.[8,68]

Intracranial hypertension is readily diagnosed when papilledema is present, but if it is absent, intracranial hypertension can mimic CDH. Intracranial hypertension may be idiopathic (IIH), with no clear identifiable cause, or symptomatic; underlying etiologies for the latter include venous sinus occlusion, a mass lesion, meningitis, trauma, radical neck dissection, hypoparathyroidism, vitamin A intoxication, systemic lupus, renal disease, or drug side effects

Table 9.8 Suggested Revised ICHD-3 β Chronic migraine criteria

A. Headache (tension-type–like and/or migraine-like) on ≥ 15 days per month for at least 3 months°
B. On ≥ 8 days per month on average ≥ 4 hours/day for at least 3 months one or more of the following criteria were fulfilled°°
   1. Criteria C and D for 1.1 *migraine without aura*
   2. Criteria B and C for 1.2 *migraine with aura*
   3. Criteria A and B for 1.5 *probable migraine*
C. Not better accounted for by another ICHD-3 β diagnosis.
D. Does not meet criteria for new *daily persistent headache* (4.7) or *hemicrania continua* (4.8)
Subtypes

- Medication overuse°
- Without medication overuse
- With medication overuse (add 8.2)
- Pattern of headache(s)°°°
- Pain-free periods (subtype A 1.3.1)
- Continuous pain (subtype A 1.3.2)

°Same as ICHD-3 β criteria; °°Same as ICHD-3 β appendix criteria; °°°Differs from ICHD-3 β appendix criteria (see)

(nalidixic acid, danazol, or steroid withdrawal). Intracranial hypertension from cerebral venous outflow obstruction can be caused by chronic otitis, head trauma, tumors, hypercoagulable states, or cerebral edema.[69] Increased intracranial pressure consequent to venous outflow hypertension can also occur without obstruction when patients have arteriovenous malformations, cardiac failure, and pulmonary failure.

Increased intracranial pressure is not always associated with either headache or papilledema, and there is no direct correlation between the degree of pressure elevation and the presence of headache. IIH, although more common in obese women, can also occur in non-obese women and in men. The presence of transient visual obscurations and intracranial noises provide clues to the diagnosis. Cerebral venous thrombosis may be difficult to diagnose. The typical features of cerebral venous thrombosis can be absent, that is, there is no history of new onset seizures, no focal neurologic deficits, no change of consciousness, no cranial nerve palsies, no bilateral cortical signs, and no evidence of papilledema on funduscopic examination.

Mosek et al.[70] prospectively measured the CSF opening pressure of 24 CDH patients without papilledema. Their average CSF opening pressure was 170 ± 41 mm: five (21%) had an opening pressure of greater than 200 mm CSF. CDH patients had a mean CSF opening pressure 13 mm higher than nonheadache patients (p = 0.05) after adjusting for body mass index, age, sex, and various non-headache disorders. The odds of having a CSF opening pressure greater than 200 mm CSF was five times greater for CDH patients than non-headache patients. These observations suggest that increased intracranial pressure may be comorbid with CDH in some patients.

Spontaneous intracranial hypotension (often due to a spontaneous CSF leak) typically presents as a daily headache with a positional component. Occasionally, orthostatic features are absent or may disappear. Patients may notice that their headaches begin after arising and gradually worsen during the day.[28] CSF hypotension may begin suddenly, with a thunderclap presentation.

Infectious causes, including fungal (coccidiomycosis), bacterial (Lyme, tuberculosis), and parasitic (neurocysticercosis) causes, should be considered in high-risk patients. Sphenoid sinusitis can present as an intractable headache that is unresponsive to analgesics and interferes with sleep. It often occurs without associated nasal symptoms. Obstructive sleep apnea can present with daily headaches upon awakening. It should be considered when patients have a snoring history, large neck size, or are obese. Cervical spine, temporomandibular joint, or dental pathology must be considered when chronic cranial, nuchal, or facial pain is present. Cervicogenic headache[34] is a unilateral pain disorder that does not switch sides,[35] occurs mainly in women, and may be associated with ipsilateral blurred vision, tinnitus, lacrimation, tingling, difficulty swallowing, photophobia, arm pain, and, when more severe, nausea and anorexia. "Neck triggers" and reduced cervical range of motion are characteristic. As it is uncertain whether cervicogenic headache is an independent entity or migraine or TTH with a cervical trigger,[71] its classification is uncertain.

MRI plus MRV (with gadolinium if needed) are the neuroimaging procedures of choice for patients suspected of having a secondary cause for CDH, since many of these disorders remain undetected even with contrast-enhanced CT. Special attention must be paid to sinus disorders, particularly the sphenoid sinus. With a normal physical examination and absence of red flags or worrisome historical features, secondary causes of CM can usually be eliminated.[72]

Once secondary headache has been excluded, frequent headache can be subdivided into two groups. When headache duration is less than 4 hours, the disorders includes cluster headache, chronic paroxysmal hemicrania, idiopathic stabbing headache, and hypnic headache. When the headache duration is greater than 4 hours, the major primary disorders to consider are CM, HC, CTTH, and NDPH (Table 9.1)[15].

Several authors have examined the relative frequency of some of these types of CDH. Mathew et al.[44] found that 77% of patients with CDH had what they called TM. Solomon et al.[73] found that most of their CDH patients had TM. Sandrini et al.[52] classified 90 consecutive CDH patients who attended an outpatient clinic in Italy. Most had CDH evolving from migraine (75.0%); 16.7% had CDH that had begun de novo, and 7.7% had CDH that had evolved from ETTH.

CTTH is described by the IHS as "[a] disorder evolving from episodic tension-type headache, with daily or very frequent episodes of headache lasting minutes to days. The pain is typically bilateral, pressing or tightening in quality and of mild to moderate intensity, and does not worsen with routine physical activity. There may be mild nausea, photophobia or phonophobia."[48] EM and CTTH can coexist. Guitera et al.[74] have suggested, based on population-based epidemiologic data, that coexistent CTTH and EM can coexist if, and only if, the current CTTH has no migrainous features and there is a remote history of migraine.

The new ICHD-3 β definition of CM relieves a problem in the differential diagnosis between CM and CTTH. Both diagnoses require headache (meeting the criteria for migraine or TTH) on at least 15 days a month. The features of the headache and the associated symptoms may change even within the same day. It was theoretically possible for a patient to have both these diagnoses. CM patients often use acute medication, making it difficult to observe the untreated characteristics of the headache. Attacks with and without aura and tension-type–like headaches now are all counted toward the headache burden. The presence of 8 migraine days (or triptan or ergot use) makes the default CM.

NDPH is characterized by the relatively abrupt onset of an unremitting primary CDH. [75,76] NDPH requires the absence of a history of evolution from migraine or ETTH. In the absence of rapid development, it is coded as CTTH or CM. NDPH may or may not be associated with medication overuse. A diagnosis of NDPH takes precedence over CM and CTTH. Two disorders can mimic NDPH: spontaneous intracranial hypotension (often due to a spontaneous CSF leak) and intracranial hypertension (due to IIH or even cerebral venous sinus thrombosis). The evaluation of NDPH (as with any new-onset headache) should include neuroimaging, specifically brain MRI with and without gadolinium (to look for diffuse pachymeningeal enhancement associated with spontaneous CSF leaks) and MRV (to diagnose venous sinus thrombosis). If these tests are negative, a lumbar puncture should be considered, especially if the patient is treatment-refractory. The lumbar puncture can rule out an indolent infection and determine CSF pressures.

HC[77,78] is an indomethacin-responsive headache disorder characterized by a continuous, moderately severe, unilateral headache that varies in intensity, waxing and waning without disappearing completely.[79] Some patients have photophobia, phonophobia, and nausea. The IHS now includes HC in the ICHD. It is described as a ". . . persistent, strictly unilateral headache responsive to indomethacin."[36] It differs from CM in that it must be unilateral and must respond to indomethacin.

Marmura et al. reviewed the records of 192 patients with the putative diagnosis of HC and divided them into groups based on their headaches' response to indomethacin. They were compared for age, gender, presence or absence of specific autonomic symptoms, medication overuse, rapidity of headache onset, and whether or not the headaches met criteria for migraine when severe. Forty-three patients had an absolute response, and 122 patients did not respond to adequate doses of indomethacin. The two groups did not differ significantly in terms of age, sex, presence of rapid-onset headache, or medication overuse. Autonomic symptoms, based on a questionnaire, did not predict response. Eighteen patients could not complete a trial of indomethacin due to adverse events. Nine patients could not be included in the HC group despite improvement with indomethacin: one patient probably had primary cough headache, another paroxysmal hemicrania; three patients improved but it was uncertain if they were absolutely pain free; and four patients dramatically improved but still had a baseline headache. They found no statistically significant differences between patients who did and did not respond to indomethacin. They concluded that all patients with continuous, unilateral headache should receive an adequate trial of indomethacin. Most patients with unilateral headache suggestive of HC did not respond to indomethacin.[80]

MEDICATION OVERUSE HEADACHE (MOH)

Medication overuse headache (MOH) was previously called rebound headache, drug-induced headache, and medication-misuse headache. Patients with frequent headaches often overuse analgesics, opioids, ergotamine, and triptans.[81] Medication overuse may be a biobehavioral disorder[82] and may be a response to both chronic pain, or, in headache-prone patients, medication overuse, which can induce the headache. Patients with MOH can develop psychological dependence, tolerance, and abstinence syndromes [43,82]. Medication overuse may be responsible, in part, for the transformation of EM to CM and for the perpetuation of the syndrome.[33] Medication overuse may make headaches refractory to prophylactic medication.[43,83–87] Although stopping the acute medication may result in withdrawal symptoms and a period of increased headache, subsequent headache improvement usually, but not always, occurs. [14,87–90] Many primary CDH patients withdrawn from ergotamine and analgesics and given no further therapy no longer had daily headaches, although about 40% still had EM attacks.[27,91] Medication overuse fulfills the criteria for physical dependency.[14]

Definition and Classification of MOH

In 1988, the ICHD-1 used the term "drug-induced headache" for MOH. [46] This terminology has been criticized because the single intake of several drugs, such as nitrates, may also lead to headache. To emphasize the regular intake of drugs, a new term, "medication overuse headache," was introduced in the 2004 ICHD-2 classification.[36] The ICHD-2 further extended the definition according to clinical symptoms caused by different drugs (Table 10, including D). The first ICHD-2 classification of MOH was confusing. It stated that a diagnosis of headache attributed to a substance becomes definite only when the headache resolves or greatly improves after exposure to the substance is terminated. An arbitrary period of 2 months after overuse cessation was stipulated; if the diagnosis was definite, improvement must occur in that time frame. Prior to cessation, or pending improvement within 2 months after cessation, the diagnosis of probable MOH was used. If improvement did not then occur within the 2-month period, the MOH diagnosis was discarded. Patients with a pre-existing primary headache who developed a new type of headache or whose migraine or TTH was made markedly worse during medication overuse were given the diagnosis of both the pre-existing headache and probable MOH.

Dissatisfaction with the ICHD-2 diagnostic criteria has led to its revision. MOH could not be diagnosed until the overuse was discontinued and the patient improved. Some patients do not improve after withdrawal and may or may not become responsive to prophylactic medication. Other patients do not improve after discontinuation of medication overuse. For these reasons *"Headache resolves or reverts to its previous pattern within 2 months after discontinuation of overused medication"* was eliminated in the revised ICHD-2R

Table 9.9 New IHS Criteria for Headache Attributed to Medication Overuse[46]

A. Headache present on > 15 days/month
B. Regular overuse for > 3 months of one or more acute/symptomatic treatment drugs as defined under sub-forms of 8.2.
   1. Ergotamine, triptans, opioids, **or** combination analgesic medications on ≥ 10 days/month on a regular basis for > 3 months
   2. Simple analgesics **or** any combination of ergotamine, triptans, analgesics opioids on ≥ 15 days/month on a regular basis for > 3 months without overuse of any single class alone
C. Headache has developed or markedly worsened during medication overuse
[**D.** *Headache resolves or reverts to its previous pattern within 2 months after discontinuation of overused medication*]***

**** Eliminated in the latest revision[58]

criteria.[58] The diagnosis of probable MOH and probable CM (or probable CTTH) no longer had to be made when a patient has medication overuse. The default diagnosis was MOH (Table 9.9). The ICHD-3 β now allows diagnosis of both CM and MOH

It was believed that MOH occurred if usage days exceeded 2 to 3 days a week, week after week, month after month,[33] emphasizing frequency and reliability of use. According to the ICHD-2R and ICHD-3 β, overuse is defined in terms of treatment days per month and emphasizes frequency and regularity of days per week. For example, the diagnostic criterion of use on 10 or more days a month (15 for simple analgesics) translates into 2 to 3 treatment days every week. Bunching treatment days and going for long periods without medication intake, as practiced by some patients, is much less likely to cause MOH. The amount of use that constitutes overuse depends on the drug. Ergotamine-overuse headache requires intake on 10 or more days a month on a regular basis for 3 or more months. The headache is often daily and constant. Triptan-overuse headache is usually frequent, intermittent, and migrainous. Triptan intake (any formulation) on 10 or more days a month may increase migraine frequency to that of CM. Evidence suggests that this occurs sooner with triptan overuse than with ergotamine overuse.[92,93]

Patients with CM, TTH, HC, and NDPH may overuse acute headache medications. MOH or, as Isler[94] called it, "painkiller headache," has been reported since the seventeenth century, with occurrences reaching epidemic proportions in Switzerland after World War II. In American subspecialty centers, most patients with MOH have a history of EM that has been converted into CM as a result

of medication overuse.[16,27,43,83,95–97] In European headache centers, 5%–10% of the patients have MOH.[16,27,43,83,95–98].

The epidemiology of MOH is uncertain, since some cases are coincidental and some are causal. In European headache centers, 5%–10% of patients have MOH. One series of 3000 consecutive headache patients reported that 4.3% had MOH.[99] Experiences in the United Kingdom (Goadsby, personal communication) suggest that drug-associated headache is more common than the literature suggests. In American specialty headache clinics, as many as 80% of patients who presented with CDH used analgesics on a daily or near-daily basis [27]. In some headache clinics, a smaller percentage, although still a majority, have had the problem.[73] MOH is less common in India.[100].

Diener and Dahlöf[98] summarized 29 studies that included 2612 patients with MOH. Migraine was the primary headache in 65% of patients, TTH in 27%, and mixed or other headaches (i.e., cluster headache) in 8%. Women had more MOH than men (3.5:1; 1533 women, 442 men). This ratio is slightly higher than one would expect because of the usual migraine frequency gender differences. The mean duration of primary headache was 20.4 years. The mean admitted time of frequent drug intake was 10.3 years in one study, and the mean duration of daily headache was 5.9 years. The number of tablets or suppositories taken daily averaged 4.9 (range 0.25 to 25). Patients averaged 2.5 to 5.8 different pharmacologic components simultaneously (range 1 to 14).[92]

Patients attending an outpatient neurology clinic in Austria reported taking, on average, 6.3 different headache pain drugs.[101] Of these, 26.5% reported using both prescription and over-the-counter medications; 31.3% used over-the-counter medications only, and 27.7% used prescription drugs only. Acetaminophen (average dose 500 mg) was the most frequently used analgesic. Most patients attending a London migraine clinic used multiple medications.[102] Acetaminophen was the most commonly used analgesic (34.9%), followed by aspirin (22.9%).

In a cross-sectional survey carried out in Tromsø in 1986–1987, 19,137 men and women (aged 12–56 years) from the general population were asked about their drug use over the preceding 14 days. On average, 28% of the women and 13% of the men had used analgesics. The most significant predictor of analgesic use was headache; a lesser association was found with infections. Drug use in women was associated with symptoms of depression. Drug use in men was associated with sleeplessness. Higher drug use was associated with smoking and high coffee consumption, but not with frequent alcohol intake.[103]

In a representative sample of the Swiss population, 4.4% of men and 6.8% of women took analgesics at least once a week; 2.3% took them daily.[104] Analgesic dependency was more frequent than dependence on tranquilizers, hypnotics, and stimulating drugs in psychiatric inpatients in Switzerland.[105] In Germany, possibly 1% of the population take up to 10 pain tablets every day.[106]

In the United States, 20.2% of a national sample survey of 20,468 individuals reported "severe headache;" 62.6% of the women and 74.6% of the men used over-the-counter medications, while prescription drugs were used by 34.5% of the women and 21.3% of the men. Over-the-counter analgesic use was greater than prescription medication use among migraineurs as well as among those suffering from undefined severe headache.[107] This could be either a cause or a result of the severe headache.

A random telephone survey of 24,159 households in Canada produced a sample of 1573 households with one or more eligible headache sufferers. Ninety percent of the IHS-diagnosed migraineurs reported using over-the-counter drugs, and 44% reported using prescription drugs. In this sample, 1.5% of migraineurs had rebound headache resulting from ergotamine tartrate or analgesic overuse. MOH is a major public health problem in both the clinic and the community.[108]

Natoli et al.[23] found that the prevalence of medication overuse among subjects with CM had wide variation. Among adults with CM, prevalence of medication overuse was 31%–69%. Determining the frequency of MOH was complicated by the fact that medication overuse in epidemiological studies is a surrogate for a diagnosis of MOH. But most studies reporting CM prevalence did not specifically mention MOH or medication overuse. Thus, they could not confirm whether MOH was truly excluded from estimates based on ICHD criteria.

Clinical Features of MOH

Wilkinson et al.[109] and Bahra et al.[110] reported that when migraine-prone patients take frequent opioid medication for non-headache reasons, headaches will escalate and MOH will occur, and that discontinuing daily low-dose caffeine frequently results in withdrawal headache.[111] Nonetheless, MOH has not been demonstrated in placebo-controlled trials. In a controlled study of caffeine withdrawal, 64 normal adults (71% women) with low-to-moderate caffeine intake (the equivalent of about 2.5 cups of coffee a day) were given a 2-day caffeine-free diet and either placebo or replacement caffeine. Under double-blind conditions, 50% of the patients who were given placebo had a headache by day 2, compared with 6% of those given caffeine. Nausea, depression, and flu-like symptoms were common in the placebo group. This study is relevant since caffeine is frequently used by headache sufferers for pain relief, often in combination with analgesics or ergotamine. The study is a model for short-term caffeine withdrawal but does not demonstrate the long-term consequences of detoxification.

In a community-based telephone survey of 11,112 subjects in Lincoln and Omaha, Nebraska, 61% reported daily caffeine consumption, and 11% of the caffeine consumers reported symptoms upon stopping coffee.[112] A group of those who reported withdrawal were assigned to one of three regimes: abrupt caffeine withdrawal, gradual withdrawal, and no change. One third of the abrupt-withdrawal group and an occasional member of the gradual-withdrawal group had symptoms that included headache and tiredness.

The actual dose limits and the time needed to develop MOH have not been defined in rigorous studies, nor is the relationship of drug half-life to rebound development known. Our clinical knowledge is derived from observing patterns of medication use in patients who present with MOH. Because there may be large individual differences in susceptibility, anecdotal data must be generalized cautiously. Overuse was believed to occur when patients took three or more simple analgesics daily more often than 5 days a week; triptans or combination analgesics containing barbiturates, sedatives, or caffeine more often than 3 days a week; or opioids or ergotamine tartrate more often than 2 days a week.[43,83–86] These limits served in part as the basis of the ICHD-2 definitions.

Specific limits are necessary to prevent analgesic, ergotamine, and triptan overuse. Clinicians [14,16,85,113] compared ergotamine intake in patients with and without CDH. In the groups without CDH, the maximum ergotamine intake was 24 mg a month. However, one patient with primary CDH consumed only 7 mg of ergotamine a month. The frequency of days of ergotamine use (treatment days per week) was emphasized as the most important variable, not the daily or monthly total dose. [14,33] MOH can develop when patients take as little as 0.5–1 mg of ergotamine three times a week.[47,85,89,114]

Scholz et al.[113] studied simple analgesic consumption in patients with and without MOH. Patients with MOH consumed between 1200 and 1500 mg of analgesics a day. Increased caffeine, but not codeine, consumption was correlated with the development of CDH. Barbiturate consumption was significantly higher in patients with primary CDH (60–500 mg a day; mean 160 mg a day) than in those without primary CDH (mean < 60 mg a day). All of the triptans are associated with MOH.[115–119] Fritsche et al.[81] reported the first cases and the specific clinical features of MOH following the frequent use of zolmitriptan and naratriptan. All patients remained responsive to triptans. Six patients had never previously used triptans or ergotamine derivatives but developed drug-induced headache within 6 months of taking the drug. Four patients consumed 7.5–10 mg of zolmitriptan or 10–12 mg of naratriptan weekly. The weekly dosages necessary to initiate drug-induced headache with the centrally penetrant triptans may be lower than with ergotamines or sumatriptan and the time of onset might be shorter. Increasing attack frequency can be the first sign that drug-induced headache is developing. We recommend limiting the use of triptans to 3 days a week.

In the presence of acute medication overuse, two diagnoses (CM and MOH) are given. Many patients develop CM without overusing medication, and others continue to have daily headaches long after the overused medication has been discontinued. Medication overuse is usually motivated by a patient's desire to treat the headaches.[120] However, some headache patients may overuse combination analgesics to treat a mood disturbance.[121,122] Certain personality types may have a predilection for certain types of medication overuse, and patients with personality disorders are likely to overuse opioids.[123]

A prospective study of 98 patients investigated the pharmacologic features, such as mean critical duration until onset of MOH, mean critical monthly intake frequencies, and mean critical monthly dosages, as well as specific clinical features of MOH after overuse, of different acute headache drugs. Triptan overuse far outnumbered ergot overuse. This reflects the fact that triptans have become much more widely used than ergots. Patients with MOH from triptans often have migraine-like daily headache or a significant increase in migraine attack frequency. Furthermore, the delay between the frequent medication intake and the development of daily headache was shortest for triptans (1.7 years), longer for ergots (2.7 years), and longest for analgesics (4.8 years). The intake frequency (single dosages per month) was lowest for triptans (18 single dosages per month), higher for ergots (37 single dosages per month), and highest for analgesics (114 single dosages per month). Triptans not only cause a different spectrum of clinical features, but are able to cause MOH faster and with lower dosages than other substance groups.[93]

Some doubted the existence of MOH.[124] When Fisher[124] failed to find analgesic rebound headache in patients who were using analgesics for arthritis, he attempted to refute the concept. His work has been reinterpreted to suggest that headache-prone patients are especially vulnerable to MOH. Headache-prone patients often develop daily headaches if they are put on analgesics for a non-headache indication.[125,126] Bahra et al. found that 8/103 patients (7.6%) attending a rheumatology-monitoring clinic developed CDH with regular analgesic use. All had a history of migraine, which preceded CDH in seven patients and began about the same time as CDH in one patient. Regular use of analgesics preceded the onset of daily headache in five patients by a mean of 5.4 years (range, 2 to 10 years). Individuals with primary headache, specifically migraine, are predisposed to developing CDH in association with regular use of analgesics. [127]

In addition to exacerbating the headache disorder, acute drug overuse has other serious effects. The overuse of acute drugs may interfere with preventive headache medications' effectiveness. Prolonged use of large amounts of medication may cause renal or hepatic toxicity in addition to tolerance, habituation, or dependence. Tolerance refers to the decreased effectiveness of the same dose of an analgesic, often leading to the use of higher doses to achieve the same degree of effectiveness. Tolerance reflects receptor hyposensitivity.[128]. Habituation and dependence are, respectively, the psychological and physical need to repeatedly use drugs.

PSYCHIATRIC COMORBIDITY OF CM

Anxiety, depression, panic disorder, and bipolar disease are more frequent in migraineurs than in non-migraine control subjects.[129,130] In clinic-based samples, depression occurs in 80% of CM patients. The Minnesota Multiphasic Personality Inventory (MMPI) was abnormal in 61% of primary CDH patients, compared with 12.2% of patients with EM. Primary CDH patients had significantly higher Zung and BDI scores than did migraine controls. [28,43,83,114] Comorbid depression often improves when the cycle of daily head pain is broken. Mongini et al.[131] found that several MMPI and State and Trait Anxiety Index 2 scores decreased after headache improvement occurred, but 12 of 20 patients continued

to have a conversion V configuration on the MMPI. Many older studies do not clearly differentiate between CDH subtypes.

Mitsikostas and Thomas[132] found that headache patients had significantly higher average Hamilton rating scores for anxiety and depression (17.4 and 14.2, respectively) than did non-headache controls (6.8 and 5.7, respectively). High headache attack frequency, a long history of headaches, and female gender correlated to the Hamilton rating elevation for both anxiety and depression. Patients with CTTH, mixed headache, or drug abuse headache had the highest Hamilton rating scores for depression and anxiety.

Verri et al.[133] found current psychiatric comorbidity in 90% of primary CDH patients, 81% of migraineurs, and 83% of chronic low back pain patients (no significant differences). Generalized anxiety disorders were the most common in each group (primary CDH 69.3%, $p \leq 0.001$; migraine 59.5%, $p \leq 0.05$; chronic low back pain 65.7%, $p \leq 0.001$). The most common mood disorder in primary CDH was major depressive disorder (25%). This was significantly more frequent than dysthymia ($p \leq 0.001$) and significantly more frequent ($p \leq 0.05$) in primary CDH than in chronic low back pain patients. Somatoform disorders (including somatization, conversion disorder, and hypochondriasis) were found in 5.7% of primary CDH patients, always concomitant with anxiety and mood disorders.

Psychiatric comorbidity is a predictor of intractability. The MMPI was abnormal in 100% of patients with primary CDH who failed to respond to aggressive management (31% of the primary CDH group), compared with 48% of the responders. Physical, emotional, or sexual abuse, parental alcohol abuse, and a positive dexamethasone suppression test also correlated highly with a poor response to aggressive management.[42] Curioso et al.[134] found that 31 of 69 (45%) primary CDH patients had an adjustment disorder, 16 (23%) had major depression, 12 (17%) were dysthymic, 6 (9%) had generalized anxiety disorder, 1 (2%) was bipolar, and 3 (4%) were normal. The risk of a bad outcome after treatment was significantly greater for patients with major depression than those without. Primary CDH patients who have major depression or have abnormal BDI scores have worse outcomes at

3 to 6 months compared with patients who are not depressed.

Monzon and Lainez,[135] using the Medical Outcomes Study Short Form (SF-36) questionnaire, found that patients with primary CDH had significantly worse scores in physical functioning, role functioning (physical), bodily pain, general health perceptions, and mental health than migraineurs.[136]

Using the SF-36, Guitera et al.[137] analyzed CDH's impact on quality of life in a population sample of 1883 individuals, 4.7% of whom met the CDH criteria established by Silberstein et al.[54] Eighty-nine healthy subjects and 89 episodic migraineurs were control groups. All the concepts evaluated by the Medical Outcome Short Form (SF-36) were significantly reduced in the CDH patients compared with the healthy subjects. There were no significant differences in quality of life between TM patients and CTTH patients. TM patients had a general reduction in quality of life compared with EM patients (significant for vitality and general and mental health). CDH patients who overused analgesics scored significantly lower than non-overusers in physical role and bodily pain. CDH's impact on quality of life depends on the chronicity of the headache disorder rather than on the severity of a given attack. The impact is worse when analgesic overuse is present. CDH patients who overused analgesics scored significantly lower than did non-overusers in physical role and bodily pain.

Puca et al.[138] evaluated psychopathologic symptoms and psychiatric disorders in 234 adult CDH patients (184 women and 50 men, mean age 43.05 ± 12.90 years). The Structured Clinical Interview for the *Diagnostic and Statistical Manual of Mental Disorders-IV* and the Symptom Check List 90R were used. At least one psychiatric disorder (anxiety disorder 45%, mood disorder 33%) was detected in 66% of the sample CDH patients. The prevalence of psychopathologic symptoms was more than 78%. At least one psychosocial stress factor was found in 42% of cases, and 64% of the whole sample overused symptomatic drugs.

Wang et al.[11] looked at the quality of life of 901 headache patients in Taiwan using the SF-36. Using the Silberstein-Lipton CDH criteria, TM was diagnosed in 310 patients and CTTH in 231; 193 had EM. The patients with TM had the worst SF-36 scores. The scores of those with CTTH and those with migraine were similar.

Juang et al.[139] investigated the frequency of depressive and anxiety disorders in 261 consecutive CDH patients seen in a headache clinic. CDH subtypes were classified according to the Silberstein-Lipton criteria. A psychiatrist evaluated the patients according to the structured Mini-International Neuropsychiatric Interview to assess the comorbidity of depressive and anxiety disorders. Mean age was 46 years, and 80% of the patients were women. TM was diagnosed in 152 patients (58%) and CTTH in 92 (35%). Seventy-eight percent of patients with TM had psychiatric comorbidity, including major depression (57%), dysthymia (11%), panic disorder (30%), and generalized anxiety disorder (8%). Sixty-four percent of patients with CTTH had psychiatric diagnoses, including major depression (51%), dysthymia (8%), panic disorder (22%), and generalized anxiety disorder (1%). The frequency of anxiety disorders was significantly higher in patients with TM after controlling for age and sex. Both depressive and anxiety disorders were significantly more frequent in women. These results demonstrate that women and patients with TM are at higher risk of psychiatric comorbidity. In their most recent review of 276 consecutive patients treated on an inpatient unit, almost all of whom suffered from CDH, Lake et al. [123], found a striking presence of psychiatric comorbidity, including anxiety, depression, and cluster B personality disorders (borderline, narcissistic, antisocial).

CDH occurs in children. Guidetti et al. [140] examined the characteristics of childhood- and adolescent-onset CDH and the prevalence of psychiatric comorbidity. Eighty-six CDH patients (60 girls, 26 boys; mean age 12.3 years; SD +2.1 years, range 7 to 18 years) were compared with 100 controls (60 girls, 40 boys; mean age 10.7 years; SD +2.6 years; range 4 to 18 years). Sixty-four patients had migraine and 36 had ETTH. All subjects underwent clinical interviews and psychometric testing. CDH was diagnosed using the Silberstein criteria:[54] CTTH was present in 40% of patients, TTH plus intermittent migraine attacks in 35%, and mixed forms in 25%. Psychiatric comorbidity was present in 90% of CDH patients, 67% of migraine patients, and 25% of TTH patients.

Zwart et al.[141] reported that the odds of depression increased as headache frequency increased. They found that in comparison with control subjects without migraine, the odds of depression in migraine sufferers occurring on 7 or fewer days per month was 2.0 (1.6 to 2.5), 7–14 days per month was 4.2 (3.2 to 5.6), and 15 or more days per month was 6.4 (4.4 to 9.3).

The American Migraine Prevalence and Prevention (AMPP) study is a longitudinal, population-based, survey. Buse et al.[13] analyzed data from the 2005 survey to assess differences in sociodemographic profiles and rates of common comorbidities between two groups of respondents: CM (ICHD-2) and EM (ICHD-2). Of 24,000 headache sufferers surveyed in 2005, 655 respondents had CM, and 11,249 respondents had EM. Compared with EM, respondents with CM had statistically significant lower levels of household income, were less likely to be employed full-time, and were more likely to be occupationally disabled. Those with CM were approximately twice as likely to have depression (depression criteria were measured by a validated depression scale, a 9-item patient health questionnaire,[PHQ-9] or by self-report of a physician diagnosis) and anxiety. They were also more likely to have bipolar disorder (CM 4.6%, EM 2.8%, OR 1.56, 95% CI [1.06–2.31], p = .024).

OTHER COMORBIDITIES

Fibromyalgia (FM) and TM are common chronic pain disorders. Peres et al.[142] estimated the prevalence of FM in 101 TM patients and analyzed its relationship to depression, anxiety, and insomnia. They enrolled 101 consecutive TM patients seen at a headache clinic in São Paulo. All had normal neuroimaging and clinical examinations. TM was diagnosed according to the 1996 Silberstein-Lipton criteria.[54] FM was diagnosed according to the American College of Rheumatology diagnostic criteria.[31] FM was diagnosed in 35.6% of cases. Patients with FM had more insomnia, were older, and their headaches were more incapacitating than patients without FM. The mean BDI score was 21.1. Fifty-seven patients (87.7%) had at least mild depression. Forty-four patients (67.7%) had state score over 46, and 51 patients (78.5%) had trait score over

46. The BDI scores correlated to pain intensity (p = 0.002) and state and trait anxiety scores ($p < 0.001$). Depression, as measured by the BDI scores, was also associated with FM (p = 0.007), insomnia (p = 0.043), and disability (p = 0.05). Predictors of FM in patients with TM included insomnia (OR 10.05, 95% CI [9.03–13.55]) and depression (OR 6.8, 95% CI [4.91–8.68]).

Fatigue is a common, frequently reported symptom in many disorders, including headache. Peres et al.[143] determined the prevalence of fatigue in 63 TM patients from the São Paulo headache clinic. TM was diagnosed using the Silberstein-Lipton criteria. FM was diagnosed according to the 1990 diagnostic criteria established by the American College of Rheumatology.[144] The Fatigue Severity Scale (FSS)[145] (cutoff of 27 defined fatigue) and the Chalder fatigue scale[146] (Likert scoring)[147] were used. The Chalder fatigue scale has two parts, physical fatigue and mental fatigue. Items related to mental fatigue include difficulty concentrating, problems thinking clearly, difficulty finding the correct word, and memory problems. Those related to physical fatigue include tiredness, need to rest more, sleepiness, drowsiness, lack of energy, and weakness or decreased muscle strength. Fifty-three patients (84.1%) had FSS scores greater than 27. Forty-two patients (66.7%) met the criteria for chronic fatigue syndrome established by the Centers for Disease Control. Thirty-two patients (50.8%) met the modified criteria of the Centers for Disease Control, in which headache was eliminated as a criterion of chronic fatigue syndrome. BDI scores correlated with FSS, mental and physical fatigue scores. Trait anxiety scores also correlated with fatigue scales. Women had higher FSS scores than men, $p < 0.05$. Physical fatigue was associated with FM, $p < 0.05$. Fatigue as a symptom and chronic fatigue syndrome as a disorder were both common in TM patients.

In a clinic-based study, Bigal et al.[45] looked for risk factors associated with CDH and its subtypes. TM without MOH (in comparison with EM) was associated with allergies, asthma, hypothyroidism, hypertension, and daily caffeine consumption.

Buse et al.[13] analyzed data from the 2005 AMPP survey of CM (ICHD-2) and EM (ICHD-2). Chronic pain disorders occurred with greater frequency in CM than EM

(31.5% vs. 15.1%), as did specific pain disorders, including arthritis (CM 33.6% vs. EM 22.2%). Respiratory disorders were also more often associated with CM. Compared with EM, respondents with CM had higher rates of allergies/hay fever (CM 59.9% vs. EM 50.7%), asthma (CM 24.4% vs. EM 17.2%), and sinusitis (CM 45.2% vs. EM 37.0%). Chronic bronchitis (CM 9.2% vs. EM 4.5%), bronchitis (CM 19.2% vs. EM 13.0%), and emphysema/chronic obstructive pulmonary disease (COPD) (CM 4.9% vs. 2.6%) also occurred with greater frequency in CM respondents.

Comorbidity rates for obesity and certain cardiovascular disorders are also significantly higher in patients with CM than EM: Obesity (BMI ≥ 30): CM 25.5%; EM 21.0%). Cardiovascular disorders including heart disease/angina (CM 9.6% vs. EM 6.3%) and stroke (CM 4.0% vs. EM 2.2%) were more often associated with CM than EM). Cardiovascular risk factors including high blood pressure (CM 33.7% vs EM 27.9%), and high cholesterol (CM 34.2% vs. EM 25.6%) occurred with greater frequency in CM. There were no significant differences in the rates of low blood pressure; however, there were significant differences in the endorsement of "circulation problems/cold hands and feet" (CM 17.2% vs. EM 11.4%).

Hagen et al.[148] evaluated the association between headache and musculoskeletal symptoms in a large cross-sectional population-based study of 92,566 adults in Nord-Trondelag County in Norway. A total of 51,050 (55%) responded to questions concerning headache and musculoskeletal symptoms. The OR for muscoskeletal symptoms (including pain) increased with increasing headache frequency. CDH prevalence was more than four times higher in those with musculoskeletal symptoms than in those without. Headache prevalence was the same in individuals with widespread musculoskeletal symptoms as in those with restricted neck pain, but chronic headache was more prevalent in those with widespread symptoms (OR = 1.7). Individuals with neck pain were more likely to have headache than those with localized musculoskeletal symptoms elsewhere. In addition, there were increased musculoskeletal symptoms in migraine subjects: women < 7 headache days/month (low frequency EM), OR 1.5; 7–14 days/month (high frequency EM), OR 3.2; ≥ 15 days/month (CM), OR 5.3. For men migraine subjects: low frequency EM, OR 1.7; high-frequency EM, OR 3.2; and CM, OR 3.6. They concluded that there was a strong association between chronic headache and musculoskeletal symptoms, which may have implications for the choice of treatment.

EPIDEMIOLOGY OF CDH AND CM

In population-based surveys performed using the Silberstein-Lipton criteria, primary CDH occurred in 4.1% of Americans, 4.35% of Greeks, 3.9% of elderly Chinese, and 4.7% of Spaniards. Population-based estimates for the 1-year period prevalence of CTTH are 1.7% in Ethiopia,[149] 3% in Denmark,[150] 2.2% in Spain,[2] 2.7% in China,[3] and 2.2% in the United States.[1]

Scher et al.[1], using a validated computer-assisted telephone interview, ascertained the prevalence of CDH in 13,343 individuals aged 18–65 years in Baltimore County, Maryland. Those reporting 180 or more headaches a year were classified as having frequent headache. Three mutually exclusive subtypes of frequent headache were identified. These included TM, CTTH, and unclassified frequent headache. The overall prevalence of CDH was 4.1% (5.0% women, 2.8% men; 1.8:1 women to men ratio). In both men and women, prevalence was highest in the lowest educational category. More than half (52% women, 56% men) met criteria for CTTH (2.2%), almost one-third (33% women, 25% men) met criteria for TM (1.3%), and the remainder (15% women, 19% men) were unclassified (0.6%). Overall, 30% of women and 25% of men who were frequent headache sufferers met IHS criteria for migraine (with or without aura). On the basis of chance, migraine and CTTH would co-occur in 0.22% of the population; the fact that TM occurred in 1.3% of this population would suggest that their co-occurrence is more than random.

Castillo et al.[2] sampled 2252 subjects older than 14 years in Cantalucia, Spain. Overall, 4.7% had CDH. Using the criteria of Silberstein et al.[15], none had HC, 0.1% had NDPH, 2.2% had CTTH, and 2.4% had

TM. Nineteen percent of CTTH patients and 31.1% of TM patients had a history of acute medication overuse. Eight patients had a previous history of migraine without aura and now had primary CDH with the characteristics of TTH only. These headaches met the criteria of CM but could have been migraine and coincidental CTTH.

In August 1993, Wang et al.[3] looked at the characteristics of primary CDH in a population of elderly Chinese (over 65 years of age) in two townships on Kinmen Island. Seventy-seven percent of the eligible population (1533/2003) participated. Sixty patients (3.9%) had CDH. Significantly more women than men had primary CDH (5.6% and 1.8%, $p < 0.001$). Of the primary CDH patients, 42 (70%) had CTTH, 15 (25%) had CM, and 3 (5%) had other CDH. Only 23% of patients had consulted a physician for headache in the previous year.

Lu et al.[151] conducted a two-stage population-based headache survey among subjects aged ≥ 15 in Taipei, Taiwan. Subjects who had had CDH in the past year were identified, interviewed, and followed up. CDH was defined as headache frequency of more than 15 days a month, with a duration of more than 4 hours a day. Of the 3377 participants, 108 (3.2%) fulfilled the criteria for CDH, with a higher prevalence in women (4.3%) than men (1.9%). TM was the most common subtype (55%), followed by CTTH (44%). Thirty-four percent of the CDH subjects overused analgesics.

Natoli et al.[23] summarized population-based studies reporting prevalence and/or incidence of CM and explored variation across studies. A systematic literature search was conducted. Sixteen publications representing 12 studies were accepted. The prevalence of CM was 0–5.1%, with estimates typically in the range of 1.4–2.2%. Seven studies used Silberstein-Lipton criteria (or equivalent), with prevalence ranging from 0.9% to 5.1%. Three estimates used migraine that occurred ≥ 15 days per month, with prevalence ranging from 0 to 0.7%. Prevalence varied by World Health Organization region and gender. The Americas had the highest prevalence of CM, with estimates up to 5.1%, but also had the largest variation across studies (1.3–5.1%).[152] The French GRIM2000 study examined three different definitions of migraine and/or migrainous disorder and found that the prevalence

ranged from 0.86% to 2.14% depending on the relative stringency of migraine definition used,[6] and three additional European studies used relatively strict criteria that required ≥ 15 migraines per month, similar to the ICHD-2, reporting very low prevalence estimates ranging from 0 to 0.7%.[153–155] Although true differences in CM prevalence may exist across countries, it is also likely that diagnostic criteria may be interpreted or applied differently.

Staube et al. analyzed the data of the German DMKG headache study, which included 7417 adults in three regions of Germany. Using the IHS definition from 2004, chronic migraine was diagnosed in 0.2% of the population. Half of these patients also fulfilled the criteria of MOH. The distribution of migraine attacks per subject was highly skewed, with only 14% of all migraine patients having more than six migraine attacks per month. Patients with CM or MOH were more often active smokers than were controls without headache. A body mass index of > 30 was present significantly more often in patients with MOH than in controls or in patients with EM.[156]

Katsavera et al. field tested different CM criteria and compared CM epidemiological profiles, which include demographic, personal, and lifestyle characteristics, with high-frequency EM (HFEM) and low-frequency EM (LFEM). They used data from the population-based survey of the German Headache Consortium (GHC) study. The GHC study was designed to investigate the prevalence and incidence of headaches within the general population of Germany from 2003 to 2005. Questionnaires were mailed to a random sample of 18,000 individuals aged 18–65 years in demographically diverse regions of Germany. Three case definitions were used for CM classification: ICHD-2, ICHD-2R, and Silberstein-Lipton (S-L) criteria. Among 9350 respondents, the prevalence of any headache occurring on ≥ 15 days per month was 2.9%. CM prevalence was lowest with ICHD-2, the most restrictive ($n = 37$, 0.4%), followed by ICHD-2R ($n = 45$, 0.5%) and S-L ($n = 185$, 2.0%). CM groups did not differ in distribution by age, gender, body mass index, education, or smoking and alcohol consumption. Compared to those with LFEM and HFEM, those with CM (S-L) had significantly different epidemiological profiles. CM prevalence varies by case definition. The epidemiological profiles of the three CM groups are similar but differ significantly from those of HFEM and LFEM.[22]

Buse et al. estimated the prevalence and distribution of CM in the US population and compared the age- and sex-specific profiles of headache-related disability in persons with CM and EM in the American Migraine Prevalence and Prevention (AMPP) Study. They mailed surveys to a sample of 120,000 US households selected to represent the US population. Data on headache frequency, symptoms, sociodemographics, and headache-related disability (using the Migraine Disability Assessment Scale) were obtained. Modified Silberstein-Lipton criteria were used to classify CM (meeting ICHD-2 criteria for migraine with a headache frequency of ≥ 15 days over the preceding 3 months). Surveys were returned by 162,756 individuals aged > 12 years; 19,189 individuals (11.79%) met ICHD-2 criteria for migraine (17.27% of females; 5.72% of males), and 0.91% met criteria for CM (1.29% of females; 0.48% of males). Relative to 12–17-year-olds, the age- and sex-specific prevalence for CM peaked in the forties at 1.89% for females and 0.79% for males. CM represented 7.68% of migraine cases overall, and the proportion generally increased with age. CM prevalence was inversely related to annual household income. Lower income groups had higher rates of CM. Individuals with CM had greater headache-related disability than those with EM and were more likely to be in the highest Migraine Disability Assessment Scale (37.96% vs. 9.50%, respectively). Headache-related disability was highest among females with CM compared with males. They concluded that in the US population, the prevalence of CM was nearly 1%. CM prevalence was highest among females, in mid-life, and in households with the lowest annual income.[157]

Risk Factors for CDH

Wang et al.[3] ascertained that significant risk factors for CDH (Table 9.10) included analgesic overuse (OR 79), a history of migraine (OR 6.6), and a Geriatric Depression Scale-Short Form score of 8 or above (OR 2.6). At follow-up, patients with persistent primary CDH had a significantly higher frequency of analgesic overuse (33% vs. 0%, p = 0.03) and major depression (38% vs. 0%, p = 0.04).

Table 9.10 **Risk Factors for CDH**

1. High headache frequency
2. Female gender
3. Obesity (BMI > 30)
4. Snoring
5. Stressful life events
6. High caffeine consumption
7. Acute medication overuse
8. Depression
9. Head trauma
10. History of migraine
11. Less than a high school education

Granella et al.[158] found that risk factors that were associated with the evolution of migraine without aura into TM included head trauma (OR 3.3), analgesic use with every attack (OR 2.8), and long duration of oral contraceptive use.

Scher et al.[159] described factors that predict CDH onset and remission in an adult population. Potential cases (180+ headaches per year, n = 1134) and controls (2 to 104 headaches per year, n = 798) (the maximum days/month is on average less than 9) were interviewed two times over an average 11 months of follow-up. Factors associated with CDH prevalence at baseline were evaluated. CDH was more common in women (OR 1.65 [1.3–2.0]), those previously married (OR 1.5 [1.2–1.9]), with obesity (BMI > 30; OR 1.27 [1.0–1.7]), and those with less education. Obesity, high baseline headache frequency, high caffeine consumption, habitual daily snoring, and stressful life events were significantly associated with new-onset CDH.[160] Snoring was a risk factor independent of headache type, sleep apnea, male gender, obesity, and increased age.[161] In a population study from the Netherlands, sleeping problems in general were also associated with CDH.[162]

In a case control study, Scher et al. looked at the association between high caffeine use (defined as being in the top quartile for dietary caffeine use or the use of a caffeine-containing medication for headache as a preferred treatment) with CDH. Pre-CDH (not current) use of caffeine was found to be a modest risk factor (OR 1.5). Pre-CDH caffeine consumption as a risk factor was most evident for those < 40 (OR 3.4), women (OR 1.9) and those with chronic episodic (vs. chronic continuous) headache (OR 1.8).[163]

Having less than a high school education was associated with a threefold increased risk of CDH (OR3.56 [2.3–5.6]).[159] At follow-up, 3% of the controls reported 180 or more headaches per year. Obesity and baseline headache frequency were significantly associated with new onset CDH. In CDH cases, the projected 1-year remission rate to less than one headache per week was 14% and to less than 180 headaches per year was 57%. A better prognosis was associated with higher education, non-white race, being married, and with diagnosed diabetes. Individuals with less than a high-school education, whites, and those who were previously married had a higher risk of CDH at baseline and reduced likelihood of remission at follow-up. New onset CDH was associated with baseline headache frequency and obesity. Existing (but not new onset) CDH was also associated with a self-reported physician diagnosis of arthritis (OR 2.50) or diabetes (OR 1.51). [164].

Bigal and Lipton assessed the influence of the body mass index (BMI) on the prevalence and severity of CDH and its most frequent subtypes, TM and CTTH, using a computer-assisted telephone interview. Among 30,215 participants, the prevalence of CDH was 4.1%; 1.3% had TM and 2.8% CTTH. In contrast with the normal weight group (3.9%), the prevalence of CDH was higher in obese (5.0%) and morbidly obese (6.8%) patients. BMI had a strong influence on the prevalence of TM, which ranged from 0.9% of the normal weighted to 1.2% of the overweight, 1.6% of the obese, and 2.5% of the morbidly obese. Adjusted analyses showed that obesity was associated with CDH and TM but not CTTH. They concluded that CDH and obesity are associated. Obesity is a stronger risk factor for TM than for CTTH.[165]

Katsarava et al. followed 532 consecutive patients with EM (< 15 days/month) for one year. Sixty-four patients (14%) developed chronic headache (≥ 15 days/month). The odds ratios for developing CDH were 20.1, comparing patients with a "critical" (10–14 days/month) versus "low" headache frequency (0–4 days/month); 6.2 in patients with an "intermediate" (6–9 days/month) versus "low" headache frequency; and 19.4 comparing patients with and without medication overuse. Incidence rates were much higher (14%) than in the Scher study, which eliminated patients who had migraine 10–14 days/month.[166]

Zwart et al.[167] examined the relationship between analgesic use at baseline and the subsequent risk of chronic pain (≥ 15 days/month) and the risk of analgesic overuse in a population-based study. In total, 32,067 adults reported the use of analgesics from 1984 to 1986 and at follow-up 11 years later (1995 to 1997). The risk ratios (RR) of chronic pain and of analgesic overuse in the different diagnostic groups (i.e., migraine, non-migrainous headache, and neck pain) were estimated in relation to analgesic consumption at baseline. Individuals who reported use of analgesics daily or weekly at baseline showed significant increased risk for having chronic pain at follow-up. The risk was most evident for chronic migraine (RR 13.3, 95% CI [9.3–19.1]), intermediate for chronic non-migrainous headaches (RR 6.2, 95% CI [5.0–7.7]), and lowest for chronic neck pain (RR 2.4, 95% CI [2.0–2.8]). Among subjects with chronic pain associated with analgesic overuse, the RR was 37.6 (95% CI [21.3–66.4]) for chronic migraine, 14.4 (95% CI [10.4–19.9]) for chronic non-migrainous headaches, and 7.1 for chronic neck pain (95% CI [5.5–9.2]). The RR for chronic headache (migraine and non-migrainous headache combined) associated with analgesic overuse was 19.6 (95% CI [14.8–25.9]) compared with 3.1 (95% CI [2.4–4.2]) for those without overuse. Analgesic overuse strongly predicts chronic pain and chronic pain associated with analgesic overuse 11 years later, especially among those with chronic migraine.

Hagen et al. estimated incidences of and identified risk factors for developing CDH and MOH in a longitudinal population-based cohort study that used data from the Nord-Trøndelag Health Surveys performed in 1995–1997 and 2006–2008. Among the 51,383 participants at baseline, 41,766 were eligible approximately 11 years later. There were 26,197 participants (responder rate 63%), among whom 25,596 did not report CDH at baseline in 1995–1997. Of these, 201 (0.8%) had MOH and 246 (1.0%) had CDH without medication overuse (CDHwoMOH) 11 years later. The incidence of MOH was 0.72 per 1000 person-years (95% CI [0.62–0.81]). In the multivariate analyses, a fivefold risk for developing MOH was found among individuals who at baseline reported regular use of tranquilizers (OR

5.2 [3.0–9.0]) or who had a combination of chronic musculoskeletal complaints, gastrointestinal complaints, and Hospital Anxiety and Depression Scale score P11 (OR 4.7 [2.4–9.0]). Smoking and physical inactivity more than doubled the risk of MOH. In contrast, these factors did not increase the risk of CDHwoO. In this large population-based 11-year follow-up study, several risk factors for MOH did not increase the risk for CDHwoO, suggesting that these are pathogenetically distinct. If the noted associations are causal, more focus on comorbid condition, physical activity, and use of tobacco and tranquilizers may limit the development of MOH.[168]

Couch et al. studied a US population sample from the Frequent Headache Epidemiology Study. Cases with CDH (≥ 180 headaches/year) and a comparison group with episodic headache (2 to 102 headaches/year) were identified. Twenty percent of male cases reported a head or neck injury the same year or the year before CDH onset (OR 3.3) The association between head or neck injury and CDH was marginally significant for women (OR 2.4). The relationship between head or neck injury and CDH did not appear to be strongly related to the proximity of the injury; that is, the risk of CDH was increased in individuals with life-time injuries to the head or neck, even if the injuries were remote to the onset of CDH. Furthermore, the severity of the injury—assessed by whether the subject reported fainting or loss of consciousness—was not related to CDH. These results suggest that head and neck injury accounts for approximately 15% of CDH cases in this non-clinical population. The lifetime risk of CDH increases with an increasing number of head and neck injuries.[169]

Non-modifiable risk factors for CDH include female sex, older age, low socioeconomic status, and non-married status. Potentially modifiable risk factors for CDH include obesity, snoring and sleep problems, comorbid pain conditions, head or neck injury, major life events, smoking, acute medication overuse, and possibly caffeine intake.[170]

PATHOPHYSIOLOGY OF CM

The pathophysiology of migraine, CM, and MOH has been discussed in Chapter 5. Recent work suggests several mechanisms that involve more than one level of the CNS contribute to the development of CM. These include the following:

1. increased peripheral nociceptive activation (perhaps due to chronic neurogenic inflammation) and activation of silent nociceptors;
2. peripheral sensitization;
3. altered sensory neuron excitability due to changes in ion-channel expression, phosphorylation, and accumulation in primary afferents;
4. central sensitization of TNC neurons due to post-translational changes in ligand- and voltage-gated ion-channel kinetics, altering excitability and strength of their synaptic inputs;
5. phenotype modulation due to alterations in the expression of receptors/transmitters/ion channels in peripheral and central neurons;
6. synaptic reorganization modification of synaptic connections caused by cell death or sprouting;
7. decreased pain modulation due to loss of local and descending input;[171] or
8. a combination of these.

Activity-independent sensitization is a possible cause of the development of CM. Such sensitization might occur during repeated migraine attacks through impaired descending inhibition and/or enhanced descending facilitation of nociception. Evidence now exists that central sensitization, defined by the presence of cutaneous allodynia, exists in CDH, including TM with and without medication overuse. [172–174]

Functional imaging studies have demonstrated abnormal brainstem activation in episodic and chronic migraine, suggesting that dysfunction of descending inhibitory pathways might facilitate migraine attacks. Functional imaging studies have also demonstrated interictal hypofunction of lateral descending pain modulatory circuits in patients with migraine.[175]

Enhanced cortical excitability, exceeding that in patients with EM or in migraine-free controls, has also been demonstrated in individuals with chronic migraine. Whether this is due to intrinsically increased excitability or to impaired intracortical inhibitory mechanisms is unclear. Overuse of acute pain medications has a major role in the development of headaches resembling chronic migraine. Animal models have revealed persistent pronociceptive adaptations following exposure to opioids and triptans, resulting in enhanced sensitivity to stimuli that trigger migraine in humans. These findings could provide insight into the adaptive changes that occur in patients who have chronic migraine associated with medication overuse, and thus further elucidate the pathophysiology of chronic migraine.

TREATMENT

Overview

Patients with CM can be difficult to treat, especially when the disorder is complicated by medication overuse, comorbid psychiatric disease, low frustration tolerance, and physical and emotional dependency.[16,114] We recommend the following steps. First, exclude secondary headache disorders; second, rule out other primary headache disorders (CTTH, HC, or NDPH); and third, identify comorbid medical and psychiatric conditions and exacerbating factors, especially medication overuse. Limit acute medications (with the possible exception of the long-acting NSAIDs and DHE). Patients should be started on preventive medication (to decrease reliance on acute medication), with the explicit understanding that the drugs may not become fully effective until medication overuse has been eliminated [102]. Some patients need to have their headache cycle terminated.[102] Patients require education and continuous support during this process. Outpatient detoxification options, including outpatient infusion in an ambulatory infusion unit, are available. If outpatient treatment proves difficult or is dangerous, hospitalization may be required.[8,176]

In some cases, CDH reverts to episodic headache when preventive medication is initiated and acute medications are limited. In other cases, there may be only moderate or no improvement. Zeeberg et al. described the treatment outcomes in patients withdrawn from medication overuse. They studied 337 outpatients who were diagnosed with MOH and were treated and dismissed from the Danish Headache Centre in 2002 and 2003.

A 46% decrease in headache frequency from the first visit to dismissal occurred ($p < 0.0001$). Patients with no improvement 2 months after complete drug withdrawal ($n = 88$) subsequently responded to pharmacologic and/or non-pharmacologic prophylaxis, with a 26% decrease in headache frequency as measured from the end of withdrawal to dismissal. At dismissal, 47% of patients were on prophylaxis. In this population, about half of MOH patients benefit from drug withdrawal alone.[177]

Contradicting the belief that patients with MOH need withdrawal of acute headache medication before they respond to prophylactic medication is the study by Hagen et al. [178] In a 1-year open-label, multicenter study, ITT analyses were performed on 56 patients with MOH. These were randomly assigned to receive prophylactic treatment from the start without detoxification, undergo a standard outpatient detoxification program without prophylactic treatment from the start, or no specific treatment (5-month follow-up). The primary outcome measure, change in headache days per month, did not differ significantly among groups. However, the prophylaxis group had the greatest decrease in headache days compared with baseline, and also a significantly more pronounced reduction in total headache index at months 3 ($p = 0.003$) and 12 ($p = 0.017$) compared with the withdrawal group. At month 12, 53% of patients in the prophylaxis group had > 50% reduction in monthly headache dayscompared with 25% in the withdrawal group ($p = 0.081$).[178]

Hagen et al. then evaluated the long-term outcome in 61 patients with MOH who 4 years previously had been included in a randomized open-label prospective multicenter study. Sixty patients still alive after 4 years were invited to a follow-up investigation. Fifty patients (83%) participated. At follow-up, the 50 had a mean reduction of 6.5 headache days/month ($p = 0.001$) and 9.5 acute headache medication days/month ($p = 0.001$) compared with baseline. Sixteen persons (32%) were considered responders due to a C>50% reduction inheadache frequency from baseline, whereas 17 persons (34%) met the criteria for MOH. None of the baseline characteristics consistently influenced all five outcome measures. At 4-year follow-up, one-third of the 50 MOH patients had C50% reduction in headache frequency from baseline. A low total Hospital Anxiety and

Depression Scale score at baseline was associated with the most favorable outcome.[179]

Diener et al. reviewed the results from two similarly designed, randomized, placebo controlled, multicenter studies of CM that were conducted in the United States and the European Union of the efficacy and safety of topiramate for the treatment of CM in patient populations both with and without MO. Topiramate was effective for the treatment of patients with CM.[180,181]

The intent-to-treat (ITT) population in the US study consisted of 306 subjects (topiramate, $n = 153$; placebo, $n = 153$); the ITT population in the EU study consisted of 59 subjects (topiramate, $n = 32$; placebo, $n = 27$).[180] A post hoc analysis in the subset of patients with MO in the US trial trended toward significance but did not reach a statistical difference between topiramate and placebo in the reduction in migraine/migrainous days ($p = 0.059$). In the EU trial, topiramate-treated patients with MO experienced a significant reduction in the mean number of migraine days versus placebo treatment ($p = 0.03$). There were several key differences between the patient populations. In the US trial, 115 of 306 (37.6%) subjects versus 46 of 59 (78%) subjects in the EU trial reported using acute medications for migraine that met the definitions of MO during the 28-day prospective baseline period. In the US trial, the most commonly overused medications were triptans and analgesics—40% of subjects overused non-steroidal anti-inflammatories and 6% overused opioids. In the EU trial, the vast majority of overused medications were triptans. Butalbital-containing analgesics were allowed in the US trial, but no butalbital-containing analgesics were available or prescribed in the EU trial.[182]

OnabotulinumtoxinA was investigated in patients with chronic migraine in two placebo-controlled trials.[51,64] Patients were prospectively stratified who overused acute medications or not (labeling these subgroups as "medication overuse yes/no") based on patient-reported frequency of acute medication use during the 28-day baseline period and not based on a diagnosis of medication overuse headache (ICHD-2 8.2). Silberstein et al. analyzed a subgroup of patients with medication overuse in the two PREEMPT trials.[183] Of 1384 patients, 65.3% ($n = 904$) were assigned to the "medication overuse-yes" stratum. Most of the patients overused triptans or combination analgesics; very few (1.7%) overused opioids. For the subgroup of patients with medication overuse, onabotulinumtoxinA was superior to placebo for most efficacy endpoints.[183]

Patients can have severe exacerbations of their migraine during detoxification. Thus patients, even if they are on preventive medication, often need additional treatment (which we call *headache terminators*) to break the cycle of CDH and/or to help with the exacerbation that occurs when overused medications are discontinued. Terminators can be given orally, by suppository, or by injection, and some can be given intravenously repetitively. The route of administration depends on both the setting and the intensity of treatment.

Patients need education and continuous support during this process. Disturbances in mood and function are common and require management with behavioral methods of pain management and supportive psychotherapy. Treatment of coexistent psychiatric illness is often necessary before CM comes under control. Chronobiologic interventions, such as encouraging regular habits of sleep, exercise, and meals, are often useful.[102]

Psychophysiologic therapy involves reassurance, counseling, stress management, relaxation therapy, biofeedback, and cognitive behavioral therapy. The use of traditional acupuncture is controversial and has not proved more effective than placebo.[184] Physical therapy consists of modality treatments (heat, cold packs, ultrasound, and electrical stimulation); improvement of posture through stretching, exercise, and traction; trigger point injections; occipital nerve blocks; and a program of regular exercise and stretching.[185] It has been our experience that treating painful trigger areas in the neck can result in the improvement of intractable CDH.

Patients who are overusing acute medication may not become fully responsive to acute and preventive treatment for 2 to 10 weeks after medication overuse is eliminated, and some may never fully respond (especially with opioids). Withdrawal symptoms include severely exacerbated headaches accompanied by nausea, vomiting, agitation, restlessness, sleep disorder, and (rarely) seizures. Barbiturates, opioids, and benzodiazepine, unless replaced with long-acting derivatives, must be tapered to avoid a serious withdrawal syndrome. The washout period may last 3 to 8 weeks; once it is over, considerable headache improvement frequently occurs.[43,53,89,186]

Outpatient treatment in an ambulatory infusion unit and home treatment options are available. If outpatient treatment proves difficult or is dangerous, hospitalization may be required.[123,187] Diener et al.[188] were able to detoxify only 1.5% of 200 patients on an outpatient basis. Hering and Steiner,[189] in contrast, successfully used outpatient detoxification in 37 of 46 patients who were taking simple analgesics or ergotamine. A recent consensus paper by the German Migraine Society recommends outpatient withdrawal for highly motivated patients who do not take barbiturates or tranquilizers with their analgesics. Inpatient treatment is recommended for patients who fail outpatient treatment, have high depression scores, or take tranquilizers, codeine, or barbiturates.[190] Hospitalization may be necessary for severe dehydration, for which inpatient parenteral therapy may be necessary; diagnostic suspicion (confirmed by appropriate diagnostic testing) of organic etiology; prolonged, unrelenting headache with associated symptoms, such as nausea and vomiting, which, if allowed to continue, would pose a further threat to the patient's welfare; status migraine; dependence on analgesics, ergots, opiates, barbiturates, or tranquilizers; pain that is accompanied by serious adverse reactions or complications from therapy wherein continued use of such therapy aggravates or induces further illness; pain that occurs in the presence of significant medical disease but appropriate treatment of headache symptom aggravates or induces further illness; failed

Table 9.11 Criteria for Hospitalization

I. Emergency or Urgent Admission
    A. Certain migraine variants (e.g., hemiplegic migraine, suspected migrainous infarction, basilar migraine with serious neurologic symptoms such as syncope, confusional migraine, etc.)
        1. When a diagnosis has not been established during a previous similar occurrence
        2. When a patient's established outpatient treatment plan has failed
    B. Diagnostic suspicion of infectious disorder involving CNS (e.g., brain abscess, meningitis) with initiation of appropriate diagnostic testing
    C. Diagnostic suspicion of acute vascular compromise (e.g., aneurysm, subarachnoid hemorrhage, carotid dissection) with initiation of appropriate diagnostic testing
    D. Diagnostic suspicion of a structural disorder causing symptoms requiring an acute setting (e.g., brain tumor, increased intracranial pressure) with initiation of appropriate diagnostic testing
    E. Low cerebrospinal fluid headache when an outpatient blood patch has failed and an outpatient treatment plan has failed or there is no obvious cause
    F. Medical emergency presenting with a severe headache
    G. Severe headache associated with intractable nausea and vomiting producing dehydration or postural hypotension, or unable to retain oral medication, and unable to be controlled in an outpatient setting or with admission to observation status
    H. Failed outpatient treatment of an exacerbation of episodic headache disorder with
        1. Failure to respond to "rescue" or backup medications or
        2. Failure to respond to outpatient treatment with IV DHE on a schedule of a minimum of twice daily
II. Non-emergent Admission
    A. Coexistent psychiatric disease documented by psychologic or psychiatric evaluation with sufficient severity of illness such that a failure to admit could pose a health risk to the patient or impair the implementation of outpatient treatment
    B. Coexistent or risk of disease (e.g., unstable angina, unstable diabetes, recent transient ischemic attack, myocardial infarction in the past 6 months, renal failure, hypertension, age > 65) necessitating monitoring for treatment of headache significant enough to warrant admission
    C. Severe chronic daily headaches involving chronic medication overuse when there is
        1. Daily use of potent opioids and/or barbiturates
        2. Daily use of triptans, simple analgesics, or ergotamine in a patient with a documented failed trial of withdrawal of these medications.
    D. Impaired daily functioning (e.g., threatened relationships, many lost days at work or school due to headache), with a failure to respond to 2 days of outpatient treatment with IV DHE, IV neuroleptics, or IV corticosteroids on a schedule of a minimum of twice daily or equivalent treatment

outpatient detoxification, for which inpatient pain and psychiatric management may be necessary; or treatment requiring co-pharmacy with drugs that may cause a drug interaction, thus necessitating careful observation (monoamine oxidase inhibitors and ß-blockers). We have proposed guidelines for hospitalization (Table 9.11).

Acute Pharmacotherapy

Choice of acute treatment depends upon the diagnosis (see Chapter 7). CM patients, who by definition are not overusing acute medication, can treat acute migrainous headache exacerbations with antimigraine drugs, including triptans and DHE, or NSAIDs. These drugs must be strictly limited to prevent superimposed MOH that will complicate treatment and require detoxification. The risk of MOH is much lower for DHE and triptans than for analgesics, opioids, and ergotamine. CTTH and NDPH can be treated with nonspecific headache medications, and HC can be treated with supplemental doses of indomethacin.

Preventive Pharmacotherapy

Patients with very frequent headaches should be treated primarily with preventive medications (see Chapter 8), with the explicit understanding that their medications may not become fully effective until the overused medication has been eliminated. It may take 3 to 6 weeks for treatment effects to develop. However, some patients remain refractory.[191]

The following principles guide the use of preventive treatment:

1. From among the first-line drugs, choose preventive agents based on their adverse event (AE) profiles, comorbid and coexistent conditions, and specific indications (e.g., indomethacin for HC).
2. Start at a low dose.
3. Gradually increase the dose until you achieve efficacy, the patient develops side effects, or the ceiling dose for the drug in question is reached.
4. Treatment effects develop over weeks and treatment may not become fully effective until rebound is eliminated.
5. If one agent fails and if all other things are equal, choose an agent from another therapeutic class.
6. Prefer monotherapy, but be willing to use combination therapy.
7. Communicate realistic expectations.[192]

Most preventive agents used for primary CDH have not been examined in well-designed double-blind studies. Table 9.12 summarizes an assessment of the efficacy, safety, and evidence for a number of agents.[102]

Antidepressants

Antidepressants are attractive agents for use in primary CDH, since many patients have comorbid depression and anxiety. The most widely used tricyclic antidepressants are nortriptyline (Aventyl, Pamelor), amitriptyline (Elavil), which has been effective in many but not all studies[193–205] and doxepin (Sinequan).[206] Descombes et al. [207] assessed the effects of amitriptyline and sudden analgesic withdrawal on headache frequency and quality of life in patients suffering from MOH related to analgesic abuse. Seventeen non-depressed patients with MOH were included in a 9-week, parallel-group, randomized, double-blind, placebo-controlled study. After abrupt analgesic withdrawal, amitriptyline or an active placebo (trihexyphenidyl) was started. The primary efficacy variable was headache frequency recorded on a headache diary in the last 4 weeks of each treatment. Headache frequency decreased by 45% in the amitriptyline group and by 28% in the trihexyphenidyl group. Amitriptyline enhanced all dimensions of quality of life and significantly improved emotional reaction and social isolation. Fluoxetine (Prozac), a selective serotonin reuptake inhibitor (SSRI), is coming into wider use for daily headaches; evidence from a double-blind study demonstrates its efficacy in CDH.[193,208] The combination of fluoxetine and amitriptyline was not more effective than amitriptyline alone. Krymchantowski et al. [209] evaluated the efficacy and tolerability of combined treatment with amitriptyline (20

Table 9.12 Summary of Prophylactic Drugs for Use in Chronic Migraine

Drug	Clinical Efficacy	Adverse Events	Clinical Evidence*
ANTIDEPRESSANTS			
Amitriptyline	+++	++	++
Duloxetine/ Venlafaxine	+++	+	++
Fluoxetine	+	+	++
ANTICONVULSANTS			
Divalproex	+++	++	++
Gabapentin	++	++	++
Topiramate	+++	++	++++
ß-BLOCKERS			
Propranolol, Nadolol, etc.	++	+	+
CALCIUM CHANNEL BLOCKERS			
Verapamil	++	+	+
MISCELLANEOUS			
Anabotulinum toxin A	++++	+	++++

All categories are rated from + to ++++ based on a combination of published literature and clinical experience. °Ratings of +++ for clinical evidence indicate at least one double-blind, placebo-controlled study. A rating of ++ indicates open well-designed studies and + indicates ratings based on clinical experience. A rating of ++++ requires at least two double-blind placebo-controlled trials.

mg bid) and fluoxetine (20 mg bid) compared with amitriptyline alone for CDH due to TM. Thirty-nine patients, 26 women and 13 men, aged 20–69 years, who fulfilled the Silberstein-Lipton criteria for TM were prospectively studied. The mean difference between the initial and final (9 weeks) headache index was 513.5 (p < .0005) for group 1 and 893 (p < .0017) for group 2. Fluvoxamine appears to be effective[210] and may have analgesic properties.[211] Other SSRIs, including paroxetine[212] and monoamine oxidase inhibitors, may have a therapeutic role, but this has not been proven to date.[213] Venlafaxine and Duloxetine, selective serotonin and norepinephrine reuptake inhibitors, may be effective for migraine, but no data exist for CM (see Chapter 8).

Beta-blockers (propranolol, nadolol) remain a mainstay of therapy for migraine[102] and are used for CM.[199,214] Clinicians fear that ß-blockers may exacerbate depression; however, this issue is controversial.[215] ß-blockers are relatively contraindicated in patients who have asthma and Raynaud's disease.

Anti-epileptic Drugs

The anticonvulsant divalproex sodium (Depakote)[216] is effective in migraine prevention.[216–219] Smaller open studies support its utility in CM.[220] In an open-label study, Edwards et al.[221] assessed the possible benefit of sodium valproate in 20 consecutive CDH patients whose headaches were refractory to multiple standard treatments. Eleven (55%) had a response (mild or no headaches within 1–4 weeks). The doses ranged from 375 mg to 1500 mg a day. Two patients (10%) discontinued medication due to side effects (nausea and difficulty thinking). Frietag et al.[222] assessed the safety and efficacy of divalproex sodium in the long-term treatment of CDH in a retrospective chart review of 642 patients treated with divalproex sodium for CDH. The mean improvement was 47%, with an improvement in migraine of about 65%. At least a 50% reduction in headache frequency was reported by 93 of the 138 patients who received treatment with only divalproex sodium. Approximately 35% of the patients experienced AEs, none of which was severe. Yurekli et al.[223] assessed the efficacy of sodium valproate in the treatment of chronic daily headache (both CM and CTTH) in a study of 70 patients. Sodium valproate was superior to placebo for a number of outcome parameters, such as general and maximum pain levels, and pain frequency. Gabapentin, structurally related to gamma-aminobutyric acid (GABA), is effective in a number of chronic pain conditions. Spira et al.[224] studied gabapentin in the treatment of CDH in a placebo-controlled study. Gabapentin was significantly superior to placebo for the primary efficacy variable for CDH prophylaxis, with a 9.1% difference in headache-free rates. Other measures were also significantly better with gabapentin, including headache-free days/months, severity, and quality of life. However, this study had limitations. First, it did not subclassify CDH. The study preceded the new IHS criteria, but did not use the Silberstein-Lipton criteria for the diagnosis of CDH subtypes. Second, the study did not take into account acute medication overuse, which is a major confounding factor in both treatment and interpretation of treatment results. Third, although the results were significant, they were modest (9.1% difference in headache-free days) and may not be clinically important. Future CDH studies require subset analysis and control for acute medication overuse.[225]

Topiramate, a D-fructose derivative, is effective in EM prevention. Shuaib et al.[226] treated 37 patients who had more than 10 migraine headaches a month with topiramate (25–100 mg a day) in an open-label study. Most patients had CDH in addition to migraine; all had failed previous preventive treatment. Over a 3- to 9-month follow-up, 11 patients (30%) had an excellent result (headache frequency decreased by over 60%), 11 patients had a good result (headache frequency decreased 40%–60%), three patients discontinued therapy due to side effects, and eight patients had no improvement. This uncontrolled study suggests that topiramate may be useful for CM. A small placebo-controlled trial of topiramate in patients with CM was also positive.

Two separate studies in Europe and the United States showed that topiramate at a dose of 100 mg daily was effective as a preventive therapy for chronic migraine.[180,181] The key difference between the two studies was that patients were allowed to take acute rescue medication as usual in the European trial,[181] but not in the US trial.[180]

Silberstein et al.[180] evaluated the efficacy and safety of topiramate (100 mg/d) compared with placebo for the treatment of CM. This was a randomized, placebo-controlled, parallel group, multicenter study consisting of 16 weeks of double-blind treatment. Subjects aged 18–65 years with 15 or more headache days per month (at least half of which were migraine/migrainous headaches) were 1:1 randomized to either topiramate 100 mg/d or placebo. Concomitant preventive migraine treatment was not allowed and acute headache medication use was not to exceed 4 days per week during the double-blind maintenance period. The intent-to-treat population included 306 of 328 randomized subjects who provided at least one efficacy assessment. Topiramate treatment resulted in a statistically significant mean reduction of migraine/migrainous headache days (topiramate –6.4 vs. placebo –4.7, $p = 0.010$) and migraine headache days relative to baseline (topiramate –5.6 vs. placebo –4.1, $p = 0.032$). Discontinuations due to AEs occurred in 18 (10.9%) topiramate subjects and 10 (6.1%) placebo subjects. There were no serious AEs or deaths. Topiramate treatment at daily doses of approximately 100 mg resulted in statistically significant improvements compared with placebo in migraine/migrainous and migraine headache days. Safety and tolerability of topiramate was consistent with experience in previous clinical trials.

Diener et al. evaluated topiramate for the prevention of CM in a randomized, double-blind, placebo controlled trial. Patients (18–65 years) who experienced CM (defined as > 15 monthly migraine days) for > 3 months prior to trial entry were randomized to topiramate or placebo for a 16-week, double-blind trial. Existing migraine preventive treatments, except for anti-epileptic drugs, were continued throughout the trial. The primary efficacy measure was the change in number of migraine days from the 28-day baseline phase to the last 28 days of the double-blind phase in the intent-to-treat population, which consisted of all patients who received at least one dose of study medication and had one outcome assessment during the double-blind phase. Eighty-two patients were screened. Thirty-two patients in the intent-to-treat population (mean age 46 years; 75% female) received topiramate. Most patients (78%) met the definition for acute medication overuse at baseline. Study completion rates for topiramate- and placebo-treated patients were 75% and 52%, respectively. Topiramate significantly reduced the mean number of monthly migraine days by 3.5, compared with placebo (–0.2). This randomized, double-blind, placebo-controlled trial showed that topiramate is effective and reasonably well tolerated when used for the preventive treatment of chronic migraine, even in the presence of medication overuse.[181]

The National Institute of Neurological Diseases and Stroke (NINDS) Clinical Research Collaboration conducted the Chronic Migraine Treatment Trial (CMTT) to examine the safety and efficacy of topiramate (up to 100 mg/day) and propranolol (up to 240 mg/day LA formulation) taken in combination, compared with treatment with topiramate (up to 100 mg/day) and placebo. This double-blind, placebo-controlled, randomized clinical trial was terminated in September 2010, when an interim analysis determined that the combination of topiramate and propranolol offered no additional advantage over topiramate alone. [227]

Neurotoxins

OnabotulinumtoxinA (Botox® [BTX-A]) is safe and effective for CM and is currently approved for use as a prophylactic therapy in more than 40 countries, including the United Kingdom and the United States. The Phase III Research Evaluating Migraine Prophylaxis Therapy (PREEMPT 1 and 2) multicenter randomized clinical trials were conducted to evaluate the efficacy and safety of botulinum toxin type A as a prophylactic treatment for adults with chronic migraine. A total of 1384 patients with chronic migraine were enrolled across both trials (Table 2). Patients were stratified into groups according to whether they were overusing acute headache medications at baseline, and were randomly assigned in a 1:1 ratio to either botulinum toxin type A or placebo injections. A total dose of botulinum toxin type A of 155 U was administered to 31 sites in seven head and neck muscles.[85–87] The studies incorporated a double-blind phase and an open-label phase, although the efficacy of blinding was not evaluated. The PREEMPT study results demonstrated significant improvements at the population level in multiple measures of headache symptoms, as well as improvements in patients' functioning, vitality, psychological distress, and overall health-related quality of life, in response to treatment with in response to treatment with botulinum toxin type A.[51,63,64]

Treatment with Limited Supporting Evidence

Levetiracetam was studied in a multicenter, randomized, placebo-controlled, crossover study that included patients with either chronic migraine or chronic tension-type headache.[88] The primary endpoint was the highly desirable, but somewhat stringent, outcome of freedom from headache. Of 96 patients recruited to the study, 73 had CM. The study failed to meet its primary efficacy endpoint, although levetiracetam was associated with a non-significant 3.9% increase in the headache-free rate versus placebo. Nevertheless, some secondary endpoints were achieved, including a reduction in the number of headache days per month, reduced disability, and reduced pain severity.[228]

Saper et al.,[229] using a placebo-controlled, double-blind format, demonstrated that tizanidine, an alpha adrenergic agonist, was effective as an adjunctive agent for the treatment of chronic daily headache.

Other Medications

NSAIDs can be used for both symptomatic and preventive headache treatment. Naproxen sodium is effective in prevention at a dose of one or two 275 mg tablets twice a day.[230] Other NSAIDs that are effective include tolfenamic acid, ketoprofen, mefenamic acid, fenoprofen, and ibuprofen.[231,232] Aspirin was found to be effective in one study [233] and equal to placebo in another.[234] We believe that the short-acting NSAIDs, such as ibuprofen and aspirin, cause MOH, and their use should be limited. The potential for MOH with the other NSAIDs is uncertain. Indomethacin is the drug of choice for HC, and the response to this medication defines the disorder. In patients with strictly unilateral headaches, we give indomethacin a therapeutic trial to rule out HC, but we otherwise limit the use of NSAIDs.

Although monotherapy is preferred, it is sometimes necessary to combine preventive medications. Antidepressants are often used with ß-blockers or calcium channel blockers, and divalproex sodium may be used in combination with any of these medications. Pascual et al.[235] found that combining a ß-blocker and sodium valproate could lead to increased benefit for patients with migraine previously resistant to either alone. Fifty-two patients (43 women) with a history of EM with or without aura, and previously unresponsive to ß-blockers or sodium valproate in monotherapy, were treated with a combination of propranolol (or nadolol) and sodium valproate in an open-label fashion. Fifty-six percent had a greater than 50% reduction in migraine days. This open trial supports the practice of combination therapy. Controlled trials are needed to determine the true advantage of this combination treatment in episodic and chronic migraine.

Opioid Maintenance

The role of maintenance opioids (daily scheduled opioid therapy) for intractable CM is controversial.[236] Some argue that chronic opioid medication is justified [237] and useful [238] when patients have truly intractable headache or alternate treatments are contraindicated (as in the senior population). Until recently, long-term studies of effectiveness, sequelae over several years, predictors of long-term benefit, comparisons of pain-related outcome measures, and prevalence of problematic drug behavior were not available. Saper et al.[239] reported the results of a treatment program of 160 sequential patients who were followed for 3 to 5 years. Seventy of the 160 remained on opioids for at least a 3-year period and qualified for inclusion in the efficacy analysis. The primary clinical efficacy variable was percentage improvement in the severe headache index (frequency X severity of severe headaches/week). Only 41 of the original 160 patients (26%) had > 50% improvement. Fifty percent of patients exhibited problem drug behavior (dose violations, lost prescriptions, multisourcing); the most common of these was dose violation. Most patients (74%) either failed to show significant improvement or were discontinued from the program for clinical reasons. This study showed that a low percentage of patients demonstrated efficacy, and there was an unexpectedly high prevalence of misuse.

Daily scheduled opioid therapy did offer significant benefit for a select group of intractable headache patients. Subsequent follow-up with many of the "benefited" patients suggests to the authors that no more than 15% of the original 160 actually did well, and that several of those reporting improvement had (via collateral information gathering) fared much more poorly than initially reported. Recently Saper and Lake[122] have recommended against opioid maintenance, except in rare circumstances. Guidelines have been provided.[122]

Non-pharmacological Treatment

For occipital nerve stimulation please see Chapter 10.

ACUPUNCTURE AND BEHAVIORAL SLEEP MODIFICATION

Three randomized controlled trials investigated non-pharmacologic treatment in patients with CDH or CM/TM.[240] In a study of 74 CDH patients randomly allocated to either medical management alone or medical management and acupuncture, only the combination therapy was associated with improved clinical outcome.[241]

A pilot trial investigated the efficacy of safflower (Carthamus tinctorius) seed extract. [242] Injections of either normal saline or safflower seed extract were administered into a series of acupuncture points in 40 patients with CDH. Compared with normal saline injections, safflower seed extract injections resulted in a significantly higher reduction in scores on the Headache Impact Test-6, which is used to assess headache-related quality of life.

In another study, 43 women with TM/CM were randomly assigned to either behavioral sleep modification, consisting of scheduled bedtimes that allowed 8 hours of time in bed; elimination of television, reading, and listening to music while in bed; visualization techniques to shorten the time to sleep onset; moving consumption of food and liquids to > 4 hours and > 2 hours before bedtime, respectively; and eliminating naps; or placebo.[243] The intervention was associated with a significant reduction in headache frequency. Owing to their small sample sizes, these studies are, at best, hypothesis generating.[240–243]

Breaking the Headache Cycle

Patients often need *headache terminators* to break the cycle of daily headache and/or help with the exacerbation that occurs when overused medications are discontinued. Terminators are given orally, by suppository or by injection, and some (DHE, neuroleptics [prochlorperazine, chlorpromazine, and droperidol], corticosteroids, valproate sodium, magnesium, and ketorolac) can be given repetitively intravenously. Outpatient home terminators include long-acting NSAIDs, COX-2 inhibitors, short courses of corticosteroids and typical (e.g., prochlorperazine suppositories) and atypical (e.g. olanzapine) neuroleptics. We also teach patients to self-inject DHE (subcutaneous or intramuscular DHE [0.25–1 mg]), ketorolac, and droperidol.

One of the original headache terminators is DHE. Patients who are not good candidates for DHE or do not respond to it can use repetitive intravenous neuroleptics, such as chlorpromazine, droperidol, prochlorperazine, and/or corticosteroids. Refractory patients can be given these agents to supplement repetitive intravenous DHE.[53] In the infusion and inpatient units, we typically insert a heplock and administer IV fluids and parenteral medications via that route. Our typical hydration mixture is D5W in 0.5 normal saline at a rate of 100–200 ml/hour, which is 3–4 L/day.

Repetitive intravenous DHE was effective in eliminating intractable headache in 89% of patients within 48 hours (with or without acute medication overuse). Silberstein et al.[53] also found that repetitive intravenous DHE was effective in eliminating prolonged migraine, cluster headache, and CM with or without medication overuse.

Repetitive intravenous DHE is often coadministered with metoclopramide,[186] which helps control nausea and is an effective antimigraine drug in its own right. Following 10 mg of intravenous metoclopramide, DHE 0.5 mg is administered intravenously. Subsequent doses are adjusted based on pain relief and side effects. Promethazine intravenously (0.15 mg/kg diluted in 50 ml of 5% dextrose or normal saline) or ondansetron (a selective 5-HT3-receptor antagonist) orally (8 mg tablet) or intravenously (4–8 mg) can be used by patients who cannot tolerate metoclopramide because of side effects. Responsiveness may be increased by using other anti-emetics and neuroleptics.

We use the neuroleptics chlorpromazine, droperidol, haloperidol, and prochlorperazine, intravenously, intramuscularly, and by suppository, as terminators for nausea, vomiting, and pain. We also use the new atypical neuroleptics, such as olanzapine. Sixteen trials (AHCPR Technical Report) compared the efficacy of rectally and parenterally administered anti-emetics. Intravenous chlorpromazine and prochlorperazine are effective in controlling intractable headache. [192,244–246] Chlorpromazine was found to be more effective than the combination of meperidine and dimenhydrinate, and prochlorperazine was more effective than placebo in treating emergency department patients.[247] Neuroleptics are locally irritating when given intravenously; they are more effective IV than when given intramuscularly or by suppository. We have found that intramuscular haloperidol (5 mg), droperidol (1–2.5 mg), and thiothixene (5 mg) are effective for severe migraine headache.[53] Intravenous haloperidol and droperidol have also been used successfully.

Prochlorperazine (Compazine) administered intramuscularly, intravenously, or rectally is relatively safe and effective for the treatment of migraine headache and associated nausea and vomiting. It can be given intravenously (7.5–15 mg over 5 to 10 minutes) via a saline drip or "slow push."[246,247] Prochlorperazine suppositories (25 mg) are used as a rescue treatment for headache and nausea and also as an outpatient terminator medication. They can be used daily, as often as three times a day, for several days. The drug is not as effective orally. Lu et al.[248] retrospectively analyzed the data of refractory CDH inpatients who received intravenous repetitive prochlorperazine. A total of 135 patients were recruited, including 95 (70%) with analgesic overuse. After intravenous prochlorperazine treatment, 121 (90%) achieved a 50% or greater reduction of headache intensity, including 85 (63%) who became headache-free. Compared with DHE, prochlorperazine seemed less effective at achieving "freedom from headache" during hospitalization, but had a similar outcome at follow-up.

Chlorpromazine (Thorazine), 10 to 50 mg three to four times a day, diluted in 20 to 30 ml of saline, can be administered intravenously by rapid drip or "slow push" over several minutes. It can also be administered intramuscularly, rectally, or orally. The oral dose is 25 to 50 mg. Hypotension may result if the patient is not adequately hydrated prior to intravenous chlorpromazine administration.

Droperidol is a parenteral neuroleptic that was effective in a pilot study of 35 patients with status migrainosus or refractory migraine in an ambulatory infusion center. Droperidol (2.5 mg) was given intravenously every 30 minutes until either three doses were given or the patient was completely or almost headache-free.[249] The success rate (headache-free or mild headache) was 88% in patients with status migrainosus and 100% in patients with refractory migraine. A double blind, placebo-controlled, randomized, parallel-group, 22-center study[250] showed intramuscular droperidol to be effective for the acute treatment of migraine with or without aura. More patients in the 2.75, 5.5, and 8.25 mg treatment groups experienced a significant reduction in headache by 2 hours (moderate or severe to none or mild; 87%, 81%, and 84%, respectively) compared with placebo (57%). AEs occurring in more than 5% of patients receiving droperidol included asthenia, anxiety, akathisia, somnolence, and injection site reactions. Most AEs were mild to moderate. Patients can successfully self-inject droperidol. We now use repetitive intravenous droperidol (1–2.5 mg every 6 hours) in combination with intravenous diphenhydramine (25–50 mg). One concern with using neuroleptics is a prolonged QTc interval on EKG. This is more likely to occur with droperidol use than with chlorpromazine or prochlorperazine. It is unlikely with olanzapine. Patients who receive daily repetitive intravenous droperidol should have an EKG before their first dose of the medication and daily thereafter. A QTc that is above 450 is considered a "gray zone" (the drug should be stopped or the dose reduced), and a QTc above 500 is a "red zone" (an absolute contraindication). Bradycardia, abnormal EKG, and a change in the QTc of more than 60 msec are the other risk factors for torsade de pointes associated with prolonged QT syndrome.

Olanzapine, a thienobenzodiazepine, is a new, "atypical" anti-psychotic drug. Olanzapine's properties suggest that it would be effective for headaches, with a low risk of acute extrapyramidal reactions and tardive dyskinesia. The oral dose is 5 to 10 mg. Olanzapine had an antinociceptive effect in the mouse tail flick pain model, which is mediated by agonistic activity at alpha2-adrenoreceptors.[251] Silberstein et al. reviewed 50 patients who had refractory headache and were treated with olanzapine for at least three months.[252] The daily dose of olanzapine varied from 2.5 to 35 mg; most patients received 5 mg (19 patients) or 10 mg (17 patients) a day. There was a statistically significant decrease in headache days, from 27.5 ± 4.9 before treatment to 21.1 ± 10.7 after treatment ($p < 0.001$, student t test). The difference in headache severity (0 to 10 scale), 8.7 ± 1.6 before treatment and 2.2 ± 2.1 after treatment) was also statistically significant ($p < 0.001$). The most common adverse events are sedation and weight gain. Quetiapine is a dibenzothiazepine derivative. In comparison with other antipsychotic agents, quetiapine has less anti-muscarinic and alpha1 antagonist receptor activity.

Krymchantowski et al.[253] evaluated Quetiapine in the preventive treatment of refractory migraine. Thirty-four consecutive patients (30 women and 4 men) with migraine (ICHD-2), fewer than 15 days of headache per month, and not overusing symptomatic medications were studied. All participants had failed the combination of atenolol (60 mg/day), nortriptyline (25 mg/day), and flunarizine (3 mg/day). Failure was defined as < 50% reduction in attack frequency after 10 weeks of treatment. After other medications were discontinued, Quetiapine was initiated at a single daily dose of 25 mg, and then titrated to 75 mg. After 10 weeks, headache frequency, consumption of rescue medications, and adverse events were analyzed. Twenty-nine patients completed the study. Among those who completed, 22 (75.9%; 64.7% of the intention-to-treat population) had greater than 50% headache reduction. The mean frequency of migraine days decreased from 10.2 to 6.2 per month. Use of rescue medications decreased from 2.3 to 1.2 days per week. AEs were reported by nine (31%) patients.[253] We use quetiapine as an acute treatment, at a dose of 50 to 100 mg. As a preventive, we use up to 100 mg bid. The sedation caused by quetiapine often limits its acute use. It may be useful at nighttime or if rest is highly desirable. It may be a better option for preventive use, as it has less tendency to cause weight gain, although somnolence is still a factor. Ziprasidone (Geodon) is another atypical neuroleptic. There is no scientific evidence for its efficacy in headache. It has the advantage of causing less weight gain and sedation than other atypical neuroleptics. Common adverse events include asthenia, akathisia, and somnolence.

Controlled studies have shown corticosteroids to be effective in the treatment of headache associated with altitude sickness. [192,244] Clinical experience suggests that corticosteroids are also effective in the treatment of other headache types. Hydrocortisone or Solu-Medrol (methyl prednisolone sodium succinate) can be given intravenously in the following manner: 100 mg via a saline drip over 10 minutes every 6 hours for 24 hours; every 8 hours for 24 hours; every 12 hours for 24 hours; and then a final dose. Dexamethasone (Decadron) can be administered intravenously or intramuscularly, starting at a dose of 8 to 20 mg per day in divided doses, rapidly tapering over 2 to 3 days. Oral dexamethasone, 1.5 to 4 mg twice daily for 2 days with a taper over 3 more days, has also proven useful for less disabled migraineurs with prolonged migraine headache.

At least five different chemical classes of NSAIDs have been used for headache treatment.[254] We use naproxen, indomethacin rectal suppositories, and selective COX-2 inhibitors. In addition, we use intramuscular or intravenous ketorolac, especially in situations where neuroleptics, narcotics, and DHE are relatively contraindicated. When we use intravenous ketorolac, we reduce the risk of gastrointestinal bleeding or renal injury by limiting the days of use (30 mg intravenously every 8 hours, for a maximum of 3 days in a row). We do not use steroids and we give gastrointestinal protection concurrently.

We occasionally use intravenous valproic acid. In an open-label study, Edwards and Santarcangelo[221] assessed the possible benefit of sodium valproate in 20 consecutive CDH patients who were refractory to multiple standard treatments. Eleven of the 20 patients (55%) had a response to mild or no headaches within 1 to 4 weeks. The dose ranged from 375 to 1500 mg a day. Two patients (10%) discontinued medication due to AEs (difficulty thinking and nausea). In a randomized, double-blind, prospective trial, Tanen et al.[255] compared IV sodium valproate to IV prochlorperazine in the acute treatment of migraine headache in the emergency department. Patients received either 10 mg of prochlorperazine or 500 mg of valproate over 2 minutes. Prochlorperazine was statistically and clinically superior to sodium valproate for the treatment of the pain and nausea of acute migraine headache. Sodium valproate, in this study, failed to significantly reduce the pain or nausea of acute migraine headache. When we use sodium valproate, we give 250 to 500 mg IV push (one-time dose, occasionally may repeat; recently published protocol every 8 hours). One can give 500 to 1000 mg IV drip.

Propofol (2,6-diidopropylphenol) is an intravenous sedative-hypnotic agent used for induction and maintenance of anesthesia or sedation. It is the active ingredient in Diprivan, an injectable emulsion. Propofol's rapid induction of hypnosis—usually within 40 seconds of injection—occurs as a result of the rapid equilibration between the plasma and the highly perfused tissue of the brain. The half-time of the blood-brain equilibration is approximately 1 to 3 minutes. Krusz et al.[256] reported that intravenous propofol was effective in treating acute headache and other headaches that were refractory to the usual therapy. Mendes et al. [257] conducted a pilot prospective study using repetitive low-dose boluses of intravenous propofol to treat patients with CDHs that were refractory to standard medications. A total of 21 trials were conducted on 18 patients. Over 90% of patients had at least some headache relief with no complications.

Hand and Stark[258] retrospectively surveyed 19 consecutive inpatients, 18 with MOH and three with status migrainosus, who were treated with intravenous lignocaine infusion. The 19 patients (16 women) received 27 lignocaine infusions. An EKG was obtained before and 30 to 60 minutes after the infusion was started. Lignocaine was infused at a rate of 2 mg/minute by a pump device. The infusion was maintained until the patients were headache-free for a minimum of 12 hours or a maximum of 14 days. Preventive medication was permitted and was started during the hospital stay. Seven minor AEs were noted during four infusions. Eighteen patients had 22 infusions for MOH, with headache resolution in 82% of infusions (17 of the 18 patients responded at least once). The median duration was 5 days. Four patients obtained lasting relief; six returned to their regular manageable pattern of migraine (two of these patients had recurrent CDH after 6 months); four were lost to follow-up; and four had no long-term benefit. Five infusions were given to three patients with status migrainosus, with four of these infusions successfully relieving the headache. Intravenous lignocaine appears to be safe and may be useful in managing severe intractable CDH and status migrainosus. It is uncertain how much of the improvement was due to the intravenous lignocaine and how much was due to discontinuing the overused acute medication and initiating preventive medication.

Rosen et al. conducted a retrospective chart review of all patients admitted to Thomas Jefferson University Hospital who received intravenous lidocaine for CDH or chronic cluster headache. All patients had failed other aggressive inpatient treatments, such as IV DHE, anti-emetics, neuroleptics, and steroidal and non-steroidal anti-inflammatory drugs (often in combination or sequentially). Patients had continuous telemetry, including continuous cardiac monitoring, during treatment. Vital signs (every 8 hours) and basic blood studies (complete blood count, basic chemistry panel, magnesium, and phosphate) and a daily 12-lead EKG were also obtained. After the initial laboratory work and initial EKG were determined to be within an acceptable range, a standard peripheral IV was placed and a lidocaine infusion was started, typically at a rate of 1 mg/min for 4 hours, after which it was raised to 2 mg/min. Some patients received doses as high as 4 mg/min after non-toxic levels were obtained. They attempted to keep the level below the upper limit of the therapeutic range for arrhythmia (1–5 microgram/ml). Lidocaine levels were obtained when indicated (eg., before going above 3 and then 4 mg/min) during treatment. Concurrent IV medications, including corticosteroids, NSAIDs, DHE, and anti-emetics, were given as needed. They found that 25.4% of patients exhibited a complete response, 57.1% exhibited a partial response, 3.2% worsened, and 14.3% exhibited no change during the lidocaine infusion. Although 50% of the patients experienced some AEs (including hallucinations, tachycardia, tremors, hypotension, light-headedness, phlebitis, line infection, and hypertension), none caused the treatment to be aborted. Most resolved after dose reduction.[259]

In a retroactive comparative study of intractable patients on an inpatient unit, Swidan et al.[260] showed that diphenhydramine delivered by intravenous infusion was as effective as dihydroergotamine.Table 9.13

Ketamine was developed in the 1960s as an anesthetic agent, and is given intravenously or intramuscularly for surgical anaesthesia. It is also used in sub-anesthetic doses as an adjuvant to opioids in the treatment of refractory pain in cancer patients, acute postoperative pain, and in the management of refractory chronic non-cancer pain. Bell reviewed the current literature, which provides evidence for acute relief of chronic non-cancer pain; information supporting the efficacy and tolerability of ketamine in the long-term treatment of chronic pain is extremely limited. Routes of administration of ketamine include intravenous, subcutaneous,

Table 9.13 Dihydroergotamine Protocol

Metoclopramide 10 mg IV		
DHE 0.5 mg IV (over 2–3 min.)		
Nausea	Head pain persists No nausea	Head pain stops No nausea
No DHE for 8 hrs. Then Give .3 or .4 mg q 8 hrs. For 3 days plus Metoclopramide 10 mg	Repeat DHE 0.5 mg IV In 1 hour (s Metoclopramide)	DHE 0.5 mg IV q 8 hrs. for 3 days plus Metoclopramide 10 mg
Nausea DHE 0.75 mg q 8 hrs. for 3 days Plus Metoclopramide 10 mg	No nausea DHE 1.0 mg q 8 hrs. for 3 days Plus Metoclopramide 10 mg	

intramuscular, epidural, intrathecal, intraarticular, intranasal, oral, and topical. Use of ketamine is limited due to psychotomimetic and other dose-dependent adverse effects, which include hallucinations, agitation, nightmares, dizziness and nausea. At higher doses (> 2 mg/kg IV), ketamine can cause delirium, impaired motor function, amnesia, anxiety, panic attacks, mania, insomnia, and high blood pressure. The current literature suggests that ketamine in sub-anesthetic doses can provide short-term relief of refractory neuropathic pain in some patients. The size and scope of controlled clinical trials to date are insufficient to support longer term use in any particular chronic pain disorder. Ketamine is a drug of addiction with neurotoxic effects and unpleasant AEs.[261]

Afridi et al. tested the hypothesis that ketamine would affect aura in a randomized controlled double-blind trial, investigating the effect of 25 mg intranasal ketamine on migraine with prolonged aura in 30 migraineurs using 2 mg intranasal midazolam as an active control. Each subject recorded data from three episodes of migraine. Eighteen subjects completed the study. Ketamine reduced the severity (p <.032) but not the duration of aura in this group, whereas midazolam had no effect. These data provide translational evidence for the potential importance of glutamatergic mechanisms in migraine aura and offer a pharmacologic parallel between animal experimental work on cortical spreading depression and the clinical problem.[262]

We have used low-dose intravenous ketamine in patients with refractory CM with mixed results. Analysis is underway.

Strategies of Treatment

OUTPATIENT

Two general outpatient strategies are in use. One approach is to taper the overused medication. The alternative strategy is to abruptly discontinue the overused drug, substitute a transitional medication to replace the overused drug, and subsequently taper the transitional drug. Serious withdrawal syndromes must be prevented. For example, if high doses of a butalbital-containing analgesic combination are abruptly discontinued, phenobarbital should be used to prevent barbiturate withdrawal syndrome. Similarly, benzodiazepines must be gradually tapered or replaced with long-acting ones. Ergotamine can be replaced with DHE and short-acting NSAIDs with long-acting ones. Terminators are used to stop the headache cycle. Drugs used for this purpose include DHE, NSAIDs, COX-2 inhibitors, corticosteroids, typical and atypical neuroleptics, and triptans.[116,205,263] Outpatient treatment is preferred for motivated patients, but it is not always safe or effective.

Patients who do not need hospital-level care but cannot be safely or adequately treated as outpatients can be considered for ambulatory infusion treatment. Outpatient ambulatory infusion treatment is effective for migraine status and uncomplicated CDH with and without MOH. It must be done in a supervised medical setting where the patient can be monitored frequently (every 15 minutes). Under these circumstances, repetitive intravenous treatment can be given twice a day for several days in a row. Although ambulatory infusion treatment is better for many patients than outpatient treatment, major concerns still exist. Contraindications to outpatient ambulatory infusion treatment include the possibility of withdrawal symptoms occurring at night when patients are withdrawn from long-acting or potent drugs; psychiatric disorders that interfere with treatment (these patients cannot be treated aggressively as outpatients); and comorbid medical illnesses that require prolonged monitoring. No long-term observation is available, and many problems manifest themselves in an intensely monitored interactive environment.

INPATIENT

The goals of inpatient headache treatment include the following:

1. acute medication withdrawal and rehydration;
2. pain control with parenteral therapy;
3. establishment of effective preventive treatment;
4. termination of the pain cycle;
5. patient education; and
6. establishment of outpatient methods of pain control.[191]

Hospitalization is also used as a time for patient education, for introducing behavioral methods of pain control, and for adjusting an outpatient program of preventive and acute therapy.

Our[53] experience with more than 300 patients has shown that repetitive IV DHE is a safe and effective means of rapidly controlling intractable headache. Of 214 patients suffering from daily headache with rebound, 92% became headache-free with an average length of stay of 7.3 days. Pringsheim and Howse[264] reported similar but less robust results (see discussion later in this chapter). Patients whose significant medical or behavioral comorbidities and/or opioid dependence are a cause of their MOH often require longer lengths of stay.[123]

Hospitalization is an essential step in achieving effective control and diagnosis for a large number of otherwise intractable headache patients. The benefits of hospitalization extend beyond IV protocols and other pharmacologic manipulations and withdrawal therapies. Observing patients' behavior in their daily interactions with staff, peers, and family, as well as being able to influence their sleeping and eating patterns, have proven enormously helpful in establishing short- and long-term treatment plans.[123,187] Moreover, observing drug-seeking behavior, tolerance or intolerance for varying levels of pain, and the accuracy of pain reporting are additional observational assets of an inpatient treatment environment and can serve as the foundation for subsequent outpatient care.

Various behavioral disturbances are more commonly seen in a hospital as opposed to an outpatient setting. Lake and Saper[123] recently reported the results of 276 consecutively discharged patients. While approximately 70% were discharged feeling moderately to significantly better than upon admission, the observation was made that patients with personality disorders were much more likely to have MOH than those without, and that certain personality disorders, such as borderline personality and narcissistic personality disorders, seemed to have a predilection for opioid misuse.[82,123,265] The authors raise the possibility that personality disorders may serve as a predisposing factor to both MOH and certain drug-specific pursuits.[122] The authors also speculated that an individuals's behavior, as imposed upon the treating physician, might prompt that physician to provide opioids defensively, even against his or her best judgment [266].

PROGNOSIS

The "natural history" of CM and MOH has never been studied and probably never will be for ethical and technical reasons. Recognition of the rebound process is probably therapeutic in and of itself and could affect the patient's behavior or the physician's approach. Retrospective analysis suggests that periods of stable drug consumption and periods of accelerated medication use may occur. Patients who are treated aggressively generally improve. There are no literature reports of spontaneous improvement of rebound headache, although this may happen. We[267] performed follow-up evaluations on 50 hospitalized primary CDH drug overuse patients who were treated with repetitive IV DHE and became headache-free. Once detoxified, treated, and discharged, most patients did not resume daily analgesic or ergotamine use. Seventy-two percent continued to show significant improvement at 3 months, and 87% continued to show significant improvement after 2 years. This would suggest at least a 70% improvement at 2 years in the initial group (35/50), allowing for patients lost to follow-up.

Our[267] 2-year success rate of 87% is consistent with the long-term success rates reported in the literature (Table 9). In a series of papers[88,89,91,158,188-190,268-270] published between 1975 and 1999, the success rate of withdrawal therapy (often accompanied by pharmacologic and/or behavioral intervention) in patients overusing analgesics, ergotamine, or both was between 48% and 91%, with the rate being reported as 77% or higher in 10 papers (Table 9.14).

Henry et al.[271] hospitalized, detoxified, and followed 22 primary CDH drug overuse patients for 4 to 24 months. Nine of 15 patients showed marked improvement, one showed slight improvement, and five did not improve. Rapoport et al.[90] studied 90 patients with primary CDH who discontinued analgesics. After 1 month, 30% were significantly improved; 67% were significantly improved within 2 months, 80% after 3 months, and 82% after 4 months. The authors suggested that an "analgesic washout period" exists and may be as long as 3 months for some patients.

Diener et al.[188] hospitalized 85 patients who were overusing analgesics or various migraine drugs (including ergotamine). The

Table 9.14 MOH: Long-Term Follow-up

Year	Author	Drug E/A/T	#PATIENTS	Follow-Up (Months)	Positive (%)	Relapse %
1975	Andersson	E	44	6	91	9
1981	Tfelt-Hansen and Krabbe	E	40	12	47.6	29
1982	Ala-Hurula	E	23	3–6	78	19
1982	Isler	A	104	1–30	77.9	58.6
1984	Diehgans	E/A	52	16	77	9
1985	Henry et al.	E/A	22	3	78	33
1986	Rapoport et al.	A	90	4	82	?
1987	Granella et al.	A	95	6	?	22
1988	Diener et al.	E/A	85	35	69	?
1988	Andersson	E	32	6	50	?
1989	Baumgartner et al.	E/A	38	16	60.5	24
1989	Diener et al.	A	139	34		
1989	Schoenen et al.	A	121	6	50	20
1990	Lake and Saper	E/A	100	3–12	87	
1990	Mathew et al.	E/A	200	3	86	?
1991	Hering and Steiner	E/A	46	6	80.4	4
1992	Silberstein and Silberstein	E/A	50	24	87	13
1996	Pini et al.	E/A/T	104	4	72	28
1996	Schnider et al.	E/A	38	60	50	39.5
1998	Pringsheim and Howse	E/A/T	132	3	56	
1998	Monzon et al.	E/A	104	12	66	?
1999	Suhr et al.	E/A/T	101	72±48		20.8
1999	Lorenzatto et al.	E/A/T	140	12	84.6%	
2005	Katsarava et al.	E/A/T	96	48	96/98*	41%/45%°8
2009	Hagen et al.	E/AT	56	12	53/25**	

° 98 detoxed/ 96 had improved at 1 month
** Prophyaxis only and withdrawal only groups
E = ergotamine tartrate; A = analgesics; T = triptans

length of admission was 14 days. They detoxified these patients and followed them for 10 to 75 months (mean = 35 months) after discharge. Sixty-nine percent had at least 50% improvement; 29.4% were unchanged, and one had deteriorated. Fifty-four patients with drug-induced headache were hospitalized by Baumgartner et al. [89] for 2 weeks. The were detoxified and started on a prophylactic drug. At an average of 16.8 months (13.6 months) after treatment and discharge, 38 patients were evaluated: 76.3% had reduced their analgesic intake and 60.5% had experienced a significant relief in headache intensity and frequency.

Lake et al.[25] reported on 100 patients who had been hospitalized with severe refractory primary CDH frequently complicated by symptomatic medication overuse. At follow-up between 3 months and 1 year after discharge, the mean number of severe headaches was reduced 64% and the mean number of dysfunctional days was reduced 70%. Overall, 87% of patients reported at least a 50% headache reduction.

Hering and Steiner[189] followed 46 migraineurs who developed primary CDH as a result of analgesic overuse. Six months after analgesic and ergotamine withdrawal, 37 (80.4%) were no longer overusing the agents and no longer had primary CDH.

Mathew et al.[43,83] studied 200 patients who were overusing daily symptomatic medication, 58% of whom were taking prophylactic medication without achieving a benefit. At the 3-month follow-up, if the analgesics had been discontinued and prophylactic medication started or modified, a reduction of approximately 86% in the weekly headache index was achieved, with a dropout rate of 10.3%. If symptomatic medication had been continued, only 21% improvement was achieved. It is interesting to note that merely discontinuing symptomatic medication resulted in 58% improvement.

Schnider et al.[272] followed 38 primary CDH inpatients who had overused ergotamine and/or analgesics and were detoxified. After 5 years, 19 patients had headache 8 or fewer days a month and 18 had no or only mild headaches. Outcome was related to headache frequency and duration of drug use. Fifteen patients (39.5%) had relapsed and were again overusing acute drugs.

Pini et al.[273] evaluated 102 primary CDH patients who were overusing ergotamine, analgesics (including butalbital combinations), and/or sumatriptan. Patients were treated as either outpatients or inpatients based on the therapeutic schedule to be followed. Both groups showed equal improvement at 1 and 4 months in the headache index, but the outpatients had a higher relapse rate (38%) than the inpatients (25%). This suggests that the more complicated and refractory patients were admitted to the hospital.

Granella et al.[158] looked for factors that were associated with the evolution of migraine without aura into CM. Risk factors included head trauma (OR 3.3), analgesic use with every attack (OR 2.8), and long duration of oral contraceptive use.

Pringsheim and Howse[264] detoxified 174 inpatients who were overusing ergotamine, analgesics, and triptans and treated them with repetitive IV DHE; 132 patients were followed after 3 months by telephone. Sixty-one percent had an immediate good result. Of these, 56% continued to do well at 3 months and 5% relapsed.

Suhr et al.[274] conducted a prospective study of 257 primary CDH patients allocated to inpatient (147) or outpatient (110) treatment, depending on the personal situation of the patient. Only 5% of the patients were headache-free at follow-up, which was up to 5 years after treatment. The total relapse to drug overuse was 20.8%, occurring in 14.0% of the outpatients and 25.0% of the inpatients. No baseline analysis of headache days a month or mean pain intensity was given, but there was no significant difference in these outcomes between groups.

Monzon et al.[275] prospectively studied the long-term (6 and 12 months) outcome of 164 consecutive primary CDH patients and analyzed various etiologic causal factors. One hundred eighteen patients (72%) had CM, 33 patients (20%) had CTTH, and 13 patients (8%) had NDPH. One hundred forty-nine patients were treated with outpatient therapy and 15 refractory patients were admitted to a comprehensive inpatient treatment. At 6 months, 54 patients had an excellent result, 64 had a good result, and 41 had a fair result; five patients continued to have CM. At 12 months, 104 patients were analyzed: 23 had an excellent result, 46 had a good result, and 28 had a fair result; seven patients continued to have CM. There were no statistically significant differences in evolution when transformation factors were analyzed. Although differences were not statistically significant, treatment was less efficacious when inpatient therapy was necessary and when patients had a history of analgesic abuse or traumatic life events. This, again, suggests that the more severe and intractable cases were admitted to the hospital.

Lorenzatto et al.[276] using the criteria proposed by Silberstein et al.[54] retrospectively studied 140 patients (101 women and 39 men aged 17 to 83) who had CDH (i.e., they overused acute drugs). The patients were taken off acute medications and were treated with preventive medications and education. After 1 month, 23.6% of patients had more than a 50% improvement in headache intensity and frequency and 56.4% had a similar improvement. Fifty percent improvement was observed after 6 months in 70.2% of patients, after 9 months in 82.6%, and after 12 months in 84.6%.

Katsarava et al. did a prospective 4-year follow-up study of 98 MOH patients following withdrawal. Two of 98 patients did not improve 1 month after withdrawal and were excluded from the study. Of the remaining 96 patients, 78 women and 18 men, with mean age of 43 years (range 23–65 years), 69 (71%) suffered from migraine, 13 (14%) from TTH, and 14 (15%) from a combination of migraine and TTH. Mean duration of primary headache was 22 years. Forty-six patients (48%) overused analgesics, 12 (13%) overused ergots, and 38 (39%) overused triptans. Twenty-six patients (31%) relapsed within the first 6 months after withdrawal. The number of relapses increased to 32 (41%) 1 year and to 34 (45%) 4 years after withdrawal. The 4-year relapse rate was lower in patients with migraine than in those with TTH (32% vs. 91%) and those with a combination of migraine and TTH (32% vs. 70%), and also lower in patients overusing triptans than those overusing analgesics (21% vs. 71%). Most relapses occurred within the first year after withdrawal; the long-term success of withdrawal depends on the type of primary headache and the type of overused medication.[277]

Hagen et al.[178] did a 1-year open-labeled, multicenter study on 56 patients with MOH. These were randomly assigned to receive prophylactic treatment from the start without detoxification, undergo a standard outpatient detoxification program without prophylactic treatment from the start, or no specific treatment (5-month follow-up). The prophylaxis group had the greatest decrease in headache days compared with baseline, and also a significantly more pronounced reduction in total headache index at months 3 (p = 0.003) and 12 (p = 0.017) compared with the withdrawal group. At 12 months, 53% of patients in the prophylaxis group had > 50% reduction in monthly headache days compared with 25% in the withdrawal group (p = 0.081).[178] Hagen et al. then evaluated their long-term outcome. Fifty patients (83%) participated. At follow-up, the 50 persons had a mean reduction of 6.5 headache days/month and 9.5 acute headache medication days/month compared to baseline. Sixteen persons (32%) were considered as responders due to a > 50% reduction in headache frequency from baseline, whereas 17 (34%) persons met the criteria for MOH. At 4-years follow-up, one-third of the 50 MOH patients had > 50% reduction in headache frequency from baseline. A low total Hospital Anxiety and Depression Scale

Table 9.15 Why Treatment Fails

The Diagnosis is Incomplete or Incorrect
- An undiagnosed secondary headache disorder is present.
- A primary headache disorder is misdiagnosed.
- Two or more different headache disorders are present.

Important Exacerbating Factors May Have Been Missed
- Medication overuse (including over-the-counter)
- Caffeine overuse
- Dietary or lifestyle triggers
- Hormonal triggers
- Psychosocial factors
- Other medications that trigger headaches

Pharmacotherapy Has Been Inadequate
- Ineffective drug
- Excessive initial doses
- Inadequate final doses
- Inadequate duration of treatment

Other Factors
- Unrealistic expectations
- Comorbid conditions complicate therapy
- Inpatient treatment required.

Modified from Lipton et al.[278]

score at baseline was associated with the most favorable outcome.[179]

Why Treatment Fails

When patients fail to respond to therapy or announce that they have already tried everything and nothing will work, it is important to try to identify the reason or reasons that treatment has failed (Table 9.15). The cause of treatment failure may be an incomplete or incorrect diagnosis.[278] For example, an undiagnosed secondary headache disorder is the major source of the head pain; a misdiagnosed primary headache disorder is present (e.g., HC is mistaken for CM, episodic paroxysmal hemicrania or hypnic headache is mistaken for cluster); or two or more different headache disorders are present. In addition, pharmacotherapy may have been inadequate, or important exacerbating factors such as medication overuse may have been missed.

PREVENTION

Headache sufferers often do not realize that excessive or frequent self-treatment may perpetuate or exacerbate their headaches. Since most headache sufferers do not seek medical advice until and unless the pain becomes frequent or intense, the opportunity for diagnosis and physician intervention to halt the cycle is often missed. Physicians need to screen CDH patients for analgesic overuse. Headache patients must be informed about the risks of analgesic overuse and rebound headache. Yet, even when patients are aware of the risks, they may still overmedicate. This requires continued vigilance on the part of the treating physician.

Because patients who overuse medication may feel ashamed and out of control, an accurate history may be difficult to obtain. To facilitate this process, the condition of medication rebound should be explained as part of the natural history of migraine. Even if the patient is not rebounding at the time, all symptomatic headache medications, with the possible exception of the long-acting NSAIDs, should be limited to prevent rebound headache.

Patients with drug-induced CDH, while difficult to treat, often return to a state of intermittent episodic headache after detoxification and treatment with a preventive medication.

REFERENCES

1. Scher AI, Stewart WF, Liberman J, Lipton RB. Prevalence of frequent headache in a population sample. *Headache*. 1998;38:497–506.
2. Castillo J, Munoz P, Guitera V, Pascual J. Kaplan Award 1998. Epidemiology of chronic daily headache in the general population. *Headache*. 1999;39:190–196.
3. Wang SJ, Fuh JL, Lu SR, et al. Chronic daily headache in Chinese elderly: prevalence, risk factors and biannual follow-up. *Neurology*. 2000;54:314–319.
4. Castillo J, Munoz P, Guitera V, Pascual J. Epidemiology of chronic daily headache in the general population. *Headache*. 1998;38:378.
5. Pascual J, Colas R, Castillo J. Epidemiology of chronic daily headache. *Curr Pain Headache Rep*. 2001;5:529–536.
6. Lanteri-Minet M, Auray JP, El Hasnaoui A, et al. Prevalence and description of chronic daily headache in the general population in France. *Pain*. 2003;102:143–149.
7. Lipton RB. Chronic migraine, classification, differential diagnosis, and epidemiology. *Headache*. 2011;51(Suppl 2):77–83.
8. Silberstein SD, Lipton RB. Chronic daily headache including transformed migraine, chronic tension-type headache, and medication overuse. In: Silberstein SD, Lipton RB, Dalessio DJ, eds. *Wolff's headache and other head pain*. 7th ed. New York: Oxford University Press, 2001:247–282.
9. D'Amico D, Usai S, Grazzi L, et al. Quality of life and disability in primary chronic daily headaches. *Neurol Sci*. 2003;24(Suppl 2):S97–100.
10. Guitera V, Munoz P, Castillo J, Pascual J. Quality of life in chronic daily headache: a study in a general population. *Neurology*. 2002;58:1062–1065.
11. Wang SJ, Fuh JL, Juang KD. Quality of life differs among headache diagnoses: analysis of SF-36 survey in 901 headache patients. *Pain*. 2001;89:285–292.
12. Bigal ME, Serrano D, Reed M, et al. Chronic migraine in the population: burden, diagnosis, and satisfaction with treatment. *Neurology*. 2008;71:559–566.
13. Buse DC, Manack A, Serrano D, et al. Sociodemographic and comorbidity profiles of chronic migraine and episodic migraine sufferers. *J Neurol Neurosurg Psychiatry*. 2010;81:428–432.
14. Saper JR, Jones JM. Ergotamine tartrate dependency: features and possible mechanisms. *Clin Neuropharmacol*. 1986;9:244–256.
15. Silberstein SD, Lipton RB, Solomon S, Mathew NT. Classification of daily and near daily headaches: proposed revisions to the IHS classification. *Headache*. 1994;34:1–7.
16. Mathew NT, Reuveni U, Perez F. Transformed or evolutive migraine. *Headache*. 1987;27:102–106.
17. Stewart WF, Wood GC, Manack A, et al. Employment and work impact of chronic migraine and episodic migraine. *J Occup Environ Med*. 2010;8–14.

18. Rasmussen BK. Migraine and tension-type headache in a general population: psychosocial factors. *Intl J Epidemiol*. 1992;21:1138–1143.

19. Sanin LC, Mathew NT, Bellmyer LR, Ali S. The International Headache Society (IHS) headache classification as applied to a headache clinic population. *Cephalalgia*. 1994;14:443–446.

20. Nappi G, Granella F, Sandrini G, Manzoni GC. Chronic daily headache: how should it be included in the IHS Classification? *Headache*. 1999;39:197–203.

21. Manack AN, Buse DC, Lipton RB. Chronic migraine: epidemiology and disease burden. *Curr Pain Headache Rep*. 2011;15:70–78.

22. Katsarava Z, Manack A, Yoon MS, et al. Chronic migraine: classification and comparisons. *Cephalalgia*. 2011;31:520–529.

23. Natoli JL, Manack A, Dean B, et al. Global prevalence of chronic migraine: a systematic review. *Cephalalgia*. 2010;30:599–609.

24. Lipton RB, Manack A, Ricci JA, Chee E, Turkel CC, Winner P. Prevalence and burden of chronic migraine in adolescents: results of the chronic daily headache in adolescents study (C-dAS). *Headache*. 2011;51:693–706.

25. Lake A, Saper J, Madden S, Kreeger C: Inpatient treatment for chronic daily headache: a prospective long-term outcome. *Headache*. 1990;30:299–300. (Abstract)

26. Brain WR. Some unsolved problems of cervical spondylosis. *Br Med J*. 1963;1:771–777.

27. Rapoport AM. Analgesic rebound headache. *Headache*. 1988;28:662–665.

28. Mathew NT. Chronic daily headache: clinical features and natural history. In: Nappi G, Bono G, Sandrini G, Martignoni E, Micieli G, eds. *Headache and depression: serotonin pathways as a common clue*. New York: Raven Press, 1991:49–58.

29. Lake AE, Saper JR, Madden SF, Kreeger C. Comprehensive inpatient treatment for intractable migraine: a prospective long-term outcome study. *Headache*. 1993;55–62.

30. Mathew NT. Transformed migraine. *Cephalalgia*. 1993;13:78–83.

31. Mathew NT, Stubits E, Nigam MR. Transformation of episodic migraine into daily headache: analysis of factors. *Headache*. 1982;22:66–68.

32. Olesen J, Tfelt-Hansen P, Welch KMA. *The headaches*. New York: Raven Press, 1993.

33. Saper JR. *Headache disorders: current concepts in treatment strategies*. Littleton, CO: Wright-PSG, 1983.

34. Sjaastad O, Saumte C, Hovdahl H. Cervicogenic headache, a hypothesis. *Cephalalgia*. 1983;3:249–256.

35. Sjaastad O. The headache challenge in our time: cervicogenic headache. *Funct Neurology*. 1990;5:155–158.

36. Headache Classification Committee. The International Classification of Headache Disorders, 2nd edition. *Cephalalgia*. 2004;24:1–160.

37. Andreoli A, Dipasquale G, Pinelli G, Grazi P, Tognetti F, Testa C. Subarachnoid hemorrhage: frequency and severity of cardiac arrhythmias. A survey of 70 cases studied in the acute phase. *Stroke*. 1987;18:558–564.

38. Messinger HB, Spierings ELH, Vincent AJP. Overlap of migraine and tension-type headache in the International Headache Society classification. *Cephalalgia*. 1991;11:233–237.

39. Saper JR, Winters M: Chronic "mixed" headaches: profile and analysis of 100 consecutive patients experiencing daily headache. *Headache*. 1982;22:145–-146.(Abstract)

40. Saper JR. Daily chronic headache. *Neurol Clin*. 1990;8:891–901.

41. Solomon S, Lipton RB, Newman LC. Evaluation of chronic daily headache-comparison to criteria for chronic tension-type headache. *Cephalalgia*. 1992;12:365–368.

42. Saper JR, VanMeter MJ: Ergotamine habituation: analysis and profile. *Headache*. 1980;20:159(Abstract).

43. Mathew NT, Kurman R, Perez F. Drug induced refractory headache: clinical features and management. *Headache*. 1990;30:634–638.

44. Mathew NT. Transformed or evolutional migraine. *Headache*. 1987;27:305–306.

45. Bigal ME, Sheftell FD, Rapoport AM, Lipton RB, Tepper SJ. Chronic daily headache in a tertiary care population: correlation between the International Headache Society diagnostic criteria and proposed revisions of criteria for chronic daily headache. *Cephalalgia*. 2002;22:432–438.

46. Headache Classification Committee of the International Headache Society. Classification and diagnostic criteria for headache disorders, cranial neuralgia, and facial pain. *Cephalalgia*. 1988;8:1–96.

47. Silberstein SD. Chronic daily headache and tension-type headache. *Neurology*. 1993;43:1644–1649.

48. Pfaffenrath V, Isler H. Evaluation of the nosology of chronic tension-type headache. *Cephalalgia*. 1993;13:60–62.

49. Bigal ME, Tepper SJ, Sheftell FD, Rapoport AM, Lipton RB. Chronic daily headache: correlation between the 2004 and the 1988 International Headache Society diagnostic criteria. *Headache*. 2004;44:684–691.

50. Lipton RB, Stewart WF, Cady R, et al. Sumatriptan for the range of headaches in migraine sufferers: results of the spectrum study. *Headache*. 2000;40:783–791.

51. Dodick DW, Turkel CC, DeGryse RE, et al. OnabotulinumtoxinA for treatment of chronic migraine: pooled results from the double-blind, randomized, placebo-controlled phases of the PREEMPT clinical program. *Headache*. 2010;50:921–936.

52. Sandrini G, Manzoni GC, Zanferrari C, Nappi G. An epidemiologic approach to nosography of chronic daily headache. *Cephalalgia*. 1993;13:72–77.

53. Silberstein SD, Schulman EA, Hopkins MM. Repetitive intravenous DHE in the treatment of refractory headache. *Headache*. 1990;30:334–339.

54. Silberstein SD, Lipton RB, Sliwinski M. Classification of daily and near-daily headaches: field trial of revised IHS criteria. *Neurology*. 1996;47:871–875.

55. Bigal M, Lipton RB, deGryse R, Dimitrova R, Silberstein SD: Similarity of chronic migraine patients with and without a history of migraine. *Cephalalgia*. 2003;23:747(Abstract).

56. Dodick DW, Mauskop A, Elkind AH, deGryse R, Brin MF, Silberstein SD. Botulinum toxin type A for the prophylaxis of chronic daily headache: subgroup analysis of patients not receiving other prophylactic medications (a randomized, double-blind, placebo-controlled study). *Headache*. 2005;45:315–324.

57. Bigal ME, Rapoport AM, Tepper SJ, Sheftell FD, Lipton RB. The classification of chronic daily headache

in adolescents: a comparison between the second edition of the international classification of headache disorders and alternative diagnostic criteria. *Headache*. 2005;45:582–589.

58. Headache Classification Committee. New appendix criteria open for a broader concept of chronic migraine. *Cephalalgia*. 2006;26:742–746.

59. Yoon MS, Obermann M, Dommes P, Diener HC, Katsarava Z: Prevalence of migraine in a population based sample in Germany: results of the GHC study. *Cephalalgia*. 2009;29(S1):56–57(Abstract).

60. Zeeberg P, Olesen J, Jensen R. Medication overuse headache and chronic migraine in a specialized headache centre: field-testing proposed new appendix criteria. *Cephalalgia*. 2009;29:214–220.

61. Bigal M, Rapoport A, Sheftell F, Tepper S, Lipton R. The International Classification of Headache Disorders revised criteria for chronic migraine-field testing in a headache specialty clinic. *Cephalalgia*. 2007;27:230–234.

62. Headache Classification of the International Headache Society. The International Classification of Headache Disorders, 3rd edition (beta version). *Cephalalgia*. 2013;33:627–808.

63. Aurora SK, Dodick DW, Turkel CC, et al. OnabotulinumtoxinA for treatment of chronic migraine: results from the double-blind, randomized, placebo-controlled phase of the PREEMPT 1 trial. *Cephalalgia*. 2010;30:793–803.

64. Diener HC, Dodick DW, Aurora SK, et al. OnabotulinumtoxinA for treatment of chronic migraine: results from the double-blind, randomized, placebo-controlled phase of the PREEMPT 2 trial. *Cephalalgia*. 2010;30:804–814.

65. Ishkanian G, Blumenthal H, Webster CJ. Efficacy of sumatriptan tablets in migraineurs self-described or physician-diagnosed as having sinus headache: a randomized, double-blind, placebo-controlled study. *Clin Ther*. 2007;29:99–109.

66. Shah AK, Freij W. Dramatic relief after sumatriptan in a patient with a pituitary macroadenona. *Headache*. 1999;39:443–445.

67. Kaniecki R, Ruoff G, Smith T. Prevalence of migraine and response to sumatriptan in patients self-reporting tension/stress headache. *Curr Med Res Opin*. 2006;22:1535–1544.

68. Bousser MG, Russell RR. Cerebral venous thrombosis. In: Bousser MG, Russell RR, eds. *Major problems in neurology*. Volume I. London: Saunders, 1997:175.

69. Wall M, Silberstein SD, Aiken RD. Headache associated with abnormalities in intracranial structure or function: high cerebrospinal fluid pressure headache and brain tumor. In: Silberstein SD, Lipton RB, Dalessio DJ, eds. *Wolff's headache and other head pain*. 7th ed. New York: Oxford University Press, 2001:393–416.

70. Mosek A, Swanson JW, O'Fallon WM, Dodick DW, Bartleson JD: CSF opening pressure in patients with chronic daily headache. *Cephalalgia*. 1999;19:323(Abstract).

71. Pfaffenrath V, Kaube H. Diagnostics of cervicogenic headache. *Funct Neurology*. 1990;5:159–164.

72. Gladstone J, Eross E, Dodick D. Chronic daily headache: a rational approach to a challenging problem. *Semin Neurol*. 2003;23:265–276.

73. Solomon S, Lipton RB, Newman LC. Clinical features of chronic daily headache. *Headache*. 1992;32:325–329.

74. Guitera V, Munoz P, Castillo J, Pascual J. Transformed migraine: a proposal for the modification of its diagnostic criteria based on recent epidemiological data. *Cephalalgia*. 1999;19:847–850.

75. Vanast WJ. New daily persistent headaches: definition of a benign syndrome. *Headache*. 1986;26:317

76. Li D, Rozen TD. The clinical characteristics of new daily persistent headache. *Cephalalgia*. 2002;22:66–69.

77. Newman LC, Lipton RB, Solomon S. Hemicrania continua: 7 new cases and a literature review. *Headache*. 1993;32:267

78. Peres MF, Silberstein SD, Nahmias A, et al. Hemicrania continua is not that rare. *Neurology*. 2001;57:948–951.

79. Bordini C, Antonaci F, Stovner LJ, Schrader H, Sjaastad O. "Hemicrania Continua": a clinical review. *Headache*. 1991;31:20–26.

80. Marmura MJ, Silberstein SD, Gupta M. Hemicrania continua: who responds to indomethacin? *Cephalalgia*. 2009;29:300–307.

81. Fritsche G, Diener HC. Drug-induced headache following the use of zolmitriptan or naratriptan. *Cephalalgia*. 1999;19:414(Abstract).

82. Saper JR, Hamel RL, Lake AE. Medication overuse headache (MOH) is a biobehavioural disorder. *Cephalalgia*. 2005;545–546(Abstract).

83. Mathew NT. Drug induced headache. *Neurol Clin*. 1990;8:903–912.

84. Diamond S, Dalessio DJ. Drug abuse in headache. In: Diamond S, Dalessio DJ, eds. The practicing physician's approach to headache. 3rd ed. Baltimore, MD: Williams & Wilkins, 1982:114–121.

85. Wilkinson M. Introduction. In: Diener HC, Wilkinson M, eds. *Drug-induced headache*. Berlin: Springer-Verlag, 1988:1–2.

86. Saper JR. Ergotamine dependence. *Headache*. 1987;27:435–438.

87. Saper JR. Chronic headache syndromes. *Neurol Clin*. 1989;7:387–412.

88. Andersson PG. Ergotism: the clinical picture. In: Diener HC, Wilkinson MS, eds. *Drug-induced headache*. Berlin: Springer, 1988:16–19.

89. Baumgartner C, Wessly P, Bingol C, Maly J. Long-term prognosis of analgesic withdrawal in patients with drug-induced headaches. *Headache*. 1989;29:510–514.

90. Rapoport AM, Weeks RE, Sheftell FD, Baskin SM, Verdi J. The "analgesic washout period": a critical variable evaluation in the evaluation of headache treatment efficacy. *Neurology*. 1986;36:100–101.

91. Dichgans J, Diener HD, Gerber WD. Analgetika-induzierter dauerkopfschmerz. *Dtsch Med Wschr*. 1984;109:369.

92. Diener HC, Dahlof CG. Headache associated with chronic use of substances. In: Olesen J, Tfelt-Hansen P, Welch KMA, eds. *The headaches*. 2nd ed. Philadelphia: Lippincott, Williams & Wilkins, 1999:871–878.

93. Limmroth V, Katsarava Z, Fritsche G, Przywara S, Diener HC. Features of medication overuse headache following overuse of different acute headache drugs. *Neurology*. 2002;59:1011–1014.

94. Isler H. Headache drugs provoking chronic headache: historical aspects and common misunderstandings. In: Diener HC, Wilkinson M, eds. *Drug-induced headache*. Berlin: Springer-Verlag, 1988:87–94.

95. Kudrow L. Paradoxical effects of frequent analgesic use. *Adv Neurol*. 1982;33:335–341.

96. Diener HC, Dichgans J, Scholz E, Geiselhart S, Gerber WD, Billie A. Analgesic-induced chronic headache: long-term results of withdrawal therapy. *J Neurol*. 1984;236:9–14.

97. Rasmussen BK, Jensen R, Olesen J. Impact of headache on sickness absence and utilization of medical services. *J Epidemiol Community Health*. 1992;46:443–446.

98. Diener HC, Tfelt-Hansen P. Headache associated with chronic use of substances. In: Olesen J, Tfelt-Hansen P, Welch KMA, eds. *The headaches*. New York: Raven Press, 1993:721–727.

99. Micieli G, Manzoni GC, Granella F, Martignoni E, Malferrari G, Nappi G. Clinical and epidemiological observations on drug abuse in headache patients. In: Diener HC, Wilkinson M, eds. *Drug-induced headache*. Berlin: Springer-Verlag, 1988:20–28.

100. Ravishankar K. Headache pattern in India: a headache clinic analysis of 1000 patients. *Cephalalgia*. 1997;17:143–144.

101. Schnider P, Aull S, Feucht M. Use and abuse of analgesics in tension-type headache. *Cephalalgia*. 1994;14:162–167.

102. Silberstein SD, Saper JR. Migraine: Diagnosis and treatment. In: Dalessio DJ, Silberstein SD, eds. *Wolff's headache and other head pain*. 6th ed. New York: Oxford University Press, 1993:96–170.

103. Eggen AE. The Tromso study: frequency and predicting factors of analgesic drug use in a free-living population (12–56 years). *J Clin Epidemiol*. 1993;46:1297–1304.

104. Gutzwiller F, Zemp E. Der Analgetikakonsum in der Bevölkerung und socioökonomische Aspekte des Analgetikaabusus. In: Mihatsch MJ, ed. *Das analgetikasyndrom*. Stuttgart: Thieme, 1986:197–205.

105. Kielholz P, Ladewig D. Probleme des medikamentenmissbrauches. *Schweis Arztezeitung*. 1981;62:2866–2869.

106. Schwarz A, Farber U, Glaeske G. Daten zu analgetikakonsum and analgetikanephropathie in der bundesrepublik. *Offentiches gesundheitswesen*. 1985;47:298–300.

107. Celentano DD, Stewart WF, Lipton RB, Reed M. Medication use and disability among migraineurs. *Headache*. 1992;32:223–228.

108. Robinson RG. Pain relief for headaches. *Can Fam Physician*. 1993;39:867–872.

109. Wilkinson SM, Becker WJ, Heine JA. Opiate use to control bowel motility may induce chronic daily headache in patients with migraine. *Headache*. 2001;41:303–309.

110. Bahra A, Walsh M, Menon S, Goadsby PJ. Does chronic daily headache arise de novo in association with regular use of analgesics? *Headache*. 2003;43:179–190.

111. Silverman K, Evans SM, Strain EC, Griffiths RR. Withdrawal syndrome after the double-blind cessation of caffeine consumption. *N Eng J Med*. 1992;327:1109–1114.

112. Potter DL, Hart DE, Calder CS, Storey JR. A double-blind, randomized, placebo-controlled, parallel study to determine the efficacy of topiramate in the prophylactic treatment of migraine. *Neurology*. 2000;54:A15(Abstract).

113. Scholz E, Diener HC, Geiselhart S, Wilkinson M. Drug-induced headache: does a critical dosage exist? In: Diener HC, ed. *Drug-induced headache*. Berlin: Springer-Verlag, 1988:29–33.

114. Saper JR. Ergotamine dependency: a review. *Headache*. 1987;27:435–438.

115. Catarci T, Fiacco F, Argentino C. Ergotamine-induced headache can be sustained by sumatriptan daily intake. *Cephalalgia*. 1994;14:374–375.

116. Diener HC, Haab J, Peters C, Ried S, Dichgans J, Pilgrim A. Subcutaneous sumatriptan in the treatment of headache during withdrawal from drug-induced headache. *Headache*. 1991;31:205–209.

117. Gaist D, Hallas J, Sindrup SH, Gram LF. Is overuse of sumatriptan a problem? A population-based study. *Eur J Clin Pharmacol*. 1996;50:161–165.

118. Diener HC, Silberstein SD. Medication overuse headache. In: Olesen J, Goadsby PJ, Ramadan NM, Tfelt-Hansen P, Welch KMA, eds. *The headaches*. 3rd ed. Philadelphia: Lippincott Williams & Wilkins, 2006:971–979.

119. Obermann M, Bartsch T, Katsarava Z. Medication overuse headache. *Expert Opin Drug Saf*. 2006;5:49–56.

120. Kaiser RS. Substance abuse and headache. 1999; 41st Annual Scientific Meeting, Boston, MA.

121. Saper JR. Approach to the intractable headache case: identifying treatable barriers to improvement. *Headache*. 2006;12:259–284.

122. Saper JR, Lake AEII. Sustained opioud therapy should rarely be administered to headache patients: clinical observations, literature review, and proposed guidelines. *Headache Currents*. 2006;3:67–70.

123. Lake AE, Saper JR, Hamel RL. Inpatient treatment of intractable headache: outcome for 267 consecutive program completers. *Headache*. 2006;46:893(Abstract).

124. Fisher CM. Analgesic rebound headache refuted. *Headache*. 1988;28:666

125. Bowdler I, Killian J, G.,nsslen-Blumberg S. The association between analgesic abuse and headache: coincidental or causal. *Headache*. 1990;30:494.

126. Lance F, Parkes C, Wilkinson M. Does analgesic abuse cause headache de novo? *Headache*. 1988;1:61–62.

127. Bahra A, Walsh M, Menon S, Goadsby PJ: Does chronic daily headache arise de novo in association with regular analgesic use? *Cephalalgia*. 2000;20:294(Abstract).

128. Mao J, Sung B, Ji RR, Lim G. Neuronal apoptosis associated with morphine tolerance: evidence for an opioid-induced neurotoxic mechanism. *J Neurosci*. 2002;22:7650–7661.

129. Merikangas KR, Angst J, Isler H. Migraine and psychopathology: results of the Zurich cohort study of young adults. *Arch Gen Psychiatry*. 1990;47:849–853.

130. Breslau N, Davis GC. Migraine, physical health and psychiatric disorders: a prospective epidemiologic study of young adults. *J Psychiatric Res*. 1993;27:211–221.

131. Mongini F, Defilippi N, Negro C. Chronic daily headache. A clinical and psychologic profile before and after treatment. *Headache*. 1997;37:83–87.

132. Mitsikostas DD, Thomas AM. Comorbidity of headache and depressive disorders. *Cephalalgia*. 1999;19:211–217.

133. Verri AP, Cecchini P, Galli C, Granella F, Sandrini G, Nappi G. Psychiatric comorbidity in chronic daily headache. *Cephalalgia*. 1998;18:45–49.

134. Curioso EP, Young WB, Shechter AL, Kaiser RS. Psychiatric comorbidity predicts outcome in chronic daily headache patients. *Neurology*. 1999;52:A471 (Abstract).

135. Monzon MJ, Lainez MJ. Quality of life in migraine and chronic daily headache patients. *Cephalalgia*. 1998;18:638–643.

136. Solomon GD, Skobieranda FG, Gragg LA. Quality of life and well-being of headache patients: measurement by the Medical Outcomes Study instrument. *Headache*. 1993;33:351–358.

137. Guitera V, Muñoz P, Castillo J, Pascual J. Impact of chronic daily headache in the quality of life: a study in the general population. *Cephalalgia*. 1999;19:412–413(Abstract).

138. Puca F, Genco S, Prudenzano MP, et al. Psychiatric comorbidity and psychosocial stress in patients with tension-type headache from headache centers in Italy. The Italian Collaborative Group for the Study of Psychopathological Factors in Primary Headaches. *Cephalalgia*. 1999;19:159–164.

139. Juang KD, Wang SJ, Fuh JL, Lu SR, Su TP. Comorbidity of depressive and anxiety disorders in chronic daily headache and its subtypes. *Headache*. 2000;40:818–823.

140. Guidetti V, Galli F. Chronic daily headache in children and adolescents: clinical features and psychiatric comorbidity. *Cephalalgia*. 1999;19:389(Abstract).

141. Zwart JA, Dyb G, Hagen K, et al. Depression and anxiety disorders associated with headache frequency: The Nord-Trondelag Health Study. *Eur J Neurol*. 2003;10:147–152.

142. Peres MF, Young WB, Kaup AO, Zukerman E, Silberstein SD. Fibromyalgia is common in patients with transformed migraine. *Neurology*. 2001;57:1326–1328.

143. Peres MF, Zukerman E, Young WB, Silberstein SD. Fatigue in chronic migraine patients. *Cephalalgia*. 2002;22:720–724.

144. Wolfe F, Smythe HA, Yanus MB. The American College of Rheumatology 1990 criteria for the classification of fibromyalgia: report of the Multicenter Criteria Committee. *Arthritis Rheum*. 1990;33:160–172.

145. Krupp LB, laRocca NG, Muir-Nash J, Steinberg AD. The fatigue severity scale. Application to patients with multiple sclerosis and systemic lupus erythematosus. *Arch Neurol*. 1989;46:1121–1123.

146. Chalder T, Berelowitz G, Pawlikowska T. Development of a fatigue scale. *J Psychosom Res*. 1993;37:147–153.

147. Morriss RK, Wearden AJ, Mullis R. Exploring the validity of the Chalder Fatigue scale in chronic fatigue syndrome. *J Psychosom Res*. 1998;411–417.

148. Hagen K, Einarsen C, Zwart JA, Svebak S, Bovim G. The co-occurrence of headache and musculoskeletal symptoms amongst 51 050 adults in Norway. *Eur J Neurol*. 2002;9:527–533.

149. Tekle Haimanot R, Seraw B, Forsgren L, Ekbom K, Ekstedt J. Migraine, chronic tension-type headache, and cluster headache in an Ethiopian rural community. *Cephalalgia*. 1995;15:482–488.

150. Rasmussen BK. Epidemiology of headache. *Cephalalgia*. 1995;15:45–68.

151. Lu SR, Fuh JL, Chen WT, Juang KD, Wang SJ. Chronic daily headache in Taipei, Taiwan: prevalence, follow-up and outcome predictors. *Cephalalgia*. 2001;21:980–986.

152. Queiroz LP, Barea LM, Blank N. An epidemiological study of headache in Florianopolis, Brazil. *Cephalalgia*. 2006;26:122–127.

153. Rasmussen BK, Jensen R, Schroll M, Olesen J. Interrelations between migraine and tension-type headache in the general population. *Arch Neurol*. 1992;49:914–918.

154. Gobel H, Petersen-Braun M, Sokya D. The epidemiology of headache in Germany: a nationwide survey of a representative sample on the basis of the headache classification of the International Headache Society. *Cephalalgia*. 1994;14:97–106.

155. Zwart JA, Dyb G, Hagen K, Svebak S, Stovner LJ, Holmen J. Analgesic overuse among subjects with headache, neck, and low-back pain. *Neurology*. 2004;62:1540–1544.

156. Straube A, Pfaffenrath V, Ladwig KH, et al. Prevalence of chronic migraine and medication overuse headache in Germany: the German DMKG headache study. *Cephalalgia*. 2010;30:207–213.

157. Buse DC, Manack AN, Fanning KM, et al. Chronic migraine prevalence, disability, and sociodemographic factors: results from the American Migraine Prevalence and Prevention Study. *Headache*. 2012;52:1456–1470.

158. Granella F, Cavallini A, Sandrini G, Manzoni GC, Nappi G. Long-term outcome of migraine. *Cephalalgia*. 1998;18:30–33.

159. Scher AI, Stewart WF, Ricci JA, Lipton RB. Factors associated with the onset and remission of chronic daily headache in a population-based study. *Pain*. 2003;106:89.

160. Scher AI, Lipton RB, Stewart W. Risk factors for chronic daily headache. *Cur Pain Headache Rep*. 2002;6:486–491.

161. Scher AI, Lipton RB, Stewart WF. Habitual snoring as a risk factor for chronic daily headache. *Neurology*. 2003;60:1366–1368.

162. Wiendels NJ, Knuistingh NA, Rosendaal FR, et al. Chronic frequent headache in the general population: prevalence and associated factors. *Cephalalgia*. 2006;26:1434–1442.

163. Scher AI, Stewart WF, Lipton RB. Caffeine as a risk factor for chronic daily headache: a population-based study. *Neurology*. 2004;63:2022–2027.

164. Scher AI, Stewart WF, Lipton RB. The comorbidity of headache with other pain syndromes. *Headache*. 2006;46:1416–1423.

165. Bigal ME, Lipton RB. Obesity is a risk factor for transformed migraine but not chronic tension-type headache. *Neurology*. 2006;67:252–257.

166. Katsarava Z, Schneeweiss S, Kurth T, et al. Incidence and predictors for chronicity of headache in patients with episodic migraine. *Neurology*. 2004;62:788–790.

167. Zwart JA, Dyb G, Hagen K, Svebak S, Holmen J. Analgesic use: a predictor of chronic pain and medication overuse headache: the Head-HUNT Study. *Neurology*. 2003;61:160–164.

168. Hagen K, Linde M, Steiner TJ, Stovner LJ, Zwart J-A. Risk factors for medication-overuse headache: an 11-year follow-up study. *Pain*. 2012;153:56–61.

169. Couch JR, Lipton RB, Stewart WF, Scher AI. Head or neck injury increases the risk of chronic daily headache: a population-based study. *Neurology*. 2007;69:1169–1177.

170. Scher AI, Midgette LA, Lipton RB. Risk factors for headache chronification. *Headache*. 2008;48:16–25.

171. Woolf CJ, Mitchell MB. Mechanism-based pain diagnosis issues for analgesic drug development. *Anesthesiology*. 2001;95:241–249.

172. Shukla P, Richardson E, Young WB. Brush allodynia in an inpatient headache unit. *Headache*. 2003;43:542(Abstract).

173. Creach C, Radat F, Laffitau M, Irachabal S, Henry P: Cutaneous allodynia in transformed migraine with medication overuse. *Cephalalgia*. 2003;23:656–657(Abstract).

174. Sobrino FE: Cutaneous allodynia in chronic migraine. *Cephalalgia*. 2003;23:750(Abstract).

175. Moulton EA, Burstein R, Tully S, Hargreaves R, Becerra L, Borsook D. Interictal dysfunction of a brainstem descending modulatory center in migraine patients. *PLoS One*. 2008;3:e3799.

176. Zed PJ, Loewen PS, Robinson G. Medication-induced headache: overview and systematic review of therapeutic approaches. *Ann Pharmacother*. 1999;33:61–72.

177. Zeeberg P, Olesen J, Jensen R. Discontinuation of medication overuse in headache patients: recovery of therapeutic responsiveness. *Cephalalgia*. 2006;26:1192–1198.

178. Hagen K, Albretsen C, Vilming ST, et al. Management of medication overuse headache: 1-year randomized multicentre open-label trial. *Cephalalgia*. 2009;29:221–232.

179. Hagen K, Albretsen C, Vilming ST, et al. A 4-year follow-up of patients with medication-overuse headache previously included in a randomized multicentre study. *J Headache Pain*. 2011;12:315–322.

180. Silberstein SD, Lipton RB, Dodick DW, et al. Efficacy and safety of topiramate for the treatment of chronic migraine: a randomized, double-blind, placebo-controlled trial. *Headache*. 2007;47:170–180.

181. Diener HC, Bussone G, Van Oene JC, Lahaye M, Schwalen S, Goadsby PJ. Topiramate reduces headache days in chronic migraine: a randomized, double-blind, placebo-controlled study. *Cephalalgia*. 2007;27:814–23.

182. Diener HC, Dodick DW, Goadsby PJ, et al. Utility of topiramate for the treatment of patients with chronic migraine in the presence or absence of acute medication overuse. *Cephalalgia*. 2009;29:1021–1027.

183. Silberstein SD, Blumenfeld AM, Cady RK, et al: OnabotulinumtoxinA for treatment of chronic migraine: PREEMPT 24-week pooled subgroup analysis of patients who had acute headache medication overuse at baseline. *J Neurol Sci*. 2013;331:48–56.

184. Tavola T, Gala C, Conte G, Invernizzi G. Traditional Chinese acupuncture in tension-type headache: a controlled study. *Pain*. 1992;48:325–329.

185. Silberstein SD. Treatment of headache in primary care practice. *Am J Med*. 1984;77:65–72.

186. Raskin NH. Repetitive intravenous dihydroergotamine as therapy for intractable migraine. *Neurology*. 1986;36:995–997.

187. Saper JR, Silberstein SD, Gordon CD, Hamel RL, Swidan S. *Handbook of headache management: a practical guide to diagnosis and treatment of head, neck, and facial pain*. 2nd ed. Baltimore, MD: Lippincott Williams & Wilkins, 1999.

188. Diener HC, Gerber WD, Geiselhart S. Short and long-term effects of withdrawal therapy in drug-induced headache. In: Diener HC, Wilkinson M, eds. *Drug-induced headache*. Berlin: Springer-Verlag, 1988:133–142.

189. Hering R, Steiner TJ. Abrupt outpatient withdrawal from medication in analgesic-abusing migraineurs. *Lancet*. 1991;337:1442–1443.

190. Diener HC, Pfaffenrath V, Soyka D, Gerber WD. Therapie des medikamenten-induzierten dauerkopfschmerzes. *Münch Med Wschr*. 1992;134:159–162.

191. Saper JR, Lake AE, III, Madden SF, Kreeger C. Comprehensive/tertiary care for headache: a 6-month outcome study. *Headache*. 1999;39:249–263.

192. Silberstein SD, Lipton RB. Overview of diagnosis and treatment of migraine. *Neurology*. 1994;44:6–16.

193. Bussone G, Sandrini G, Patruno G, Ruiz L, Tasorelli C, Nappi G. Effectiveness of fluoxetine on pain and depression in chronic headache disorders. In: Nappi G, Bono G, Sandrini G, Martignoni E, Micieli G, eds. *Headache and depression: serotonin pathways as a common clue*. New York: Raven Press, 1991:265–272.

194. Couch JR, Ziegler DK, Hassainein R. Amitriptyline in the prophylaxis of migraine. *Arch Neurol*. 1976;26:121–127.

195. Diamond S, Baltes B. Chronic tension headache treated with amitriptyline: a double blind study. *Headache*. 1971;11:110–116.

196. Holland J, Holland C, Kudrow L. Low dose amitriptyline prophylaxis in chronic scalp muscle contraction headache. Proceedings of the First International Headache Congress. Munich, September 1983.

197. Lance JW, Curran DA. Treatment of chronic tension headache. *Lancet*. 1964;1:1236–1239.

198. Pluvinage R. Le traitement des migraines et des cephalees psychogenes par l'amitriptyline. *Sem Hop*. 1978;54:713–716.

199. Pfaffenrath V, Kellhammer U, Pollmann W. Combination headache: practical experience with a combination of beta-blocker and an antidepressive. *Cephalalgia*. 1986;6:25–32.

200. Holroyd KA, Nash JM, Pingel JD. A comparison of pharmacologic (amitriptyline HCl) and nonpharmacologic (cognitive-behavioral) therapies for chronic tension headaches. *J Consulting Clin Psychology*. 1991;59:387–393.

201. Gobel H, Hamouz V, Hansen C, et al. Chronic tension-type headache: amitriptyline reduces clinical headache-duration and experimental pain sensitivity but does not alter pericranial muscle activity readings. *Pain*. 1994;59:241–249.

202. Pfaffenrath V, Diener HC, Isler H, et al. Efficacy and tolerability of amitriptylinoxide in the treatment of chronic tension-type headache: a multicentre controlled study. *Cephalalgia*. 1994;14:149–155.

203. Cerbo R, Barbanti P, Fabbrini G, Pascali MP, Catarci T. Amitriptyline is effective in chronic but not in episodic tension-type headache: pathogenic implications. *Headache*. 1998;38:453–457.

204. Mitsikostas DD, Gatzonis S, Thomas A, Ilias A. Buspirone vs amitriptyline in the treatment of

chronic tension-type headache. *J Neurol Scand.* 1997;96:247–251.

205. Bonuccelli U, Nuti A, Lucetti C, Pavese N, Dellagnello G, Muratorio A. Amitriptyline and dexamethasone combined treatment in drug-induced headache. *Cephalalgia.* 1996;16:197–200.

206. Morland TJ, Storli OV, Mogstad TE. Doxepin in the prophylactic treatment of mixed "vascular" and tension headache. *Headache.* 1979;19:382–383.

207. Descombes S, Brefel-Courbon C, Thalamas C, et al. Amitriptyline treatment in chronic drug-induced headache: a double-blind comparative pilot study. *Headache.* 2001;41:178–182.

208. Saper JR, Silberstein SD, Lake AE, Winters ME. Double-blind trial of fluoxetine: chronic daily headache and migraine. *Headache.* 1994;34:497–502.

209. Krymchantowski AV, Silva MT, Barbosa JS, Alves LA. Amitriptyline versus amitriptyline combined with fluoxetine in the preventative treatment of transformed migraine: a double-blind study. *Headache.* 2002;42:510–514.

210. Manna V, Bolino F, DiCicco L. Chronic tension-type headache, mood depression and serotonin. *Headache.* 1994;34:44–49.

211. Palmer KJ, Benfield P. Fluvoxamine: an overview of its pharmacologic properties and a review of its use in nondepressive disorders. *CNS Drugs.* 1994;1:57–87.

212. Foster CA, Bafaloukos J. Paroxetine in the treatment of chronic daily headache. *Headache.* 1994;34:587–589.

213. Langemark M, Olesen J. Sulpiride and paroxetine in the treatment of chronic tension-type headache. *Headache.* 1994;34:20–24.

214. Mathew NT. Prophylaxis of migraine and mixed headache: a randomized controlled study. *Headache.* 1981;21:105–109.

215. Bright RA, Everitt DE. Beta-blockers and depression: evidence against association. *JAMA.* 1992;267:1783

216. Jensen R, Brinck T, Olesen J. Sodium valproate has a prophylactic effect in migraine without aura. *Neurology.* 1994;44:647–651.

217. Mathew NT, Saper JR, Silberstein SD, et al. Migraine prophylaxis with divalproex. *Arch Neurol.* 1995;52:281–286.

218. Hering R, Kuritzky A. Sodium valproate in the prophylactic treatment of migraine: a double-blind study versus placebo. *Cephalalgia.* 1992;12:81–84.

219. Klapper J Divalproex sodium in the prophylactic treatment of migraine. *Headache.* 1995;35:290(Abstract).

220. Mathew NT, Ali S. Valproate in the treatment of persistent chronic daily headache. An open label study. *Headache.* 1991;31:71–74.

221. Edwards K, Santarcangelo V, Shea P, Edwards J. Intravenous valproate for acute treatment of migraine headaches. *Cephalalgia.* 1999;19:356(Abstract).

222. Freitag FG, Diamond S, Diamond M, Urban G. Divalproex in the long-term treatment of chronic daily headache. *Headache.* 2001;41:271–278.

223. Yurekli VA, Akhan G, Kutluhan S, Uzar E, Koyuncuoglu HR, Gultekin F. The effect of sodium valproate on chronic daily headache and its subgroups. *J Headache Pain.* 2008;9:37–41.

224. Spira PJ, Beran RG. Gabapentin in the prophylaxis of chronic daily headache: a randomized, placebo-controlled study for the Australian Gabapentin

Chronic Daily Headache Group. *Neurology.* 2003;61:1753–1759.

225. Silberstein SD. Gabapentin in the treatment of chronic daily headache (Commentary). *Neurology.* 2003;61:1637

226. Shuaib A, Ahmed F, Muratoglu M, Kochanski P. Topiramate in migraine prophylaxis: a pilot study. *Cephalalgia.* 1999;19:379–380(Abstract).

227. Silberstein SD, Dodick DW, Lindblad AS, et al. Randomized, placebo-controlled trial of propranolol added to topiramate in chronic migraine. *Neurology.* 2012;78:976–984.

228. Beran RG, Spira PJ. Levetiracetam in chronic daily headache: a double-blind, randomised placebo-controlled study. (The Australian KEPPRA Headache Trial [AUS-KHT]). *Cephalalgia.* 2011;31:530–536.

229. Saper JR, Lake AE, III, Cantrell DT, Winner PK, White JR. Chronic daily headache prophylaxis with tizanidine: a double-blind, placebo-controlled, multicenter outcome study. *Headache.* 2002;42:470–482.

230. Miller DS, Talbot CA, Simpson W, Korey A. A comparison of naproxen sodium, acetaminophen and placebo in the treatment of muscle contraction headache. *Headache.* 1987;27:392–396.

231. Johnson ES, Tfelt-Hansen P. Nonsteroidal antiinflammatory drugs. In: Olesen J, Tfelt-Hansen P, Welch KMA, eds. *The headaches.* New York: Raven Press, 1993:391–395.

232. Mylecharane EJ, Tfelt-Hansen P. Miscellaneous drugs. In: Olesen J, Tfelt-Hansen P, Welch KMA, eds. *The headaches.* New York: Raven Press, 1993:397–402.

233. Kangasniemi PJ, Nyrke T, Lang AH, Petersen E. Femoxetine—a new 5HT uptake inhibitor—and propranolol in the prophylactic treatment of migraine. *Acta Neurol Scand.* 1983;68:262–267.

234. Scholz E, Gerber WD, Diener HC, Langohr HD. Dihydroergotamine vs flunarizine vs nifedipine vs metoprolol vs propranolol in migraine prophylaxis: a comparative study based on time series analysis. In: Scholz E, Gerber WD, Diener HC, Langohr HD, eds. *Advances in headache research.* London: John Libbey, 1987:139–145.

235. Pascual J, Leira R, Lainez JM. Combined therapy for migraine prevention? Clinical experience with a beta-blocker plus sodium valproate in 52 resistant migraine patients. *Cephalalgia.* 2003;23:961–962.

236. Harden RN. Chronic opioid therapy: another reappraisal. APS Bulletin 2002;12:1–12.

237. Ziegler DK. Opioids in headache treatment: is there a role? *Neurol Clin.* 1997;15:199–207.

238. Robbins L. Long-acting opioids for severe chronic daily headache. *Headache Quarterly.* 1999;10:135–139.

239. Saper JR, Lake AE, Hamel RL, et al. Daily scheduled opioids for intractable head pain: long-term observations of a treatment program. *Neurology.* 2004;62:1687–1694.

240. Nicholson RA, Buse DC, Andrasik F, Lipton RB. Nonpharmacologic treatments for migraine and tension-type headache: how to choose and when to use. *Curr Treat Options Neurol.* 2011;13:28–40.

241. Coeytaux RR, Kaufman JS, Kaptchuk TJ, et al. A randomized, controlled trial of acupuncture for chronic daily headache. *Headache.* 2005;45:1113–1123.

242. Park JM, Park SU, Jung WS, Moon SK. Carthami-Semen acupuncture point injection for chronic daily

headache: a pilot, randomised, double-blind, controlled trial. *Complement Ther Med.* 2011;19:S19–S25.

243. Calhoun AH, Ford S. Behavioral sleep modification may revert transformed migraine to episodic migraine. *Headache.* 2007;47:1178–1183.

244. Silberstein SD, Saper JR, Freitag F. Migraine: Diagnosis and treatment. In: Silberstein SD, Lipton RB, Dalessio DJ, eds. *Wolff's headache and other head pain.* 7th ed. New York: Oxford University Press, 2001:121–237.

245. Bell R, Montoya D, Shuaib A, Lee MA. A comparative trial of three agents in the treatment of acute migraine headache. *Ann Emerg Med.* 1990;19:1079–1082.

246. Callaham M, Raskin N. A controlled study of dihydroergotamine in the treatment of acute migraine headache. *Headache.* 1986;26:168–171.

247. Jones J, Sklar D, Dougherty J, White W. Randomized double-blind trial of intravenous prochlorperazine for the treatment of acute headache. *JAMA.* 1989;261:1174–1176.

248. Lu SR, Fuh JL, Juang KD, Wang SJ. Repetitive intravenous prochlorperazine treatment of patients with refractory chronic daily headache. *Headache.* 2000;40:724–729.

249. Wang SJ, Silberstein SD, Young WB. Droperidol treatment of status migrainosus and refractory migraine. *Headache.* 1997;37:377–382.

250. Silberstein SD, Young WB, Mendizabal J, Rothrock J, Alam A. Efficacy of intramuscular droperidol for migraine treatment: a dose response study. *Headache Quarterly.* 1999;10:55–57.

251. Schreiber S, Getslev V, Backer MM, Weizman R, Pick CG. The atypical neuroleptics clozapine and olanzapine differ regarding their antinociceptive mechanisms and potency. *Pharmacol Biochem Behav.* 1999;64:75–80.

252. Silberstein SD, Peres MF, Hopkins MM, Shechter AL, Young WB, Rozen TD. Olanzapine in the treatment of refractory migraine and chronic daily headache. *Headache.* 2002;42:515–518.

253. Krymchantowski AV, Jevoux C, Moreira PF. An open pilot study assessing the benefits of quetiapine for the prevention of migraine refractory to the combination of atenolol, nortriptyline, and flunarizine. *Pain Medicine.* 2010;11:48–52.

254. Pradalier A, Clapin A, Dry J. Treatment review: nonsteroid antiinflammatory drugs in the treatment and long-term prevention of migraine attacks. *Headache: The Journal of Head and Face Pain.* 1988;28(8):550–557.

255. Tanen DA, Miller S, French T, Riffenburgh RH. Intravenous sodium valproate versus prochlorperazine for the emergency department treatment of acute migraine headaches: a prospective, randomized, double-blind trial. *Ann Emerg Med.* 2003;41:847–853.

256. Krusz JC, Belanger J. Propofol: a highly effective treatment for acute headaches. *Cephalalgia.* 1999;19:358(Abstract).

257. Mendes PM, Silberstein SD, Young WB, Rozen TD, Paolone MF. Intravenous Propofol in the Treatment of Refractory Headache. *Headache.* 2002;42:638–641.

258. Hand PJ, Stark RJ. Intravenous lignocaine infusions for severe chronic daily headache. *Med J Aust.* 2000;172:157–159.

259. Rosen NL, Abbas MA, Silberstein SD. Effects of intravenous lidocaine in the treatment of refractory chronic daily headache. 2007(UnPub).

260. Swidan SZ, Lake AE, III, Saper JR. Efficacy of intravenous diphenhydramine versus intravenous DHE-45 in the treatment of severe migraine headache. *Curr Pain Headache Rep.* 2005;9:65–70.

261. Bell RF. Ketamine for chronic non-cancer pain. *Pain.* 2009;141:210–214.

262. Afridi SK, Giffin NJ, Kaube H, Goadsby PJ. A randomized controlled trial of intranasal ketamine in migraine with prolonged aura. *Neurology.* 2013;80:642–647.

263. Drucker P, Tepper S. Daily sumatriptan for detoxification from rebound. *Headache.* 1998;38:687–690.

264. Pringsheim T, Howse D. Inpatient treatment of chronic daily headache using dihydroergotamine: a long-term followup study. *Can J Neurol Sci.* 1998;25:146–150.

265. Saper JR, Lake AE, III. Borderline personality disorder and the chronic headache patient: review and management recommendations. *Headache.* 2002;42:663–674.

266. Saper JR, Lake AE, III. Medication overuse headache: type I and type II. *Cephalalgia.* 2006;26:1262

267. Silberstein SD, Silberstein JR. Chronic daily headache: prognosis following inpatient treatment with repetitive IV DHE. *Headache.* 1992;32:439–445.

268. Tfelt-Hansen P, Aebelholt-Krabbe A. Ergotamine abuse: do patients benefit from withdrawal? *Cephalalgia.* 1981;1:27–32.

269. Schoenen J, Lenarduzzi P, Sianard-Gainko J. Chronic headaches associated with analgesics and/or ergotamine abuse: a clinical survey of 434 consecutive outpatients. In: Rose FD, ed. *New advances in headache research.* London: Smith-Gordon, 1989:29–43.

270. Isler H. Migraine treatment as a cause of chronic migraine. In: Rose FC, ed. *Advances in migraine research and therapy.* New York: Raven Press, 1982:159–164.

271. Henry P, Dartigues JF, Benetier MP. Ergotamine—and analgesic-induced headache. In C. Rose (ed.), Migraine: Proceedings from the Fifth International Migraine Symposium, London, 1984;197.

272. Schnider P, Aull S, Baumgartner C. Long-term outcome of patients with headache and drug abuse after inpatient withdrawal: five-year followup. *Cephalalgia.* 1996;16:481–485.

273. Pini LA, Bigarelli M, Vitale G, Sternieri E. Headaches associated with chronic use of analgesics: a therapeutic approach. *Headache.* 1996;36:433–439.

274. Suhr B, Evers S, Bauer B, Gralow I, Grotemeyer KH, Husstedt IW. Drug-induced headache: long-term results of stationary versus ambulatory withdrawal therapy. *Cephalalgia.* 1999;19:44–49.

275. Monzon MJ, Lainez MJA, Morales F, Sancho J: Long-term prognosis of chronic daily headache. *Cephalalgia.* 1999;19:410(Abstract).

276. Lorenzatto WS, Cheim CF, Adriano M, Barbosa JS, Christino PS, Krymchantowski AV. Long-term outcome in chronic daily headache. *Cephalalgia.* 1999;19:413(Abstract).

277. Katsarava Z, Muessig M, Dzagnidze A, Fritsche G, Diener HC, Limmroth V. Medication overuse headache: rates and predictors for relapse in a 4-year prospective study. *Cephalalgia.* 2005;25:12–15.

278. Lipton RB, Silberstein SD, Saper JR, Bigal ME, Goadsby PJ. Why headache treatment fails. *Neurology.* 2003;60:1064–1070.

Chapter 10

Neuromodulation

PERIPHERAL NERVE STIMULATION
Occipital Nerve Stimulation
Sphenopalatine Ganglion Stimulation
Supraorbital Nerve Stimulation
Vagal Nerve Stimulation

CENTRAL NEUROSTIMULATION
Single-Pulse Transcranial Magnetic

Stimulation
Repetitive Transcranial Magnetic
  Stimulation (rTMS)
Transcranial Direct Current
  Stimulation (tDCS)

REFERENCES

Neuromodulation has emerged as a potentially promising therapeutic modality and treatment approach for many headache disorders. Neurostimulation therapies for headache may be separated into peripheral nerve neurostimulation (PNS) and central neurostimulation (CNS) strategies. PNS strategies include occipital nerve stimulation (ONS), vagal nerve stimulation (VNS)—both implanted and portable transcutaneous VNS, and other extracranial nerve stimulation procedures that target the supraorbital and sphenopalatine ganglion stimulation. CNS strategies include hypothalamus deep brain stimulation (hDBS) (for patients with medically intractable trigeminal autonomic cephalalgias), transcutaneous direct current stimulation (tDCS), and single pulse transcranial magnetic stimulation (sTMS). The evidence base to support each of these modalities is highly variable. However, controlled studies are gradually emerging. The

evidence in migraine is most robust for ONS and sTMS; hDBS will not be discussed in this chapter, as this modality has been evaluated only in patients with trigeminal autonomic cephalalgias (primarily cluster headache) and not migraine.

PERIPHERAL NERVE STIMULATION

Occipital Nerve Stimulation

RATIONALE AND POTENTIAL MECHANISM(S)

The use of anesthetic blockade of the greater occipital nerve (GON) has been employed in clinical practice to treat the pain associated with a variety of primary and secondary headache disorders for decades.[1] Experimentally, anesthetic blockade of the greater occipital nerve inhibits the nociceptive specific blink reflex,[2,3] and a number of placebo-controlled studies have demonstrated the efficacy of anesthetic blockade or corticosteroid injections in the area of the occipital nerves for treatment of cluster headache.[4,5] The ability to acutely relieve the pain that frequently resides in the anterior (first division of trigeminal nerve) part of the head and to modulate the frequency of headache attacks led to anatomic and physiological studies that have provided a basis for therapies directed toward the occipital nerves. [1,6–11] It is now established that there is anatomical and physiological convergence of nociceptive input from dural and C-2 afferents. [12–14] Sensory nociceptive information from the dura mater to the first synapse in the brainstem is transmitted via small-diameter A- and C-fiber afferents in the ophthalmic division of the trigeminal nerve via the trigeminal ganglion to nociceptive second-order neurons in the superficial and deep layers of the medullary dorsal horn of the trigeminocervical complex. [13] The nociceptive sensory traffic from suboccipital structures is also mediated by small-diameter afferent fibers in the upper cervical roots, terminating in the dorsal horn of the cervical spine and extending from the C_2 segment up to the medullary dorsal horn.[12,13,15] The major afferent contribution is mediated by the spinal root C_2 that is peripherally represented by the GON. These cervical neurons show a high convergence of input from neck muscles and skin.

It is also now established that the nociceptive inflow to second-order neurons in the spinal cord and the trigeminocervical complex is subject to modulation by descending projections from the pain-matrix; supratentorial and brainstem structures, including the periaqueductal gray (PAG); nucleus raphe magnus (NRM); and the rostroventral medulla (RVM).[16–22]

The mechanism by which ONS mediates a reduction in the frequency and severity of headache in patients with primary headache disorders is not clear. Based on the anatomical convergence and influence of the pain-matrix on activity of second-order sensory transmission neurons within the trigeminal nucleus caudalis (TNC), one hypothesis by which peripheral nerve stimulation reduces centrally transmitted pain is based upon the ideas of Melzack and Wall.[23] The Melzack–Wall gate-control theory suggests that there

is an inverse relationship between activity in small-diameter nociceptive afferents and large-diameter nerve fibers, in that stimulation of large-diameter fibers leads to suppression of small-diameter fiber nociceptive input and elevation of pain thresholds. However, in a study of ONS in subjects with chronic cluster headache (CCH), no significant change in pain thresholds was demonstrated, which argues against a diffuse analgesic effect.[24] In fact, the nociceptive blink reflex increased with longer durations of ONS, and it was suggested that the delay of 2 months or more between implantation and significant clinical improvement suggests that the procedure acts via slow neuromodulatory processes at the level of upper brainstem or diencephalic centers.

It has also been speculated that ONS might exert its action by decreasing the excitability of second-order nociceptors in the TNC on which converge cervical, somatic, trigeminal, and visceral trigeminovascular afferents. [13] However, the nociception-specific blink reflex, mediated by spinal trigeminal nucleus interneurons, was unchanged or increased, rather than decreased, in this same study in subjects with CCH and chronic migraine (CM), and it remained unchanged in healthy subjects after short, low-frequency transcutaneous stimulation of the greater occipital nerve.[25]

An alternative explanation for the therapeutic effect of ONS in headache comes from recent evidence from FDG-PET study in subjects with drug-resistant CCH, where ONS generated slow neuromodulator processes within the pain-matrix, specifically the ipsilateral hypothalamus, midbrain, and ipsilateral caudal pons.[26] Selective activation of the perigenual anterior cingulated cortex (PACC), a pivotal structure in the endogenous opioid system, suggests that ONS may restore balance within dysfunctional pain control centers. The authors of this study suggested that ONS is a symptomatic treatment and does not change disease outcome, based on persistent hypothalamic hypermetabolism, which may explain why cranial autonomic features persist in the absence of pain in some patients[27] and the return of painful attacks if stimulation is discontinued.[28] In a H2O-PET study in chronic migraine, similar activation patterns were demonstrated in the pain-matrix, including the dorsal rostral pons, anterior cingulate cortex, and cuneus, directly correlated to pain scores, and in the left pulvinar, inversely correlated to pain scores.[28]

CHRONIC MIGRAINE

In 1999, Weiner and Reed reported the beneficial effects of subcutaneous ONS in 12 of 13 patients who they believed had occipital neuralgia.[29,30] Leads were placed in the subcutaneous tissue superficial to the cervical musculature and fascia transversing the occipital nerves at the level of C1. These patients, after a careful clinical and functional imaging interrogation, were found to have CM.[28] The results from this and other open-label observational studies of ONS in patients with CM—though definitions of improvement vary—appear promising, with approximately 80% of patients achieving at least a 50% improvement.[24,31–37]

Popenoy published a series of 25 subjects with medically refractory CM, having failed an average of seven migraine medications prior to ONS.[38] Headache frequency was reduced from 76/90 days pre-ONS to 38/90 days with ONS ($p < .001$). The responder rate (> 50% reduction in headache frequency or severity) was 88%. Acute medication consumption was substantially reduced, as was migraine-related disability. Nine patients experienced lead migrations, and one patient developed an infection.

In another open-label series, Oh and colleagues reported on 10 patients who underwent ONS who had experienced migraine for up to 25 years.[39] A robust response to anesthetic nerve block of the GON was used as a criterion for ONS. More than 90% relief was achieved by seven of nine patients available for follow-up at 6 months. Two patients developed infections.

Schwedt and colleagues reported the long-term follow-up (mean 17.8 months) in a series of 15 patients with refractory headache. Eight of the 15 patients had CM with pain that involved the C2 distribution.[31] Headache frequency was reduced to 60/90 days from 90/90 days ($p = 0.04$), and headache severity was reduced to 4.5 (scale of 1 to 10) from 6.75 ($p = 0.009$). Headache-related disability and depression scores were also meaningfully reduced in these subjects. Three patients had lead migration, one patient needed surgical revision for an impulse generator revision, and one patient had persistent incision-site pain.

Matharu and colleagues reported the results of eight patients who underwent ONS.[28] Four patients had an excellent response (complete suppression or rare breakthrough headaches), two patients had very good response (complete suppression most of the time with breakthrough headaches on ~ 10 days/month), and the final two patients had a good response (continued constant headaches but with severity reduced by 50%–75%). [28] All patients substantially reduced or eliminated headache medication consumption. Similar to other series, more than one-third (3/8) of patients had lead migration, and a single patient had surgical site complications (abdominal hematoma related to IPG implant).

Three controlled trials of ONS in patients with CM have been performed. Subjects in the ONSTIM study (Occipital Nerve Stimulation for the Treatment of Chronic Migraine Headache) had suffered from migraine for an average of 22 years and CM for 10 years, had approximately 23 days per month with headache, had pain in the distribution of the occipital nerves, were intractable to prophylactic medications from at least two standard classes, and had transient relief of pain following occipital nerve block.[40] These subjects were randomized to one of three groups: adjustable stimulation (AS) ($n = 33$); sham stimulation (SS) (pre-set stimulation for one minute daily) ($n = 17$); or continued medical management (MM) ($n = 17$). In order to assess whether or not response to occipital nerve block was a useful predictor for response to occipital nerve stimulation, a subset of subjects who did not benefit from the blocks was placed into an ancillary group that also received treatment with adjustable stimulation ($n = 8$). Safety and efficacy data were derived from 3 months of follow-up. The study was not designed to yield conclusive results regarding this treatment modality. Many of these outcomes showed numerical superiority (although not necessarily statistically significant superiority) of adjustable stimulation over sham stimulation and over continued medical management. Despite the small sample size, adjustable stimulation was associated with statistically superior benefit for a few disability and quality-of-life outcomes when independently analyzed. Seventy-five of 110 subjects were assigned to a treatment group. A responder was defined as a subject who achieved a 50% or greater reduction in number of headache days per month or a three-point or greater reduction in average overall pain intensity compared with baseline. Three-month responder rates were 39% for AS, 6% for PS, and 0% for MM. No unanticipated adverse device events occurred. Lead migration occurred in 12 of 51 (24%) subjects. In an accompanying editorial, several limitations of the study, including the significant potential for unblinding regarding treatment group assignment, confounding factors such as the inclusion of subjects using prophylactic medications and the exclusion of subjects overusing acute medication overuse, limit the generalizability since many patients in practice with recalcitrant CM overuse acute medications.[41] The author also underscored the fact that 61% of patients did not respond, highlighting the need for more effective therapies for this highly disabled group of patients.

In another prospective randomized multicenter double-blind controlled study, 125 subjects with CM were implanted with a neurostimulation system (St. Jude Medical Neuromodulation Division, Plano, TX) and randomized to an active or control group for 12 weeks.[42] Patients then continued in an open-label phase. Reduction in the number of headache days, scores for MIDAS, Zung Pain and Distress Scale (PAD), VAS, quality of life (QoL), and satisfaction are presented for a subset of patients that met the criteria for intractable CM (defined as 15 or more days per month with headache of at least 4 hours of pain with peak intensity that is at least of moderate severity, failure of 3 or more preventative drugs, and at least moderate disability determined using a validated migraine disability instrument [e.g., MIDAS or HIT-6]). Most patients (122/125) completed the 12-week visit. Although there was not a significant group difference in the number of patients with a 50% reduction on the VAS (primary endpoint), there was a significant difference at 30% (p < 0.05), which is considered clinically significant. Significant group differences for reduction in number of headache days, MIDAS, Zung PAD, VAS, QoL, and satisfaction at 12 weeks were observed (p < 0.05). In the active and control groups, number of headache days (defined as at least 4 hours of pain with peak intensity that is at least of moderate intensity) decreased by 7.0 and 2.7,

total MIDAS scores improved by 72.9 and 27.2, PAD scores improved by 14.6 and 5.5, and a 30% reduction in VAS was achieved in 36.4% and 13.5% of patients, respectively. In addition, 64.8% of patients in the active group reported improved QoL, whereas only 18.9% of patients in the control group reported this result. For satisfaction, 46.6% of patients in the active group reported being satisfied, whereas only 16.2% in the control group reported being satisfied. The authors concluded that these results provide evidence to support the safety and efficacy of PNS of the occipital nerves for the management of headache pain and disability associated with intractable CM. In a 52-week outcome analysis of this study, headache days were significantly reduced by 6.7 (8.4) days in the ITT population (p < 0.001) and by 7.7 (8.7) days in the group classified as having intractable chronic migraine (ICM) population (p < 0.001). The percentages of patients who achieved a 30% and 50% reduction in headache days and/or pain intensity were 59.5% and 47.8%, respectively. Excellent or good headache relief was reported by 65.4% of the ITT population and 67.9% of the ICM population. A total of 70% of patients experienced an adverse event and a total of 183 device/procedure-related adverse events occurred during the study, of which 18 (8.6%) required hospitalization and 85 (40.7%) required surgical intervention. The authors concluded that these results confirmed the 12-month efficacy of PNS of the occipital nerves for headache pain and disability associated with chronic migraine, but that more emphasis on adverse event mitigation is needed.[42a]

In a third prospective, double-blind, randomized, controlled, multicenter trial, 139 patients were randomized to receive either active stimulation (250 us pulses, 60Hz, -12.7mA) or sham (10us, 2Hz, < 1mA, 1s on / 90 min off duty cycle) stimulation. The full study results are only available in abstract form. [43] Prior to permanent implant, all subjects received 5–10 days of percutaneous trial stimulation (with randomized settings) to evaluate predictive value on 12-week outcome. The primary endpoint was the change from baseline in migraine days per month, evaluated 12 weeks after implantation. ONS did not produce statistically significant benefits in relation to sham stimulation on the primary endpoint. Subgroup analysis identified several candidate predictors of a favorable response, including the absence of medication overuse, no opioid use, and a positive response to a trial of percutaneous stimulation. In those randomized to the active group who derived a positive response to trial stimulation compared with those who had no response during the trial stimulation period, the reduction in migraine days was –8.8 compared to –0.7 ($p < 0.001$). In the study, there were two deaths; both were determined to be unrelated to the device or procedure. The most frequent device-related safety events over 2 years included non-target area sensory symptoms (18%), implant site pain (17.3%), infection requiring either antibiotics, (15.1%), explant (8.6%), or hospitalization.2] Incision site pain was seen in 7.9% of patients, and lead migration in 6.8%.

CHRONIC CLUSTER HEADACHE

A number of observational studies have demonstrated promising efficacy of ONS for the treatment of chronic cluster headache. Burns et al.[32] and Magis et al.[24] reported their experiences with eight subjects in each of their series. Subjects were stimulated bilaterally in the series by Burns et al. and unilaterally in the series by Magis et al. In the series by Burns et al., the median follow-up was 20 months. Subjective self-assessment of benefit was graded as substantial (≥ 90%) by two patients, moderate (≥ 40%) by three, mild (≥ 25%) by one, and nonexistent by two. Notably, five of eight patients continued to have daily attacks of cluster headache, and six of eight patients reported that they would recommend the use of ONS to similarly afflicted patients. There were no complications in four patients, and six complications in the other four: excessive pain at incision site (1), electrode migration (3), electrode fracture (1), and shock-like sensation due to kinking of wires (1). Four patients reported battery depletion, which required surgery for replacement.

In a long-term follow-up study in a larger cohort, Burns et al. reported on 14 patients with drug-resistant CCH who were implanted with bilateral electrodes.[36] At a median follow-up of 17.5 months (range 4–35 months), 10 of 14 patients reported improvement, and 9 of these recommended ONS. Three patients noticed a marked improvement of > 90%, three reported moderate improvement of > 40% or

better, and four reported mild improvement of 20%–30%. Improvement occurred within days to weeks for those who responded, and patients consistently reported that their attacks returned within hours to days when the device was off. One patient found that ONS helped abort acute attacks. Adverse events of concern were lead migrations and battery depletion. The authors concluded that ONS offers a safe, effective option for some patients with drug-resistant and highly disabling CCH.

In the series by Magis et al., at a mean follow-up of 15.1 months, two of eight patients were pain-free, three had an approximate 90% reduction in headache frequency, two had an approximate 40% reduction, and one experienced no benefit.[24] The cluster attacks shifted sides in two patients, requiring suboccipital steroid injections. One patient had electrode migration, one had lead displacement after a fall, two had thoracic discomfort or tingling, four had battery depletion, and one had the stimulator turned off due to lack of efficacy and unbearable paresthesias (some patients had more than one complication). In a long-term follow-up study from this group of 15 patients followed for a mean of 36.8 months after surgery (range 11–64 months), 11/14 (80%) had at least a 90% improvement, with 60% becoming pain-free for prolonged periods. One patient had an immediate postoperative infection of the device. Two patients did not respond or described mild improvement. The intensity of residual attacks was not modified by ONS. Four patients (29%) were able to reduce their prophylaxis. The major technical problems were battery depletion due to the use of high current intensities (n = 9/14, 64%) and immediate or delayed material infection (n = 3/15, 20%). Significant electrode migration was seen in only one patient. Clinical peculiarities during the ONS follow-up period were side-shift with infrequent contralateral attacks (n = 5/14, 36%) and/or isolated ipsilateral autonomic attacks without pain (n = 5/14, 36%). Two patients considered ONS-related paresthesias unbearable: one had his stimulator removed, and the other switched it off although he was objectively ameliorated. Subjectively, nine patients were very satisfied with ONS and three were moderately satisfied. Effective stimulation parameters varied between patients. The authors concluded that their long-term follow-up cohort confirms the efficacy of ONS in drug-resistant CCH, which remains a safe and well-tolerated technique, and that the occurrence of contralateral attacks and isolated autonomic attacks in nearly 50% of ONS responders may have therapeutic and pathophysiological implications.

In an abstract report by Lainez et al., three of five patients with CCH obtained excellent responses, one obtained a partial response, and one was unresponsive 24 months after the initiation of bilateral ONS.[44] No adverse events were reported. A study of three cluster patients with a mean follow-up of 20 months reported less benefit. Headache frequency was unchanged in two subjects and increased in one, and headache severity decreased in two subjects and was not changed in one. Two patients required revisions for lead migration.

Fontaine and colleagues reported 13 patients with medically intractable CCH lasting for longer than 2 years who underwent ONS.[37] During a mean follow-up of 14 months, the mean attack frequency and intensity decreased by 68% and 49%, respectively. At last follow-up, 10/13 patients were considered to be responders (improvement > 50%). Prophylactic treatment could be stopped or reduced in 8/13 cases. One patient experienced local infection, and had the hardware removed. The authors concluded that their data confirmed the 36 similar cases reported in the literature, suggesting that ONS may act as a prophylactic treatment in CCH.

In a prospective study involving 27 patients with CCH(23) or CM(3), bilateral ONS leads were implanted for those patients responding to a trial stimulation period.[45] Over a mean follow-up period of 20 months (range 5–47 months), 25/27 patients (93%) responded to treatment. All three CM patients responded to therapy. Twenty-one of 27 patients reported satisfaction with the outcome compared to their preoperative status, and 22/27 would recommend the procedure to other patients. Twenty-one complications in 14 patients were identified, necessitating re-operation in 13 cases. Most complications were local infection, leading to explantation of the hardware in four patients (15%). Of these patients, two experienced recurrent infections that required several surgical interventions.

In a prospective study, four patients with medically refractory CCH underwent implantation of a unilateral Bion microstimulator.[46]

The Bion microstimulator (Boston Scientific Neuromodulation Corporation, Valencia, CA) is a cylindrical, rechargeable, telemetrically programmable, self-contained, lithium ion battery-powered device. It includes an integrated electrode and battery that are encased in a device that measures 27.5 mm × 3.2 mm. In-person follow-up was conducted for 12 months after implantation, and a prospective follow-up chart review was carried out to assess long-term outcome. Three of the participants returned their headache diaries for evaluation. The mean duration of CCH was 14.3 years (range 3–29 years). Pain was predominantly or exclusively retro-ocular/periocular. One participant demonstrated a positive response (> 50% reduction in cluster headache frequency) at 3 months post-implant, while two responders demonstrated a positive response at 6 months. At least one of the participants continued to show > 60% reduction in headache frequency at 12 months. A chart review showed that at 58–67 months post-implant, all three participants reported continued use and benefit from stimulation. No side-shift in attacks was noted in any participant. Only two participants reported adverse events (neck pain and/or cramping with stimulation at high amplitudes); one required revision for a faulty battery.

Several authors report that the beneficial effects of ONS for the treatment of cluster headache may be delayed, reaching their maximum after several months of stimulation. [24,25] This observation must be considered if one is using a beneficial response to a short trial with a percutaneous stimulator as a prerequisite for permanent implantation, determining the role for continued stimulation in an individual patient, and setting outcomes in prospective clinical trials.

HEMICRANIA CONTINUA AND OTHER TRIGEMINAL AUTONOMIC CEPHALALGIAS

A cross-over prospective study was performed in six patients with hemicrania continua (HC) who underwent ipsilateral implantation of a suboccipital Bion microstimulator.[34] The stimulator was on for the first 3 months, off for the fourth month, and on again during long-term follow-up. Detailed prospective headache diaries were kept for 1 month before implantation and for 5 months after. Long-term data were obtained from patients' estimates of their outcome. The outcome of this study was assessed by a comparison of headache pain severity before and after ONS. At a median follow-up of 13.5 months (range 6–21 months), five of six patients reported sufficient benefit to recommend the device to other patients with HC. At long-term follow-up, four of six patients reported a substantial improvement (80%–95%), one patient reported a 30% improvement, and one patient reported that his pain was worse by 20%. The onset of the benefit of ONS was delayed by days to weeks, and headaches did not recur for a similar period when the device was switched off. These findings were very similar to two patients with hemicrania continua reported by Schwedt et al.[27,31]

OTHER TRIGEMINAL AUTONOMIC CEPHALALGIAS

Nine patients with medically intractable short-lasting unilateral neuralgiform headache with conjunctival injection and tearing (SUNCT) and three with short-lasting unilateral neuralgiform headache attacks with autonomic symptoms (SUNA) achieved more than 50% improvement with ONS, and four patients were nearly pain-free after around 14 months of follow-up.[47,48] Four patients with primary stabbing headache have been reported in abstract form to have responded to ONS. Three patients experienced complete resolution, while one patient had a substantial reduction in attack frequency.[49] More evidence for the efficacy of ONS in these less common primary headache disorders is needed, but compared to the invasiveness and potential for morbidity associated with deep brain stimulation, ONS should be considered first for medically recalcitrant TAC patients.

Sphenopalatine Ganglion Stimulation

The sphenopalatine ganglion (SPG), which contains parasympathetic efferents destined for meningeal blood vessels, the lacrimal gland, and nasal mucosa, has been implicated in the pathogenesis of the headache and cranial autonomic features associated with cluster headache and other trigeminal autonomic cephalalgias, as well as migraine. Cranial autonomic features have been reported in up to 73% of adults and 62% of children and adolescents with migraine. These symptoms reflect activation of and increase outflow from parasympathetic efferents within the SPG. The SPG has also been a therapeutic target in patients with cluster headache and serves as the basis for the use of the use of intranasal lidocaine in primary headache disorders.[50–59]

In a recent review of SPG stimulation, Khan and colleagues speculated that SPG stimulation may work by either interrupting SPG parasympathetic outflow by interfering with preganglionic SSN to SPG efferents or postganglionic outflow, or modulating the sensory processing in TNC via slow neuromodulatory changes to the pain processing structures of the brainstem.[60]

A small, open-label study using an on-demand neurostimulation system (Autonomic Technologies, Inc.) for electrical stimulation of the SPG indicated that this modality may be effective in patients with CCH.[55] SPG stimulation resulted in resolution of headache in 11 of 18 CH attacks, with partial improvement (> 50% improvement in VAS) in three others. Pain relief was noted within several minutes of stimulation. SPG stimulation has also been attempted in 10 migraine patients (2 episodic; 8 chronic) during attacks triggered by alcohol and odors.[54] One patient responded to sham stimulation, making it difficult to interpret the response. Two patients (one EM and one CM) had complete pain relief within 3 minutes of SPG stimulation, three had reduction in pain, and five had no response. Five patients had no pain relief. As in the cluster study, accurate placement of the stimulation needle and electrode was the most important predictor of clinical success. In a recent multicenter, controlled study, an implantable on-demand SPG neurostimulator was evaluated in 32 patients suffering from drug-resistant CCH.[61] Each CH attack was randomly treated with full, sub-perception, or sham stimulation. Pain relief was achieved in 67.1% of full-stimulation-treated attacks compared with 7.4% of sham-treated and 7.3% of sub-perception-treated attacks ($p < 0.0001$). Nineteen of 28 patients (68%) experienced a clinically significant improvement: seven (25%) achieved pain relief in > 50% of treated attacks and 10 (36%), achieved a > 50% reduction in attack frequency. Five SAEs occurred, and most patients (81%) experienced transient, mild/moderate loss of sensation within distinct maxillary nerve regions. Most patients (65%) had resolution of these adverse events within 3 months.

A multicenter (Pathway M1—Sphenopalatine Ganglion Stimulation for the Treatment of Chronic or High Frequency, High Disability Migraine Headache) randomized, sham-controlled, prospective study to evaluate the use of an implanted SPG neurostimulator for the treatment of migraine headache pain, migraine headache symptoms, and migraine frequency in high-disability migraineurs (clinicaltrial.gov: NCT01540799) is active but no longer recruiting. In addition, a US multicenter randomized sham-controlled study evaluating an implanted SPG neurostimulator for the treatment of cluster headache is currently recruiting subjects. (NCT02168764).

Supraorbital Nerve Stimulation

Since the distribution of pain may either be isolated to the anterior head region or present both anteriorly and posteriorly, the potential for bilateral supraorbital nerve stimulation (SONS) in combination with ONS was explored in seven patients with CM.[62] Five patients were able to eliminate their headache medications, and the remaining two patients markedly reduced their headache medications; disability was substantially reduced in all patients. One patient had lead migration, one had infection, and one had a titanium allergic reaction. Patients were able to switch between combined stimulation and ONS alone. All seven patients preferred the combined setting and used it almost exclusively. Six of the seven patients reported a 90%–100% reduction in pain. The remaining patient had a 60% reduction. Five of the seven no longer required medication. The follow-up period ranged from 1 to 35 months. In another study, 44 patients with CM underwent dual supraorbital and occipital nerve stimulation and were followed for a mean duration of 3 months.[63] In this group, the frequency of severe headaches decreased by 81%, and 50% of patients reported near-elimination of headache. Adolescents who ranged in age from 12 to 17 years and had treatment-resistant CM underwent a similar dual stimulation procedure; 60% were rendered pain-free.

The variables that are predictive of the need for SONS are unclear. The question of whether ONS can effectively ameliorate anterior pain is important. The efficacy of ONS alone for the treatment of anterior pain was evaluated in 33 patients who had undergone implantation of unilateral or bilateral ONS leads for the treatment of medically resistant chronic headache, 19 of whom had CM.[64] Thirty-one patients had both anterior and posterior pain (posterior/anterior to vertex). Overall, 26.33 patients responded (> 30% subjective global improvement). The average patient subjective global improvement was 73%. Nine of 24 patients felt that ONS was more effective for the posterior pain, while 15/24 patients considered ONS equally effective for both anterior and posterior pain. Therefore, while posterior pain was preferentially improved in one-third of patients, two-thirds experienced significant and equal relief of both anterior and posterior pain. The authors concluded that these results support a role for central inhibition of sensory trigeminal pathways from peripheral ONS. Future studies should address the magnitude of response from ONS in those with posterior-only versus anterior-plus-posterior pain, as well as the differential response between ONS alone and ONS plus SONS in those with anterior and posterior pain.

The efficacy of a transcutaneous supraorbital stimulator (Cefaly, STX-Med., Herstal, Belgium) in migraine prevention was looked at in a pilot study of 10 patients, and it was found to be an effective acute treatment option in 43% of attacks.[65] The device was then tested in a double-blinded, randomized, sham-controlled trial; 67 patients with two or more migraine attacks a month were randomized equally to active or sham stimulation.[66] Stimulation was applied for 20 minutes per day over a 3-month period. The primary outcome measures were change in monthly migraine days and 50% responder rate. Between the baseline period and the end of the third month of treatment, the mean number of migraine days decreased significantly in the active (6.94 vs. 4.88; $p < 0.023$), but not in the sham group (6.54 vs. 6.22; $p < 0.608$). The 50% responder rate was significantly greater ($p < 0.023$) in the active group (38.1%) than in the sham group (12.1%). Monthly migraine attacks ($p < 0.044$), monthly headache days ($p < 0.041$), and monthly acute anti-migraine medication intake ($p < 0.007$) were also significantly reduced in the stimulation but not in the sham group. There were no adverse events in either group. While blinding is an issue in all peripheral neurostimulation trials, this appears to be a less invasive modality than percutaneous stimulation, and should be considered in those with episodic migraine before considering more invasive stimulation approaches.

Vagal Nerve Stimulation

Stimulation of the vagus nerve (VNS) has received some interest as a treatment for migraine and other primary headache disorders. However, the evidence thus far is sparse, retrospective, and mainly derived from patients who had undergone placement of a percutaneous vagal nerve stimulator for treatment of refractory epilepsy. In three retrospective studies with small numbers of patients, at least 50% reported a substantial (> 50%) reduction in migraine frequency after at least 6 months of stimulation.[67,68]

In a recent open-label, single-arm, multiple-attack study study evaluating the efficacy and safety of an external vagal nerve stimulator for the acute treatment of migraine with and without aura, 27 subjects treated 80 painful migraine attacks with two 90-second doses, at 15-minute intervals. Stimulation was delivered to the right cervical branch of the vagus nerve. An adverse event was reported in 13 patients, notably: neck twitching, raspy voice, and redness at the device site. No unanticipated, serious or severe adverse events were reported. The pain-free rate at two hours was four of 19 (21%) for the first treated attack with a moderate or severe headache at baseline. For all moderate or severe attacks at baseline, the pain-free rate was 12/54 (22%).

External vagal nerve stimulation was also recently reported as being effective in an open-label, observational cohort study in 19 cluster headache patients (11 chronic, 8 episodic). [69a] Fifteen patients reported an overall improvement in their condition. Of all attacks treated, 47% were terminated within an average of 11 minutes of commencing stimulation. Ten patients reduced their acute use of high-flow oxygen by 55% with 9 reducing triptan use by 48%. Prophylactic use of the device resulted in a substantial reduction in estimated mean attack frequency from 4.5/24 hours to 2.6/24 hours (p < 0.0005) post-treatment.

In a prospective, open-label, randomised study that compared adjunctive prophylactic nVNS (n = 48) with standard of care (SoC) alone (control [n = 49]), subjects were treated during a 4-week randomization phase (SoC plus nVNS vs control) and a 4-week extension phase (SoC plus nVNS).[69b] The primary end point was the reduction in the mean number of CH attacks per week. During the randomised phase, subjects in the intent-to-treat population treated with SoC 12 plus nVNS (n = 45) had a significantly greater reduction in the number of attacks per week versus 13 control (n = 48) (–5.9 vs –2.1, respectively). Higher ≥50% response rates were also observed with SoC plus 15 nVNS (40% [18/45]) vs control (8.3% [4/48]; P (8.3% [4/48]; P < 0.001). No serious treatment adverse events were documented.

The potential mechanism of action of VNS in the treatment of migraine and other primary headache disorders has not been fully elucidated. However, emerging evidence indicates that VNS has the potential to suppress the development of central trigeminal sensitization. Using a rat model of trigeminal allodynia, nVNS was evaluated as a modality to suppress the behavioral response and neurotransmitter changes following the induction of trigeminal pain by infusing an inflammatory cocktail onto the dura in awake rats three times per week for 4 weeks.[70] The 1-minute nVNS stimulation paradigm consisted of 1 ms bursts of a 5 kHz sine wave repeated at 25 Hz and a peak voltage of 22 V. The control for nVNS was electrode placement, without stimulation. The rise in extracellular glutamate was blocked by 2 minutes of nVNS stimulation and both behavioral (withdrawal thresholds) and physiological (rise in extracellular glutamate) measures of trigeminal pain and allodynia were suppressed by 1 to 2 minutes of nVNS. These and other potential mechanisms will need to be more fully explored and, of course, the efficacy of VNS for migraine still awaits properly designed, randomized, sham-controlled studies.

CENTRAL NEUROSTIMULATION

Single-Pulse Transcranial Magnetic Stimulation

Single-pulse transcranial magnetic stimulation (sTMS) is a noninvasive method by which weak electrical currents are induced in the brain by a rapidly changing magnetic field. More than 20 years of clinical experience with sTMS have shown it to be a low-risk technique with promise in diagnosing, monitoring, and treating neurologic and psychiatric disease in adults. Thousands of subjects have been exposed to sTMS for diagnostic, investigational, and therapeutic intervention purposes, with minimal adverse events or side effects. No discernible evidence exists to suggest that sTMS causes harm to humans.[71] When sTMS is applied to the head, the magnetic field passes through the skull, inducing mild electric currents in the brain that excite and depolarize neurons in the brain. STMS (0.8–1.3 Tesla) has been shown in animal models to inhibit cortical spreading depression and to significantly decrease spontaneous neuronal firing of third-order thalamic neurons and C-fiber activity in response to dural vessel stimulation. Pre-treatment with naloxone blocks the inhibitory actions of sTMS on both the spontaneous neuronal firing and on C-fiber–induced activity.

The authors of this study concluded that the mechanism of action of sTMS in migraine treatment may involve modulation of third-order thalamic neurons, possibly through a corticothalamic relay, and endogenous opioid transmission is one of the neurotransmitter pathways involved in this modulation.[72]

TMS was tested in individuals with migraine based on the hypothesis that a fluctuating magnetic field delivered by the device would, when applied to the back of the head, induce electrical current and disrupt cortical spreading depression, the physiological substrate of cortical spreading depression. To date, only a few studies have been done that specifically assess the effects of TMS in migraine with table-top devices and in-clinic treatment. Upton and colleagues undertook a small pilot study with a Cadwell stimulator (model MES-10) that provided TMS pulses to 42 patients with migraine for treatment of 75 attacks.[73] Pain was measured on the five-point Likert-type scale. TMS was associated with a mean decrease in pain of 70% and was well tolerated. In a second study, 42 patients with migraine were treated with sTMS (n = 23) or placebo (n = 19). About 69% of the participants had relief from headache within 2 hours of active treatment compared with 48% in the placebo group. Treatment was well tolerated.

In an effort to ensure blinding for a placebo-controlled study, Lipton et al. undertook a pilot study to assess the adequacy of masking of the sham device to ensure blinding of treatment.[74,75] They enrolled 60 patients and showed that 50% of those treated with sTMS and 60% of those administered the sham device believed they had received genuine sTMS. Results from this study suggest that the treatment effect of TMS is not due to unblinding of the device after administration of treatment. This led to a randomized, double-blind, parallel-group, multicenter, two-phase, sham-controlled study that enrolled 267 adults.[75] All individuals had to meet ICHD-2 criteria for migraine with aura, with visual aura preceding at least 30% of migraines, followed by moderate or severe headache in more than 90% of those attacks. Sixty-six patients dropped out during phase one. In phase two, 201 individuals were randomly allocated by computer to either sham stimulation (n = 99) or sTMS (n = 102). We instructed participants to treat up to three attacks over 3 months while experiencing an aura. The primary outcome was pain-free response 2 hours after the first attack, and co-primary outcomes were non-inferiority at 2 hours for nausea, photophobia, and phonophobia. Thirty-seven patients did not treat a migraine attack and were excluded from outcome analyses. One hundred and sixty-four patients treated at least one attack with sTMS (n = 82) or sham stimulation (n = 82; modified intention-to-treat analysis set). Pain-free response rates after 2 hours were significantly higher with sTMS (32/82 [39%]) than with sham stimulation (18/82 [22%]), for a therapeutic gain of 17% (95% CI [3–31%], p = 0.0179). Sustained pain-free response rates significantly favored sTMS at 24 hours and 48 hours post-treatment. Non-inferiority was shown for nausea, photophobia, and phonophobia. No device-related serious adverse events were recorded, and the incidence and severity of adverse events were similar between sTMS and sham groups.

Repetitive Transcranial Magnetic Stimulation (rTMS)

Repetitive transcranial magnetic stimulation (rTMS) is able to activate or inhibit the underlying cortex depending on whether high

(5–20 Hz) or low (≤1 Hz) frequency stimulations are used.[76,77] rTMS may provide a therapeutic effect for patients with migraine via multiple potential mechanisms.

RTMS (10Hz) normalizes the habituation of visual evoked potentials in migraine subjects and has been shown to induce long-lasting changes in cortical excitability and VEP habituation pattern.[78] High-frequency somatosensory oscillations (HFOs), which reflect thalamocortical activation, are decreased in subjects with migraine between attacks, and high-frequency rTMS can normalize the habituation deficit of VEPs. In migraineurs, 10Hz rTMS can normalize habituation in migraine patients. This normalization is accompanied by an early HFO increase, which is thought to reflect thalamocortical activity. The authors of this study concluded that these findings support the hypothesis that dysfunctional thalamocortical loops may be responsible for the interictal habituation deficit in migraine.[79]

RTMS was delivered on the hot spot of the right abductor digiti minimi on alternate days for 3 days in eight patients with episodic migraine and 17 with CM. Each session consisted of 600 pulses at 10 Hz. Beta-endorphin level pre-rTMS was significantly reduced in EM compared with controls and in CM compared with both EM and control subjects. Following rTMS, the headache frequency, severity, functional disability, and analgesic intake were significantly reduced on the seventh day of rTMS and remained significant until the fourth week compared with baseline. The clinical improvement was associated with increase in b-endorphin level.[80]

Based on the assumption that the dorsolateral prefrontal cortex is the rostral and pivotal beginning of the descending inhibitory antinociceptive system and is hypoactive in CM, rTMS has been applied to prevent CM. Brighina et al. applied high-frequency rTMS to this area (20 Hz, 12 sessions, 400 pulses per session, 90% of motor output) in six CM sufferers and sham-stimulation to another five patients.[81] RTMS significantly reduced attack frequency, headache index, and acute treatment medication, and this effect lasted up to 2 months. Brighina et al. also demonstrated that rTMS conditioning normalized excitability in migraineurs with aura using high-frequency

rTMS by increasing intracortical inhibition and reversing the paradoxical effects of 1 Hz rTMS. [82] In another study involving 51 patients with more than seven attacks/month that were refractory to at least two prophylactic drugs, three sessions of alternate day 10 Hz rTMS comprising 600 pulses in 10 trains were delivered to the left frontal cortex. The response was evaluated at the end of the session and weekly for 4 weeks.[83] Fifty patients (98%) had more than 50% reduction of headache frequency at the end and one week after rTMS treatment, and the improvement persisted until the fourth week in 80.4% patients. Headache frequency, severity, functional disability, migraine index, and rescue medication use were significantly reduced at all time points, but the maximum benefit was observed in the first 2 weeks. There were no serious adverse events. The authors concluded that rTMS in the left frontal cortex is effective and well tolerated for migraine prophylaxis.

Based on the assumption that the brain is hyperexcitable between attacks and that low-frequency rTMS might normalize this hyperexcitability, Teepker et al. used low-frequency rTMS 1Hz frequency rTMS (2 trains of 500 pulses at motor threshold on five consecutive days) over the vertex for prevention in 27 patients suffering from episodic migraine with or without aura.[84] Twenty-seven migraineurs completed the study and were treated with rTMS on five consecutive days. The active treatment group was exposed to two trains of 500 pulses with a frequency of 1 Hz applied over the vertex with a round coil, while the placebo group was exposed to a figure-of-eight sham coil. While there was a decrease in migraine attacks in the TMS group, there was no statistical difference between active and placebo groups, nor were there significant differences for secondary outcome measures (migraine days and total migraine hours), pain intensity, or analgesic consumption. The effects of rTMS may depend on the baseline activation level of the underlying cortex where in migraine; the cortical preactivation level seems to be reduced. rTMS can promote long-lasting plastic changes, leading to a functional reorganization of the underlying cortex, and even sTMS can engage multiple brain networks functionally connected to the visual system, which might be relevant for its effects in migraine.[85]

Transcranial Direct Current Stimulation (tDCS)

Transcranial direct current stimulation (tDCS), a noninvasive and safe neurostimulation modality, uses weak currents to alter the modulation of cortical excitability. Cathodal tDCS inhibits, while anodal tDCS increases neuronal firing, and motor cortex tDCS may be effective in managing a variety of chronic pain syndromes. [85–87] Pre-clinical animal models have shown that tDCS may inhibit cortical spreading depression.[88] In addition, cathodal tDCS of the primary motor cortex (M1) results in an 18% decrease in pain-related evoked potentials (PREPs), while anodal tDCS lead to increased PREPs by 35%. The decreased PREPs suggest an inhibition of trigeminal and extracranial pain processing induced by tDCS of the M1. These results may provide a physiological rationale for the effectiveness of tDCS as a therapeutic modality in migraine.[89]

Both tDCS (unknown polarity) and sham stimulation resulted in a 54% decrease in headache intensity in migraine subjects.[90] The effects of cathodal tDCS and sham stimulation applied three times per week for 6 weeks over the primary visual cortex were evaluated in 26 patients with episodic migraine.[91] While mean headache intensity was reduced in the tDCS group, there was no significant difference in migraine days or migraine duration between the two groups. In a sham-controlled trial, the analgesic effects of a 4-week treatment of tDCS over the primary motor cortex were evaluated in 13 patients with CM.[92] The subjects were randomized to receive 10 sessions of active or sham tDCS for 20 minutes with 2 mA over 4 weeks. Significant effect on pain intensity and length of migraine episodes was noted, and a post hoc analysis showed a significant improvement in the follow-up period for the active tDCS group. The authors concluded that their findings provided preliminary evidence that patients with CM have a positive but delayed response to anodal tDCS of the primary motor cortex.

CONCLUSION

The evidence that peripheral and central neurostimulation treatment strategies may be effective for the acute and/or preventive management of migraine and other primary headache disorders has accumulated from centers and investigators around the world over the past decade. The response to the initial efficacy reports has been measured, and the results of observational studies from different investigators have been very similar. Sham-controlled studies that have been performed for ONS, transcutaneous SONS, sTMS, and tDCS show early promise.

The ability to blind several of these modalities has proven to be uniquely challenging, as has finding sensitive outcome measures that capture the improvement seen at the bedside, particularly in the most highly disabled and medically intractable patient populations. In addition, adverse events rates, especially lead migration, battery failure, and infection, were relatively high in early studies. Nevertheless, the clinical community has been persistent, and key learnings from early controlled studies are being used to design better randomized controlled trials and refinements in procedural technique that will reduce the incidence of adverse events.

Cost is and will likely continue to be an issue, since many neurostimulation modalities and the procedure required to implant them (with the exception of transcranial stimulation devices) may be substantial.[93,94] Cost-effectiveness studies will be necessary if pivotal phase III studies confirm the efficacy and long-term safety of implantable neurostimulation devices.

For patients who are disabled and suffer intensely and have failed to respond to conventional and evidence-based pharmacologic and non-drug therapies, the emergence of peripheral and central neurostimulation offers hope for a safe and effective long-term strategy to reduce the suffering associated with intractable headache pain.

REFERENCES

1. Anthony M. Arrest of attacks of cluster headache by local steroid injection of the occipital nerve. In: Rose FC, ed. *Migraine clinical and research aspects.* London: Karger, 1985:169–173.
2. Busch V, Jakob W, Juergens T, Schulte-Mattler W, Kaube H, May A. Functional connectivity between trigeminal and occipital nerves revealed by occipital nerve

blockade and nociceptive blink reflexes. *Cephalalgia.* 2006;26:50–55.

3. Busch V, Jakob W, Juergens T, Schulte-Mattler W, Kaube H, May A. Occipital nerve blockade in chronic cluster headache patients and functional connectivity between trigeminal and occipital nerves. *Cephalalgia.* 2007;27:1206–1214.

4. Leroux E, Valade D, Taifas I, et al. Suboccipital steroid injections for transitional treatment of patients with more than two cluster headache attacks per day: a randomised, double-blind, placebo-controlled trial. *Lancet Neurol.* 2011;10:891–897.

5. Ambrosini A, Vandenheede M, Rossi P, et al. Suboccipital injection with a mixture of rapid- and long-acting steroids in cluster headache: a double-blind placebo-controlled study. *Pain.* 2005;118:92–96.

6. Gale GD, Caputi CA, Firetto V. Therapeutic blockade of the greater occipital and supraorbital nerves in migraine patients. *Headache.* 1998;38:57.

7. Piovesan EJ, Werneck LC, Kowacs PA, Tatsui CE, Lange MC, Vincent M. Anesthetic blockade of the greater occipital nerve in migraine prophylaxis. *Arq Neuropsiquiatr.* 2001;59:545–551.

8. Inan N, Ceyhan A, Inan L, Kavaklioglu O, Alptekin A, Unal N. C2/C3 nerve blocks and greater occipital nerve block in cervicogenic headache treatment. *Funct Neurol.* 2001;16:239–243.

9. Peres MF, Stiles MA, Siow HC, Rozen TD, Young WB, Silberstein SD. Greater occipital nerve blockade for cluster headache. *Cephalalgia.* 2002;22:520–522.

10. Afridi SK, Shields KG, Bhola R, Goadsby PJ. Greater occipital nerve injection in primary headache syndromes: prolonged effects from a single injection. *Pain.* 2006;122:126–129.

11. Cook BL, Malik SN, Shaw JW, Oshinsky ML, Young WB. Greater occipital nerve (GON) block successfully treats migraine within five minutes. *Neurology.* 2006;66:A42(Abstract).

12. Bartsch T, Goadsby PJ. Stimulation of the greater occipital nerve induces increased central excitability of dural afferent input. *Brain.* 2002;125:1496–1509.

13. Bartsch T, Goadsby PJ. Increased responses in trigeminocervical nociceptive neurons to cervical input after stimulation of the dura mater. *Brain.* 2003;126:1801–1813.

14. Bartsch T, Goadsby PJ. Stimulation of the greater occipital nerve (GON) enhances responses of dural responsive convergent neurons in the trigeminocervical complex in the rat. *Cephalalgia.* 2001;21:401–402.

15. Goadsby PJ, Hoskin KL, Knight YE. Stimulation of the greater occipital nerve increases metabolic activity in the trigeminal nucleus caudalis and cervical dorsal horn of the cat. *Pain.* 1997;73:23–28.

16. Knight YE, Bartsch T, Kaube H, Goadsby PJ. P/Q-type calcium channel blockade in the PAG facilitates trigeminal nociception: a functional genetic link for migraine? *J Neurosci.* 2002;22(5):RC213.

17. Holland P, Goadsby PJ. The hypothalamic orexinergic system: pain and primary headaches. *Headache.* 2007;47:951–962.

18. Goadsby PJ, Charbit AR, Andreou AP, Akerman S, Holland PR. Neurobiology of migraine. *Neuroscience.* 2009;161:327–341.

19. De FM, Sanoja R, Wang R, et al. Engagement of descending inhibition from the rostral ventromedial medulla protects against chronic neuropathic pain. *Pain.* 2011;152(12):2701–2709.

20. Basbaum AI, Fields HL. Endogenous pain control mechanisms: review and hypothesis. *Neuroscience.* 1978;42:183–200.

21. Heinricher MM, Morgan MM, Tortorici V, Fields HL. Disinhibition of off-cells and antinociception produced by an opioid action within the rostral ventromedial medulla. *Neuroscience.* 1994;63:279–288.

22. Fields HL, Basbaum AI. (1994). Central nervous system mechanisms of pain modulation. In P. D. Wall & R. Melzack (Eds.), *Textbook of pain.* 3rd ed. Edinburgh: Churchill-Livingstone, 1994:245–257.

23. Melzack R, Wall PD. Evolution of pain theories. *Int Anesthesiol Clin.* 1970;8:3–34.

24. Magis D, Allena M, Bolla M, dePasqua V, Remacle JM, Schoenen J. Occipital nerve stimulation for drug-resistant chronic cluster headache: a prospective pilot study. *Lancet Neurol.* 2007;6:314–321.

25. Jurgens TP, Busch V, Opatz O, Schulte-Mattler WJ, May A. Low-frequency short-time nociceptive stimulation of the greater occipital nerve does not modulate the trigeminal system. *Cephalalgia.* 2008;28:842–846.

26. Magis D, Bruno MA, Fumal A, et al. Central modulation in cluster headache patients treated with occipital nerve stimulation: an FDG-PET study. *BMC Neurol.* 2011;11:25.

27. Schwedt TJ, Dodick DW, Trentman TL, Zimmerman RS. Occipital nerve stimulation for chronic cluster headache and hemicrania continua: pain relief and persistence of autonomic features. *Cephalalgia.* 2006;26:1025–1027.

28. Matharu MS, Bartsch T, Ward N, Frackowiak RS, Weiner R, Goadsby PJ. Central neuromodulation in chronic migraine patients with suboccipital stimulators: a PET study. *Brain.* 2004;127:220–230.

29. Matharu MS, Goadsby PJ. Bilateral paroxysmal hemicrania or bilateral paroxysmal cephalalgia, another novel indomethacin-responsive primary headache syndrome? *Cephalalgia.* 2005;25:79–81.

30. Weiner RL, Reed KL. Peripheral neurostimulation for control of intractable occipital neuralgia. *Neuromodulation.* 1999;2:217–222.

31. Schwedt TJ, Dodick DW, Hentz J, Trentman TL, Zimmerman RS. Occipital nerve stimulation for chronic headache: long-term safety and efficacy. *Cephalalgia.* 2007;27:153–157.

32. Burns B, Watkins L, Goadsby PJ. Treatment of medically intractable cluster headache by occipital nerve stimulation: long-term follow-up of eight patients. *Lancet.* 2007;369:1099–1106.

33. Ambrosini A. Occipital nerve stimulation for intractable cluster headache. *Lancet.* 2007;369:1063–1065.

34. Burns B, Watkins L, Goadsby PJ. Treatment of hemicrania continua by occipital nerve stimulation with a bion device: long-term follow-up of a crossover study. *Lancet Neurol.* 2008;7:1001–1012.

35. Goadsby PJ, Bartsch T, Dodick DW. Occipital nerve stimulation for headache: mechanisms and efficacy. *Headache.* 2008;48:313–318.

36. Burns B, Watkins L, Goadsby PJ. Treatment of intractable chronic cluster headache by occipital nerve stimulation in 14 patients. *Neurology.* 2009;72:341–345.

37. Fontaine D, Christophe SJ, Raoul S, et al. Treatment of refractory chronic cluster headache by chronic occipital nerve stimulation. *Cephalalgia*. 2011;31:1101–1105.

38. Popeney CA, Alo KM. Peripheral neurostimulation for the treatment of chronic, disabling transformed migraine. *Headache*. 2003;43:369–375.

39. Oh MY, Ortega J, Belotte JB. Peripheral nerve stimulation for the treatment of occipital neuralgia and transformed migraine using a C-1-2-3 subcutaneous paddle style electrode: a technical report. *Neuromodulation*. 2004;7:103–112.

40. Saper JR, Dodick DW, Silberstein SD, McCarville S, Sun M, Goadsby PJ. Occipital nerve stimulation for the treatment of intractable chronic migraine headache: ONSTIM feasibility study. *Cephalalgia*. 2011;31:271–285.

41. Schwedt TJ. Occipital nerve stimulation for chronic migraine: interpreting the ONSTIM feasibility trial. *Cephalalgia*. 2011;31:262–263.

42. Silberstein SD, Dodick DW, Saper J, et al. Safety and efficacy of peripheral nerve stimulation of the occipital nerves for the management of chronic migraine. Results from a randomized, multicenter, double-blinded, controlled study. *Cephalalgia*. 2012;32:1165–1179.

42a. Dodick DW, Silberstein SD, Reed KL, Deer TR, Slavin KV, Huh B, et al. Safety and efficacy of peripheral nerve stimulation of the occipital nerves for the management of chronic migraine: Long-term results from a randomized, multicenter, double-blinded, controlled study. *Cephalalgia*. 2015;35:344–358.

43. Lipton RB, Goadsby PJ, Cady RK, et al. PRISM study: occipital nerve stimulation for treatment-refractory migraine. *Cephalalgia*. 2009;29:30(Abstract PO47).

44. Lainez MJA, Piera A, Salvador A, Roldan P, Gonzales-Darder J. Efficacy and safety of occipital nerve stimulation for treatment of chronic cluster headache. *Headache*. 2008;S15(Abstract).

45. Mueller O, Diener HC, Dammann P, et al. Occipital nerve stimulation for intractable chronic cluster headache or migraine: A critical analysis of direct treatment costs and complications. *Cephalalgia*. 2013;33:1283–1291.

46. Strand NH, Trentman TL, Vargas BB, Dodick DW. Occipital nerve stimulation with the Bion microstimulator for the treatment of medically refractory chronic cluster headache. *Pain Physician*. 2011;14:435–440.

47. Marin JC, Goadsby PJ. Response of SUNCT (short-lasting unilateral neuralgiform headaches with confunctival injection and tearing), SUNA (short-lasting unilateral neuralgiform headaches with autonomic symptoms) and primary stabbing headaches to occipital nerve stimulation (ONS). *Cephalalgia*. 2010;74(Supp 2):P04.006(Abstract).

48. Shanahan P, Watkins L, Matharu M. Treatment of medically intractable short-lasting unilateral neuralgiform headache attacks with conjunctival injection and tearing (SUNCT) and short-lasting unilateral neuralgiform headache attacks with autonomic symptoms (SUNA) with occipital nerve stimulation (ONS) in 6 patients. *Cephalalgia*. 2009;29(Suppl1):50 (Abstract).

49. Marin JC, Goadsby PJ. Response of primary stabbing headache to occipital nerve stimulation (ONS). *Cephalagia*. 2009;29(Suppl 1):110(Abstract).

50. Sluder G. The syndrome of sphenopalatine ganglion neurosis. *Am J Med*. 1910;140:868–878.

51. Meyer JS, Binns PM, Ericsson AD. Sphenopalatine ganglionectomy for cluster headache. *Arch Otolaryngol*. 1970;92:475–484.

52. Delepine L, Aubineau P. Plasma protein extravasation induced in the rat dura mater by stimulation of the parasympathetic sphenopalatine ganglion. *Exp Neurol*. 1997;147:389–400.

53. Narouze S, Kapural L, Casanova J, Mekhail N. Sphenopalatine ganglion radiofrequency ablation for the management of chronic cluster headache. *Headache*. 2009;49:571–577.

54. Tepper SJ, Rezai A, Narouze S, Steiner C, Mohajer P, Ansarinia M. Acute treatment of intractable migraine with sphenopalatine ganglion electrical stimulation. *Headache*. 2009;49:983–989.

55. Ansarinia M, Rezai A, Tepper SJ, et al. Electrical stimulation of sphenopalatine ganglion for acute treatment of cluster headaches. *Headache*. 2010;50:1164–1174.

56. Morelli N, Mancuso M, Felisati G, et al. Does sphenopalatine endoscopic ganglion block have an effect in paroxysmal hemicrania? A case report. *Cephalalgia*. 2010;30:365–367.

57. Ivanusic JJ, Kwok MM, Ahn AH, Jennings EA. 5-HT(1D) receptor immunoreactivity in the sphenopalatine ganglion: implications for the efficacy of triptans in the treatment of autonomic signs associated with cluster headache. *Headache*. 2011;51:392–402.

58. DeMaria S Jr, Govindaraj S, Chinosorvatana N, Kang S, Levine AI. Bilateral sphenopalatine ganglion blockade improves postoperative analgesia after endoscopic sinus surgery. *Am J Rhinol Allergy*. 2012;26:e23–e27.

59. Oomen KP, van Wijck AJ, Hordijk GJ, de Ru JA. Effects of radiofrequency thermocoagulation of the sphenopalatine ganglion on headache and facial pain: correlation with diagnosis. *J Orofac Pain*. 2012;26:59–64.

60. Khan S, Schoenen J, Ashina M. Sphenopalatine ganglion neuromodulation in migraine: What is the rationale. *Cephalalgia*. 2014;34:382–391.

61. Schoenen J, Jensen RH, Lanteri-Minet M, et al. Stimulation of the sphenopalatine ganglion (SPG) for cluster headache treatment. Pathway CH-1: a randomized, sham-controlled study. *Cephalalgia*. 2013;33:816–830.

62. Reed KL, Black SB, Banta CJ, Will KR. Combined occipital and supraorbital neurostimulation for the treatment of chronic migraine headaches: initial experience. *Cephalalgia*. 2010;30:260–271.

63. Reed KL, Will KR, Chapman J, Richter E. Combined occipital and supraorbital neurostimulation for chronic migraine headache: an extended case series. *Cephalalgia*. 2011;31(Suppl1):98(Abstract).

64. Yancy HM, Trentman TL, Dodick DW. The effect of occipital nerve stimulation on anterior pain in primary headache disorders. *Headache*. 2013;52:897(Abstract).

65. Gerardy PY, Fabry D, Fumal A, Schoenen J. A pilot study on supra-orbital surface electrotheraphy in migraine. *Cephalalgia*. 2009;29:134(Abstract).

66. Schoenen J, Vandersmissen B, Jeangette S, et al. Migraine prevention with a supraorbital transcutaneous stimulator. *Neurology*. 2013;80(8):697–704 (Abstract).

67. Lenaerts ME, Oommen KJ, Couch JR, Skaggs V. Can vagus nerve stimulation help migraine? *Cephalalgia.* 2008;28:392–395.

68. Mauskop A. Vagus nerve stimulation relieves chronic refractory migraine and cluster headaches. *Cephalalgia.* 2005;25:82–86.

69. Goadsby PJ, Grosberg BM, Mauskop A, Cady R, Simmons KA. Effect of noninvasive vagus nerve stimulation on acute migraine: An open-label pilot study. *Cephalalgia.* 2014;34(12) 986–993.

69a. Nesbitt AD, Marin JCA, Tompkins E, Ruttledge MH, Goadsby PJ. Initial use of a novel noninvasive vagus nerve stimulator for cluster headache treatment. *Neurology.* 2015;84:1249–1253.

69b. Gaul C, Diener HC, Silver N, Magis D, Reuter U, Andersson A, et al. Non-invasive Vagus Nerve Stimulation for Prevention and Acute Treatment of Chronic Cluster Headache (PREVA): A Randomised Controlled Study. *Cephalalgia.* 2015; doi: 10.1177/0333102415607070.

70. Oshinsky ML, Murphy AL, Hekierski H Jr, Cooper M, Simon BJ. Noninvasive vagus nerve stimulation as treatment for trigeminal allodynia. *Pain.* 2014;155(5):1037–1042.

71. Dodick DW, Schembri CT, Helmuth M, Aurora SK. Transcranial magnetic stimulation for migraine: a safety review. *Headache.* 2010;50:1153–1163.

72. Andreou AP, Fredrick J, Goadsby PJ. Endogenous opiouds mediate the sTMS effects in the sensory thalamous of migraine models. *Cephalalgia.* 2013;33:11(Abstract).

73. Clarke BM, Upton AR, Kamath MV, Al-Harbi T, Castellanos CM. Transcranial magnetic stimulation for migraine: clinical effects. *J Headache Pain.* 2006;7:341–346.

74. Lipton RB, Dodick DW, Silberstein SD, et al. Single-pulse transcranial magnetic stimulation for acute treatment of migraine with aura: a randomised, double-blind, parallel-group, sham-controlled trial. *Lancet Neurol.* 2010;9:373–380.

75. Lipton RB, Dodick DW, Goadsby PJ, et al. Transcranial magnetic stimulation (TMS) using a portable device is effective for the acute treatment of migraine with aura: results of a double-blind, sham controlled, randomized study. *Headache.* 2008;48:S1–S72.

76. Hallett M. Transcranial magnetic stimulation and the human brain. *Nature.* 2000;406:147–150.

77. Kobayashi M, Pascual-Leone A. Transcranial magnetic stimulation in neurology. *Lancet Neurol.* 2003;2:145–156.

78. Fumal A, Coppola G, Bohotin V, et al. Induction of long-lasting changes of visual cortex excitability by five daily sessions of repetitive transcranial magnetic stimulation (rTMS) in healthy volunteers and migraine patients. *Cephalalgia.* 2006;26:143–149.

79. Coppola G, DePasqua VPF, Schoenen J. Effects of repetitive transcranial magnetic stimulation on somatosensory evoked potentials and high frequency oscillations in migraine. *Cephalalgia.* 2011;32:700–709.

80. Misra UK, Kalita J, Tripathi GM, Bhoi SK. Is beta endorphin related to migraine headache and its relief? *Cephalalgia.* 2013;33:316–322.

81. Brighina F, Piazza A, Fierro B. Can high-frequency repetitive transcranial magnetic stimulation (HF-rTMS) of the left dorsolateral prefrontal cortex (DLPFC) ameliorate chronic refractor migraine? *Cephalalgia.* 2002;22:609(Abstract).

82. Brighina F, Palermo A, Daniele O, Aloisio A, Fierro B. High-frequency transcranial magnetic stimulation on motor cortex of patients affected by migraine with aura: a way to restore normal cortical excitability? *Cephalalgia.* 2010;30:46–52.

83. Misra UK, Kalita J, Bhoi SK. High frequency repetitive transcranial magnetic stimulation (rTMS) is effective in migraine prophylaxis: an open labeled study. *Neurol Res.* 2012;34:547–551.

84. Teepker M, Hotzel J, Timmesfeld N, et al. Low-frequency rTMS of the vertex in the prophylactic treatment of migraine. *Cephalalgia.* 2010;30:137–144.

85. Magis D, Schoenen J. Advances and challenges in neurostimulation for headaches. *Lancet Neurol.* 2012;11:708–719.

86. Antal A, Terney D. Anodal transcranial direct current stimulation of the motor cortex ameliorates chronic pain and reduces short intracortical inhibition. *J Pain Symp Manage.* 2010;39:890–903.

87. Kutschenko A, Liebetanz D. Meningioma causing gabapentin-responsive secondary SUNCT syndrome. *J Headache Pain.* 2010;11:359–361.

88. Liebetanz D, Fregni F, Monte-Silva KK, et al. After-effects of transcranial direct current stimulation (tDCS) on cortical spreading depression. *Neurosci Lett.* 2006;398:85–90.

89. Hansen N, Obermann M, Poitz F, et al. Modulation of human trigeminal and extracranial nociceptive processing by transcranial direct current stimulation of the motor cortex. *Cephalalgia.* 2011;31:661–670.

90. Obodescu S, ptaru L, oldovanu I, otaro V, ursky N. Non-pharmacologic acute treatment of chronic migraine patients by transcranial cerebral electrical stimulation vs. placebo. *Cephalalgia.* 2011;31(Suppl 1):101(Abstract).

91. Antal A, Kriener N, Lang N, Boros K, Paulus W. Cathodal transcranial direct current stimulation of the visual cortex in the prophylactic treatment of migraine. *Cephalalgia.* 2011;31:820–828.

92. DaSilva AF, Mendonca ME, Zaghi S, et al. tDCS-induced analgesia and electrical fields in pain-related neural networks in chronic migraine. *Headache.* 2012;52:1283–1295.

93. Leone M, Franzini A, Cecchini AP, Mea E, Broggi G, Bussone G. Costs of hypothalamic stimulation in chronic drug-resistant cluster headache: preliminary data. *Neurol Sci.* 2009;30(Suppl 1):S43–S47.

94. Mueller O, Diener HC, Dammann P, et al. Occipital nerve stimulation for intractable chronic cluster headache or migraine: a critical analysis of direct treatment costs and complications. *Cephalalgia.* 2013;33:1283–1291.

Chapter 11

Hormones

INTRODUCTION

Hormonal factors greatly influence the expression of headache. Migraine occurs more frequently in adult women (18%) than in men (6%), although prevalence is equal in children.[1–3] Migraine prevalence and disability are highest in women of childbearing age. Prevalence is also high in male-to-female transsexuals who utilize hormone therapy.[4] Migraine develops most frequently in the second decade, with the peak incidence occurring in adolescence.[5,6] Menstrual migraine (MM) begins at menarche in 33% of affected women.[6] More than half of women with migraine experience MM mainly at the time of menses (menstrually related migraine), and some experience it exclusively with menses (true menstrual migraine [TMM]). [6] MM can be associated with other somatic complaints, such as nausea, backache, breast tenderness, and cramps, that arise before and often persist into menses, and, like these complaints, it appears to be the result of falling sex hormone levels.[2,7,8] In addition, premenstrual migraine can be associated with premenstrual syndrome (PMS), which is distinct from the physical symptoms of the perimenstrual period and is probably not directly driven by declining progesterone levels.[9] Migraine that occurs during (rather than prior to) menstruation is usually not associated with PMS. Premenstrual dysphoric disorder differs from PMS in its characteristic pattern of symptoms, their severity, and the impairment that results.[8]

259

Migraine may worsen during the first trimester of pregnancy, and although many women become headache-free during the last two trimesters, 25% have no change in their migraine. [10–12] MM typically improves with pregnancy, perhaps due to sustained high estrogen levels.[10–12] Hormonal replacement with estrogens can exacerbate migraine, and oral contraceptives (OC) can change its character and frequency.[13,14] Migraine prevalence decreases with advancing age but may regress or worsen at menopause.[1,15,16] Changes in the headache pattern with OC use and during menarche, menstruation, pregnancy, or menopause are related to changes in estrogen levels. [17] These phenomena suggest a relationship between migraine headaches and changes in sex hormone levels.[18]

MENSTRUATION AND MIGRAINE

The connection between the menstrual cycle and migraine is important. Migraine can occur before or during menstruation. When migraine occurs before menstruation, features of PMS, including depression, anxiety, crying spells, difficulty in thinking, lethargy, backache, nausea, and breast tenderness and swelling, may also be present.[6] MM is often associated with dysmenorrhea and may frequently be longer in duration[19] and more refractory to treatment.[20]

Based on clinical experience, the frequency of MM is as high as 60%–70%. Based on retrospective analysis, prevalence ranges from 26% to 60% in headache clinic patients. The prevalence is lower in patients not attending a headache clinic. The frequency of MM depends on the means of ascertainment.[19]

In order to define the relationship between the menstrual cycle and the frequency of migraine attacks, MacGregor et al.[21] prospectively followed 55 migraineurs. They defined true menstrual migraine (TMM) as attacks that occurred regularly on or between days –2 to +3 of the menstrual cycle and at no other time, and menstrually related migraine (MRM) as attacks that occurred at any time during the cycle, with an increased frequency during menstruation. Using these criteria, 7.2% of the patients had TMM (if –4 to +4 days was used as the interval, 10.9% had TMM). None had migraine with aura. Another 34.5% had increased attack frequency with MRM, while 32.7% did not.

In a follow-up study, MacGregor et al. [22] prospectively assessed 100 migraineurs to determine if their attacks were related to menstruation. Eighty-four women were still menstruating; 50.6% thought that their attacks were related to menstruation, while 49.4% did not. Women with MRM noticed a relationship between migraine and menarche. Premenstrual symptoms of weight gain, abdominal distension, depression, and irritability were reported more frequently by women with MRM. Twenty women completed the 3-month diary. From this self-selected group, three women (15%) fulfilled the criteria for TMM, and three women (15%) fulfilled the criteria for MRM. Most of the attacks were migraine without aura.

Johannes et al.[19] studied 79 women who were screened for migraine with aura in Washington County, Maryland. They completed daily diaries and recorded information regarding their menstrual-cycle phase, time of headache occurrence, and attack characteristics. Headache was classified into four categories: (1) migraine with aura; (2) migraine without aura; (3) tension-type headache; and (4) other headache types. Headache occurred on 30% of the study days. All headache types occurred more frequently during the first 3 days of the menstrual cycle, but this was statistically significant only for migraine without aura (66% higher), despite the fact that the entry criteria required a history of migraine with aura.

Stewart et al.[23] followed up their Washington County, Maryland study[19] to see if it is true that migraines are more common and severe around the time of menses (Figure 11.1). In a population-based sample, 81 menstruating women who had clinically diagnosed migraine (with or without aura) were enrolled in a 98-day diary study. An excess risk of headache occurred perimenstrually and was highest on days 0 and 1 of the cycle (day 0 being the first day of menses). A significantly elevated risk of headache on days 0 and 1 was observed for migraine without aura (odds ratio [OR] 2.04) and for tension-type headache (OR 1.67). Elevated risks were also observed in the two days before the onset of menses for migraine without aura (OR 1.80). Migraine headache intensity was slightly greater during

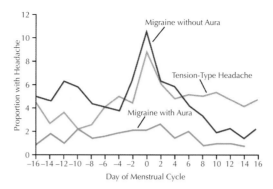

Figure 11.1. Incidence of headache by type of headache and the menstrual cycle.Solid line – migraine with aura; large dashes = migraine without aura; dashed line = tension-type headache. Source: Reference 13.

the first 2 days of menses. Attacks of migraine without aura, but not migraine with aura, were more likely to occur 2 days before the onset of menses and on the first 2 days of menses. Migraine headaches were slightly but significantly more painful during the first 2 days of menses.

MacGregor and Hackshaw analyzed diary data from 155 women from the City of London Migraine Clinic using within-woman analysis. Compared with all other times of the cycle, migraine was 1.7 times more likely to occur during the 2 days before menstruation and 2.1 times more likely to be severe, and 2.5 times more likely to occur during the first 3 days of menstruation and 3.4 times more likely to be severe. In this study, migraine at menstruation was different from non-menstrual attacks within individuals and was more severe.[24]

Granella et al.[25] tried to determine if menstrual attacks differed from non-menstrual attacks in clinical features or response to acute treatment in women with MRM. Sixty-four women with MRM were enrolled in a 2-month diary study. Perimenstrual attacks were split into three groups (premenstrual, menstrual, and late menstrual attacks) and compared to non-menstrual attacks. Perimenstrual attacks were significantly longer than non-menstrual attacks. Work-related disability was significantly greater in premenstrual and menstrual attacks than in non-menstrual attacks. Acute attack treatment was less effective in perimenstrual attacks. In this clinic-based study, perimenstrual attacks were longer and less responsive to acute attack treatment than were non-menstrual attacks.

Couturier et al.[26] assessed the prevalence of menstrual migraine and its effects on daily activities in a representative Dutch population sample of 1181 women aged 13 to 55 years. Oral contraceptive (OC) use seemed to reduce the occurrence of menstrual complaints, but not the occurrence of headache and migraine. In this study, attacks of menstrual migraine were more severe, of longer duration, and more resistant to treatment than migraine attacks at other times of the month.

Using a questionnaire, Dzoljic et al.[27] determined the prevalence and characteristics of MRM and non-migraine headache in women who were students at Belgrade University. Among 1298 students with headache, 245 (12.6%) had migraine and 1053 (54.2%) had non-migraine headaches. Female students with migraine had menstrually related attacks more frequently than did students with non-migraine headaches (67.7% versus 29.5%). Exacerbation of migraine during menstruation was slightly more severe and more complex than exacerbation of non-migraine headaches.

Dowson et al. investigated the disability of women who had migraine and other headaches during and outside the menstrual period. Menstrual attacks were more likely to be migraine than were non-menstrual attacks ($p < 0.05$). Migraine attacks related to menstruation were significantly more severe and disabling ($p < 0.05$). They were also associated with a greater productivity loss ($p = .01$).[28]

Mattsson[29] investigated some of the relationships between IHS migraine and hormonal factors. A neurologist clinically assessed 728 women, aged 40–74, who attended a population-based mammography screening program. Twenty-one percent of women with migraine without aura and 4% of women with migraine with aura reported that they experienced more than 75% of their attacks within –2 to +3 days of the menstrual cycle. A small but significant proportion (12%, p = .04) of women with migraine without aura also had premenstrual disorder. During pregnancy, women experienced less frequent or less intense attacks of both migraine without aura and migraine with aura.

Using a within-woman analysis, MacGregor et al. compared the severity, duration, and relapse of menstrual versus non-menstrual episodes of migraine during treatment with usual migraine therapy. They did a post hoc within-woman analysis of the usual-care phase (month 1) of a 2-month, multicenter, prospective, open-label study at 21 US medical practices. Participants were women ≥ 18 years of age with regular, predictable menstrual cycles. Women (n = 153) reported 212 menstrual (59.2%) and 146 non-menstrual (40.8%) migraine treatment episodes. Compared with non-menstrual treatment episodes, menstrual treatment episodes were more impairing, longer lasting, and more likely to relapse in this selected population of women with frequent MM. Most of the variability in these outcomes is due to differences between headache types and not within-patient differences for a given type of headache.[30]

The 2009 American Migraine Prevalence and Prevention Study, a population-based study, included 1697 females aged 18–60, who met criteria for episodic migraine, had a menstrual cycle, and fit one of three group definitions based on the self-reported association of menses and migraine: menstrual-only migraine (MOM), menstrually associated migraine (MAM), and menstrually unrelated migraine (MUM). Migraine cases were classified as follows: MOM (5.5%), MAM (53.8%), or MUM (40.7%). MOM cases had an older age of onset. Measures of headache impact were consistently higher and statistically significant for MOM cases compared to MUM cases, but less so for MAM cases versus MUM cases. The findings from this population-based study indicate that MOM is relatively uncommon, MAM is commoner, and both appear to have greater impact on functioning than MUM. Previous population-based diary studies included all

migraine headache sufferers and may have had insufficient power to detect the higher impact of headaches among MOM cases; the number of participating MOM cases would have been low, and MOM headaches that occurred perimenstrually could have been lumped with perimenstrual headaches, contributed by cases not triggered by menses.[31]

Most women have increased headache and migraine attacks (usually without aura) at the time of menses. Women pre-selected on the basis of PMS have more headaches prior to the onset of menses, but most women have more headaches during or just before menstruation. Some women have migraine (usually without aura) only with menses. Menstrual migraine can be defined by looking at attacks that are regularly triggered by menstruation. The quality of the attacks, their response to treatment, and patients' hormonal changes could then be analyzed based on this association.

The new IHS classification (ICHD-3 β) includes menstrual migraine in the appendix. It defines *pure menstrual migraine (PMM) without aura (A1.1.1)* as attacks, in a menstruating woman, that fulfill criteria for migraine without aura and occur exclusively on day 1±2 (i.e., days –2 to +3) of menstruation in at least 2 of 3 menstrual cycles and at no other times of the cycle (Table 11.1). (The first day of menstruation is day 1 and the preceding day is day –1; there is no day 0.) This replaces the term *true menstrual migraine*. The IHS classification defines *menstrually related migraine*

Table 11.1 Pure Menstrual Migraine Without Aura

Diagnostic criteria

A. Attacks, in a menstruating woman, fulfilling criteria for 1.1 *migraine without aura*

B. Attacks occur exclusively on day 1 ± 2 (i.e., days –2 to +3) of menstruation in at least two out of three menstrual cycles and at no other times of the cycle.

The first day of menstruation is day 1 and the preceding day is day –1; there is no day 0.

Menstruation is considered to be endometrial bleeding resulting from either the normal menstrual cycle or from the withdrawal of exogenous progestogens, as in the use of combined oral contraceptives or cyclical hormone replacement therapy.

Table 11.2 Menstrually Related Migraine Without Aura

Diagnostic criteria
A. Attacks, in a menstruating woman, fulfilling criteria for 1.1 *migraine without aura*
B. Attacks occur on day 1 ± 2 (i.e., days –2 to +3) of menstruation in at least two out of three menstrual cycles and additionally at other times of the cycle.

without aura (A1.1.2) as attacks, in a menstruating woman, that fulfill criteria for migraine without aura and occur on day 1±2 (i.e., days –2 to +3) of menstruation in at least two out of three menstrual cycles and additionally at other times of the cycle[32] (Table 11.2).

TREATMENT OF HEADACHES ASSOCIATED WITH THE MENSTRUAL CYCLE

Overview

Recall is an unreliable way to determine a connection between headaches and the menstrual period. Recorded diary information about headaches and the menstrual cycle can confirm a diagnosis of menstrual-related headache and plan treatment. Attacks of menstrual migraine may differ from non-menstrual attacks in the same woman. Menstrual attacks are less likely to be associated with aura and may be longer, more difficult to treat, or more prone to recur after an initial acute response.[33] In women who have frequent headaches, however, the onset of menstruation is responsible for only a small proportion of attacks overall.[19] In the general population, the differences between menstrual and non-menstrual headaches are much less apparent.[23] Women who have headache throughout their menstrual cycle should be treated with reassurance, education, and pharmacologic intervention. Behavioral intervention may be useful in selected instances.[34] The two major pharmacologic approaches to treatment are acute treatment and preventive treatment. Women who have migraine predominantly with their menses can just be treated perimenstrually with short-term mini-prophylaxis.

Acute Treatment

Drugs that are proven effective or are commonly used for the acute treatment of migraine work well for MM. These include non-steroidal anti-inflammatory drugs (NSAIDs), the combination of aspirin, acetaminophen, and caffeine (AAC),[35] dihydroergotamine (DHE), and the triptans. NSAIDs must be used in adequate doses.[36,37] If the first NSAID is ineffective, other classes of NSAIDs should be tried.

DHE, available in parenteral form and as a nasal spray, is effective for the treatment of MRM.[38,39] In an open study, patients with MRM responded as well to 1 mg of intramuscular dihydroergotamine, as did patients with non-menstrual migraine.[40] Headache, nausea, and vomiting were all well controlled.

The triptans that have been studied appear to be equally as effective for non-menstrual attacks and attacks that coincide with menstruation as for non-MRM[41] and, in addition, control the nausea and vomiting associated with attacks.[41–51,52] In patients who fail to achieve an optimal response or often develop headache recurrence, the use of dexamethasone or an NSAID along with a triptan may be useful. In a randomized, double-blind, crossover study, rizatriptan 10 mg, dexamethasone 4 mg, or the combination were used in patients with MRM attacks, and the combination was superior for the 24-hour sustained pain-free endpoints (51% combination vs. 32% rizatriptan alone; $p < 0.05$).[53] In addition, the sumatriptan-naproxen combination has also been shown to be effective for MRM attacks.

If severe MRM cannot be controlled with NSAIDs, DHE, or triptans, then analgesics combined with opioids, opioids alone,[54] high-dose corticosteroids, neuroleptics (chlorpromazine, haloperidol, thiothixene, droperidol), or a course of intravenous DHE can be tried.[39,54] Women with frequent, severe MRM are candidates for preventive therapy (either continuous or short-term), and they often respond better to acute therapy when they are on preventive treatment.

PREVENTIVE TREATMENT

Women who are already using preventive medication and continue to have MRM can increase the medication dose perimenstrually, although this strategy has not been validated in clinical trials. Women who do not use preventive medicine or have migraine mainly with their menses can just be treated perimenstrually with short-term prophylaxis for 5 to 7 days.[7,54,55] Regular periods and a predictable relationship between the attacks and the menses are essential for this strategy to succeed. The use of an ovulation predictor kit may help women with irregular cycles to time their treatment. Since the interval from ovulation to the onset of menstrual bleeding is generally fixed at around 14 days, the expected onset of headache can often be surmised.[56] Treatment of coexistent PMS may help control premenstrual headache.

Drugs that have been used perimenstrually for short-term prophylaxis include NSAIDs, ergotamine, DHE, methergine, triptans, and magnesium. NSAIDs in adequate doses can be used preventively 1–2 days before the expected onset of headache and continued for the duration of vulnerability. The optimal dose and duration of treatment can be determined through trial and error over several months. The most commonly used NSAID for this purpose is naproxen sodium 550 mg po bid.[57] If the first NSAID fails, a different NSAID from another chemical class should be tried.

DHE can be used prophylactically at the time of menses without significant risk of developing ergot dependence.[7,55,58,59] DHE nasal spray, given every 8 hours for 6 days, beginning 3 days before the expected onset of headache, was used in a placebo-controlled, double-blind, short-term trial for the treatment of MM. The mean pain severity rating for DHE nasal spray was lower than placebo for 67.5% of the 40 evaluable patients.[60]

Newman et al.[61] used oral sumatriptan (25 mg tid) 2–3 days before the expected headache onset and continued for a total of 5 days in an open-label study of 20 women with MRM. In 126 sumatriptan-treated cycles, headache was absent in 52.4% of patients and reduced in severity by 50% or more in 42%. Breakthrough headaches were rare and significantly reduced in severity compared with baseline headache.

Newman et al.[62] found that naratriptan 1 mg significantly reduced the number of MRMs and MRM days compared with placebo (2.0 MRMs vs. 4.0 MRMs, $p = 0.011$; 4.0 days vs. 7.0 days, $p = 0.001$). In other studies, however, naratriptan's beneficial effect on MRM was only slightly superior to that of placebo.[63]

Zolmitriptan was studied for the prevention of MM in a randomized, double-blind, parallel-group, placebo-controlled, multicenter, phase II study. Patients received either zolmitriptan 2.5 mg three times daily or twice daily or placebo three times daily. Both regimens of zolmitriptan were superior to placebo in reducing both the mean number of headaches (three times daily = 0.56, twice daily = 0.75, placebo = 0.95) and the frequency of headaches compared with placebo (three times daily = 58.6%, $p = 0.0007$; twice daily = 54.7%, $p = 0.002$; placebo = 37.8%). Zolmitriptan was well tolerated when used for the prevention of MM headaches.[64]

Silberstein et al.[65] examined frovatriptan's efficacy in the prevention of MRM in 546 women. Frovatriptan was given in two doses: 2.5 mg once daily (qd) and 2.5 mg twice daily (bid). Treatment was started 2 days before the anticipated start of the MRM headache and continued for 6 days. A double loading dose was given the first day. Women treated three perimenopausal periods. The incidence of MRM headache was 67%, 52%, and 41% for placebo, frovatriptan 2.5 mg qd and frovatriptan 2.5 mg bid, respectively. Frovatriptan also significantly reduced migraine severity and duration and the use of rescue medications.

A second double-blind, placebo-controlled study of 415 women (MAM02) was similar to MAM01 except that patients had to have documented evidence of previous treatment failure with at least one triptan. The benefit over placebo in the mean number of MM–headache-free periods was 64% and 119% in the frovatriptan once daily and twice daily groups, respectively.[66] The mean number of periods with ≤ 1 day of mild MM headache per patient was 0.7, 1.1, and 1.3 for placebo, frovatriptan once a day, and frovatriptan twice a day, respectively. The percentage of patients who failed to have any periods with ≤ 1 day of mild MM headache was 60%, 38%, and 35%, respectively. The total migraine burden and use of rescue medication was reduced in frovatriptan-treated patients.[66]

Patients were recruited into an open-label supportive study (MAM03). Frovatriptan reduced the incidence, severity, and duration of MM headaches and associated symptoms over a 12-month period. There was no suggestion that patients developed tolerance, as efficacy was maintained over the entire 12-period study period. There was no evidence of an increased risk of cardiovascular adverse events (AEs) relative to acute treatment, and rebound headache was not evident. A short-term regimen with frovatriptan may be a safe and viable treatment option for preventing predictable migraine such as MM.[67]

Hu et al. systematically assessed the efficacy and tolerability of triptans compared with placebo as short-term prophylaxis of MM. They searched Cochrane CENTRAL, MEDLINE, and EMBASE for randomized, double-blind, placebo-controlled trials of triptans for MM until October 1, 2012. A total of six RCTs were identified. A total of 633 participants received frovatriptan 2.5 mg qd, 584 received frovatriptan 2.5 mg bid, 392 received naratriptan 1 mg bid, 70 received naratriptan 2.5 mg bid, 80 received zolmitriptan 2.5 mg bid, 83 received zolmitriptan 2.5 mg tid and 1104 received placebo. Overall, triptans are effective, short-term, prophylactic treatments for MM. Considering MM frequency, severity, and adverse events, frovatriptan 2.5 mg bid and zolmitriptan 2.5 mg tid tend to be the preferred regimens.[68]

A placebo-controlled, double-blind study of 24 women with PMS and migraine has shown that oral magnesium (360 mg of magnesium pyrrolidone carboxylic acid) decreases the severity of the PMS symptoms and the duration and intensity of MRM that occurs prior to the onset of menstruation.[69,70]

There is no evidence that diuretics or vitamins help with menstrual migraine. Diuretics may help with fluid retention and other premenstrual symptoms, but do not have an impact on migraine.[18,71–73] The efficacy of pyridoxine to treat both PMS and menstrual migraine has not been proven in double-blind studies.[74,75] In fact, high doses of pyridoxine have been reported to cause a sensory neuropathy.[76] Phytoestrogens have been studied for menstrual migraine prophylaxis, but trial methods make it impossible to reach a conclusion about their efficacy.[77,78]

If severe MM cannot be controlled by standard acute and preventive treatment, hormonal therapy may be indicated. Successful hormonal or hormonal modulation therapy of MRM has been reported with estrogens[79] (alone or combined with progesterone or testosterone),[80] combined oral contraceptives (COCs), synthetic androgens, estrogen modulators and antagonists,[81] and medical oophorectomy with GnRH analog with or without add-back therapy and prolactin release inhibitors.[82] Progesterone is not effective in the treatment of headache or the symptoms of PMS,[83] despite many favorable anecdotal reports.[84,85]

The decrease in estrogen levels during the late luteal phase of the menstrual cycle is a trigger for migraine.[86] Estrogen replacement prior to menstruation has been used to prevent migraine.[87] In a double-blind, crossover study, DeLignières[79] used percutaneous estradiol gel perimenstrually with significant (30.8% vs. 96.3%) headache reduction. In a double-blind trial of percutaneous estradiol gel, Dennerstein[88] reported similar excellent results. Magos found estradiol implants (available investigationally in the US) and cyclic progesterones to be effective in MRM in both an open study[89] and a double-blind study. [80] Somerville[86] attempted MM prophylaxis with estradiol implants. These implants did not produce stable plasma estrogen levels and caused severe menstrual disturbance, loss of headache periodicity, and unpredictable headache improvement. In contrast, the cutaneous gel[79] and the estradiol implant used by Magos[80] provide stable blood estrogen levels.

The estradiol cutaneous patch provides a relatively stable plasma-estrogen level over the time of application.[90–92] Levels are less stable with higher-dose patches. Serum estrogen levels rise within 4 hours of applying the transdermal patch and are proportional to the dose (patch transdermal therapeutic system [TTS]) (patch 25~serum level of 23pg/ml; TTS 50~39ng/ml; and TTS 100~74pg/ml).[93]

A dose threshold appears to exist. A study using a TTS 25 patch from 4 days before to 4 days after menstruation showed that it was not as effective as the same regimen with a TTS 100 patch.[94] A serum estradiol level of 60–80 pg/ml is needed during the crucial week to prevent MM.[95] Pfaffenrath,[96] using TTS 50 patches (TTS = 39pg/ml), did not find a significant difference from placebo in a placebo-controlled, double-blind trial. Similarly, Smits et al.[97] found minimal benefit of TTS 50 in a placebo-controlled trial. Women receiving transdermal estradiol (2 × 100 mg patches) to suppress ovulation, supplemented by norethisterone 5 mg on days 19 to 26 to ensure withdrawal bleeding, showed significant improvement in PMS symptoms at 6 months compared with those receiving placebo.[98] The patches can be used for both contraception and treatment of PMS and MRM in younger women when estrogens are not contraindicated or when natural estrogens are preferred.

Guidotti et al., in a pilot, open-label, non-randomized, parallel-group study in 38 women with a history of MM, compared the efficacy of frovatriptan (n = 14) 2.5 mg po or transdermal estrogens (n = 10) 25 µg or naproxen sodium (n = 14) 500 mg po once daily for the short-term prevention of MM. All treatments were administered in the morning for 6 days, beginning 2 days before the expected onset of menstrual headache. All women reported at least one episode of MM at baseline. During treatment, all patients taking transdermal estrogens or naproxen sodium, and 13 of the 14 patients (93%) taking frovatriptan, had at least one migraine attack (p = 0.424). Daily incidence of migraine was significantly lower (p = 0.045) with frovatriptan than with transdermal estrogens or nasal spray. Treatment differences were particularly evident for the subgroup of patients with TMM (n = 22) and for frovatriptan versus naproxen sodium. This study suggests that short-term prophylaxis of MM with frovatriptan may be more effective than that based on transdermal estrogens or naproxen sodium. However, the dose of transdermal estrogens may have been too low.[99]

Combinations of estrogens and progestogens, or progestogens alone in the form of OCs, may be a reasonable approach for some patients with intractable MRM, particularly if it is associated with severe dysmenorrhea. [100] Most OCs are packaged as a 21/7 cycle (21 days of active tablets and 7 days of placebo), resulting in 13 withdrawal bleeding episodes each year. Women on OCs who have menstrual-related problems can extend the active OCs for 6–12 weeks and delay the menstrually related symptoms. Sulak et al.[101] prospectively analyzed 50 women who were on OCs and had menstrual-related problems (including 76% with MRM); 74% stabilized on an extended regimen of 6–12 weeks of consecutive days of active OCs, while 26% either discontinued OCs or reverted to the standard regimen of 3 weeks of active pills and 1 week

of placebo. Two other OCs (Seasonique and Seasonale) have a 91-day cycle with only four withdrawal bleeds per year. Lybrel is the first FDA-approved low-dose combination OC taken 365 days a year without a placebo or pill-free interval. All tablets contain low doses of levonorgestrel (0.09 mg) and ethinyl estradiol (20 mcg).

A Cochrane review compared extended-duration contraceptive regimens to traditional regimens. Three out of four studies that reported on menstruation-associated headache showed a benefit.[102] Cachrimanidou et al. showed decreased headache frequency in the continuous-dosing group compared with traditional (p < 0.05).[103] Miller and Notter found that headache was less severe in women receiving a 49-day cycle regimen compared with those on a traditional cyclic regimen (p = 0.04).[104] Anderson and Hait found fewer headaches in the continuous group than the cyclic group (OR 0.7; 95% CI [0.5–1.0]). [105] However, Kwiecien et al. did not find a significant difference in headache between the two groups.[106]

Danazol (Danocrine™),[81,107] an androgen derivative, suppresses the pituitary-ovarian axis by binding to androgen and progestogen receptors and by inhibiting ovarian steroidogenesis. It may be effective in preventing MM at a dose of 200–600 mg a day, starting before the expected onset of the headache and continuing through the menses.

Tamoxifen (Nolvadex™),[108,109] a selective estrogen receptor modulator that binds to a cytosol ER, may be effective in resistant MRM. Its long-acting nuclear retention time results in estrogen antagonism by down-regulation of an estrogen receptor and inhibition of messenger RNA transcription in some tissues. In other tissues, such as the uterus, it has estrogen-like action. A dose of 5–15 mg per day for days 7–14 of the luteal cycle has provided significant relief of menstrual headache without side effects. The effectiveness of raloxifene, a new selective estrogen receptor modulator with a different profile, on MRM is unknown.[110]

Ferrante et al.[78] assessed the efficacy of the combination of two phytoestrogens as perimenstrual preventive treatment of MM and tested their effect on cerebral hemodynamic. Eleven women with a history of MM (i.e., attacks occurring exclusively on day 1+/−2 days of menstruation and at no other time of the cycle) were included. They underwent a 3-month cyclic treatment with 56 mg of genisteine and 20 mg of diadzeine per day. Transcranial doppler evaluation was performed at baseline and after treatment. Ten women completed the study. The average number of days with migraine during the baseline period decreased significantly after 3 months of therapy ($p < 0.005$). There were no major side effects. Therapy did not affect cerebral blood flow velocities.

Burke et al. assessed the efficacy of a phytoestrogen combination in the prophylactic treatment of MM.[77] Forty-nine patients were randomized to receive either placebo, or a daily combination of 60 mg soy isoflavones, 100 mg dong quai, and 50 mg black cohosh, with each component standardized to its primary alkaloid. Patients received study medication for 24 weeks. The average frequency of menstrually associated migraine attacks during weeks 9–24 was reduced from 10.3 +/–2.4 (mean +/– SEM) in placebo-treated patients to 4.7 +/–1.8 ($p < 0.01$) in patients treated with the phytoestrogen preparation. It is uncertain which ingredient was responsible for the effect. Phytoestrogens may be an effective treatment in MM prevention. Placebo-controlled trials on larger number of patients are necessary to confirm these findings.

Neither hysterectomy nor oophorectomy has been proven to be effective in unselected cases in the treatment of migraine. Other methods of suppressing ovulation have been studied for the treatment of PMS. Medical ovariectomy using GnRH analogues to suppress ovulation are effective in refractory PMS.[111–113 GnRH, isolated and characterized in 1971,[114,115] has a short half-life and is rapidly degraded by endopeptidases. GnRH agonists are produced by altering the amino acids in position 6 and/or 10, resulting in compounds with high affinity for the GnRH receptor[116,117] and a long half-life due to their resistance to cleavage by endopeptidases.[118] GnRH agonists are initially stimulatory, releasing supraphysiologic amounts of LH and FSH.[119] The initial rise in estradiol may be associated with worsening of disease symptoms. Continued exposure results in down-regulation of pituitary GnRH receptors, with resultant hypogonadotrophic hypogonadism and decreased serum LH and FSH levels.[120] FSH falls abruptly within 2 weeks, whereas LH suppression tends to be

slower and more gradual. Estradiol concentrations decrease to menopausal levels within 3–5 weeks, leading to hypoestrogenemic side effects, including hot flashes (91%), insomnia (55%), vaginal dryness (37%), and headache (39%).[121]

In two placebo-controlled, double-blind studies, GnRH was significantly better than placebo in controlling both behavioral and physical symptoms of PMS (headache, breast fullness and tenderness, bloating, and fatigue). [112,113] GnRH analogues may be effective in severe MRM. Since GnRH analogues induce hypogonadism, with many of the same short-term and long-term side effects as menopause, treatment is usually limited to 6 months unless replacement estrogens are used.[111,122]

Add-back therapy can be used to limit these side effects and is not usually detrimental to effective GnRH agonist treatment.[122] Add-back treatment prevents bone mineral loss and minimizes the adverse effects of hypoestrogenism. Combined add-back regimens are lipid neutral,[123–125] protect against bone loss,[123,124,126–130] diminish vasomotor symptoms,124,126,131–134] decrease symptoms and blood loss in women with dysfunctional uterine bleeding,[82] and improve symptoms associated with ovarian hyperandrogenism.[122,123,135,136]

In an open study, five women who had repetitive, severe migraine headaches limited to the perimenstrual period were followed for 2 months, then received a GnRH agonist (leuprolide acetate depo formulation, 3.75 mg IM) monthly for 10 months. Beginning with the fifth month, "add-back" therapy (transdermal estradiol, 0.1 mg daily and oral medroxyprogesterone acetate, 2.5 mg daily) was initiated. The mean headache scores for the GnRH agonist treatment months (4.0 ± 1.5) and for the GnRH agonist and add-back treatment months (3.1 ± 0.7) were significantly lower than for the control months (15.3 ± 2.4). Both treatments were well tolerated and effective. GnRH agonist administration, alone or with add-back therapy, may be an effective treatment for carefully selected patients with severe perimenstrual migraine headaches.[137]

Schmidt et al.[138] gave women with PMS the GnRH agonist leuprolide. Only 10 of 18 women responded. These results were consistent with most other studies, which show the efficacy of short-term GnRH agonist therapy in some, but not all, women.[139] Most PMS symptom scores for week 4 were significantly lower than those for both the baseline period and week 4 in the women with PMS who were receiving placebo. Women with PMS had significant increases in symptoms during treatment with leuprolide plus replacement hormone, either estradiol (transdermal 0.1) or progesterone (200 mg a day vaginal suppositories), compared with treatment with leuprolide alone.[138] The deleterious effects of add-back therapy attenuated during the last week of estradiol or progesterone replacement. Long-term (or low-dose) hormonal replacement therapy may not continue to precipitate adverse mood symptoms. These results are consistent with observations that changes in gonadal steroids early in the menstrual cycle are correlated with symptoms that appear later in the cycle in women with PMS.[140,141]

Martin et al.142] attempted to determine the preventive benefit of "medical oophorectomy" and transdermal estradiol in women with migraine. Twenty-one migraineurs with regular menstrual cycles were enrolled. After a 2.5-month placebo run-in phase, all patients received a subcutaneous goserelin (a GNRH agonist) implant to induce a medical oophorectomy. One month later, while continuing goserelin, participants were randomized to receive a transdermal patch containing 100 µg of estradiol-17 β (GNRH/estradiol group, $n = 9$) or a placebo patch (GNRH/placebo group, $n = 12$) during a 2-month treatment phase. The primary outcome measure was the headache index, which was defined as the mean of pain-severity ratings (0 to 10 scale) recorded three times a day in a daily diary. The headache index was significantly lower during the treatment period in the GNRH/estradiol group than in the GNRH/placebo group ($p = .025$). Similar improvements were observed in the GNRH/estradiol group for all secondary outcome measures with the exception of headache frequency, which was unchanged between the groups. Within the GNRH/estradiol group, there was a 33.7% reduction in the headache index during the treatment phase compared with the placebo run-in phase; no difference was seen between those phases within the GNRH/placebo group. Minimization of hormonal fluctuations with GNRH therapy alone is inadequate to prevent headache in women migraineurs who are premenopausal.

The addition of transdermal estradiol to existing GNRH therapy provides a modest preventive benefit.

PMS sufferers who have had a hysterectomy without an oophorectomy continue to have cyclic mental and physical symptoms during the late luteal phase of the menstrual cycle, demonstrating that neither the presence of the uterus nor the occurrence of menstruation is necessary for PMS maintenance. [143] Some physicians are again advocating the use of hysterectomy and oophorectomy for women with severe intractable PMS or MRM who respond to medical ovariectomy. [144,145] There are no long-term follow-up or controlled studies to prove the effectiveness of this radical procedure. One retrospective study[146] reported oophorectomy in 14 women who responded to ovulation suppression with Danazol. Postoperatively they were given conjugated estrogens without progestin. At 48-month followup, they were improved compared to their preoperative status. In another study,[145] 14 women with intractable PMS had total abdominal hysterectomy, bilateral salpingo-oophorectomy, and postoperative continuous estrogen replacement. At 6-month follow-up, none of the women had scores diagnostic of PMS.

The ability to gauge and interpret the effects of ovariectomy and hysterectomy on PMS and headache is contaminated by the postoperative use of daily estrogen. No study is placebo-controlled, and women with PMS are very sensitive to placebo. The use of continuous estrogen alone could account for the positive results.[98] Until more conclusive data are available, we do not recommend oophorectomy for MRM; instead, GnRH agonists should be used as a last resort, supplemented by estrogens, preferably in a patch or depo formulation, and low-dose progestins.

Another strategy is the use of a dopamine receptor agonist, short-term or continuously. Bromocriptine (Parlodel™),[147–150] a dopamine D2 receptor agonist, is an inhibitor of prolactin release. A dose of 2.5–5 mg a day during the luteal phase of the menstrual cycle may decrease the premenstrual symptoms of breast engorgement, irritability, and headache. In an open trial,[151] 24 women with severe, disabling MRM (occurring within 3 days of menstruation) were treated with continuous bromocriptine 2.5 mg three times

Table 11.3 **Preventive Treatment of Menstrual Migraine**

1. Perimenstrual use of standard preventive drugs
2. Perimenstrual use of non-standard preventive drugs
   - NSAIDs
   - DHE
   - Triptans
3. Hormonal therapy
   - Estrogens (with or without androgens or progestin): patch
   - Combined oral contraceptives
   - Synthetic androgens (Danazol™)
   - Antiestrogen (Tamoxifen™)
   - Medical oophorectomy (GnRH analogues)
4. Dopamine agonists (Bromocriptine™)

Table 11.4 **Hormonal Methods of Contraception**

Method		Primary Mode of Action
Combined hormonal contraceptives	Combined pill	Inhibit ovulation
	Ring	
	Patch	
Progestin-only methods	Progestin-only minipill	Thicken cervical mucus
	Desogestrel pill	Inhibit ovulation
	DMPA injection	Inhibit ovulation
	Implant	Inhibit ovulation
	LNG-IUS	Endometrial suppression and thicken cervical mucus

daily. Seventy-five percent of the women had at least a 25% reduction in headache compared to baseline. Overall headache frequency decreased 72%. No patients had less than a 10% increase in headache; three could not tolerate bromocriptine, and three did not benefit.

A sequential approach to the treatment of menstrual migraine is outlined in Table 11.3.

MIGRAINE ASSOCIATED WITH HORMONAL CONTRACEPTIVE USE

Introduction

Contraception can be hormonal or non-hormonal (copper intrauterine device, condoms, withdrawal, natural family planning, and sterilization). Hormonal methods include combined hormonal contraceptives (COCs, vaginal rings, and transdermal combination patches) and progestin-only methods (oral, subcutaneous implants, and depo-injections) (Table 11.4). [92,98,152,153]

There are three major types of OC formulations: two are COCs (fixed-dose and phasic combinations) and one is progestin only. The OCs most commonly used in the United States contain combinations of synthetic estrogen (ethinyl estradiol [10–50 mcg] or mestranol) and synthetic progestin (Table 11.5). In an attempt to minimize the associated androgenic side effects, the type of synthetic progestin has been changed. The sequential formulations use

fixed amounts of estrogen and progestin taken 21 days each month, followed by a steroid-free period of 7 days.[154,155] Some combinations add back estrogen during the placebo week (10 µg of ethinyl estradiol for 5 of 7 days). Two others (Seasonique and Seasonale) have a 91-day cycle with only four withdrawal bleeds per year. Another formulation (Lybrel) is the first FDA-approved low-dose COC that is taken 365 days a year without a placebo or a pill-free interval.

The combination multiphasic formulations contain two or three different amounts of the same estrogen and progestin. Each dosage combination is given for intervals that vary from 5 to 11 days during the 21-day medication period. The multiphasic combinations have not been shown to have fewer AEs than the fixed-dose combination formulations. The third type of OC formulation is a progestin alone, taken daily, without a steroid-free interval.[147] The progestin-only contraception would be expected to have fewer systemic AEs, but it is less effective and is associated with a high incidence of irregular bleeding.[153,156] It must be taken daily and meticulously, because contraceptive efficacy can be lost by 27 hours after the last dose. The COCs interfere with the midcycle gonadotropin surge at both the hypothalamic and pituitary levels, thus preventing ovulation,[147] while the progestin-only OC inhibits the LH surge. All the OC formulations

Table 11.5 Oral Contraceptives

Pill Type		Estrogen (mcg)	Progestin (mcg)	Cycle-Cycles/ Year
Monophasic				
EE/ethynodiol diacetate	1/35, 1/50	35, 50	1000	21/7–13
EE/norethindrone	1/10 Fe	10	1000	24/4–13
	1/20, Fe 1/20, 1/25	10	0 (2 tbs)	21/7–13
	1.5/30, Fe 1.5/30,	20	1000	21/7–13
	0.4/35	30	1500	21/7–13
	0.5/35	35	400	21/7–13
	1/35,	35	500	21/7–13
	1/50	35	1000	21/7–13
		50	1000	
EE/levonorgestrel		20	90	28/0–continuous
		20	100	21/7–13
		20	100 (84 tabs)	84/7–4
		10	0 (7 tbs)	21/7–13
		30	150	84/7–4
		30	150 (84 tbs)	84/7–4
		10	0 (7 tbs)	
EE/norgestrel		30	300	300
		50	250	
				21/7–13
				500
EE/norgestimate		35	250	21/7–13
EE/desogestrel		20	150 (21 tbs)	21/7–13
		10	0 (5 tbs)	21/7–13
		30	150	
EE/drospirenone		20	3000	24/4–13
		30	3000	
Mestranol/ norethindrone	1/50	50°	1000	21/7–13
Estradiol valerate				
Estradiol valerate/ dienogest		3000	0 (2 tbs)	22/6–13
		2000	2000 (5 tbs)	
		2000	3000 (17 tbs)	
		1000	0 (2 tbs)	
		0	0 (2 tbs)	
Biphasic				
EE/norethidrone	10/11	35	500 (10 tbs)	21/7–13
		35	1000 (11 tbs)	
Triphasic				
EE/norethidrone acetate		20 (5)/ 30 (7)/ 35 (10 TABS)	1000	21/7–13
	,	35	500 (7 tbs)	21/7–13
		35	1000 (9 tbs)	
		35	500 (5 tbs)	

(continued)

Table 11.5 **Continued**

Pill Type	Estrogen (mcg)	Progestin (mcg)	Cycle-Cycles/ Year
	35	500 (7 tabs)	21/7–13
	35	750 (7 tabs)	
	35	1000 (7 tabs)	
EE/levonorgestrel	30	50 (6 tbs)	21/7–13
	40	75 (5 tbs)	
	30	125(10 tbs)	
EE/norgestimate	25	180 (7 tbs)	21/7–13
	25	215 (7 tbs)	
	25	250 (7 tbs)	
	35	180 (7 tabs)	21/7–13
	35	215 (7 tabs)	
	35	250 (7 tabs)	
EE/desogestrel	25	100 (7 tbs)	21/7–13
	25	125 (7 tbs)	
	25	150 (7 tbs)	
Progestin-only Norethindrone		350	

Type	PROGESTIN (mg)/ETHINYL ESTRADIOL (µg)
© COMBINATION MONOPHASIC	1/30,1/35,1/50
Second Generation	0.1/20, 0.15/30
Ethynodiol diacetate	0.4/35, 0.5/35, 1/20, 1/35, 1/50, 1.5/30, 1/50°
Levonorgestrel°	0.05/35, 0.1/20, 0.1/35, 0.15/30
Norethindrone	0.3/30, 0.5/50
Norethindrone acetate	0.15/30
Norgestrel	0.25/35
Third Generation	3.0/20, 3.0/30
Desogestrel	
Norgestimate	
Drospirenone	
© BIPHASIC	0.5/35 and 1/35
Norethindrone	.15/20, placebo, & .15/10; .15/20, placebo, & 0.0/10
Desogestrel	
© TRIPHASIC	1/20, 1/30, 1/35; .5/35, .75/35, 1/35; .5/35, 1/35, .5/35
Norethindrone	0.05/30, .075/40, .125/30
Levonorgestrel	0.18/35, 0.215/35, 0.25/35
Norgestimate	
© PROGESTIN ONLY	0.5 Most oral contraceptives are packaged
Ethynodiol diacetate	as a 21/7 cycle (21 days of active tablets and
Levonorgestrel	7 days of placebo), resulting in 13 withdrawal bleeding
Norethindrone	episodes each year.
Norgestrel	0.030
	0.35
	0.075

°equivalent to 35 mcg EE= Ethinylestradiol
°available as 84 active tablets and 7 placebo tablets (Seasonale)
°Mestranol

alter the cervical mucus, making it thick, viscid, and scanty, which retards sperm penetration. They also alter the motility of the uterus and oviduct, impairing transport of both ova and sperm.

Advantages of COCs include high efficacy, rapid reversibility, and additional noncontraceptive benefits. Side effects, including nausea and headaches, are less common with the low-dose pills (<50 μg ethinyloestradiol) and are mostly limited to early cycles of use. By eliminating most, if not all, pill-free intervals, long-cycle regimens with infrequent bleeds are a variable option.[157] This is now available commercially. Two synthetic estrogens are used in OCs: ethinyl estradiol and its 3-methyl ether, mestranol. These have different biologic activity. Mestranol must be demethylated to ethinyl estradiol to become biologically active, with consequent lower levels of derived ethinyl estradiol. Ethinyl estradiol has an ethinyl radical on carbon 17. This inhibits 17 β hydroxylation, which initiates estradiol metabolism in the intestinal wall, the hepatocyte, and most target tissues. Because of its potency and strong anti-gonadotropic effect with a single daily oral dose, it is the most popular estrogen used in oral contraception. Two major types of synthetic progestins are derivatives of 19-nortestosterone and derivatives of 17 α-acetoxyprogesterone (C21 progestins, called pregnanes). The 19-nortesterone progestins have a C19 methyl group replaced by a hydrogen atom. Those used in OCs are of two major subtypes: estranes (norethindrone acetate and ethynodiol diacetate) and gonanes (del-norgestrel and its active isomer, levonorgestrel), which have an ethyl group attached to the 13 carbon. Gonanes have more intrinsic progestational activity than do estranes, and thus a lower dose is used in OC formulations. The progestins, desogestrel, gestodene, and norgestimate, are gonanes and are less androgenic and have less effect on carbohydrate and lipid metabolism, but may increase the risk of thromboembolic disease compared to the older progestins.[156] They appear to produce relatively minor effects on the coagulation system.[153] Drospirenone, a pregnene progestogen derived from spironolactone, shares many of the pharmacodynamic features of progesterone. It is an anti-mineralocorticoid with less water retention, less weight gain, and fewer breast symptoms.[158] The progestins are combined with varying dosages of either of the estrogens, ethinyl estradiol, or mestranol. There are large intraindividual differences in ethinyl estradiol and progestin plasma concentration, with means of around 100–1000 pg/ml for 50 μg ethinyl estradiol and 1–5 ng/ml for the usual dose of the various progestins. Progestins are also available as monotherapy for hormonal contraception.

The ethinyl estradiol content in COCs has progressively decreased: most now contain 20–35 μg. Formulations with 50 μg or more of estrogen are called first-generation OCs, and those with less than 50 mg of estrogen are called second-generation OCs. Formulations with the new progestins (desogestrel, norgestimate, gestodene, and drospirenone) are called third-generation OCs. Formulations containing 35 μg of ethinyl estradiol and one of the new progestins are comparable in efficacy to each other and to established agents.[153,156,159–162] In addition, they may be associated with stronger suppression of ovarian activity. These properties have allowed a further reduction in the estrogenic content of OCs to 20 μg; no data show that further decreases in the estrogen dose confer any added benefit.[163] One formulation uses low-dose desogestrel (.15 mg) in combination with 20 μg of ethinyl estradiol for 21 days followed by placebo for 2 days, then desogestrel (.15 mg) in combination with ethinyl estradiol (10μg) for 5 days.[164] Another formulation uses 15 μg ethinyloestradiol and 60 μg gestodene with a shortened pill-free interval of 4 days.[165] A fourth-generation combination pill has a nortestosterone-derived progestogen, dienogest. It has low androgenicity, allowing even lower doses of estrogen.[166] Drospirenone (3 mg), a pregnene progestogen, is available in combination with ethinyl estradiol (30 μg).

OCs have many non-contraceptive benefits. Users have less menorrhagia, irregular menstruation, and intermenstrual bleeding.[167] Other non-contraceptive medical benefits of OCs result from their main action: the inhibition of ovulation. The Royal College of General Practitioners study[168] showed that OC users had 63% less dysmenorrhea and 29% less premenstrual tension than did controls. OC users are less likely to develop rheumatoid arthritis or acquire salpingitis (pelvic inflammatory disease).[163] Absolute contraindications to OC use include a history of vascular disease, including thromboembolism, thrombophlebitis, atherosclerosis, and stroke, and systemic disease that may affect the vascular system, such as lupus erythematosus or diabetes with retinopathy or nephropathy. Cigarette smoking by OC users over age 35 and uncontrolled hypertension are also contraindications.

Transdermal Contraceptive Patch

A transdermal contraceptive patch (Ortho Evra) containing an ethinyloestradiol/orelgestromin (17-diacetyl nogestimate) was approved by the FDA in 2001. It delivers 150 µg of norelgestromin and 20 µg of ethinyl estradiol daily to the systemic circulation. Patients use one patch for 3 weeks and follow with a patch-free week. Audet et al., in a randomized controlled trial, compared the contraceptive efficacy, cycle control, compliance, and safety of a transdermal contraceptive patch and an OC.[169] Overall and method-failure Pearl Indices (number of unintentional pregnancies per 100 women years) were numerically lower with the patch (1.24 and 0.99, respectively) than the OC (2.18 and 1.25, respectively); this difference was not statistically significant (P –.57 and .80, respectively). The incidence of breakthrough bleeding and/or spotting was significantly higher only in the first two cycles in the patch group, but the incidence of breakthrough bleeding alone was comparable between treatments in all cycles. The mean proportion of participants' cycles with perfect compliance was 88.2% (811 total participants, 4141 total cycles) with the patch and 77.7% (605 total participants, 4134 total cycles) with the OC (< .001). Only 1.8% (300/16,673) of patches completely detached. The contraceptive patch is comparable to a COC in contraceptive efficacy and cycle control. Failures occurred more commonly in women weighing more than 90 kg (196 lb).[170] Compliance was better with the weekly contraceptive patch than with the OC.

Vaginal Rings

The contraceptive vaginal ring (CVR) is made of soft flexible silicone rubber with hormones implanted in the core of the ring. Various ring prototypes have been evaluated, including progestin-only rings and combined progestin-estrogen rings, as well as combination of progestins and estrogens. The progestin-only ring is intended for continuous use, whereas the combined ring has been designed for cyclic 3-week in/1-week out use, although several studies have explored alternative schemes of extended use. In 2001, the FDA approved Organon's CVR (NuvaRing), a 1-month combined ring that releases 150 mg etonogestrel and 15 mg ethinyl estradiol into the systemic circulation each day. The steroids are absorbed through the vaginal epithelium, and the ring does not require placement in a certain area of the vagina. It is used for one cycle consisting of 3 weeks of continuous ring use and a 1-week ring-free period. The ring is effective, easy to use, well-tolerated, and well-accepted; adherence with the regimen is high (90.8%). A multicenter clinical study found that menstrual irregularities and device-related problems (frequent expulsion) account for most discontinuations.[171]

Progering is a three-month progesterone-releasing ring for use by lactating women. A one-year Nestorone/ethinyl estradiol CVR is approaching the final stages of development, as the Population Council is preparing to submit a new drug application to the FDA. The main advantages of CVRs are their effectiveness (similar or slightly better than the pill), ease of use without the need of remembering a daily routine, user ability to control initiation and discontinuation, nearly constant release rate (allowing for lower doses), greater bioavailability, and good cycle control with the combined ring, in comparison with OCs.

It has been postulated that administering estrogens through the vaginal route would avoid the approximately 60% first-pass of the steroid through the liver that occurs after oral administration. Unfortunately, studies comparing the effect of equivalent dosages of orally and vaginally administered EE on hepatic proteins, hemostasis variables, and lipids have failed to show any difference between delivery routes. The effects of combined hormonal contraceptives on clotting factors and markers of coagulation and fibrinolysis are largely due to the EE component (with its high potency and slow metabolism) and independent of the route of administration.[172]

Injectable and Implantable Hormonal Contraception

Three types of injectable, long-acting steroid formulations are currently in use for contraception throughout the world. These include depo-medroxyprogesterone acetate, given in a dose of 150 mg every 3 months; norethindrone enanthate, given in a dose of 200 mg every 2 months; and several once-a-month injections of combinations of different progestins and estrogens. Only depo-medroxyprogesterone acetate is currently available in the United States. Medroxyprogesterone acetate is a 17-acetoxy progesterone compound and is the only progestin used for contraception that is not a 19-nortesosterone derivative. The 17-acetoxy progestins, which do not have androgenic activity and are structurally related to progesterone instead of testosterone, were used in OC formulations about 30 years ago. The exact frequency of headache associated with the use of medroxyprogesterone acetate suspension is uncertain.

Norethindrone enanthate is another injectable progesterone that has been approved for contraceptive use in more than 40 countries (but not in the US). It is administered in an oily suspension and thus its pharmacodynamics differ from those of depo-medroxyprogesterone acetate. Several combined progestin-estrogen injectables consist of a low dose of a long-acting progestin plus a small amount of an estradiol ester.

Subdermal progestin implants are effective long-acting contraceptives. The first subdermal system, Norplant, used six silastic capsules filled with 216 mg of crystalline levonorgestrel (LNG) released at an average of 30 mg daily to achieve typical serum concentrations of 175 to 250 pg/mL. It is no longer available in the United States because of litigation involving difficulty removing the rods. Low concentrations of LNG do not inhibit ovulation; contraception is due to creating an inhospitable fertilization environment, with cervical mucus that is scant, thick, and hostile to sperm penetration and an endometrium not supportive of sperm capacitation or implantation. At higher concentrations of LNG, ovulation is inhibited, but follicles still enlarge and produce near-normal amounts of estradiol.[173] The primary AEs are irregular menstrual bleeding and headaches. Headache, the primary reason cited for removal other than menstrual disturbance, occurs in about 5%–20% of patients. The cumulative headache rate was 6.4/100 by the end of the second year.[174] In one study, headache was a complaint of 4% of women at 3 months compared with 2% of women using a copper IUD.[175]

Because of the removal problems and AEs of the six-rod Norplant system, new one- and two-implant systems[176] have been developed and compared with the six-rod Norplant. Jadelle, the new name for Norplant-2®, uses two implanted rods.[177] It is made of an elastomer with improved drug release capability and has the same rate of LNG release as the six-rod Norplant® system. Sivin et al.[178] reported a 5-year trial of a two-rod LNG contraceptive implant (Jadelle). The 5-year cumulative pregnancy rate was 0.8 per 100; the annual average pregnancy rate was less than two per 1000 women. Prolonged bleeding or spotting (8.2% of subjects) and irregular bleeding (5.6%) were the most frequently cited medical reasons for removal. Removal because of headache (4.7%) and weight change (4.0%) were the next most frequent medical reasons. In a direct comparison of the two-rod Jadelle system with the six-rod Norplant system, efficacy, bleeding, and other side effects were similar, but the two-rod system was twice as fast to insert and remove as the six-rod Norplant.[179]

Chompootaweep et al.[180] prospectively studied the two-rod LNG (Jadelle) contraceptive subdermal implants. The 3-year cumulative termination rate for personal reasons (divorce, husband having vasectomy, moving away from the study area) was 7.2%. The other leading causes for termination were acne, headache, and pain at the implant site. (The termination rate was 4.6%.)

Coukell and Balfour[181] reviewed the contraceptive efficacy and acceptability of LNG subdermal implants. LNG implant use was associated with idiopathic intracranial hypertension.[182,183] After 1 year, the incidence of increased appetite, perceived weight gain, emotional problems, and headaches did not differ significantly between US adolescents who chose LNG implants and those who chose OCs.[184]

A new implantable form of contraception containing 68 mg of etonogestrel (Implanon®) is now available in the United States. Etonogestrel is the active metabolite of desogestrel. It is a single-rod contraceptive implant that is inserted under the skin of the upper arm and provides highly reliable protection against pregnancy for as long as 3 years. It consists of a non-biodegradable rod that measures 40 mm in length and 2 mm in diameter. The average hormone release rate is 40 micrograms per day. Frequent or prolonged bleeding is the most frequent reason for discontinuation. Funk et al. investigated Implanon's safety and efficacy in a multicenter clinical trial of 330 sexually active American women who used the implant for up to 2 years.[185] No pregnancies occurred. Besides bleeding irregularities, common AEs leading to discontinuation were emotional lability (6.1%), weight increase (3.3%), depression (2.4%), and acne (1.5%). Headaches related to study medication occurred in 42 women (12.7%). Implanon was compared with six-rod Norplant in a multinational randomized trial. [176] Implanon was more effective, had fewer prolonged episodes of bleeding, and was faster to insert and remove. Ovulation was more frequently suppressed and the incidence of follicular cysts was decreased in the Implanon users.

ADVERSE EVENTS

The most common dose-dependent AEs seen with estrogen OCs are nausea, breast tenderness, fluid retention, and depression. Depression occurs with high, but not with low (<50 μg), estrogen formulations. Physiologic doses of estrogen alone (less than the pharmacologic dose used in OCs) improve mood, while an added progestin may provoke depression, irritability, tension, and fatigue.[168] Weight gain, breakthrough bleeding, nausea, headache, breast tenderness, mood swings, acne, and hirsutism are the most common causes of premature OC discontinuation.[167] Older progestins, structurally related to testosterone, produce adverse androgenic effects, including weight gain, acne, and nervousness. Estrogen causes an increase in HDL cholesterol, a decrease in LDL levels, and an increase in total cholesterol and triglyceride levels. Progestin causes a decrease in HDL and an increase in LDL levels while causing a decrease in both total cholesterol and triglyceride levels.

Because of the low clearance rate and the first-pass hepatic effect, liver cells metabolize around 60% of the ethinyl estradiol dose,[186] resulting in estrogen stimulation comparable to that observed during pregnancy. This stimulation modifies lipids and coagulation factors: triglycerides, HDL cholesterol, Factor VII, and resistance to activated protein-C increase and antithrombin decrease.[187] The addition of norethisterone or norgestrel, first- and second-generation progestins that have mild androgenic activity, attenuates the changes in liver metabolism induced by ethinyl estradiol; HDL cholesterol and triglyceride levels tend to decrease in comparison with those of individuals who use ethinyl estradiol alone, and even in low ethinyl estradiol dose users in comparison with nonusers. The third-generation progestins, such as desogestrel and gestodene, do not modify the ethinyl estradiol-induced changes in liver metabolism. Thus, mean HDL cholesterol and triglyceride levels and pro-coagulant effects (specifically, acquired resistance to protein C) are higher in users of third generation OCs than in users of second generation OCs. [188–191] The potential consequences of the pro-coagulant effect may be particularly worrisome in women who are older, who smoke, who are hyperlipidemic, diabetic, obese, or hypertensive, or have a past personal or family history of venous or arterial thromboembolic accidents. These woman should not use any formulation containing oral ethinyl estradiol. [192,193] Even reduced ethinyl estradiol doses in a young, selected, and controlled population of women have an increased risk of thromboembolic accident, in particular, phlebitis and perhaps ischemic stroke, in comparison with past users[194] or never users.[167,195–197]

The safety of COCs has been confirmed with the publication of a 25-year follow-up of 23,000 COC users and age-matched controls. [198] Despite the cohort being mainly users or ex-users of high-dose pills, there were no excess deaths overall and no effect of past use 10 years after stopping COCs. The Cancer and Steroid Hormone (CASH) study[199] did not show any association between OC use and breast cancer (relative risk, 1.0; 95% CI [0.9–1.1]). However, a 1996 metaanalysis of data from 54 epidemiologic studies of OC use and the risk of breast cancer showed that women had a slightly increased risk of breast cancer while taking OCs, as compared with the risk among non-users (relative risk, 1.24; 95% CI [1.15–1.33]).[200]

The results of the Women's Contraceptive and Reproductive Experiences study are similar to those of the CASH analysis. No association between past or present use of OCs and breast cancer was observed in this well-conducted, population-based study of 4575 women with breast cancer and 4682 controls. [201] Among women from 35 to 64 years of age, current or former OC use was not associated with a significantly increased risk of breast cancer.[202]

OCs reduce the risk of both endometrial and ovarian cancer. For example, in the CASH study, there was a 40% reduction in the risk of endometrial cancer (OR, 0.6; 95% CI [0.3–0.9]) after 12 months of OC use. Furthermore, there was a 40% reduction in the risk of ovarian cancer after as short a period as 3–6 months of use, and 10 or more years of use was associated with an 80% reduction in the risk (OR, 0.2; 95% CI 0.1–0.4).[203] Chasan-Taber and Stampfer[204–206] searched the MEDLINE database for all English-language epidemiologic studies of OCs and cardiovascular disease published between 1967 and 1997 and concluded that the current use of OCs increases the risk for myocardial infarction, but most of the excess risk is attributable to an interaction with cigarette smoking. Current OC users who are younger than 40 years of age and do not smoke have little or no increased myocardial infarction risk. The newest progestogen-containing OCs may carry lower relative risks for myocardial infarction than did earlier preparations. Progestin-only OCs are an alternative to COCs in women at risk of thrombosis. [205,207] There is no increased myocardial infarction risk among former OC users. The incidence of cardiovascular disease is also not correlated with the duration of OC use.

There is persistent controversy concerning OCs and the risk of stroke in migraineurs. [14] Studies of OCs and stroke are often small, typically do not discriminate between hemorrhagic and thromboembolic stroke, and often do not control for major risk factors for stroke. Retrospective studies have looked at the influence of OCs on the risk of cerebral thromboembolic events. Many were conducted during a period when pills (first-generation OCs) were widely used. These data suggest that OCs containing more than 50 mg, 50 mg, and 30–40 mg of estrogen are associated with odds ratios for cerebral thromboembolic attacks of about

8–10, 2–4, and 1.5–2.5, respectively, whereas those containing a progestin only are not associated with any increased risk. Smoking was associated with an odds ratio of 1.5–1.6 independent of age and use or non-use of OCs. [197] The Collaborative Group for the Study of Stroke in Young Women did not confirm reports that migraine may increase the risk of stroke in women using OCs.[208] Migraine itself may be a risk factor for stroke in younger women. The Physicians' Health Study,[209] based on 22,071 US male physicians, found an increased risk of stroke in migraineurs, with a relative risk of 2–2.5, but since it included only men, it found no sex difference. In a large cohort study that included 12,220 subjects (both men and women), migraine was associated with increased risk for stroke.[210] The migraine-associated risk for stroke decreased with increasing age (from a risk ratio of 2.8 at age 40 to 1.7 at age 60).

Tzourio et al.,[211] in a 1993 case-control study of 212 patients with stroke and an equal number of controls, found that the odds ratio for any migraine type in women under the age of 45 with stroke was 4.3 (1.2–16.3). There was no increased risk in men or in older women. The risk for stroke was even higher in younger women migraineurs who smoked.[211] In their 1995 study, Tzourio et al.[212] found that migraine without aura had an odds ratio of 3.0 (1.5–5.8) and migraine with aura had an odds ratio of 6.2 (2.1–18.0) for stroke in women younger than 45 years. Migraine prevalence was similar in patients with proven arterial lesions, such as dissection, cardiac abnormalities, or anticardiolipin antibodies. Chang et al. [213] conducted a retrospective case-control study that included 291 women with stroke and 736 age-matched controls. Migraine was associated with an increased risk of ischemic stroke (OR 3.54 for all migraines; 3.81 for MA, 2.97 for MO) but not of hemorrhagic stroke. The coexistence of migraine, hypertension, smoking, and OC use was associated with a more-than-multiplicative risk of ischemic stroke. Stroke risk was associated with migraine of more than 12 years' duration, initial migraine with aura, and attack frequency of > 12/year or an increasing attack frequency.[214] Since the prevalence of stroke in young women is low, the absolute stroke risk in young female migraineurs is still low (17–19/100,000 women-years) in the absence of other risk factors.[215]

Kurth et al. conducted a prospective cohort study among 39,754 US health professionals age 45 and older who participated in the Women's Health Study.[216] A total of 385 strokes (309 ischemic, 72 hemorrhagic, and 4 undefined) occurred. Compared with non-migraineurs, those with migraine overall or migraine without aura had no increased risk of any stroke type. Those with migraine with aura had increased adjusted hazards ratios (HR) of 1.53 (95% CI [1.02–2.31]) for total stroke and 1.71 (95% CI [1.11–2.66]) for ischemic stroke, but no increased risk for hemorrhagic stroke. Participants with migraine with aura who were < 55 years old had a greater increase in risk of total (HR 1.75; 95% CI [1.02–3.00]) and ischemic (HR 2.25; 95% CI [1.30–3.91]) stroke. The absolute risk increase was with 3.8 additional cases per year per 10,000 women.

Kurth et al. further evaluated the association between migraine with and without aura and the subsequent risk of overall and specific cardiovascular disease (CVD) in the Women's Health Study, in women who were free of CVD and angina at study entry.[217,218] During a mean of 10 years of follow-up, 580 major CVD events occurred. Compared with women with no migraine history, women who reported active (within the last year) migraine with aura had multivariable-adjusted HRs of 2.15 (95% CI [1.58–2.92]. p = .001) for major CVD, 1.91 (95% CI [1.17–3.10], p = .01) for ischemic stroke, 2.08 (95% CI [1.30–3.31], p = .002) for myocardial infarction, 1.74 (95% CI [1.23–2.46], p = .002) for coronary revascularization, 1.71 (95% CI [1.16–2.53], p = .007) for angina, and 2.33 (95% CI [1.21–4.51], p = .01) for ischemic CVD death. Women who reported active migraine without aura did not have increased risk of any vascular events or angina. Women with active migraine with (but not without) aura had increased risk of major CVD, myocardial infarction, ischemic stroke, and death due to ischemic CVD, as well as with coronary revascularization and angina.

Most recent prospective studies have not shown an increased risk for stroke among either past users of OCs or persons who had ever used OCs. Studies of stroke in current users have yielded inconsistent results. One case was seen in the Group Health Cooperative Study[219] and a relative risk of 0.6 (CI 0.1–2.9) was seen in the Royal College of General Practitioners study.[220] Hannaford et al.[220]

examined the data obtained between 1968 and 1990 during the Royal College of General Practitioners OC study to determine the relationship between OC use and the risk of first-ever stroke, including the diagnosis of sub-arachnoid hemorrhage, cerebral hemorrhage, or thromboembolic stroke. Women using OCs containing a high estrogen dose (more than 50 µg) had a nearly sixfold increase in the risk of stroke, while women ingesting OC formulations containing 30–35 µg estrogen did not have an increased risk.

No significant increased thromboembolic or hemorrhagic stroke risk in OC users was seen in the study performed by Pettiti et al. in a large California Health Management Organization from 1991 to 1994.[221] The relative risk of thromboembolic stroke was 0.65 and hemorrhagic stroke 1.01 for OC users compared with women who never used OCs, and 1.18 and 1.13, respectively, compared with newer users and past users.[163] In a hospital-based, case-control study, the risk of ischemic stroke in current COC use was assessed in 697 women, aged 20–44 years, and 1962 age-matched hospital controls in 21 centers in Africa, Asia, Europe, and Latin America.[205] The overall OR of ischemic stroke was 2.99 (95% CI [1.65–5.40]) in Europe and 2.93 (2.15–4.00) in the non-European countries. ORs were lower in younger women and those who did not smoke, and less than 2 in women with normal blood pressure who reported that their blood pressure had been checked before the current episode of OC use. Among current OC users with a history of hypertension, the OR was 10.7 (2.04–56.6) in Europe and 14.5 (5.36–39.0) in the developing countries. In Europe, the OR associated with current use of low-dose OCs (< 50 µg estrogen) was 1.53 (0.71–3.31), whereas for higher-dose preparations it was 5.30 (2.56–11.0). In the developing countries, there was no significant difference between overall estimates of risk associated with use of low-dose or higher-dose OCs (3.26 [2.19–4.86] vs. 2.71 [1.75–4.19]). In this study, the incidence of ischemic stroke was low in women of reproductive age, and any risk attributable to OC use was small. The risk can be further reduced if users are younger than 35, do not smoke, do not have a history of hypertension, and have blood pressure measured before the start of OC use; in these women, OC preparations with low estrogen doses may be associated with even lower risk.

The WHO collaborative case-control study also assessed the risk of hemorrhagic stroke from the use of COCs in 1068 cases, aged 20 to 44 years, and 2910 age-matched controls.[222] Current COC use was associated with slightly increased risk of hemorrhagic stroke, which was significant in the developing countries (OR 1.76, 95% CI [1.34–2.30]) but not in Europe (1.38 [0.84–2.25]). OC use did not increase the risk of hemorrhagic stroke in women younger than 35, but in women older than 35, OR was greater than 2. Current OC users with a history of hypertension outside of pregnancy had a 10- to 15-fold increased risk of hemorrhagic stroke compared with non-OC users without a history of hypertension. OR among current OC users who were also current cigarette smokers was greater than 3. In both groups of countries, past use of OCs, the dose of estrogen, and the dose and type of progestogen had no effect on risk, and risks were similar for subarachnoid and intracerebral hemorrhage.[222]

The ORs for any type of stroke associated with current use of low-dose (<50μ:g estrogen) and higher-dose OCs were 1.41 (0.90–2.20) and 2.71 (1.70–4.32), respectively, in Europe and 1.86 (1.49–2.33) and 1.92 (1.48–2.50) in the developing countries. This is about 13% and 8% of all strokes in women aged 20–44 in Europe and the developing countries, respectively, and are attributable to the use of OCs. The risk of hemorrhagic stroke attributable to OC use is not increased in younger women and is only slightly increased in older women. The estimated excess risk of all stroke types associated with the use of low-estrogen and higher estrogen dose OCs in Europe was about 2 and 8, respectively, per 100,000 women-years of OC use.[222]

Chang et al., in the European subset of the World Health Organization Collaborative Study of Cardiovascular Disease and Steroid Hormone Contraception, compared 291 women aged 20–44 years who had ischemic, hemorrhagic, or unclassified arterial stroke with 736 age- and hospital-matched controls.[213] Adjusted OR associated with a personal history of migraine was 1.78 (95% CI [1.14–2.77]), 3.54 (1.30–9.61), and 1.10 (0.63–1.94) for all stroke, ischemic stroke, and hemorrhagic stroke, respectively. OR for ischemic stroke was similar for migraine with aura 3.81 (1.26–11.5) and migraine without aura 2.97 (0.66–13.5). A family history of migraine,

regardless of personal history, was also associated with increased OR, not only for ischemic stroke but also hemorrhagic stroke. Migrainous women with coexistent use of OCs or a history of high blood pressure or smoking had greater than multiplicative effects on the OR for ischemic stroke associated with migraine alone. Change in the frequency or type of migraine with OC use did not predict subsequent stroke. Between 20% and 40% of strokes in women with migraine seemed to develop directly from a migraine attack, but there was no evidence that a change in migraine type predicted stroke.[14] The rates of conversion from migraine with aura to migraine without aura were essentially the same among all cases of stroke and their controls (difference of 2.3%, 95% CI [9.7%–14.3%]). The findings of an OR of 34.4 (3.3–361) for ischemic stroke among migrainous women who use OCs and smoke is of considerable concern, even though the rate of cases of stroke fulfilling the eligibility criteria of the study (estimated from one of the European collaborative centers to be 5.5 per 100,000 woman years) was relatively low.

Schwaag et al. designed a case-control study of a homogeneous group of patients with juvenile cerebral ischemia as part of a larger German epidemiologic research project looking at the association of IHS migraine with CVD.[223] They enrolled 160 consecutive patients under the age of 46 with first-ever ischemic stroke or transient ischemic attack, and 160 strictly sex- and age-matched controls. Patients suffering from arterial dissection, brain hemorrhage, cranial sinus thrombosis, lacunar stroke, or migrainous infarction were excluded. Migraine was a significant risk factor for juvenile stroke for the total sample, with an OR of 2.11 (CI 1.16–3.82). The OR was even higher in the subgroup under the age of 35 (3.26) and in the female subgroup (2.68). Their data suggest that migraine is a significant risk factor for stroke in patients under the age of 35 independent of other vascular risk factors.

Gillum et al. published a large meta-analysis of 16 case-control and cohort studies. Among the case-control studies (published between 1993 and 1999), the RR was still elevated among those using low-dose (< 50 μg) estrogen (OR 2.08, 95% CI [1.55–2.80]) but was significantly lower than among those using higher doses (<50 μg) of estrogen (OR 4.53, 95% CI [2.17–9.50]). The overall RR, regardless of the OC dose, was 2.75 (95% CI [2.24–3.38]). OC use appeared to impart a similar ischemic stroke risk among smokers and non-smokers. Furthermore, there was no difference in the risk imparted by OC use according to hypertensive status, presence or absence of migraine history, and age. This translates to an additional 4.1 ischemic strokes per 100,000 non-smoking, normotensive women using low-estrogen OCs, or one additional ischemic stroke per year per 24,000 such women.[224]

In a Dutch study that included women aged 18–49 years, OC use (of any type) was associated with an increased risk of ischemic stroke (OR 2.3).[225] The risk was higher for older (ages 40–49) compared with younger (ages 18–29) women (OR 2.6 vs. 1.3). The risks with second-generation (containing levonorgestrel) and third-generation (containing desogestrel or gestodene) OCs were similar. Smoking, hypertension, hypercholesterolemia, and obesity further increased the stroke risk associated with OC use. Lidegaard et al. studied 626 cases (women with cerebral thromboembolic attacks [CTA]) and 4054 controls.[226] The use of OCs containing 50 μg, 30–40 μg, and 20 μg EE implied adjusted ORs for CTA of 4.5, 1.6, and 1.7, respectively. Unlike the results of the Dutch study, third-generation pills were associated with a lower CTA risk (OR 1.4) compared with second-generation pills (OR 2.2). Progestin-only pills were not associated with an increased CTA risk.

In a case-control study from Australia, the use of low-dose OCs was not associated with a significantly increased risk for ischemic stroke. Siritho et al. identified consecutive women between 15 and 55 years of age with ischemic stroke from four Melbourne hospitals. Neighborhood-based control subjects (227) were individually age and geographically matched to subject cases (227). Compared with non-current use, current use of the OCP, in doses of < 50 μg estrogen, was not associated with an increased risk of ischemic stroke (OR 1.76, 95% CI [0.86–3.61], p = 0.124). Factors associated with an increased risk of ischemic stroke were a history of hypertension (OR 2.18, 95% CI [1.22–3.91]); transient ischemic attack (OR 8.17, 95% CI [1.69–39.6]); previous myocardial infarction (OR 5.64, 95% CI [1.04–30.61]); diabetes mellitus (OR 5.42, 95% CI [1.42–20.75]); family history of stroke (OR 2.22, 95% CI [1.12–4.43]); and smoking

> 20 cigarettes per day (OR 3.68, 95% CI [1.22–11.09]).[227]

In a 15-year Danish historical cohort study, Lidegaard et al. followed non-pregnant women, 15–49 years old, with no history of cardiovascular disease or cancer. Data on use of hormonal contraception, clinical endpoints, and potential confounders were obtained from four national registries. A total of 1,626,158 women contributed 14,251,063 person-years of observation, during which 3311 thrombotic strokes (21.4 per 100,000 person-years) and 1725 myocardial infarctions (10.1 per 100,000 person-years) occurred. As compared with non-use, current use of oral contraceptives that included EE at a dose of 30–40 μg was associated with the following relative risks for thrombotic stroke and myocardial infarction, according to progestin type: norethindrone, 2.2 (1.5–3.2) and 2.3 (1.3–3.9); levonorgestrel, 1.7 (1.4–2.0) and 2.0 (1.6–2.5); norgestimate, 1.5 (1.2–1.9) and 1.3 (0.9–1.9); desogestrel, 2.2 (1.8–2.7) and 2.1 (1.5–2.8); gestodene, 1.8 (1.6–2.0) and 1.9 (1.6–2.3); and drospirenone, 1.6 (1.2 –2.2) and 1.7 (1.0 –2.6), respectively. With EE at a dose of 20 μg, the corresponding relative risks according to progestin type were as follows: desogestrel, 1.5 (1.3 –1.9) and 1.6 (1.1–2.1); gestodene, 1.7 (1.4 –2.1) and 1.2 (0.8–1.9); and drospirenone, 0.9 (0.2–3.5) and 0.0. For transdermal patches, the corresponding relative risks were 3.2 (0.8–12.6) and 0.0, and for a vaginal ring, 2.5 (1.4–4.4) and 2.1 (0.7–6.5). They concluded that although the absolute risks of thrombotic stroke and myocardial infarction associated with the use of hormonal contraception were low, the risk was increased by a factor of 0.9 to 1.7 with OCs that included EE at a dose of 20 μg and by a factor of 1.3 to 2.3 with those that included EE at a dose of 30–40 μg, with relatively small differences in risk according to progestin type.[228]

The results of these clinical studies were supported by neuroimaging findings. In a population-based MRI study from The Netherlands, patients with migraine had a higher prevalence of silent cerebellar infarcts compared with age- and sex-matched controls.[229] The risk of silent cerebellar infarcts was higher in patients with migraine with aura and those with higher attack frequency. Migraine was also associated with an increase in deep white matter lesions in women, but not in men.

The mechanism by which migraine increases stroke risk is not known. Several hypotheses have been raised, including vasospasm, endothelial dysfunction, and increased platelet aggregation.[215] Migraine is associated with cardiac abnormalities, such as patent foramen ovale.[230] Scher et al. have shown that migraineurs, particularly those who have migraine with aura, have a higher cardiovascular risk profile than individuals without migraine.[231] Compared with controls, migraineurs were more likely to smoke (OR 1.43), less likely to consume alcohol (OR 0.58), and more likely to report a parental history of early myocardial infarction. Migraineurs with aura were more likely to have an unfavorable cholesterol profile, have elevated BP (systolic BP > 140 mm Hg or diastolic BP > 90 mm Hg [OR 1.76 (1.04–3.0)]), and report a history of early onset CHD or stroke (OR 3.96 [1.1–14.3]); female migraineurs with aura were more likely to be using oral contraceptives (OR 2.06 [1.05–4.0]). The odds of having an elevated Framingham risk score for CHD were approximately doubled for the migraineurs with aura.

High-dose (≥ 50 μg estrogen) OCs increase the risk of ischemic stroke in young women, with an average RR of 4.1 compared with non-users.[197,205,212,225,226] The studies of low-dose (< 50 μg estrogen) OCs suggest that these drugs produce little increase in risk for ischemic stroke, but a two- to three-fold increase in risk cannot be ruled out.[232,233] Occlusive stroke in young women has an estimated rate of 5.4 per 100,000 person-years.[221] Fatal occlusive stroke is even rarer, with rates less than 0.5 per 100,000 for women younger than 45 years of age.[234] Therefore, any attributable risk for death from occlusive stroke associated with the use of OCs is small. Smokers may be particularly susceptible.[221] A positive interaction between OCs, smoking, and stroke exists. The Royal College of General Practitioners study found no evidence to support the existence of an increased risk for stroke among past users of OCs, with the exception of smokers (RR 1.8 [CI 1.1–2.8]).

Bousser and Kittner reviewed the relationship between OCs and stroke. Since 1962, more than 25 studies have been devoted to the relationship between OCs and stroke.[233] They are all case-control or cohort epidemiologic studies and thus contain the difficulties and biases that are inherent in these types of studies. The following conclusions can be drawn from these studies: high estrogen content (≥ 50 μg) increases the risk of stroke, all stroke subtypes, and stroke death; low estrogen content (< 50 μg) carries a very low or no risk of stroke; there are no data on progestogen-only OCs; stroke risk is greatly increased if associated risk factors are present, in particular, hypertension, cigarette smoking, and migraine; OCs, even at low doses, significantly increase the risk of cerebral venous thrombosis, which is further enhanced if congenital thrombophilia is present; and the attributable risk of stroke in young women using OCs is about one per 200,000 woman-years. The contraceptive and non-contraceptive benefits of low-dose OCs vastly outweigh their risks, provided that other risk factors are absent or well controlled.

Curtis et al. conducted a systematic review to evaluate whether women with headaches who use COCs have a greater risk of stroke than women with headaches who do not use COCs. Evidence from six case-control studies suggested that COC users with a history of migraine were two to four times as likely to have an ischemic stroke as non-users with a history of migraine. The odds ratios for ischemic stroke ranged from 6 to almost 14 for COC users with migraine compared with non-users without migraine. The studies that provided evidence on hemorrhagic stroke reported low or no risk associated with migraine or with COC use.[217,218]

Gerstman et al. showed a dose-response relation between estrogen and venous thromboembolism by comparing OCs that contain high levels of estrogen (≥ 50 μg) with OCs that contain intermediate (50 μg) and low (< 50 μg) levels of estrogen.[235] Bottiger et al. noted a marked decline of approximately 80% in reports of non-fatal thromboembolism per 100,000 users when low-dose estrogen OCs replaced high-dose preparations in Sweden.[236] Recent studies[237–240] suggest an increased risk of venous thromboembolism for users of the most recent progestogens compared with persons who do not use OCs, but confounding and bias may account for some of the apparent differences in the incidence of venous thromboembolism.[163]

Factor V Leiden mutation carriers (about 3% of the general population) have a sevenfold increase in thrombosis[193,241] compared with non-carriers. Factor V Leiden greatly increases the risk of venous thrombosis associated with OC use. As compared with the baseline risk for women who do not use OCs and do not carry factor V Leiden, the risk is increased by a factor of 4 in those who use OCs but do not carry factor V Leiden, by a factor of 7 in carriers of the factor V mutation who do not use OCs, and by a factor of 35 in women who carry the mutation and also use OCs. This susceptibility is even higher in the few women who are homozygous for this mutation.[242] Similarly, users of the newest progestogens have about a sixfold increased risk for thrombosis compared to an increased risk of 2 to 4 for the older progestogens. The increased risk for thromboembolic disease with the newest compared with older progestogens is modest. The baseline rate of thromboembolic disease in the United States is 5 or less per 100,000 person-years among women of reproductive age,[196,219,243] and the rate with the newest progestogens is approximately 30 per 100,000 person-years.[163]

Contraceptive Use

Women of reproductive potential, especially if they are taking drugs, require contraceptive counseling. Hormonal contraceptive failure can occur when drugs, especially anti-epileptic drugs, are used. Among 307 responders to a Johns Hopkins survey, 27% of the neurologists and 21% of the obstetricians reported contraceptive failure.[244] The anti-epileptic drugs phenobarbital, primidone, phenytoin, and carbamazepine induce the hepatic cytochrome P_{450} system of mixed function oxidizes, resulting in a reduction of exogenous estradiol and progesterone levels. Steroid hormone-binding globulins may also be increased, resulting in a decrease in free hormone levels.

The failure rate of OCs is 0.7 per 100 women-years. This rate is increased to 3.1 per 100 women-years in women who use high-dose estrogen-containing OCs (50 μg or more) and enzyme-inducing anticonvulsants.[245] Since the failure rate is higher when the more commonly used lower estrogen-dose OCs are used, an OC containing 50 μg or more of ethinyl estradiol or mestranol is recommended.[246] In contrast, valproic acid inhibits the hepatic microsomal enzyme system; the new anti-epileptic drugs, gabapentin, vigabatrin, lamotrigine, and topiramate (< 200 mg/day), have no effect. Since these anti-epileptic drugs have not been reported to result in hormonal contraceptive failure, they could be used if oral contraception is desired.[247] Intramuscular medroxyprogesterone (Depo-Provera®) and etonorgestrel implants (Implanon®) are not viable alternatives. Both are progestins whose efficacy is reduced by anti-epileptic drugs. (248) Women who use enzyme-inducing drugs or have epilepsy that requires medication

---

Table 11.6 **Headache Attributed to Exogenous Hormone**

Diagnostic criteria
A. Any headache fulfilling criterion C
B. Regular intake of one or more exogenous hormones
C. Evidence of causation demonstrated by both of the following:
    1. Headache has developed in temporal relation to the commencement of hormone intake
    2. One or more of the following:
        a) Headache has significantly worsened after an increase in dosage of the hormone.
        b) Headache has significantly improved or resolved after a reduction in hormone dosage.
        c) Headache has resolved after cessation of hormone intake.
D. Not better accounted for by another ICHD-3 β diagnosis.

Estrogen-Withdrawal Headache

Diagnostic criteria
A. Headache or migraine fulfilling criteria C
B. Daily use of exogenous estrogen for ≥ 3 weeks, which has been interrupted
C. Evidence of causation demonstrated by both of the following:
    1. Headache or migraine has developed within 5 days after the last use of estrogen.
    2. Headache or migraine has resolved within 3 days of its onset.
D. Not better accounted for by another ICHD-3 β diagnosis.

probably should be treated with formulations containing 50 μg of estrogen, because a higher incidence of abnormal bleeding has been reported when lower-dose-estrogen formulations are used. This is due to lower circulating levels of ethinyl estradiol caused by the action of most antiepileptic medications.

The IHS classification acknowledges that both the use of exogenous hormones and the withdrawal of estrogen can induce or exacerbate headaches[32](Table 11.6). The older combined OCs can induce, change, or alleviate headache.[14] OCs can trigger the first migraine attack, most often in women with a family history of migraine.[13,14,249] Existing migraine may exacerbate and headaches may occur on the days off the OC.[14,15,249,250] The headache pattern may become more severe and frequent and may be associated with neurologic symptoms.[208,249,251] Most women, however, have no change in the headache pattern, and some women have a distinct improvement in their headaches.[252,253] New onset of migraine usually occurs in the early cycles of OC use, but it can occur after prolonged OC usage.[249] Stopping the OC may not bring immediate headache relief; there may be a delay of one-half to 1 year or no improvement.[16,55,251]

Studies from neurologic or migraine clinics show increased incidence and severity of migraine in users of the older OCs (Table 11.7).

Table 11.7 Oral Contraceptives and Headaches: Neurologic and Migraine Clinics

Study	Year	Country	Type	Number Studied	Effect of Contraceptive
Whitty et al.[252]	1966	United Kingdom	Retrospective	50	Decreased attack frequency in many women. Remaining migraine attacks increased in severity in days off OC.
Phillips[250]	1968	United Kingdom	Retrospective	41	21 patients reported new migraine on OC. 78% of migraine patients had increased severity and frequency of headache on OC.
Carroll[254]	1971	United Kingdom	Retrospective	290	Increased frequency or intensity of migraine in 49%.
Kudrow[13]	1975	United States	Retrospective	60	Increased migraine frequency in OC users versus non-users. Stopping OC decreased migraine frequency in 70% of patients.
Dalton[251]	1976	United Kingdom	Retrospective	886	Increased migraine frequency in 34% of OC users and 60% of exOC users. New migraine in 5%. Stopping OC decreased migraine in 39% of exOC users.
Ryan[249]	1978	United States	Prospective, 4 months	40	40 migraine patients treated with OC: 12 better, 28 worse.

OC = oral contraceptives

[250,251,254] While headaches frequently occur on the days off the OC, Whitty[252] found that many women had relief with certain OCs, and Ryan[249] found that 12 of 40 of his patients improved. Studies from contraceptive clinics and general practitioners (Table 11.8) are more favorable toward the older OCs. Larrson-Cohen and Lundberg,[253] Diddle,[255] Ramchurian,[256] Kappius,[100] and others[257–259] reported either improvement or no worsening of migraine in OC users. The headaches that occurred appeared to cluster around the menses. Aznar-Ramos gave placebo to 147 women who believed they were getting an OC and found a headache incidence of 15.6% of the months.[260] A study from the Philippines of 1800 women using three different low-dose estrogen OCs reported headache incidence between 5.2% and 8.0%, significantly below that reported with placebo.[261] Five double-blind, placebo-controlled studies showed no difference in headache incidence between OC and placebo. [262–266] Both groups had decreasing headache incidence with continued observation. Some uncontrolled studies show an increase in headache frequency in women on OCs. [267–270] A third-generation OC containing 35 mg of the new third-generation progestin, Norgestimate (Ortho-Cyclen), was associated with a low incidence of headaches over three cycle intervals (5% after the third cycle, 3% after the sixth cycle) in an open prospective study.[160] A review of studies for the new COC containing 150 mg of desogestrel and 30 mg of ethinyl estradiol found headache to be low (approximately 5% at the sixth cycle).[271]

An OC containing 150 μg desogestrel and 20 μg ethinyl estradiol (Mircette®), given for 21 days, and then 10 μg ethinyl estradiol for five days, was evaluated in a large, open-label, 18-month, multicenter trial. The most common drug-related AEs included headache (8.5%), breast pain (7.3%), dysmenorrhea (4.2%), and menstrual disorder (4.2%). There were no reports of venous thromboembolic events or significant changes in blood pressure, lipid metabolism, or serum glucose level.[272]

Archer et al. evaluated the efficacy and safety of a low-dose 21-day COC containing 100 μg levonorgestrel and 20 μg ethinyl estradiol.[273] The two most common AEs cited as reasons for discontinuation were headache (2% of subjects) and metrorrhagia (2% of subjects).

The incidence of general symptoms seen in this study (headache, sinusitis, flulike symptoms, and abdominal pain) approximated those seen in the population of women who do not use OCs.

Coney et al. pooled data from two placebo-controlled, randomized trials in a general contraceptive-seeking population. They assessed weight change and other AEs that were attributable to an OC that contained 20 mg of ethinyl estradiol and 100 mg of levonorgestrel in 684 women. Subjects kept daily diary cards. Over the course of this 6-month study, 31% of the women in the OC group and 32% of the women in the placebo group reported headache as an AE, a difference that was not statistically significant. In this study, headache incidence was similar between groups.[266]

Aegidius et al.[274] examined the prevalence of headache and migraine among women using OCs in a large, cross-sectional, population-based study in Norway. Among 14,353 premenopausal women, 13,944 (97%) responded to questions regarding contraceptive use. A significant association existed between headache and reported use of estrogen-containing OCs in premenopausal women, both for migraine (OR 1.4, 95% CI [1.2–1.7]) and for non-migrainous headache (OR 1.2, 95% CI [1.0–1.4]). A significant dose relationship between headache and the amount of estrogen in the OCs could not be demonstrated. A significant association between headache and OCs containing only gestagen was not found. In this study, headache, especially migraine, was more likely among premenopausal women using oral contraceptives containing estrogen.

Headaches occur during the pill-free interval and may resolve with the use of daily, continuous COCs (long-cycle treatment). [154,155] Some newer COCs add back estrogen during the placebo week (10 μg of ethinyl estradiol for 5 of 7 days). A new formulation (Seasonale) is packaged with an 84-day dosing regimen that results in only four menses per year. Phasic OCs cannot be used continuously because the variation in steroid levels may cause breakthrough bleeding.[103] In two noncomparative multicenter clinical trials, 13% and 9.9% of women, respectively, reported headache prior to use of either norgestimate/ EE or desogestrel/EE.[275,276] Headache incidence declined as the women continued to take the OCs; at cycle three, 9.9% and 6.9% of

Table 11.8 Oral Contraceptives and Headaches: Contraceptive Clinics and General Practitioners

Study	Year	Country	Type	Number Studied	Effects of Contraceptive
Nilsson et al.[268]	1967	Sweden	R	281	Increased headache symptoms, 20.2% of OC users. Decreased headache symptoms, 14.7% of OC users.
Nilsson & Solwell[262]	1967	Sweden	P; 12 mo; DB CO	159	Headache incidence: 50% during treatment with placebo and OC.
Grant[269]	1968	United Kingdom	P; 12 mo	532	Headache incidence: 17% pretreatment; 295 on OC.
Aznar-Ramos et al.[260]	1969	Mexico	P; 12 mo; placebo only	147	Headache incidence: 15.6% on placebo.
Cullberg et al.[267]	1969	Sweden	P; 6 mo	99	New headache in 2% of OC users.
Diddle et al.[255]	1969	United States	P	10,889	Headache incidence: 8% of controls; 3.2% of OC users. New headaches in 0.8% of OC users.
Herzberg & Coppers[257]	1970	United Kingdom	P; 11mo; IUD controls	163	Headache incidence (moderate to severe): 5 wk—4% on OC, 0% on IUD; 11 mo—2% on OC, 0% on IUD.
Larsson-Cohn & Lundberg[253]	1970	Sweden	P; 12 mo	1676	New migraine in 10% of OC users. Migraine patients: 36% improved, 18% worsened on OCs.
Herzberg et al.[258]	1971	United Kingdom	P; 12 mo; IUD controls	272	Headache incidence: 5 mo, OC = IUD; 10 mo, OC>IUD.
Goldzieher et al.[263]	1971	United States	P; 6 mo; DB placebo CO	398	Headache incidence decreased 68% with both placebo and OC.
Silbergeld et al.[264]	1971	United States	P; 4 mo; DB placebo CO	8	No increase in headache with OC.
Cullberg[265]	1972	Sweden	P; 2 mo; DB placebo CO	332	No difference in headache frequency between OC and placebo.
Desrosiers[270]	1973	Canada	P	125	Headache incidence: 27.4% pretreatment; 36.8% on OC.
Royal College of General Prac-titioners[259]	1974	United Kingdom	P; 48 mo	46,000	No evidence that headache is a pharmacologic side effect of OC use.
Ramchurian et al.[256]	1980	United States	P; 96 mo	16,638	No evidence of increased frequency of migraine or tension headache in OC users.
Kappius & Goolkasian[100]	1987	United States	P; 2 mo	78	Headache on OCs less severe, less frequent, clustered around menses.
Ramos et al.[261]	1989	Philippine Island	P; 12 mo	1800	Headache incidence on OC: 0–3 mo, 6%; 10–12 mo, 2%; 2.7% stopped OC because of headache.
Coney et al.[266]	2001	United States	P; SB; PC; 6 mo	684	No increase in headache with OC.

R = retrospective; P = prospective; OC = oral contraceptive; DB = double blind; SB = Single blind; CO = crossover; IUD = intrauterine device; PC = Placebo controlled[292–294] the women, respectively, reported headache. Many of these women inappropriately attributed their headaches to OC use. It is important to counsel patients during cycle three about the probability of their headaches diminishing, because by cycle six, 6.2% and 2.8%, respectively, reported headache. OC use did not influence tension-type headache, frequency, or intensity.[277] Wimberly et al. assessed 218 women to determine whether expectations about AEs were associated with having them. [278] Twenty-five subjects (15%) anticipated having more headaches before taking OCs; 32 women (19%) reported more headaches at 3 months, a correlation no greater than that expected by chance alone. Most participants had previously used OCs.

Loder et al. conducted a two-part systematic review of published studies to examine the evidence that combination oral contraceptives can aggravate or cause headache.[279] They concluded that there is little indication that OCs have a clinically important effect on headache activity. Headache that occurs during early cycles of OC use tends to improve or disappear with continued use. No evidence supports the common clinical practice of switching OCs to treat headache; however, manipulating the extent or duration of estrogen withdrawal may provide benefit.

Contraception with progestins alone is a hormonal alternative to the use of the COC, but the progestin-only contraceptives are associated with a higher incidence of headache. [280,281] They are the contraceptive of choice for hypertensive women.[153] Progestins decrease endogenous estradiol production and were initially believed to be free of increased thromboembolic risk.[197] Some studies suggest that atherogenesis can be enhanced by progestogen in a hypoestrogenic animal. Some progestins may also alter endothelium function and reduce estrogen's physiologic vasodilating effects on the brain, the muscle vasculature, and the coronary arteries.[282] The risk for aneurysmal bleeding and hemorrhagic stroke may be increased in norgestrel users.[194] Progestin-only OCs are also associated with an increased risk of diabetes.[283] Suppressing ovarian estradiol secretion may induce early menopause-like consequences, such as osteoporosis,[284] reduced quality of life, impaired vaginal secretions, dyspareunia, and increased risk of sexually transmitted diseases.[285,286]

Women need to be told that hormonal contraception may generate new headaches or aggravate or even ameliorate pre-existing headaches. This variability is also noted with pregnancy and menopause and may be a consequence of a variation in intrinsic estrogen or progestin neuronal response. The risks and benefits of the different types of contraception, including hormonal contraception, should be discussed with the patient. Women who are given OCs must be followed for headache aggravation or neurologic symptoms. Women should not use OCs if they smoke or have uncontrolled hypertension or other cardiovascular disease, such as thromboembolism, thrombophlebitis, stroke, vasculitis, or diabetes with retinopathy or nephropathy. Progestins can be used for contraception when estrogens have caused increased headaches or are contraindicated.

Migraine itself may be a risk factor for stroke in women under the age of 45. Migraine with aura may be associated with double the risk compared with migraine without aura. The risk for stroke is higher in women over the age of 35, and these women should use OCs with caution, particularly when other risk factors are present. OC use is relatively safe for women under the age of 35 who have migraine without aura. Women with intractable menstrual migraine or a history of headache relief with OCs are particularly good candidates for a trial of OC. OCs are probably safe for women under the age of 35 who have migraine with typical aura, but they should be used with caution. It is an unproven belief that women with prolonged aura or hemiplegic, basilar, or confusional migraine should not use OCs. Patients should be started on a formulation that contains less than 50 µg of ethinyl estradiol (unless cytochrome P450 system inducing drugs are being used), and formulations with the lowest androgenic potency of progestin should be used. Progestin-only formulations have a lower incidence of adverse metabolic effects than do the combination formulations. The incidence of thromboembolism in women ingesting the new progestin is probably increased, but blood pressure is not affected, nausea and breast tenderness are eliminated, and milk production and quality are unchanged. Women who want to continue OC but whose headaches increase when they start on a COC should consider switching to a lower estrogen dose preparation

Table 11.9 **Medical Eligibility Criteria for Contraceptive Use of Combined Hormonal Contraceptives (Based on US, WHO, and UK MEC)[114–116]**

Condition	Subcondition		CHC UK MEC	CHC US MEC & WHO MEC
Age	Menarche to menopause		✓	✓
DVT/PE	Personal current or past history		✗	✗
	Family history (first-degree relatives)	Age < 45	✗	✓
		Age ≥ 45	✓	✓
Diabetes	Nonvascular disease		✓	✓
	Nephropathy/retinopathy/ neuropathy		✗	✗
	Other vascular disease or diabetes of > 20 years' duration			
Headaches	Non-migraine		✓	✓
	Migraine	Without aura, age < 35	✓	✓/✗
		Without aura, age ≥ 35	✓	✗
		With aura, any age	✗	✗
Hypertension	Systolic 140–159 or diastolic 90–99		✗	✗
	Systolic ≥ 160 or diastolic ≥ 100		✗	✗
	Vascular disease		✗	✗
	Adequately controlled hypertension		✗	✗
Ischemic heart disease	Current and past history		✗	✗
Multiple risk factors for arterial CVD	Such as older age, smoking, diabetes, and hypertension		✗	✗
Obesity	BMI	≥ 30–34 kg/m2	✓	✓
		≥ 35 kg/m2	✗	✓
Smoking	Age < 35, any smoking		✓	✓
	Age ≥ 35	< 15 cigarettes/day	✗	✗
		≥ 15 cigarettes/day	✗	✗
Stroke			✗	✗
Thrombogenic mutations			✗	✗

✓ = MEC 1 or 2; ✗ = MEC 3 or 4; ✓/✗ = MEC 2 for initiation/MEC 3 for continuation.
MEC 1: no restriction for use of the method.
MEC 2: advantages generally outweigh theoretical or proven risks.
MEC 3: theoretical or proven risks usually outweigh the advantages.
MEC 4: unacceptable health risk.
CHC = combined pill, patch, ring; CVD = cardiovascular disease; DVT = deep venous thrombosis; MEC= Medical Eligibility Criteria; PE = pulmonary embolism; WHO = World Health Organization.

with a different progestin in the absence of neurologic symptoms.

The World Health Organization (WHO) group determined that women with non-migrainous headaches can use COCs (WHO Category 1), women who have migraine without aura and are less than 35 years of age can generally use COCs (WHO Category 2), women who have migraine without aura and are 35 years or older generally should not use COCs (WHO Category 3), and women who have migraine with aura, at any age, should not use COCs (WHO Category 4).[287] WHO recommended that women who experience new headaches or a marked change in existing headaches while using COCs should be evaluated. If a woman develops non-migrainous headaches while taking COCs, she can generally continue COC use (WHO Category 2); if a woman develops migraine without aura while she is taking COCs and is less than 35 years of age, she should generally not continue to use COCs (WHO Category 3); and if she develops migraine without aura at 35 years of age or older, or if she develops migraine with aura at any age while taking COCs, she should not continue to use COCs (WHO Category 4).

The International Headache Society Task Force concluded that OCs are not contraindicated if migraineurs do not have migraine aura or other risk factors.[288] It can be difficult to apply these guidelines to individual patients. Clinical judgment is needed to weigh the risks and benefits of hormonal contraception for a particular woman.[289] In contrast to the WHO, the International Headache Society Task Force believes that migraine with aura is not an absolute contraindication to the use of OCs. Women should be counseled and regularly assessed for additional risk factors. There is a potentially increased risk of ischemic stroke in migraineurs who are using COCs and have additional risk factors. Risk factors should be identified and evaluated: migraine type, particularly migraine with aura, should be diagnosed; women who have migraine and are smokers should stop smoking before starting COCs; other risk factors, such as hypertension and hyperlipidemia, should be treated; and nonethinylestradiol methods should be considered for women who are at increased risk of ischemic stroke, particularly if they have multiple risk factors. Non-hormonal or progestin-only contraception have no adverse effects on the risk of ischemic stroke and can be used without restriction by women with migraine with or without aura.[152] Progestin-only hormonal contraception, while safer, may aggravate headache.[290,291]

No specific tests need to be undertaken other than those that are routinely performed or are indicated by the patient's history or the presence of specific symptoms, for example, a patient with a relative who experienced arterial disease at or before age 45. Migraine-related symptoms that may necessitate further evaluation and/or cessation of COCs include a new persisting headache, new onset of migraine aura, increased headache frequency or intensity, or the development of unusual aura symptoms, particularly prolonged aura.

REFERENCES

1. Goldstein M, Chen TC. The epidemiology of disabling headache. In: Critchley M, editor. *Advances in Neurology*, Volume 33. New York: Raven Press, 1982:377–90
2. Waters WE, O'Connor PJ. Epidemiology of headache and migraine in women. *J Neurol Neurosurg Psychiatry*. 1971;34:148–153.
3. Lipton RB, Stewart WF, Diamond S, Diamond ML, Reed M. Prevalence and burden of migraine in the United States: data from the American Migraine Study II. *Headache*. 2001;41:646–657.
4. Pringsheim T, Gooren L. Migraine prevalence in male to female transsexuals on hormone therapy. *Neurology*. 2004;63:593–594.
5. Selby G, Lance JW. Observation on 500 cases of migraine and allied vascular headaches. *J Neurol Neurosurg Psychiatry*. 1960;23:23–32.
6. Epstein MT, Hockaday JM, Hockaday TDR. Migraine and reproductive hormones throughout the menstrual cycle. *Lancet*. 1975;1:543–548.
7. Silberstein SD, Merriam GR. Estrogens, progestins, and headache. *Neurology*. 1991;41:775–793.
8. American Psychiatric Association. *Diagnostic and statistical manual of mental disorders*. 4th ed. Washington, DC: American Psychiatric Association, 1994.
9. Mortola JF. Premenstrual syndrome: pathophysiologic considerations. *N Engl J Med*. 1998;338:256–257.
10. Lance JW, Anthony M. Some clinical aspects of migraine: a prospective survey of 500 patients. *Arch Neurol*. 1966;15:356–361.
11. Ratinahirana H, Darbois Y, Bousser MG. Migraine and pregnancy: a prospective study in 703 women after delivery. *Neurology*. 1990;40:437.
12. Somerville BW. A study of migraine in pregnancy. *Neurology*. 1972;22:824–828.
13. Kudrow L. The relationship of headache frequency to hormone use in migraine. *Headache*. 1975;15:36–49.
14. Bickerstaff ER. *Neurological complications of oral contraceptives*. Oxford: Clarendon Press, 1975.
15. Neri I, Granella F, Nappi RM, Facchinetti F, Genazzani AR. Characteristics of headache at menopause: a clinico-epidemiologic study. *Maturitas*. 1993;17:31–37.
16. Whitty CWM, Hockaday JM. Migraine: a followup study of 92 patients. *Br Med J*. 1968;1:735–736.
17. Welch KMA, Darnley D, Simkins RT. The role of estrogen in migraine: a review. *Cephalalgia*. 1984;4:227–236.
18. Lundberg PO. Endocrine headaches. In: Rose FC, ed. *Handbook of clinical neurology*, Volume 48. New York: Elsevier, 1986:431–440.
19. Johannes CB, Linet MS, Stewart WF, Celentano DD, Lipton RB, Szklo M. Relationship of headache to phase of the menstrual cycle among young women: a daily diary study. *Neurology*. 1995;45:1076–1082.
20. Solbach P, Sargent J, Coyne L. Menstrual migraine headache: results of a controlled, experimental,

20. outcome study of nondrug treatments. *Headache*. 1984;24:75–78.

21. MacGregor EA, Chia H, Vohrah RC, Wilkinson M. Migraine and menstruation: a pilot study. *Cephalalgia*. 1990;10:305–310.

22. MacGregor EA, Igarashi H, Wilkinson M. Headaches and hormones: subjective versus objective assessment. *Headache Quarterly*. 1997;8:126–136.

23. Stewart WF, Lipton RB, Chee E, Sawyer J, Silberstein SD. Menstrual cycle and headache in a population sample of migraineurs. *Neurology*. 2000;55:1517–1523.

24. MacGregor EA, Hackshaw A. Prevalence of migraine on each day of the natural menstrual cycle. *Neurology*. 2004;63:351–353.

25. Granella F, Sances G, Allais G, et al. Characteristics of menstrual and nonmenstrual attacks in women with menstrually related migraine referred to headache centres. *Cephalalgia*. 2004;24:707–716.

26. Couturier EG, Bomhof MA, Neven AK, van Duijn NP. Menstrual migraine in a representative Dutch population sample: prevalence, disability and treatment. *Cephalalgia*. 2003;23:302–308.

27. Dzoljic E, Sipetic S, Vlajinac H, et al. Prevalence of menstrually related migraine and nonmigraine primary headache in female students of Belgrade University. *Headache*. 2002;42:185–193.

28. Dowson AJ, Kilminster SG, Salt R, Clark M, Bundy MJ. Disability associated with headaches occurring inside and outside the menstrual period in those with migraine: a general practice study. *Headache*. 2005;45:274–282.

29. Mattsson P. Hormonal factors in migraine: a population-based study of women aged 40 to 74 years. *Headache*. 2003;43:27–35.

30. MacGregor EA, Victor TW, Hu X, et al. Characteristics of menstrual vs nonmenstrual migraine: a post hoc, within-woman analysis of the usual-care phase of a nonrandomized menstrual migraine clinical trial. *Headache*. 2010;50:528–538.

31. Buse DC, Loder EW, Gorman JA, et al. Sex differences in the prevalence, symptoms, and associated features of migraine, probable migraine and other severe headache: results of the American Migraine Prevalence and Prevention (AMPP) Study. *Headache*. 2013;

32. Headache Classification Committee. The International Classification of Headache Disorders, 2nd Edition. *Cephalalgia*. 2004;24:1–160.

33. MacGregor EA. Oestrogen and attacks of migraine with and without aura. *Lancet Neurol*. 2004;3:354–361.

34. Silberstein SD, Lipton RB. Chronic daily headache. In: Goadsby PJ, Silberstein SD, eds. *Headache*. Newton: Butterworth-Heinemann, 1997:201–225.

35. Silberstein SD, Armellino JJ, Hoffman HD, et al. Treatment of menstruation-associated migraine with the nonprescription combination of acetaminophen, aspirin, and caffeine: results from three randomized, placebo-controlled studies. *Clin Therapeutics*. 1999;21:475–491.

36. Sargent J, Solbach P, Damasio H. A comparison of naproxen sodium to propranolol hydrochloride and a placebo control for the prophylaxis of migraine headache. *Headache*. 1985;25:320–324.

37. Robinson K, Huntington KM, Wallace MG. Treatment of the premenstrual syndrome. *Br J Obstet Gynecol*. 1977;84:784–788.

38. D'Alessandro R, Gamberini G, Lozito A, Sacquegna T. Menstrual migraine, intermittent prophylaxis with a timed-release pharmacological formulation of dihydroergotamine. *Cephalalgia*. 1983;3:156–158.

39. Silberstein SD, Schulman EA, Hopkins MM. Repetitive intravenous DHE in the treatment of refractory headache. *Headache*. 1990;30:334–349.

40. Winner P, Sheftell F, Sadowsky C, Dalessio D. A profile of menstrual migraine sufferers. *Cephalalgia*. 1993;13:242.

41. Solbach MP, Waymer RS. Treatment of menstruation-associated migraine headache with subcutaneous sumatriptan. *Obstet Gynecol*. 1993;82:769–772.

42. Sheftel F, Silberstein SD, Rapoport A. Pharmacological treatment of chronic headache. *Drug Therapy*. 1992;22:47–59.

43. Facchinetti F, Bonellie G, Kangasniemi P, Pascual J, Shuaib A. The efficacy and safety of subcutaneous sumatriptan in the acute treatment of menstrual migraine. The Sumatriptan Menstrual Migraine Study Group. *Obstet Gynecol*. 1995;86:911–916.

44. Silberstein SD, Watson C, O'Quinn S. Sumatriptan tablets and injection are effective in the treatment of menstrually associated migraine: a review. *Neurology*. 1998;50:406.

45. Loder E, Silberstein SD. Clinical efficacy of 2.5 and 5mg Zolmitriptan (Zomig™) in migraine associated with menses or in patients using nonprogestogen oral contraceptives. *Neurology*. 1998;50:341.

46. Loder E, Silberstein SD, bu-Shakra S, Mueller L, Smith T. Efficacy and tolerability of oral zolmitriptan in menstrually associated migraine: a randomized, prospective, parallel-group, double-blind, placebo-controlled study. *Headache*. 2004;44:120–130.

47. Tuchman M, Hee A, Emeribe U, Silberstein SD. Oral zolmitriptan demonstrates high efficacy and good tolerability in the acute treatment of menstrual migraine. *CNS Drugs*. 2006;20:1019–1026.

48. Silberstein SD, Massiou H, leJeunne C, Pratt LJ, McCarroll KA, Lines CR. Rizatriptan in the treatment of menstrual migraine. *Ob Gyn*. 2000;96:237–242.

49. Silberstein SD, Massiou H, McCarroll KA, Lines CR. Further evaluation of rizatriptan in menstrual migraine: retrospective analysis of long-term data. *Headache*. 2002;42:917–923.

50. MacGregor EA, Keywood C. Frovatriptan is effective in menstrually associated migraine. Poster presented at Headache World 2000, London, 2000.

51. Hettiarachichi J, Pitei D. Oral eletriptan is effective in treating menstrually associated migraine and migraine in women on oral contraceptives or hormone replacement. *Headache*. 2000;40:411(Abstract).

52. Allais G, Acuto G, Cabarrocas X, Esbri R, Benedetto C, Bussone G. Efficacy and tolerability of almotriptan versus zolmitriptan for the acute treatment of menstrual migraine. *Neurol Sci*. 2006;27(Suppl 2):S193–S197.

53. Bigal M, Sheftell F, Tepper S, Tepper D, Ho TW, Rapoport A. A randomized double-blind study comparing rizatriptan, dexamethasone, and the combination of both in the acute treatment of menstrually related migraine. *Headache*. 2008;48:1286–1293.

54. Silberstein SD, Saper JR. Migraine: Diagnosis and treatment. In: Dalessio DJ, Silberstein SD, eds. *Wolff's headache and other head pain*. 6th ed. New York: Oxford University Press, 1993:96–170.

55. Raskin NH. *Headache.* 2nd ed. New York: Churchill-Livingstone, 1988.
56. MacGregor EA, Frith A, Ellis J, Aspinall L. Predicting menstrual migraine with a home-use fertility monitor. *Neurology.* 2005;64:561–563.
57. Sances G, Martignoni E, Fioroni L, Blandini F, Facchinetti F, Nappi G. Naproxen sodium in menstrual migraine prophylaxis: a double-blind placebo controlled study. *Headache.* 1990;30:705–709.
58. Edelson RN. Menstrual migraine and other hormonal aspects of migraine. *Headache.* 1985;25:376–379.
59. Silberstein SD. Treatment of headache in primary care practice. *Am J Med.* 1984;77:65–72.
60. Silberstein SD. DHE-45 in the prophylaxis of menstrually related migraine. *Cephalalgia.* 1996;16:371.
61. Newman LC, Lipton RB, Lay CL, Solomon S. A pilot study of oral sumatriptan as intermittent prophylaxis of menstruation-related migraine. *Neurology.* 1998;51:307–309.
62. Newman LC, Mannix LK, Landy SH, et al. Naratriptan as short-term prophylaxis for menstrually associated migraine: a randomized, double-blind, placebo-controlled study. *Headache.* 2000;41:248–256.
63. Mannix LK. Naratriptan Studies II, III, and Extension on the tolerability of naratriptan for prophylaxis. Presented at Headache Update: Managing the Difficult Patient. Orlando, FL, 2003.
64. Tuchman M, Hee A, Emeribe U. Oral zolmitriptan 2.5 mg demonstrates high efficacy and good tolerability in the prophylactic treatment of menstrual migraine headaches. *Headache.* 2005;45:771(Abstract).
65. Silberstein SD, Elkind AH, Schreiber C, Keywood C. Randomized trial of frovatriptan for the intermittent prevention of menstrual migraine. *Neurology.* 2004;63:261–269.
66. Brandes JL, Poole A, Kallela M, et al. Short-term frovatriptan for the prevention of difficult-to-treat menstrual migraine attacks. *Cephalalgia.* 2009;29:1133–1148.
67. MacGregor EA, Brandes JL, Silberstein S, et al. Safety and tolerability of short-term preventive frovatriptan: a combined analysis. *Headache.* 2009;49:1298–1314.
68. Hu Y, Guan X, Fan L, Jin L. Triptans in prevention of menstrual migraine: a systematic review with meta-analysis. *J Headache Pain.* 2013;14:7.
69. Facchinetti F, Montorsi S, Borella P, et al. Magnesium prevention of premenstrual migraine: a placebo controlled study. In: Rose FC, ed. *New advances in headache research.* 2nd ed. London: Smith-Gordon, 1991: .
70. Facchinetti F, Borella P, Sances G, Fioroni L, Nappi G, Genazzani A. Oral magnesium successfully relieves premenstrual mood changes. *Obstet Gynecol.* 1991;78:177.
71. Vellacott ID, O'Brien PM. Effect of spironolactone on premenstrual syndrome symptoms. *J Reprod Med.* 1987;32:429–434.
72. Wang M, Hammarback S, Lindhe BA, Backstrom T. Treatment of premenstrual syndrome by spironolactone: a double-blind, placebo-controlled study. *Acta Obstet Gynecol Scand.* 1995;74:803–808.
73. Reid RL, Yen SSC. Premenstrual syndrome. *Am J Obstet Gynecol.* 1981;139:85–104.
74. Williams MJ, Harris RI, Dean BC. Controlled trial of pyridoxine in the premenstrual syndrome. *J Int Med Res.* 1985;1:174–179.
75. Hagen I, Nesheim B, Tuntland t. No effect of vitamin B-6 against premenstrual tension: a controlled clinical study. *Acta Obstet Gynecol Scand.* 1985;64:667–670.
76. Schaumburg H, Kaplan J, Windebank A, et al. Sensory neuropathy from pyridoxine abuse. *N Eng J Med.* 1983;309:445–458.
77. Burke BE, Olson RD, Cusack BJ. Randomized, controlled trial of phytoestrogen in the prophylactic treatment of menstrual migraine. *Biomed Pharmacother.* 2002;56:283–288.
78. Ferrante F, Fusco E, Calabresi P, Cupini LM. Phytoestrogens in the prophylaxis of menstrual migraine. *Clin Neuropharmacol.* 2004;27:137–140.
79. DeLigniŠresB, Vincens M, Mauvais-Jarvis P, Mas JL, Touboul PJ, Bousser MG. Prevention of menstrual migraine by percutaneous estradiol. *Br Med J.* 1986;293:1540.
80. Magos AL, Brincat M, Studd JWW. Treatment of the premenstrual syndrome by subcutaneous estradiol implants and cyclical oral noresthisterone: placebo controlled study. *Br Med J Clin Res.* 1986;292:1629–1633.
81. Calton GJ, Burnett JW. Danazol and migraine. *N Eng J Med.* 1984;310:721–722.
82. Thomas EJ, Okuda KJ, Thomas NM. The combination of depot gonadotropin releasing hormone agonist and cyclical hormone replacement therapy for dysfunctional uterine bleeding. *Br J Obstet Gynecol.* 1991;98:1155–1159.
83. Freeman E, Rickels K, Sondheimer SJ, Polansky M. Ineffectiveness of progesterone suppository treatment for premenstrual syndrome. *JAMA.* 1990;264:349–353.
84. Dalton K. Progesterone suppositories and pessaries in the treatment of menstrual migraine. *Headache.* 1973;13:151–159.
85. Bancroft J, Backstrom T. Premenstrual syndrome. *Clin Endocrinol.* 1985;22:313–136.
86. Somerville BW. Estrogen-withdrawal migraine. I. Duration of exposure required and attempted prophylaxis by premenstrual estrogen administration. *Neurology.* 1975;25:239–244.
87. Moskowitz MA. The neurobiology of vascular head pain. *Ann Neurol.* 1984;16:157–168.
88. Dennerstein L, Morse C, Burrows G, Oats J, Brown J, Smith M. Menstrual migraine: a double-blind trial of percutaneous estradiol. *Gynecol Endocrinol.* 1988;2:113–120.
89. Magos AL, Zilkha KJ. Treatment of menstrual migraine by estradiol implants. *Gynecol Endocrinol.* 1988;2:113–120.
90. Anonymous. Transdermal estrogen. *Med Lett Drugs Therap.* 1986;28:119–120.
91. Judd H. Efficacy of transdermal estradiol. *Obstet Gynecol.* 1987;156:1326–1331.
92. Stumpf PG. Pharmacokinetics of estrogen. *Obstet Gynecol.* 1990;75:9–17.
93. Schwartz J, Freeman R, Frishman W. Clinical pharmacology of estrogens: cardiovascular actions and cardioprotective benefits of replacement therapy in postmenopausal women. *J Clin Pharmacol.* 1995;35:1–16.
94. Pradalier A, Vincent D, Beaulieu PH, Baudesson G, Launay JM. Correlation between estradiol plasma level and therapeutic effect on menstrual migraine. In: Rose FC, ed. *New advances in headache research.* 4th ed. London: Smith-Gordon, 1994:129–132.
95. Dennerstein L, Laby B, Burrows GD, Hyman GJ. Headache and sex hormone therapy. *Headache.* 1978;18:146–153.

96. Pfaffenrath V. Efficacy and safety of percutaneous estradiol vs. placebo in menstrual migraine. *Cephalalgia*. 1993;13:168(Abstract).

97. Smits MG, VanderMeer YG, Pfeil JP, Rijnierse JJ, Vos AJ. Perimenstrual migraine: effect of estraderm TTS and the value of contingent negative variation and exteroceptive temporalis muscle suppression test. *Headache*. 1993;34:103–106.

98. Watson NR, Studd JW, Savvas M, Garnett T, Baber RJ. Treatment of severe premenstrual syndrome with estradiol patches and cyclical oral norethisterone. *Lancet*. 1989;2:730–732.

99. Guidotti M, Mauri M, Barrila C, Guidotti F, Belloni C. Frovatriptan vs. transdermal oestrogens or naproxen sodium for the prophylaxis of menstrual migraine. *J Headache Pain*. 2007;8:283–288.

100. Kappius REK, Goolkasian P. Group and menstrual phase effect in reported headaches among college students. *Headache*. 1987;27:491–494.

101. Sulak PJ, Cressman BE, Waldrop E, Holleman S, Kuehl TJ. Extending the duration of active oral contraceptive pills to manage hormone withdrawal symptoms. *Obstet Gynecol*. 1997;89:179–183.

102. Edelman A, Gallo MF, Nichols MD, Jensen JT, Schulz KF, Grimes DA. Continuous versus cyclic use of combined oral contraceptives for contraception: systematic Cochrane review of randomized controlled trials. *Hum Reprod*. 2006;21:573–578.

103. Cachrimanidou AC, Hellberg D, Nilsson S. Long-interval treatment regimen with a desogestrel-containing oral contraceptive. *Contraception*. 1993;48:205–216.

104. Miller L, Notter KM. Menstrual reduction with extended use of combination oral contraceptive pills: randomized controlled trial. *Obstet Gynecol*. 2001;98:771–778.

105. Anderson FD, Hait H. A multicenter, randomized study of an extended cycle oral contraceptive. *Contraception*. 2003;68:89–96.

106. Kwiecien M, Edelman A, Nichols MD, Jensen JT. Bleeding patterns and patient acceptability of standard or continuous dosing regimens of a low-dose oral contraceptive: a randomized trial. *Contraception*. 2003;67:9–13.

107. Sarno AP, Miller EJ, Lundblad EG. Premenstrual syndrome: beneficial effects of periodic, low-dose danazol. *Obstet Gynecol*. 1987;70:33–36.

108. O'Dea PK, Davis EH. Tamoxifen in the treatment of menstrual migraine. *Neurology*. 1990;40:1471.

109. Powles TJ. Prevention of migrainous headaches by tamoxifen. *Lancet*. 1986;2:1344.

110. Delmas PD, Bjarnason NH, Mitlak BH, et al. Effects of raloxifene on bone mineral density, serum cholesterol concentrations, and uterine endometrium in postmenopausal women. *N Engl J Med*. 1997;337:16411647.

111. Conn PM, Crowley WF. Gonadotropin-releasing hormone and its analogues. *N Eng J Med*. 1991;324:93–103.

112. Muse KN, Cetel NS, Fitterman LA, Yen SC. The premenstrual syndrome: effects of "medical ovariectomy." *N Eng J Med*. 1984;311:1345–1349.

113. Hammarback S, Backstrom T. Induced anovulation as a treatment of premenstrual tension syndrome: a double-blind cross-over study with GnRH-agonist

114. Matsuo H, Baba Y, Nair RM, Arimura A, Schally AV. Structure of porcine LH and FSH releasing hormone 1. The proposed amino acid sequence. *Biochem Biophys Res Commun*. 1971;43:1334–1349.

115. Burgus R, Butcher M, Amoss M. Primary structure of the ovine hypothalamic luteinizing hormone-releasing hormone factor (LHRF). *Proc Natl Acad Sci USA*. 1972;69:278–282.

116. Perrin MH, River JE, Vale WW. Radiologand assay for gonadotropin-releasing hormone: relative potencies of agonists and antagonists. *Endocrinology*. 1980;106:1289–1296.

117. Loumaye E, Naor Z, Catt KJ. Binding affinity and biological activity of gonadotropin-releasing hormone agonists in isolated pituitary cells. *Endocrinology*. 1982;111:730–736.

118. Swift AD, Crighton DB. Relative activity, plasma elimination and tissue degradation of synthetic luteinizing hormone releasing hormone and certain of its analogues. *J Endocrinol*. 1979;80:141–152.

119. Vaughan-Williams CA, McNeilly AS, Baird DT. Comparison of single and repeated applications of long-acting synthetic analogue of LHRGH[D-Ser(TBU)⁶EA¹⁰LHRH] in the assessment of pituitary gonadotropin secretory capacity. *Clin Endocrinol*. 1980;13:51–56.

120. Filicori M, Flamigni C. GnRH agonists and antagonists: current clinical status. *Drugs*. 1988;35:63–82.

121. Shaw RW. The role of GnRH analogues in the treatment of endometriosis. *Br J Obstet Gynecol*. 1988;99:9–12.

122. Pickersgill A. GnRH agonists and add-back therapy: is there a perfect combination? *Br J Obstet Gynecol*. 1998;105:475–485.

123. Lemay A, Faure N. Sequential estrogen-progestin addition to gonadotropin-releasing hormone agonist suppression for the chronic treatment of ovarian hyperandrogenism: a pilot study. *J Clin Endocrinol Metab*. 1994;79:1716–1722.

124. Howell R, Crook D, Edmonds DK, Lees B, Dowsett M, Stevenson J. Gondotrophin-releasing hormone analogue (goserelin) plus hormone replacement therapy for the treatment of endometriosis: a randomized control trial. *Fertil Steril*. 1995;64:474–481.

125. Surrey ES, Voigt B, Fournet N, Judd HL. Prolonged gonadotropin-releasing hormone agonist treatment of symptomatic endometriosis: the role of cyclic sodium etidronate and low-dose norethindrone add-back therapy. *Fertil Steril*. 1995;63:747–755.

126. Maheux R, Lemay A. Treatment of perimenopausal women: potential long-term therapy with a depot GnRH agonist combined with hormone replacement therapy. *Br J Obstet Gynecol*. 1992;99:13–17.

127. Simberg N, Titinen A, Silfvast A, Viinikka L, Ylikorkala O. High bone density in hyperandrogenic women: effect of gonadotropin-releasing hormone agonist alone or in conjunction with estrogen-progestin replacement. *J Clin Endocrinol Metab*. 1996;81:646–651.

128. Leather AT, Studd JWW, Watson NR, Holland EFN. The prevention of bone loss in young treated with GnRH analogues with add-back estrogen therapy. *Obstet Gynecol*. 1993;81:104–107.

versus placebo. *Acta Obstet Gynecol Scand*. 1988;67:159–166.

129. Moghissi KS. Add-back therapy in the treatment of endometriosis: the North America experience. *Br J Obstet Gynecol*. 1996;103:14.

130. Maheux R, Lemay A, Blanchet P, Friede J, Pratt X. Maintained reduction of uterine leiomyoma following addition of hormonal replacement therapy to a monthly luteinizing hormone-releasing hormone agonist implant: a pilot study. *Hum Reprod*. 1991;6:500–505.

131. Kiiholma P, Tuimala R, Kivinen S, Korhonen M, Hagman E. Comparison of the gonadotropin-releasing hormone agonist goserelin acetate along verus goserelin combined with estrogen-progestogen add-back therapy in the treatment of endometriosis. *Fertil Steril*. 1995;64:903–908.

132. Friedman AJ, Daly M, Juneau-Norcross M, Gleason R, Rein MS, LeBoff M. Long-term medical therapy for leiomyomata uteri: a prospective, randomized study of leuprolide acetate depot plus either estrogen-progestin or progestin add-back for 2 years. *Hum Reprod*. 1994;9:1618–1625.

133. Kiesel L, Schweppe KW, Sillem M, Siebzehnrubl E. Should add-back therapy for endometriosis be deferred for optimal results? *Br J Obstet Gynecol*. 1996;103:15–17.

134. Friedman AJ, Daly M, Juneau-Norcross M. A prospective, randomized trial of gonadotropin-releasing hormone agonist plus estrogen-progestin or progestin 'add-back' regimes for women with leiomyomata uteri. *J Clin Endocrinol Metab*. 1993;76:1439–1445.

135. Elkind-Hirsch KE, Anania C, Mack M, Malinak R. Combination gonadotropin-releasing hormone agonist and oral contraceptive therapy improves treatment of hirsute women with ovarian hyperandrogenism. *Fertil Steril*. 1995;63:970–978.

136. Azziz R, Ochoa TM, Bradley EL, Potter HD, Boots LR. Leuprolide and estrogen versus oral contraceptive pills for the treatment of hirsutism: a prospective randomized study. *J Clin Endocrinol Metab*. 1995;80:3406–3411.

137. Murray SC, Muse KN. Effective treatment of severe menstrual migraine headaches with gonadotropin-releasing hormone agonist and "add-back" therapy. *Fertil Steril*. 1997;67:390–393.

138. Schmidt PJ, Nieman LK, Danaceau MA, Adams LF, Rubinow DR. Differential behavioral effects of gonadal steroids in women with and in those without premenstrual syndrome. *N Eng J Med*. 1998;338:209–216.

139. West CP, Hillier H. Ovarian suppression with the gonadotropin-releasing hormone agonist goserelin (Zoladex) in management of the premenstrual tension syndrome. *Hum Reprod*. 1994;9:1058–1063.

140. Halbreich U, Endicott J, Goldstein S, Nee J. Premenstrual changes and changes in gonadal hormones. *Obstet Gynecol*. 1986;74(6):576–586.

141. Wang MI, Seippel LE, Purdy RH, Bäckström T. Relationship between symptom severity and steroid variation in women with premenstrual syndrome: study on serum pregnenolone, pregnenolone sulfate, 5 alpha-pregnane-3, 20-dione and 3 alpha-hydroxy-5 alpha-pregnan-20-one. *J Clin Endocrinol Metab*. 1996;Mar;81(3):1076–1082.

142. Martin V, Wernke S, Mandell K, et al. Medical oophorectomy with and without estrogen add-back therapy in the prevention of migraine headache. *J Head Face Pain*. 2003;43:309–321.

143. B,,kstr"nm CT, Boyle HB. Persistence of symptoms of premenstrual tension in hysterectomized women. *Br J Obstet Gynecol*. 1981;88:530–536.

144. Casson P, Hahn PM, VanVugt DA, Reid RL. Lasting response to ovariectomy in severe intractable premenstrual syndrome. *Obstet Gynecol*. 1990;162:99–105.

145. Casper RF, Hearn MT. The effect of hysterectomy and bilateral oophorectomy in women with severe premenstrual syndrome. *Am J Obstet Gynecol*. 1990;162:105–109.

146. Alvarez WC. The migrainous scotoma as studied in 618 persons. *Am J Opthalmol*. 1960;49:489–504.

147. Wentz AC. Management of the menopause. In: Jones HW, Wentz AC, Burnett LS, eds. *Novak's textbook of gynecology*. 11th ed. Baltimore, MD: Williams and Wilkins, 1985:397–442.

148. Andersch B, Hahn L, Wendestam C, Ohman R, Abrahamsson L. Treatment of premenstrual syndrome with bromocriptine. *Acta Endocrinol*. 1978;88:165–174.

149. Ylostalo P, Kauppila A, Puolakka J, Ronnberg L, Janne O. Bromocriptine and noresthisterone in the treatment of premenstrual syndrome. Obstet Gynecol 1982;58:292–298.

150. Andersen AN, Larsen JF, Steenstrup OR, Svendstrup B, Nielsen J. Effect of bromocriptine on the premenstrual syndrome: a double-blind clinical trial. *Br J Obstet Gynecol*. 1977;84:370–374.

151. Herzog AG. Continuous bromocriptine therapy in menstrual migraine. *Neurology*. 1995;48:101–102.

152. MacGregor EA. Contraception and headache. *Headache*. 2013;53:247–276.

153. Baird DT, Glasier AF. Hormonal contraception. *N Eng J Med*. 1993;328:1543–1549.

154. Wentz AC. Contraception and family planning. In: Jones HW, Wentz AC, Burnett LS, eds. *Novak's textbook of gynecology*. 11th ed. Baltimore, MD: Williams and Wilkins, 1985:204–239.

155. Derman R. Oral contraceptives: a reassessment. *Obstet Gyn Survey*. 1989;44:662–668.

156. Speroff L, DeCherney A, The Advisory Board for the New Progestins. Evaluation of a new generation of oral contraceptives. *Obstet Gynecol*. 1993;81:1034–1047.

157. Thomas SL, Ellertson C. Nuisance or natural and health: should monthly menstruation be optional for women? *Lancet*. 2000;2000:922–924.

158. Fuhrmann U, Krattenmacher R, Slater EP, Fritzemeier KH. The novel progestin drospirenone and its natural counterpart progesterone: biochemical profile and antiandrogenic potential. *Contraception*. 1996;54:243–251.

159. Corson SL. Contraceptive efficacy of a monophasic oral contraceptive containing desogestrel. *Am J Obstet Gynecol*. 1993;168:1017–1020.

160. Huber J. Clinical experience with a new norgestimate-containing oral contraceptive. *Int J Fertil*. 1992;32:47–53.

161. Dunson TR, McLaurin VL, Israngkura B, et al. A comparative study of two low-dose combined oral contraceptives: results from a multicenter trial. *Contraception*. 1993;48:109–119.

162. Shoupe D. Effects of desogestrel on carbohydrate metabolism. *Am J Obstet Gynecol*. 1993;168:1041–1047.

163. Mishell DR. Family planning: contraception, sterilization, and pregnancy termination. In: Mishell DR, Stenchever MA, Droegemueller W, Herbst AL, eds. *Comprehensive gynecology*. 3rd ed. St. Louis: Mosby, 1997:283–352.

164. Medical Economics Company. *Physicians' desk reference*. 53rd ed. Montvale, NJ: Medical Economics Company, 1999.

165. Sullivan H, Furniss H, Spona J, Elstein M. Effect of 21-day and 24-day oral contraceptive regimens containing gestodene (60mcg) and ethinyl estradiol (15mcg) on ovarian activity. *Fertil Steril*. 1999;72:115–120.

166. Zimmermann t, Dietrich H, Wisser KH, Hoffmann H. The efficacy and tolerability of Valetter: a postmarketing surveillance study. *Eur J Contraception Reprod Health Care*. 1999;4:155–164.

167. Silberstein SD, Merriam GR. Sex hormones and headache. In: Goadsby PJ, Silberstein SD, eds. *Headache*. Newton: Butterworth-Heinemann, 1997:143–173.

168. Kay CR. The Royal College of General Practitioners' Oral contraception study: some recent observations. *Clin Obstet Gynecol*. 1984;11:759.

169. Audet MC, Moreau M, Koltun WD, et al. Evaluation of contraceptive efficacy and cycle control of a transdermal contraceptive patch vs an oral contraceptive: a randomized controlled trial for the Ortho EVRA/EVRA 004 Study Group. *JAMA*. 2001;285:2347–2354.

170. Zieman M, Guillebaud J, Weisberg E. Contraceptive efficacy and cycle control with the Ortho Evra/Evra transdermal system: the analysis of pooled data. *Fertil Steril*. 2002;77:S13–S18.

171. Mishell DR, Stenchever MA, Droegemueller W, Herbst AL. Menopause: endocrinology, consequences of estrogen deficiency, effects of hormonal replacement therapy, treatment regimens. In: Mishell DR, Stenchever MA, Droegemueller W, Herbst AL, eds. *Comprehensive gynecology*. 3rd ed. St. Louis: Mosby, 1997:1159–1198.

172. Brache V, Pavan LJ, Faundes A. Current status of contraceptive vaginal rings. *Contraception*. 2013;87:264–272.

173. Shulman LP, Nelson AL, Darney PD. Recent developments in hormone delivery systems. *Am J Obstet Gynecol*. 2004;190:S39–S48.

174. Lopez G, Rodriguez A, Rengifo J, Sivin I. Two-year prospective study in Columbia of Norplant implants. *Obstet Gynecol*. 1985;68:204–208.

175. Shaaban MM, Salah M, Zarzour A, Abdullah SA. A prospective study of NORPLANT[R] implants and the Tcu 380Ag IUD in Assiut, Egypt. *Stud Fam Plan*. 1983;14:163–169.

176. Zheng SR, Zheng HM, Qian SZ, Sang GW, Kaper RF. A randomized multicenter study comparing the efficacy and bleeding pattern of a single-rod (Implanon) and a six-capsule (Norplant) hormonal contraceptive implant. *Contraception*. 1999;60:1–8.

177. Buckshee K, Chatterjee P, Dhall GI, et al. Phase III clinical trials with Norplant[R] II (two covered rods): report on five years of use. *Contraception*. 1993;48:120–132.

178. Sivin I, Alvarez F, Mishell DR, et al. Contraception with two levonorgestrel rod implants: a five year study in the United States and Dominican Republic. *Contraception*. 1998;58:275–282.

179. Sivin I, Campodonico I, Kiriwat O, et al. The performance of levonorgestrel rod and Norplant contraceptive implants: a 5 year randomized study. *Hum Reprod*. 1998;13:3371–3378.

180. Chompootaweep S, Kochagarn E, Usaha JT, Theppitaksak B, Dusitsin N. Experience of Thai women in Bangkok with Norplant-2r implants. *Contraception*. 1998;58:221–225.

181. Coukell AJ, Balfour JA. Levonorgestrel subdermal implants: a review of contraceptive efficacy and acceptability. *Drugs*. 1998;55:861–887.

182. Cravioto MC, Alvarado G, DeCetina CT. A multicenter comparative study on the efficacy, safety, and acceptability of the contraceptive subdermal implants Norplantr and Norplantr II. *Contraception*. 1997;55:359–367.

183. Alder JB, Fraunfelder FT, Edwards R. Levonorgestrel implants and intracranial hypertension. *N Eng J Med*. 1995;332:215–219.

184. Berenson AB, Wiemann CM, Rickerr VI. Contraceptive outcomes among adolescents prescribed Norplant implants versus oral contraceptives after one year of use. *Am J Obstet Gynecol*. 1997;176:586–592.

185. Funk S, Miller MM, Mishell DR, Jr., et al. Safety and efficacy of Implanon, a single-rod implantable contraceptive containing etonogestrel. *Contraception*. 2005;71:319–326.

186. Humpel M, Nieuweber B, Wendt H, Speck U. Investigations of pharmacokinetics of ethinylestradiol to specific consideration of a possible first-pass effect in women. *Contraception*. 1979;19:421–432.

187. Crook D, Goldsland IF, Wynn V. Oral contraceptives and metabolic risk markers for coronary heart disease. *Int J Fertil*. 1991;36:38–46.

188. Kauppinen-Makelin R, Kuusi T, Ylikorkala O, Tikkanen MJ. Contraceptives containing desogestrel or levonorgestrel have different effects on serum lipoproteins and postheparin plasma lipase activities. *Clin Endocrinol*. 1992;36:203–209.

189. Rosing J, Tans G, Nicolaes GA. Oral contraceptives and venous thrombosis: different sensitivities to activate protein C in women using second and third generation oral contraceptives. *Br J Haematol*. 1997;97:233–238.

190. Prasad RN, Koh S, Ratnam SS. Effects of three types of combined OC pills on blood coagulation, fibrinolysis and platelet function. *Contraception*. 1989;39:369–383.

191. Lobo RA, Slinner JB, Lippman JS, Cirillo SJ. Plasma lipids and desogestrel and ethinyl estradiol: a meta-analysis. *Fertil Steril*. 1996;65:1100–1109.

192. Bloemenkamf KW, Rosendaal FR, Helmerhorst FM. Enhancement by factor V Leiden mutation of risk of deep vein thrombosis associated with oral contraceptives containing a third generation progestagen. *Lancet*. 1995;346:1593–1596.

193. Vandenbroucke JP, Koster T, Briet E, Reitsma PH, Bertina RM, Rosendaal FR. Increased risk of venous thrombosis in oral-contraceptive users who are carriers of factor V Leiden mutation. *Lancet*. 1994;344:1453–1457.

194. Schwartz SM, Siscovick DS, Longstreth WT. Use of low-dose oral contraceptives and stroke in young women. *Ann Intern Med*. 1997;127:596–603.

195. Andersen BS, Olsen J, Nielsen GL. Third generation oral contraceptive and heritable thrombophilia as risk factors of nonfatal venous thromboembolism. *Thromb Haemost*. 1998;79:28–31.

196. Jick H, Derby LE, Myers MW, Vasilakis C, Newton KM. Risk of hospital admission for idiopathic venous thromboembolism among users of postmenopausal estrogens. *Lancet*. 1996;348:981–983.

197. Lidegaard O. Oral contraception and risk of a cerebral thromboembolic attack: results of a case-control study. *Br Med J Clin Res*. 1993;306:956–963.

198. Beral V, Hermon C, Kay C, Hannaford P, Darby S, Reeves G. Mortality associated with oral contraceptive use: 25 year followup of 46,000 women from Royal College of general Practitioners' oral contraception study. *Br Med J*. 1999;318:96–100.

199. The Centers for Disease Control and The National Institute of Child Health and Human Development. Oral contraceptive use and the risk of breast cancer: The Cancer and Steroid Hormone Study. *N Engl J Med*. 1986;315:405–411.

200. Collaborative Group on Hormonal Factors in Breast Cancer. Breast cancer and hormonal contraceptives: collaborative reanalysis of individual data of 53,297 women with breast cancer and 100,239 women without breast cancer from 54 epidemiological studies. *Lancet*. 1996;347:1713–1727.

201. Hatcher RA, Guillebaud J. The pill: combined oral contraceptives. In: Hatcher RA, Trussel J, Stewart F, eds. *Contraceptive technology*. New York: Ardent Media, 1998:405–466.

202. Marchbanks PA, McDonald JA, Wilson HG, et al. Oral contraceptives and the risk of breast cancer. *N Engl J Med*. 2002;346:2025–2032.

203. Davidson NE, Helzlsouer KJ. Good news about oral contraceptives (Editorial). *N Engl J Med*. 2002;346:2078–2079.

204. Chasan-Taber L, Stampfer MJ. Epidemiology of oral contraceptives and cardiovascular disease. *Ann Intern Med*. 1998;128:467–477.

205. World Health Organization Collaborative Study of Cardiovascular Disease and Steroid Hormone Contraception. Ischemic stroke and combined oral contraceptives: results of an international, multicenter, case-control study. *Lancet*. 1996;348:498–505.

206. World Health Organization Collaborative Study of Cardiovascular Disease and Steroid Hormone Contraception. Hemorrhagic stroke, overall stroke risk, and combined oral contraceptives: results of an international, multicenter, case-control study. *Lancet*. 1996;348:505–510.

207. Heinemann LA, Assman A, Dominh T, Garbe E. Oral progestogen-only contraceptives and cardiovascular risk: results from the Transnational Study on Oral Contraceptives and the Health of Young Women. *Eur J Contracept Reprod Health Care*. 1999;4:67–73.

208. Collaborative Group for the Study of Stroke in Young Women. Oral contraceptives and stroke in young women. *JAMA*. 1975;231:718–722.

209. Buring JE, Hebert P, Romero J, et al. Migraine and subsequent risk of stroke in the Physicians' Health Study. *Arch Neurol*. 1995;52:129–134.

210. Merikangas KR, Fenton B, Cheng SH, Stolar MJ, Risch N. Association between migraine and stroke in a large-scale epidemiological study of the United States. *Arch Neurol*. 1997;54:362–368.

211. Tzourio C, Iglesias S, Hubert JB. Migraine and risk of ischemic stroke: a case-control study. *Br Med J*. 1993;307:289–292.

212. Tzourio C, Tehindrazanarivelo A, Iglesias S. Case-control study of migraine and risk of ischemic stroke in young women. *Br Med J*. 1995;310:830–833.

213. Chang CL, Donaghy M, Poulter N. Migraine and stroke in young women: case-control study. The World Health Organization Collaborative Study of Cardiovascular Disease and Steroid Hormone Contraception. *Br Med J*. 1999;318:13–18.

214. Donaghy M, Chang CL, Poulter N. Duration, frequency, recency, and type of migraine and the risk of ischaemic stroke in women of childbearing age. On behalf of the European Collaborators of the World Health Organization Collaborative Study of Cardiovascular Disease and Steroid Hormone Contraception. *J Neurol Neurosurg Psychiatr*. 2002;73:747–750.

215. Tzourio C, Kittner SJ, Bousser MG, Alperovitch A. Migraine and stroke in young women. *Cephalalgia*. 2000;20:190–199.

216. Kurth T, Slomke MA, Kase CS, et al. Migraine, headache, and the risk of stroke in women: a prospective study. *Neurology*. 2005;64:1020–1026.

217. Curtis KM, Mohllajee AP, Peterson HB. Use of combined oral contraceptives among women with migraine and nonmigrainous headaches: a systematic review. *Contraception*. 2006;73:189–194.

218. Kurth T, Gaziano JM, Cook NR, Logroscino G, Diener HC, Buring JE. Migraine and risk of cardiovascular disease in women. *JAMA*. 2006;296:283–291.

219. Porter JB, Hunter JR, Jick H, Stergachis A. Oral contraceptives and nonfatal vascular disease. *Obstet Gynecol*. 1985;66:1–4.

220. Hannaford PC, Croft PR, Kay CR. Oral contraception and stroke. Evidence from the Royal College of General Practitioners' Oral Contraception Study. *Stroke*. 1994;25:935–942.

221. Petitti DB, Sidney S, Bernstein A, Wolf S, Quesenberry C, Ziel HK. Stroke in users of low-dose oral contraceptives. *N Eng J Med*. 1996;335:8–15.

222. Poulter NR, Chang CL, Farley TM, Meirik O, Marmot MG. Hemorrhagic stroke, overall stroke risk, and combined oral contraceptives: results of an international, multicenter, case-control study (The Writing Committee for the World Health Organization Collaborative Study of Cardiovascular Disease and Steroid Hormone Contraception). *Lancet*. 1996;348:505–510.

223. Schwaag S, Nabavi DG, Frese A, Husstedt IW, Evers S. The association between migraine and juvenile stroke: a case-control study. *Headache*. 2003;43:90–95.

224. Gillum LA, Mamidipudi SK, Johnston SC. Ischemic stroke risk with oral contraceptives: a meta-analysis. *JAMA*. 2000;284:72–78.

225. Kemmeren JM, Tanis BC, van den Bosch MA, et al. Risk of arterial thrombosis in relation to oral contraceptives (RATIO) study: oral contraceptives and the risk of ischemic stroke. *Stroke*. 2002;33:1202–1208.

226. Lidegaard O, Edstrom B, Kreiner S. Oral contraceptives and venous thromboembolism: a five-year national case-control study. *Contraception*. 2002;65:187–196.

227. Siritho S, Thrift AG, McNeil JJ, You RX, Davis SM, Donnan GA. Risk of ischemic stroke among users of the oral contraceptive pill: The Melbourne Risk Factor Study (MERFS) Group. *Stroke*. 2003;34:1575–1580.

228. Lidegaard O, Lokkegaard E, Jensen A, Skovlund CW, Keiding N. Thrombotic stroke and myocardial infarction with hormonal contraception. *N Engl J Med*. 2012;366:2257–2266.

229. Kruit MC, vanBuchem MA, Hofman PA, et al. Migraine as a risk factor for subclinical brain lesions. *JAMA*. 2004;921:427–434.

230. Bousser MG. Estrogens, migraine, and stroke. *Stroke*. 2004;35:2652–2656.

231. Scher AI, Terwindt GM, Picavet HS, Verschuren WM, Ferrari MD, Launer LJ. Cardiovascular risk factors and migraine: the GEM population-based study. *Neurology*. 2005;64:614–620.

232. Becker WJ. Use of oral contraceptives in patients with migraine. *Neurology*. 1999;53:519–525.

233. Bousser MG, Kittner SJ. Oral contraceptives and stroke. *Cephalalgia*. 2000;20:183–189.

234. US Department of Health and Human Services. Vital statistics of the United States, Centers for Disease Control and Prevention, National Center for Health Statistics, 1992, Hyattsville, MD. *Mortality*. 1996;1:24–27.

235. Gerstman BB, Piper JM, Tomita DK, Ferguson WJ, Stadel BV, Lundin FE. Oral contraceptive estrogen dose and the risk of deep venous thromboembolitic disease. *Am J Epidemiol*. 1991;133(1):32–37.

236. Böttiger LE, Boman G, Eklund G, Westerholm B. Oral contraceptives and thromboembolic disease: effects of lowering estrogen content. *Lancet*. 1989;8178:1097–1101.

237. Jick H, Jick SS, Myers MW, Vasilakis C, Gurewich V. Risk of idiopathic cardiovascular death and nonfatal venous thromboembolism in women using oral contraceptives with differing progestagen components. *Lancet*. 1995;346(8990):1589–1593.

238. Spitzer WO, Lewis MA, Heinemann LA, Thorogood M, MacRae KD. Third generation oral contraceptives and risk of venous thromboembolic disorders: an international case-control study. Transnational Research Group on Oral Contraceptives and the Health of Young Women. *Br Med J*. 1996;312:83–88.

239. World Health Organization Collaborative Study of Cardiovascular Disease and Steroid Hormone Contraception. Venous thromboembolic disease and combined oral contraceptives: results of international multicenter case-control study. *Lancet*. 1995;346:15751581.

240. Farmer RD, Lawrenson RA, Thompson CR, Kennedy JG, Hambleton IR. Population-based study of risk of venous thromboembolism associated with various oral contraceptives. *Lancet*. 1997;83–88.

241. Rosendaal FR, Koster T, Vandenbroucke JP, Reitsma PH. High risk of thrombosis in patients homozygous for factor V Leiden (activated protein C resistance). *Blood*. 1995;85:1504–1508.

242. Vandenbroucke JP, Rosing J, Bloemenkamp KW, et al. Oral contraceptives and the risk of venous thrombosis. *N Engl J Med*. 2001;344:1527–1534.

243. Porter JB, Jick H, Walker AM. Mortality among oral contraceptive users. *Obstet Gynecol*. 1987;70:29–32.

244. Krauss GL, Brandt J, Campbell M, Plate C. Reproductive issues in epilepsy are poorly understood by US. neurologists and obstetricians. *Epilepsia*. 1995;36:12(Abstract).

245. Mattson RH, Cramer JA, Darney PD, Naftolin F. Use of oral contraceptives by women with epilepsy. *JAMA*. 1986;256:238–240.

246. So EL. Update on epilepsy. *Med Clin N Amer*. 1993;77:203–214.

247. Shuster EA. Epilepsy on women. *Mayo Clin Proc*. 1996;71:991–999.

248. Haukkamaa M. Contraception by Norplant subdermal capsules is not reliable in epileptic patients on anticonvulsant therapy. *Contraception*. 1986;33:559–565.

249. Ryan RE. A controlled study of the effect of oral contraceptives on migraine. *Headache*. 1978;17:250–252.

250. Phillips bM. Oral contraceptive drugs and migraine. *Br Med J Clin Res*. 1968;2:99.

251. Dalton K. Migraine and oral contraceptives. *Headache*. 1976;15:247–251.

252. Whitty CWM, Hockaday JM, Whitty M. The effect of oral contraceptives on migraine. *Lancet*. 1966;1:856–859.

253. Larrson-Cohn U, Lundberg PO. Headache and treatment with oral contraceptives. *Acta Neurol Scand*. 1970;46:267–278.

254. Carroll JD. Migraine and oral contraception. Sandoz Conference Proceeding, 1971:45–46.

255. Diddle AW, Gardner WH, Williamson PJ. Oral contraceptive medications and headache. *Am J Obstet Gynecol*. 1969;105:507–511.

256. Ramchurian S, Pellegrin FA, Ray RM, Hsu JP. The Walnut Creek contraceptive drug study. *J Reprod Med*. 1980;25:346–371.

257. Herzberg B, Coppen A. Changes in psychological symptoms in women taking oral contraceptives. *Br J Psychiatry*. 1970;116:161–164.

258. Herzberg BN, Draper KC, Johnson AL, Nicol GC. Oral contraceptives, depression, and libido. *Br Med J Clin Res*. 1971;3:495–300.

259 Royal College of General Practitioners. Oral Contraceptives and Health: an interim report from the oral contraception study of the Royal College of General Practitioners. Pitman; 1974.

260. Aznar-Ramos R, Giner-Velazquez J, Lara-Ricalde R, Martinez-Manautou J. Incidence of side effects with contraceptive placebo. *Am J Obstet Gynecol*. 1969;105:1144–1149.

261. Ramos R, Apelo R, Osteria T, Vilar E. A comparative analysis of three different dose combinations of oral contraceptives. *Contraception*. 1989;39:165–177.

262. Nilsson L, Solvell L. Clinical studies on oral contraceptives: a randomized, double-blind, cross-over study of four different preparations (AnovlarR mite, LyndiolR mite, OvulenR, and VolidanR). *Acta Obstet Gynecol Scand*. 1967;46:3–31.

263. Goldzieher JW, Moses LE, Averkin E, Scheel C, Taber BZ. A placebo-controlled double-blind cross-over investigation of the side effects attributed to oral contraceptives. *Fertil Steril*. 1971;22:623.

264. Silbergeld S, Brast N, Noble EP. The menstrual cycle: a double-blind study of symptoms, mood and

behavior, and biochemical variables using enovid and placebo. *Psychosom Med.* 1971;33:411–428.

265. Cullberg J. Mood changes and menstrual symptoms with different gestagen/estrogen combinations: a double-blind comparison with a placebo. *Acta Psychiatr Scand.* 1972;236:259–276.

266. Coney P, Washenik K, Langley RG, diGiovanna JJ, Harrison DD. Weight change and adverse event incidence with a low-dose oral contraceptive: two randomized, placebo-controlled trials. *Contraception.* 2001 Jun 30;63(6):297–302.

267. Cullberg J, Celli MG, Jonsson CO. Mental and sexual adjustment before and after six months use of an oral contraceptive. *Acta Psychiatr Scand.* 1969;45:259–276.

268. Nilsson A, Jacobson L, Ingemanson CA. Side-effects of an oral contraceptive with particular attention to mental symptoms and sexual adaptation. *Acta Obstet Gynecol Scand.* 1967;46:537–556.

269. Grant ECG. Relation between headaches from oral contraceptives and development of endometrial arterioles. *Br Med J Clin Res.* 1968;3:402–405.

270. Desrosiers JJJ. Headaches related to contraceptive therapy and their control. *Headache.* 1973;13:117–124.

271. Fotherby K. Twelve years of clinical experience with an oral contraceptive containing 30æg ethinyloestradiol and 150æg desogestrel. *Contraception.* 1995;51:3–12.

272. The MircetteT Study Group. An open-label, multicenter, noncomparative safety and efficacy study of MircetteT, a low dose estrogen-progestin oral contraceptive. *Am J Obstet Gynecol.* 1998;179:S2–S8.

273. Archer DF, Maheux R, delConte A, O'Brien FB, North American Levonorgestrel Study Group. Efficacy and safety of a low-dose monophasic combination oral contraceptive containing 100æg levonorgestrel and 20 æg ethinyl estradiol (Alesser). *Am J Obstet Gynecol.* 1999;181:S39–S44.

274. Aegidius K, Zwart JA, Hagen K, Schei B, Stovner LJ. Oral contraceptives and increased headache prevalence: the Head-HUNT Study. *Neurology.* 2006;66:349–353.

275. Runnebaum B. The androgenicity of oral contraceptives: the young patient's concerns. *Int J Fertil.* 1992;37:211–217.

276. Bilotta P, Favilli S. Clinical evaluation of a monophasic ethinyl-estradiol/desogestrel-containing oral contraceptive. *Drug Res.* 1988;38:932934.

277. Mraz M, Aull S, Feucht M. Tension headache: new evaluation of symptomatology based on International Headache Society diagnostic criteria. *Wien Klin Wochenschr.* 1993;105:42–52.

278. Wimberly YH, Cotton S, Wanchick AM, Succop PA, Rosenthal SL. Attitudes and experiences with levonorgestrel 100 microg/ethinyl estradiol 20 microg among women during a 3–month trial. *Contraception.* 2002;65:403–406.

279. Loder EW, Buse DC, Golub JR. Headache as a side effect of combination estrogen-progestin oral contraceptives: a systematic review. *Am J Obstet Gynecol.* 2005;193:636–649.

280. Schwallie PC, Assenzo JR. Contraceptive use-efficacy study utilizing medroxyprogesterone acetate administered as an intramuscular injection once every 90 days. *Fertil Steril.* 1973;24:331–339.

281. Darney PD, Atkinson E, Tanner S. Acceptance and perceptions of Norplantr among users in San Francisco, USA. *Stud Fam Plan.* 1990;21:152–160.

282. Clarkson T. Progestogens and cardiovascular disease: a critical review. *J Reprod Med.* 1999;44:180–184.

283. Kjos SL, Peters RK, Xiang A. Contraception and the risk of type 2 diabetes mellitus in Latina women with prior gestational diabetes mellitus. *JAMA.* 1998;280:533–538.

284. Scholes D, Lacroix AZ, Ott SM. Bone mineral density in women using depo-medroxyprogesterone acetate for contraception. *Ob Gyn.* 1999;93:233–238.

285. Marx PA, Spira AI, Gettie A. Progesterone implants enhance SIV vaginal transmission and early virus load. *Nature Med.* 1996;2:1084–1089.

286. Kaushic C, Mrdin AD, Underdown BJ, Wira CR. Chlamydia trachomatis infection in the female reproductive tract of the rat: influence of progesterone on infectivity and immune response. *Infect Immun.* 1998;66:893–898.

287. World Health Organization. *Medical eligibility criteria for contraceptive use.* Geneva: World Health Organization, 2004.

288. Bousser MG. International Headache Society (IHS) Task Force on oral contraceptives (OCs) and hormone replacement therapy (HRT) used in migraine sufferers. *Cephalalgia.* 2000;20:147.

289. Loder EW, Buse DC, Golub JR. Headache and combination estrogen-progestin oral contraceptives: integrating evidence, guidelines, and clinical practice. *Headache.* 2005;45:224–231.

290. Archer B, Irwin D, Jensen K, Johnson ME, Rorie J. Depot medroxyprogesterone. Management of side-effects commonly associated with its contraceptive use. *J Nurse Midwifery.* 1997;42:104–111.

291. Harel Z, Biro FM, Kollar LM. Depo-Provera in adolescents: effects of early second injection or prior oral contraception. *J Adolesc Health.* 1995;16:379–384.

292. Centers for Disease Control and Prevention (CDC). United States Medical Eligibility Criteria (US MEC) for Contraceptive Use, 2010. Cited 2013-12-16. Available from: URL: http://www.cdc.gov/reproductivehealth/unintendedpregnancy/usmec.htm.

293. Faculty of Sexual and Reproductive Healthcare. UK medical eligibility criteria for contraceptive use. http://www.fsrh.org/pages/Clinical_Guidance_1.asp. 2012. 9-4-2012.

294. World Health Organization. Medical eligibility criteria for contraceptive use. http://www.who.int/reproductivehealth/publications/family_planning/9789241563888/en/index.hyml (4th). 2009. World Health Organization. 9-19-2012.

295. MacGregor, EA Contraception and Headache, *Headache*, 2013;53:247–276.

Index